EVOLUTION OF THE MOLECULAR BIOLOGY OF BRAIN TUMORS AND THE THERAPEUTIC IMPLICATIONS

Edited by **Terry Lichtor**

Evolution of the Molecular Biology of Brain Tumors and the Therapeutic Implications
http://dx.doi.org/10.5772/50198
Edited by Terry Lichtor

Contributors

Bruno Costa, Chunzhi Zhang, Martin Jadus, Satoshi Utsuki, Almos Klekner, Hassan Mahmoud Fathallah-Shaykh, Elza Tiemi Sakamoto-Hojo, Geraldo Passos, Paulo Roberto D´Auria Vieira Godoy, Flávia Donaires, Patrícia Carminati, Ana Paula Montaldi, Jarah Meador, Adayabalam Balajee, Mine Erguven, Phanithi Prakash Babu, Giuseppe Raudino, Mariella Caffo, Gerardo Caruso, Concetta Alafaci, Federica Raudino, Valentina Marventano, Alberto Romano, Francesco Montemagno, Massimo Belvedere, Francesco Maria Salpietro, Francesco Tomasello, Anna Schillaci, Wenbo Zhu, Guangmei Yan, Sihan Wu, Stephano Spano Mello, Eduardo Donadi, James Rutka, ANDRES CARDONA, LEON DARIO ORTIZ, Toshiyuki Ishiwata, Yoko Matsuda, Hisashi Yoshimura, Petr Busek, Aleksi Sedo, Davide Schiffer, Lee Roy Morgan, Joonas Haapasalo, Kristiina Nordfors, Hannu Haapasalo, Seppo Parkkila, Albert Magro, Nic E. Savaskan, Valeria Barresi, Francesca Granata, Mario Venza, Jerzy Trojan

Published by InTech

Janeza Trdine 9, 51000 Rijeka, Croatia

Publishing Process Manager Iva Simcic
Technical Editor InTech DTP team
Cover InTech Design team

Additional hard copies can be obtained from orders@intechopen.com

Evolution of the Molecular Biology of Brain Tumors and the Therapeutic Implications, Edited by Terry Lichtor
p. cm.
ISBN 978-953-51-0989-1

For EU product safety concerns:
IN TECH d.o.o., Prolaz Marije Krucifikse Kozulić 3, 51000 Rijeka, Croatia,
info@intechopen.com or visit our website at intechopen.com.

Meet the editor

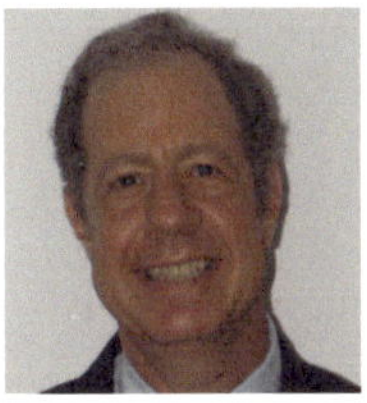

Dr. Lichtor is a practicing neurosurgeon. He has a number of research interests, and his brain tumor work is largely focused on the development of a DNA vaccine for treatment of primary and metastatic intracerebral tumors. In particular Dr. Lichtor has shown that vaccines prepared by transfer of DNA from the tumor into a highly immunogenic cell line can encompass the array of tumor antigens that characterize the patient's neoplasm. Poorly immunogenic tumor antigens, characteristic of malignant cells, can become strongly antigenic if they are expressed by highly immunogenic cells. The introduction of the vaccine directly into the tumor bed of animals with an intracerebral tumor stimulates a systemic cellular anti-tumor immune response associated with a prolongation of survival. It is hopeful that this vaccine strategy will be efficacious in the treatments of patients with brain tumors. Dr. Lichtor is a member of the neurosurgery faculty at Rush University Medical Center in Chicago, Illinois.

Contents

Preface

Although technical advances have resulted in marked improvements in the ability to diagnose and surgically treat primary and metastatic brain tumors, the incidence and mortality rates of these tumors is increasing. Particularly affected are young adults and the elderly. The present standard treatment modalities following surgical resection including cranial irradiation and systemic or local chemotherapy each have limited efficacy and serious adverse side effects. Furthermore the relatively few long-term survivors are inevitably left with cognitive deficits and other disabilities. The difficulties in treating malignant gliomas can be attributed to several factors. Glial tumors are inherently resistant to radiation and standard cytotoxic chemotherapies. The existence of blood-brain and blood-tumor barriers impede drug delivery to the tumor and adjacent brain infiltrated with tumor. In addition the low therapeutic index between tumor sensitivity and toxicity to normal brain severely limits the ability to systemically deliver therapeutic doses of drugs or radiation therapy to the tumor. New treatment strategies for the management of patients with these tumors are urgently needed.

A number of emerging treatment strategies currently being developed are outlined in this book. In particular advances in the molecular biology of brain tumors including the evolution of stem cell biology, microRNAs along with angiogenesis and tumor invasion patterns are reviewed in this book. Another emerging strategy in the treatment of brain tumors involves the stimulation of an immunologic response against the neoplastic cells. Although in most instances proliferating tumors do not provoke anti-tumor cellular immune responses, the hope is that the immune system can be called into play to destroy malignant cells. In addition the tumors display a particular resistance to radiation therapy and chemotherapy. Some of the mechanisms that enable antigenic neoplasms to escape host immunity or develop a resistance to radiation therapy or chemotherapy are reviewed in this book. Hopefully this information coupled with advances in the understanding of the pathophysiology and molecular biology of brain tumors which are outlined in this book will translate into novel therapeutic treatment strategies with an emphasis on molecular targeting that should lead to the prolongation of survival without a decline in cognitive functions or other side effects in patients with brain tumors.

Dr. Terry Lichtor
Rush Medical College,
Department of Neurosurgery,
Chicago, United States

Section 1

Angiogenesis and Tumor Invasion

Chapter 1

Brain Tumor Invasion and Angiogenesis

Almos Klekner

Additional information is available at the end of the chapter

http://dx.doi.org/10.5772/50198

1. Introduction

It is a well-known fact that effectiveness of oncotherapy in brain tumors remains under the expectations in comparison to anaplastic tumors of other organs. Knowing the very modest survival rates enormous efforts of neuro-oncological researches has been made, but only partial success is produced. Beside the extremely high proliferation rate of high grade glioma cells researches established the highly intensive invasiveness and angiogenesis as the main reasons of treatment failure. In this chapter the main molecular mechanisms of brain tumor invasion and angiogenesis will be discussed followed by the hopeful treatment possibilities that are already in studies and will be achievable in the near-future.

2. General a spects of glioma invasion

Malignant gliomas are the most common primary brain tumors. They are associated with the shortest survival time explained by their early recurrence due to their deep invasion of the normal brain, which makes them practically impossible to remove completely. Invasive anaplastic gliomas are almost invariably fatal, recurring close to the resection margin in almost all cases. Interestingly, primary brain tumors have a strong tendency to invade their environment, but with rare exceptions, do not metastasize outside the brain. [1-3].

To understand the invasion behaviour of gliomas, the cellular and molecular events of peritumoral infiltration have to be discussed. The most important medium for this process is the extracellular matrix (ECM). The ECM comprises a considerable proportion of the normal brain volume. The extracellular space (ECS) of the healthy brain tissue volume is approximatley 20%. The extracellular volume fraction in the majority of primary brain tumors is significantly increased, representing about 48% of the total tumor tissue volume especially in high grade gliomas. The structure and compounds of the ECM of the brain tissue have many specific differences from other human organs. The ECM of the brain contains mainly macromolecules like glycosaminoglycans (GAGs) and proteoglycans (PGs), and only moderately express fibrillary glycoproteins (e.g. collagens, fibronectin, elastin or reticulin). The compounds of ECM glycoproteins play a crucial role in peritumoral invasion forming structural elements for cellular attachment and migration. There is much evidence that ECM components can modulate brain tumor growth, proliferation, and invasion by many different mechanisms. Thus extracellular matrix plays a pivotal role in the tumorous infiltration of the surrounding tissue. The presence and functions of hyaluronic acid (hyaluronan, HA), PGs and various types of GAGs have already been intensively investigated to clarify the molecular mechanisms of invasion, and a positive correlation has been established many times. To allow cell adhesion and migration, the ECM components interact with specific receptors on the cell membrane, such as integrins, CD44, or CD168. Some proteases and synthases also strongly influence invasiveness because of their capacity to alter the actual levels of the ECM molecules or to degrade the pericellular network. [4-16]

Using the ECM macromolecules to their active movement, glioma cells infiltrate the enviroment and form it similar to the tumor tissue. The process of the peritumoral invasion depends on the confrontation zone of the tumor cells and the non-neoplastic cells and ECM. Glioma cells express mainly adhesion receptors and proteases, while host cells produce macromolecules to maintain original structure and to inhibit invading cell movement. Since brain ECM has no strong fibrillar, collagen-rich network, the brain parenchyma remains soft, that can not hinder significantly the migration of tumor cells.

In case of glial cell tumors there are two main factors that significantly promote peritumoral infiltration. First is the normal structure of the brain parenchyma composed mainly by tracts in the white matter and basement membranes, which are suitable for guiding cell migration. Second is the increased ability of glia cells to migration. Both factors are special for the brain and they can be easily understood knowing the connection of development, structure and function. [17, 18]

From neuro-oncological point of view the increased glioma cell mobility and extensive peritumoral infiltration leads to the following problems:

a. A. Total extirpation of a low grade tumor is not an easy and evident technical tool of therapy. This is one main reason why these tumors are "semi-benign" tumors. Thus in spite of the macroscopically radical surgical removal, the recurrence rate of these tumors is very high, and full recovery is not a general event.

b. B. In case of high grade tumors, neither open surgery, nor stereotactic radiosurgery can achieve radical tumor removal. This experience can explain the local recurrence that appears in almost every case.

c. C. Local chemotherapeutical treatment (intraparenchymal or post operatively administered intracavital drug) has low effectiveness.

http://dx.doi.org/10.5772/50198

3. Molecular aspects of glioma invasion

Molecules that are responsible for the cell migration are divided in three groups:

1. Cell-membrane associated molecules (receptors and adhesion molecules).
2. Extracellular matrix (ECM) components (targets for the receptors).
3. Enzymes that are synthesizing or lysating the ECM components.

3.1. Cell-membrane associated molecules (receptors and adhesion molecules)

Molecules with evident role in peritumoral invasion are located either on the cell surface, or form transmembrane structure. The main representatives of this group are the receptors and adhesion molecules as detailed below.

The **Ig superfamily** contains molecules in the cell membrane consisted of immunoglobulin-like and fibronectin type III domains involved in cell–cell adhesion. The superfamily includes the integrins, a variety of cell adhesion molecules (CAMs) with distinct ligand-binding specificities, namely ICAM (intercellular), NCAM (neural), Ep-CAM (epithelial), L1-CAM, VCAM (vascular), ALCAM (activated leukocyte), and JAM (junctional adhesion molecule), among others. [19]

The **integrins** are the most common molecules that serve for glioma cells to adhere to ECM. These molecules are heterodimeric transmembrane glycoproteins consisting of non-covalently linked α and β chains, which both determine ligand binding strength and specificity. Eight distinct α and 18 β chains combine to form about 24 different heterodimers. They can interact with two groups of ligands: some of the ECM proteins, such as fibrinogen, fibronectin, vitronectin, and cell surface molecules, that are members of the immunoglobulin superfamily. Regarding the many different heterodimers, each cell type maintains a specific and activation-dependent integrin repertoire and consequence ligand preference. The cytoplasmic integrin domains connect to signalling proteins and to the actin-cytoskeleton mediating intracellular signal transduction and cell movement. This function definietly demonstrate the dynamics of cell–ECM interaction as cells move along a substrate. Thus, integrins are prominently important mediators for cell adhesion and migration. They also interact with growth hormone receptors and contribute to cell–cell contacts due to direct interactions with counterpart cell receptors. On the other hand, focal contacts mainly depend on the ECM-compartment and on the cell type. Different integrins are known to be involved in that process. Integrin $\alpha5\beta1$ binds to fibronectin, $\alpha6\beta1$ or $\beta4$ binds to laminin, $\alpha v\beta3$ binds to fibronectin, vitronectin and tenascin-C and $\alpha2\beta1$ binds to fibrillar collagen. Some of the integrins are directly connected to malignant behavior of gliomas. Neutralizing antibodies to $\beta1$- and $\alpha v\beta5$-integrin lead to decreased glioma migration in vitro. It was also demonstrated, that tenascin increases in vitro motility of human gliomas through interaction with $\beta1$-integrins. Inhibition of $\beta1$-integrins leads also to decreased motility, whereas inhibition of αv-integrin causes increased motility. The integrin $\alpha v\beta3$ plays a central role in glioma invasion. Increased expression of integrin $\alpha v\beta3$ results in increased motility of glioma cells with a decrease in apoptosis sensitivity. Furthermore, inhibition of integrin αvβ3 decreases glioma cell motility. Integrins αvβ3 and αvβ6 interacting with tenascin was proved to mediate adhesion rather than migration. Expression of β5-integrin is correlated with in vitro invasiveness and migration of human glioma cells. However α-actin expression and linkage of integrins to the cytoskeleton is related to glioma aggressiveness and poor prognosis in WHO II and III astrocytoma. [20-33]

Integrins mediate also activation of **focal adhesion kinase (FAK) that** associates with β1- and β3-integrins, which can trigger FAK phosphorylation. It is a non receptor tyrosine kinase overexpressed in invasive glioma cells, and its expression correlates with tumor recurrence and invasiveness in many tumor types. FAK is activated either by integrin mediated adhesion to ECM or by growth factor stimulation and it induces cell migration. Induction of FAK can protect cells from apoptosis. [34-41]

The **neural cell adhesion molecule (NCAM)** is expressed mainly by developing neurons. It is downregulated during embryogenesis and re-expressed again once differentiation is initiated. Overexpression of NCAM decreases glioma cell motility in vitro. In drug-resistant glioma cell lines NCAM expression is reduced and integrin-expression is increased that help to explain decreased chemosensitivity in invading glioma. [42- 45]

CD44 is the most important HA-receptor expressed by every nucleated cells in vertebrates. CD44 is a transmembrane glycoprotein belonging to the immunoglobulin receptor superfamily. Besides the standard form (CD44s), multiple splice variants encoded by variable exons v1–10 (CD44v1–10) can be identified depending on the cell differentiation and activation state. Interactions of CD44 with numerous other molecules, such as collagens, laminins and fibronectin, have been proved in vitro. CD44 is consisted of four functional domains: amino terminal domain, stem structure, transmembrane domain and cytoplasmic domain. The amino terminal domain can link to the ECM components such as HA and other GAGs. The stem structure domain binds the amino-terminal domain and transmembrane domain. The transmembrane region is probable responsible for the association of CD44 with lipid rafts. The cytoplasmic domain of CD44 is connected to the cytoskeleton via ankyrin and other proteins that is necessary to cell adhesion and motiliy. CD44 can be cleaved to two parts, and both the extracellular and intracellular components of CD44 promote cell migration. CD44 also interacts with various regulatory mediators to cell signaling pathways. Through these connections CD44 promotes MMP-mediated matrix degradation, tumor cell growth, migration and invasion and its expression correlates well with invasion potential of glioblastoma. [46-54]

The **receptor for hyaluronate-mediated motility (RHAMM)** is also a HA-binding protein expressed on the cell surface and also in the cytoplasm, cytoskeleton and nucleus. Interaction of HA with RHAMM induces many cellular signaling pathways in connection to protein kinase-C, FAK, MAP kinases, NFκB, RAS, phosphatidylinositol kinase (PI3K), tyrosine kinases and cytoskeletal components. CD44 and RHAMM probably have redundant or overlapping functions, but it is evident that interactions of HA with CD44 and RHAMM are necessary for tumorigenesis and tumor progression. [55-58]

Syndecans are a family of transmembrane heparan sulphate proteoglycans with four members, syndecans 1 to 4. Syndecans are co-receptors by binding their ECM ligands in conjunction with other receptors, mainly integrins. Through their heparan sulphate side chains, syndecans may further take part in other ligand binding, like VEGF, fibronectin and antithrombin-1. Linking syndecan to fibronectin is modulated by tenascin-C. Syndecan-1, -3, and syndecan -2, -4 bild two different structural subgroups. Syndecan-1 is expressed generally in fibroblasts and epithelial cells (especially in keratinocytes), but normally there is only a moderate presence in endothel and neural cells. Syndecan-3 dominates in neural cells, but not in epithelial cells, and syndecan-4 can be found mainly in epithel cells and fibroblasts, while it is poorly expressed by endothel and neural cells. Syndecans have four main function: 1. activation of growth hormon receptors; 2. cell adhesion to ECM components such as collagens type I, III, V, fibronectin, thrombospondin and tenascin; 3. cell-to-cell adhesion (e.g. syndecan-4 and integrin linkage takes part in intercellular interactions; 4. tumor suppression (anti-invasive effect by keeping tumor cells together) or tumor progression (depending on tumor histology and growth phase). [59-62]

Cadherin superfamily is also an important group of adhesion molecules regarding glioma invasion. Cadherins are transmembrane proteins compound of several tandemly repeated cadherin domains that interact in calcium-dependent homophilic cell–cell contacts. The cadherin superfamily consists of more than 100 different members, with E- (epithelial) and N- (neural) and P-cadherin, most intensively expressed in epithelial and neural tissues, respectively. Desmosomal cadherins (desmoglein and desmocollin) provide a linkage to the intermediate filament network through connection with cytosolic proteins (desmoplakin, plakoglobin and plakophilin). Adherens junctions play a pivotal role in embryonic development as well as in the maintenance of tissue architecture in adults. Cadherins are linked to the actin-cytoskeleton network through catenins (α-, β-catenin, plakoglobin and p120ctn), thereby providing molecular lines of communication to other cell–cell junctions and to cell-substratum junctions. Cadherin cluster forms a transmembrane core of adherens junctions at sites of the cell–cell contacts. During tumor progression decreased cadherin function is correlated with de-differentiation, metastasis and poor prognosis. In glioblastoma N-cadherin cleavage is regulated by ADAM-10 that promotes tumor cell migration. Furthermore, aberrantly processed proN-cadherin promotes cell migration and invasion in vitro, and in human glioma the level of proN-cadherin is elevated that directly correlates with the invasion potential. [63-68]

Dystroglycan is a transmembrane glycoprotein expressed mainly in sceletal muscle cells, but it can be also found in brain tissue as well. Its main function is to creat contact between the ECM macromolecules and the intracellular cytosceleton. It is linked intracellularly to dystrophin, a protein coded on the X-chromosome (lack of dystrophin causes the herediter muscle disease named dystrophia musculorum Duchenne). Dystroglycan is a heterodimeric complex consisting of non-covalently associated α and β subunits. The α-subunit connects α2-laminin, agrin and perlecan (components of the lamina basalis), the β-subunit is the transmembrane part that binds to dystrophin. Overexpression of dystroglycan decreased the growth rate of glioma cell lines so it was found to be involved in the progression of primary brain tumors. [69-71]

3.2. Extracellular Matrix (ECM) components (targets for the receptors)

Various components of brain ECM, like GAGs and PGs are overexpressed in gliomas. These molecules are binding sites for tumor cell receptors or they can inhibit cell migration, so they take an important part in peritumoral glioma invasion, and consequently could also serve as targets for anti-tumor therapy.

Proteoglycans (PGs) are composed of a protein core and **glycosaminoglycan side chains (GAGs)**. GAGs are carbohydrate polymers containing N-acethylglucosamine or N-acethylgalactosamine and uronic acid (glycuronacid or iduronacid).

Depending on the GAG side chains the main types of PGs are chondroitin-sulphate (glycuronacid and N-acethylgalactosamine polymer and protein core), dermatan-sulphates (former name chondroitin-sulphate-B, composed of iduronacid and N-acethylgalactosamine polymer and protein core), heparansulphate (glycuronacid and N-sulphoglucosamine polymer and protein core) and keratansulphate (galactose and N-acethylgalactosamine polymer and protein core). Hyaluronic acid (hyaluronan, HA) is consisted of only GAGs (glycuronacid and N-acethylglucosamin polymer) that has no covalent bind to a protein, so it is not a PG by definition, but due to its tight relation to the PGs in general it is discussed together with them.

One of the most frequent adhesion glycoprotein in the ECM is **fibronectin**. It has a pivotal role in cell attachment, migration, differentiation and proliferation. Although its protein fragment is coded by only one gene, more isoform exits due to alternative splicing. The main cell surface receptors for fibronectin are the integrins, but it can also bind collagens, fibrin and heparan-sulphates. It is structured of two different subunits linked by disulphid bridges to each other. Fibronectin appears in two different forms: the solubile molecule can be found in the plasma, produced by hepatocytes, it accumulates at wessel wall damage and has an evident role in clot-building. The insolubile form of fibronectin is expressed by fibroblasts and mainly localized in the intercellular ECM. In tumor stroma production of fibronectin is reduced and its degradation is increased. Paralel to these changes on tumor cell surface, the expression of the fibronectin receptor $\alpha5\beta1$ integrin is also decreased. ECM components such as fibronectin and collagen type IV are mostly produced by the host tissue and are associated dominantly with the vessel walls in gliomas. Fibronectin is mainly degraded by MMP-2 that is specifically active in gliomas explaining partly the moderate presence of extracellular fibronectin in glioma ECM. [72-74]

Another common component of the ECM is the molecular family of **laminins**. This glycoprotein has many variants, and it is the main component of lamina basalis. It is thought to take part in cell differentiation, adhesion, migration and cell survival. Each molecule of laminin consits three different chains (α, β, and γ chain) which has 5, 4 and 3 genetic variants, respectively. Recently at least fifteen different chain-combinations have been detected in human tissues. In the lamina basalis laminins promote cell-to-cell linkage, and it forms a spe-

http://dx.doi.org/10.5772/50198

cific network with connection to enactin, fibronectin and perlecan. These molecules can also bind to cell surface receptors such as integrins or dystroglycans, etc. Laminins regulate glioma cell adhesion to ECM proteins in specific manner leading to cell proliferation or cell migration and up-regulation of laminin is associated with the invasiveness activity. [75-77]

Agrin is also an ECM forming PG with the capability to collect acetylcholin receptors. Normally it is indispensible in developing neuromuscular junctions during embryogenesis. Agrin is secretaed at the end of the moto-neurons, and it is also a main component of membrana basalis in various human organs taking part in cell-ECM interactions. Together with neurocan, tenascin-C and versican it is responsible for the peritumoral infiltration of gliomas. [78]

Hyaluronan(HA) is a non-sulphated, linear, high-molecularweight GAG. It differs evidently of other GAGs, because of its extremely large molecular weight (103–104 kDa) composed of 10,000 or more disaccharide repeating units, the lack of sulfate groups or epimerized uronic acid residues and because HA is synthesized at the inner face of the plasma membrane as a free linear polymer without any protein core. It has a significant waterbinding capacity, so it controls the water content of the brain interstitium. HA comprises a substantial fraction of brain ECM and is involved in many physiological and pathological processes. In normal ECM, HA sustain tissue homeostasis, biomechanical integrity, structure and some kind of tissue cohesion. In malignant tumor tissues, HA transmit signals into cytoplasm and induces cell proliferation, motility and invasion. HA binds tenascins, lecticans, the cell surface receptors including CD44, RHAMM or ICAM-1, which together contribute to ECM organization and cell–matrix interaction. Through elevating the level of MMP-9 HA also promotes peritumoral invasion by activating the protease system. Glial tumors have increased amounts of HA which facilitates invasion activity of glioma cells. [79-84]

Lecticans comprise also a family of chondroitin sulphate proteoglycans with four members (brevican, versican, neurocan, and aggrecan), whereby brevican and neurocan are brain-specific molecules. Lecticans contain HA and tenascin binding sites and thus mediates linkage in protein–PG-GAG networks. [85-86]

Brain enriched hyaluronan binding (BEHAB) molecule,also known as **brevican**, a brain-specific chondroitin sulfate PG shows dramatic upregulation in gliomas and it is also induced during periods of increased glial cell motility in development and following brain injury. Gliomas express unique brevican isoforms and the processing of this specific isoform is important for its proinvasive role. In experimentally induced tumors brevican accumulates at the invasive borders and it associates with high infiltrative profiles. Furthermore, brevican up-regulation correlates well with short survival periods of patients with high grade gliomas. Brevican expression in gliomas is restricted to membrane localization, and its presence in high-grade gliomas suggests that it plays a significant role in glioma progression. Brevican promotes activation of epidermal growth factor receptor (EGFR), increases the synthesis of cell adhesion molecules and facilitate fibronectin microfibrill presence on the cell membrane. The effect of brevican on glioma cells motility is mediated not only via EGFR signaling but also by fibronectin-dependent adhesion, and increased expression of CAMs. This motogenic signals could not be worked in the normal neural ECM, where fibronectin is almost absent but it is effective in the microenvironment of glioma cells, which co-express large amounts of brevican and fibronectin in vivo. This interaction explains the distinct ability of these tumors spreading in the central nervous system. Overexpression of brain-specific isoforms of brevican proved to be correlated with ability to peritumoral invasion of gliomas. [73, 87-89]

Neurocan is a large brain specific chondroitin-sulphate PG that interacts with heparan-sulphate proteoglycan (HSPG) molecules, such as syndecan-3 and glypican-1. It has influence on cell adhesion and migration. Neurocan has two HSPG-binding domain with different affinity. In cell culture neurit outgrowth is increased by C-terminal part of neurocan. HSPGs serve also as cell-surface receptors for neurocan, and connection of neurocan to the HSPGs is necessary for the neurit growth. It was found on clinical samples that higher expression of neurocan is associated with the invasive activity of astrocytomas. [89-90]

The ECM glycoprotein **tenascin**, which forms a hexabrachion structure, can be detected in both the ECM and the perivascular tissues of high-grade gliomas. Tenascin R, a brain-specific member of the tenascin family comprising also tenascin C, X, and W, is a homotrimer with both lectican and integrin binding sites forming an adhesion link between the ECM and cells. The developed brain does not contains tenascin, but in normal brain tissue distinguishable deposits of this glycoprotein can be found in the glia limitans externa, and some tenascin was also detected in the ECS of white matter. Theres is a positive correlation between tenascin production and the malignancy or angiogenesis of astrocytomas and there is a prognostic utility of its immunohistochemical detection in ependymomas. The accumulation of tenascin in the ECS in high grade glial tumors can be one of the major factors leading to the critical increase in ECS tortuosity and the simultaneous enlargement of the ECS. It has been arised that the ECM distribution is modified at the brain-tumor zone of confrontation and the presence of tenascin in this zone represents a negative prognostic factor in pediatric ependymomas. Tenascin-C is overexpressed in both low and high grade astrocytomas as well. In cultured brain-tissue tenascin-C is produced by the endothelial cells. It takes an important part in various cellular mechanisms like heamagglutination, T-cell immunsuppression, angiogenesis, chondrogenesis and it also has some antiadhesive effect. Tenascin subunits contain EGF- and fibronectin-like repeated sequences that are responsible for the growth inducing effect. Tenascin-C enhances migration of endothelial cells and phosphorylation of focal adhesion kinase (FAK). Tenascin-C signaling is mainly mediated by integrin-β1 which interacts with FAK. Tenascin-C is produced by the glioma cells rather than by the invaded brain and it improves aggressive behaviour and invasion activity of grade II astrocytoma cells in vitro and in vivo. Furthermore, expression of tenascin-C can be used as prognostic factor in grade II astrocytomas showing correlation with ability of tumor recurrence. Beside this, low tenascin-C expression was found to be associated with prolonged average survival time in glioblastomas and highest tenascin-C expression could be detected at the border of the malignant gliomas. [91-104]

Versican (also known as VCAN or CSPG2), a chondroitin sulfate PG, is one of the main components of the ECM, expressed almost in all human tissues. Versican takes part in normal tissue development, but its increased expression can be also detected in most malignan-

http://dx.doi.org/10.5772/50198

cies. Elevated versican production occurs in either the tumor cells or the stromal cells surrounding the tumor. Increased versican expression strongly correlates with poor outcomes for many different tumor types. Versican regulates a wide variety of intracellular processes including cell adhesion, proliferation, apoptosis, migration and invasion via the chondroitin and dermatan sulfate side chains. In addition, the versican G1 and G3 domains can interact with various intracellular or extracellular molecules. In addition to HA, versican associates with tenascin-R, fibulin-1 and -2, fibrillin-1, fibronectin, P- and L-selectin, and many chemokines. It also binds to cell surface proteins including epidermal growth factor receptor (EGFR), CD44, and integrin β1.

A number of proteinase families are capable of generating the proteolytic fragments of versican. Matrix metalloproteinase (MMP)-1, -2, -3, -7, and -9, ADAMTS-1, -4, -5 and -9 cleave versican and generates proteolytic fragments.The accumulation of proteolytic fragments of versican play an important role in cancer progression. The regulation of G1 and G3 versican levels by proteases is known to be important in regulating cancer cell motility and metastasis. Through the EGF-like motifs in the G3 domain versican can stimulate cell proliferation and its G1 domain destabilizes cell adhesion and promotes cell growth. Versican expression is associated with a high rate of proliferation and it is localized in HA-rich tissues and also accumulated in perivascular elastic tissues involved in peritumoral invasion. These features of versican make it a proliferative, anti-adhesive and pro-migratory molecule that facilitates tumor cell motility. In clinical samples the association of versican to invasiveness of astrocytoma could be evidently demonstrated. On the other side, the decreased expression of versican V0 and V1 isoforms in glioma ECM can be related to the marked local invasivity and rarity of extracranial metastasis of gliomas. [105-111]

3.3. Enzymes that are synthesizing or lysating the ECM components

Matrix metalloproteinases (MMPs) are the most common proteases that degrade ECM to create the space for invading glioma cells. MMPs belong to the zinc-dependent endopeptidase together with adamalysins, serralysins and astacins. MMPs take part in remodelling after tissue damage, cell migration, differentiation and angiogenesis. At least 28 different types of MMPs are identified composing a protease family that is able to degrade practically every component of the ECM. Due to their function, MMPs also play evident role of activating mechanism by cleavage metabolits of inactive molecules. MMPs are overexpressed in glioma cells compared with normal brain tissue. MMP-2, MMP-3 and MMP-9 activity correlates well with glioma cell migration and invasion. [46, 112, 113]

Cathepsin-B is a cystein protease involved in protein degradation primarily within intracellular lysosomes but it takes evidently part in degradation of ECM-proteins. In order to be able to interact with ECM proteins, the lysosomal enzyme is secreted from its intracellular localization. Thus cathepsin B appears on the surface of glioma cells, where the enzyme can interact with the surrounding matrix components. Cathepsin-B is overexpressed in gliomas. Downregulation of cathepsin B in human glioma cells leads to decreased invasiveness in matrigel-assay and coculture experiments. Furthermore, downregulation of cathepsin-L in human glioma cells correlates with decreased invasiveness and increased sensitivity to apoptotic stimuli. [114-118]

4. Invasion process of tumor cells

Knowing the invasion potential of primary brain tumors, many of the molecular mechanisms of peritumoral infiltration have been already studied and some of the invasion processes have been defined. During malignant transformation, invasiveness is determined by the complex functions of tumor cells of distinct histological types. A four-step model of invasion has been applied, that is also valid for brain tumors. This model contains the following steps: 1) the tumor cells at the invasive site detach from the growing primary tumor mass; 2) they adhere to the extracellular matrix (ECM) via specific recebptors; 3) proteases secreted by the glioma cells locally degrade the ECM components, forming a pathway migration into the surrounding tissue, and 4) tumor cell movement due to cytosceletal processes. Each step of the peritumoral invasion requires a harmonized cooperation of numerous molecules resulted in active cellular movement into the normal brain parenchyma. [119, 120]

The detachment of invading glioma cells from the primary tumor mass is a complex process comprising the following steps: 1) Destabilization and disorganization of the cadherin mediated junctions that hold the primary mass together. 2) Decrease expression of cell adhesion molecule which provides adhesion to the primary tumor mass. This leads to a reduction in gap junction formation. Cell–cell communication is necessary for growth control and differentiation, and it is mainly achieved through gap junctions. Increased malignancy of gliomas is accociated with reduced in situ gap junction formation, and invasion of gliomas. 3) Cleavage of CD44, which anchors the primary mass to the ECM. This process is mediated by metalloproteinase ADAM. [119-123]

Tumor cell adherence to the ECM components is mediated by specific cell surface or transmembrane receptors like integrins binding to laminins, fibronectins and collagens or CD44 to hyaluronan.

Degradation of ECM components occurs due to the local enhancement and activation of protease suc as MMPs, hyaluronidase, cathepsins and chondroitin suphatase.

Due to migration the glioma cell must interact with the surrounding ECM, which forms a mechanical barrier to the cells, and serves as a substratum for traction for the moving cells. For cell movement changes in cell morphology occur: the cell becomes polarized and membrane protrusions develop, including the extensions at the leading edge of pseudopodia, lamellipodia, filopodia, and invadopodia. These extensions contain filamentous actin and various structural and signaling molecules. The formation of membrane anchors needs cytoskeletal contraction, which finally results a cell forward displacement. Glioma cell motility and contractility also require A and B isoforms of myosin II. Myosin II is the major source of cytoplasmic contractile force. Myosin II allows glioma cells to squeeze through pores smaller than their nuclear diameter, which is especially important for gliomas because the human

http://dx.doi.org/10.5772/50198

brain tissue has particularly narrow extracellular spaces. The connection of ECM macromolecules and cytosceleton is mediated by dystroglycans. [69, 124]

5. The possible agents for antiinvasive therapy

Tumor cell invasion into the surrounding brain tissue is mainly responsible for the failure of radical surgical resection and successful treatment, with tumor recurrence as microdisseminated disease. ECM related molecules and their receptors predominantly participate in the invasion process, including the cell adhesion to the surrounding microenvironment and cell migration. Determination of the key molecules of invasion process can help toprovide possible targets for antiinvasive therapy. Regarding peritumoral infiltration activity of glioma cells, the following molecules are supposed to serve as antitumor agents.

Cilengitide is a cyclic peptide targeting the RGD-motif of integrins blocking $\alpha v\beta 3$- and $\alpha v\beta 5$-integrin mediated interaction between endothelial cells and ECM. By targeting these integrins cilengitide could inhibit both glioma invasion and angiogenesis. Cilengitide causes significant regression of glioma xenograftsand induces apoptosis in U87 glioma cells cultured on tenascin and vitronectin. In clinical trials targeting glioma invasion, in a randomized phase II study cilengitide proved to be safe and was associated with a median survival of 10 months in recurrent glioma patients. The North American Brain Tumor Consortium (NABTC) study aimed to determine cilengitide penetration rate into GBM in human patients. This study confirmed that cilengitide is effectively delivered into primary human GBM tumors with good retention. The effect of combination therapy, such as cilengitide with XRT or with another chemotherapeutic agent, is likely to be cumulative. [125-129]

Knowing the evident role of versican proteolytic fragments in cancer progression, its possible role as target for anti-cancer therapy has been arised. Although there are only a few results regarding anti-versican therapy in glioma patients, some possible agents are notable to mention for their potential future role.The tyrosine kinase inhibitor **genistein** has been shown to block versican expression in malignant mesothelioma cell lines and in vascular smooth muscle cells. Versican G3 fragments facilitate cancer cell growth, invasion and metastasis through EGFR signaling. The selective EGF receptor inhibitor, **AG1478** prevents G3 fragment enhanced cell growth, migration, invasion and chemical resistance in vitro. **Galardin,** an antibody against the ADAMTS specific versican cleavage site inhibits glioma cell migration. **GM6001**, a MMP and ADAMT proteases inhibitor, also decreases cancer cell invasion and metastasis in several kinds of carcinoma. Other protease inhibitors such as **catechin gallate esters**, present in natural sources (green tea) selectively inhibit ADAMTS-1, -4 and -5 catabolism. [130-137]

Tumor formation of the pericellular matrix with HA and versican can be inhibited by treatment with **HA oligomers,** which can block the interaction between HA and versican, serving as inhibitors of cancer dissemination. Furthermore, disruption of the HA CD44 interaction with HA oligomers could also inhibit the growth of B16F16 melanoma cells, Therefore the application of HA oligomers can be an effective agent for inhibiting the formation of vesicant-HA-CD44 complexes, providing valuable targets against tumor progression. [138-140]

Emodin (3-methyl-1,6,8-trihydroxyanthraquinone) has evident anti invasive effect on HA-induced glioma invasion. In glioma cells emodin inhibits the TGFbeta and FGF-2 induced expression of syndecan-1. It decreses the expression of MMP-2 and MMP-9 at both transcriptional and translational levels suggesting that emodin can be a clinically valuable anti-cancer agent against glioma invasion. [141, 142]

Since increased MMP levels are associated with glioma invasion and angiogenesis, **marimastat**, an orally active drug that can reduce MMP levels in patients with gliomas could inhibit growing of tumor. A phase II study evaluated marimastat combined with temozolomide (TMZ) in patients with recurrent malignant glioma and good outcome was documented, but joint and tendon pain was reported in 47% of patients. [143, 144]

6. General aspects of angiogenesis

Rapidly growing tumors need to develop their own vasculature. The hypervascularisation of high grade gliomas can be visualized well on radioimaging and it can be a preoperative characteristic of glioblastoma. Furthermore, glioma angiogenesis is necessary for tumor expansion and survival, so its inhibition could be a potential tool in anti-tumor therapy.

There are two main angiogenic and invasive glioma phenotypes. Clusters of glioma cells perform single cell infiltrations into normal parenchyma independent of vasculature. Another group of glioma cells can be found around newly developed vessels in the normal brain parenchyma near to the tumor margin. These two different angiogenic and invasive phenotypes are called angiogenesis-dependent and angiogenesis independent invasions. High grade astrocytomas content both invasion phenotypes in a mixture of subclones present in different intratumoral regions. Molecular mechanisms of single cell migration were detailed above, but the role of neo-angiogenesis forms also a very important way to glioma expansion. [145]

In expanding, highly proliferate gliomas angiogenesis is activated when the pro-angiogenic stimuli dominates over the anti-angiogenic stimuli. These stimuli are mediated by factors secreted from glioma, endothelial or microglia cells, or arise from the extracellular matrix or other environmental sources like hypoxia induced cell productions. The pro- and anti-angiogenic forces are influenced strongly by tissue hypoxia and genetic alterations. The summation of these stimulileads to the so-called "angiogenic switch" in glioma angiogenesis.The most effective activator of angiogenesis in brain tumors is hypoxia that downregulates anti-angiogenic pathways and induces many pro-angiogenic ones. A well-known pathway is the HIF-1/VEGF-A pathway, which play a significant role in endothelial cell proliferation and migration. Another pathway mediator is interleukin-8, which is produced by microglia cells as a reaction to hypoxia. It is important to mention, that genetic instability of high grade gliomas provides the way of angiogenesis independently of hypoxia (such as chronic HIF activation via phosphoinositide 3-kinase (PI3K) or mitogenactivated protein kinase (MAPK) pathways. [146-152]

After activating the "angiogenic switch", the tumor produces new vessels. The modes of new blood vessel formation in glioma occur by one of three different methods: 1) angiogenesis; 2) vasculogenesis; or 3) arteriogenesis. Angiogenesis is the formation of new blood vessels by rerouting or remodeling existing tumor vessels, and is supposed to be the main stream of neo-angiogenesis. Vasculogenesis means de novo production of blood vessels from circulating marrow-derived endothelial progenitor cells originally as the method of vasculature development in embryonic process. Since these progenitor cells have been also identified in tumors, they role in tumor angiogenesis cannot be denied. Vasculogenesis is probably regulated by tumor-secreted stromal-derived factor 1 under the control of the hypoxia-induced transcription factor hypoxia-inducible factor 1α (HIF1α). Arteriogenesis is the third mode of arteriolar networks formation representing a moderate proportion of tumor angiogenesis. [153-156]

6.1. Neoangiogenesis

The most significant way to form new blood vessels in gliomas is neoangiogenesis. Formation of new vessels from native vessels begins with breaking down the original vessel wall. The process of blood vessel breakdown is composed of three main phases. The first event in forming new vessels from existing ones is the disintegration of the vessel wall. Angiopoietin-1 (Ang-1) and its receptor Tie-2 play a pivotal role in this phase. Normally, Ang-1 binds to Tie-2 achieving a close association between pericytes and endothelial cells that is necessary for vasculature stability. In rapidly proliferating tumors like glioblastoma, tissue hypoxia increases and it induces Ang-2 upregulation in endothelial cells whereas Ang-1 is accumulated tumor cells. Increased Ang-2 expression, which is an antagonist of Tie-2, leads to the initial regression of blood vessels. Beside these, matrix-metalloproteinase (MMP)-2 expression is induced via Tie-2 signaling, and in conjunction with VEGF promotes angiogenesis. The second phase is the breakdown of ECM to provide place for the migration of endothel cells to form new blood vessels. Following dissolution of native vessel wall, degradation of the vessel basement membrane and relating ECM is the necessary condition for endothelial cells for invasion the surrounding microenvironment. MMPs play an integral role in this phase. In case of glioma angiogenesis, the collagenases MMP-2 and MMP-9 are involved in this process and their expression correlates with a poor prognosis in gliomas. Expression of MMP-2 and MMP-9 is also induced by hypoxia and through their proteolytic activity interaction of endothelial cells and tumor-ECM contents like VEGF and fibroblast growth factor (FGF) occurs. [157-166]

The third phase to form new blood vessels is the migration of endothelial cells. After dissolution of the basement membrane of the blood vessels and decomponent ECM, endothelial cells begins to proliferate and migrate toward tumor cells that expresses pro-angiogenic factors. Due to this process cell surface adhesion and migration molecules, such as integrins and CD44 upregulates.The activated endothelial cells secrets platelet-derived growth factor (PDGF) that induces pericytes to participate in creating a new basement membrane. For this reason beside migration of endothelial cells, pericyte migration also occurs as a necessary event of vasculogenesis. [167-169]

At the end of tumor blood vessel formation a significant change occurs in the extracellular environment, caused by increased expression of embryonic ECM molecules, such as tenascin-C. Elevation of VEGF and Ang-2 levels can be also detected, that probably explains the leakiness and pathologic structure of the new vessels. The result of glioma angiogenesis are highly tortuous dilated vessels and lots of small diameter vessels with alterations in endothelial cell adhesion molecule expression and disrupted basement membrane. [170-174]

7. Molecular aspects of glioma angiogenesis

Angiogenesis is mainly induced through growth hormone receptors, especially through the **vascular endothel growth factor receptor (VEGFR)**. This is a transmembrane receptor with an extracellular antibody-binding domain (for vascular endothel growth factor (VEGF)) and an intracellular tyrosin kinase domain stimulating the PI3K/Akt pathway. In tumor angiogenesis the effect of VEGFR can be increased either by receptor overexpression on the cell surface or by mutation of the receptor that without a hormone-ligand or by only a moderate ligand connection it keeps on a permanent stimulus.

Regarding glioma angiogenesis not only VEGFR but the hormone ligand **VEGF** has also an evident role in the process. There are more types of VEGF. Specifically, VEGF-A is upregulated in glioblastoma and it is produced by many cell types, such as tumor cells, stromal, and inflammatory cells. VEGF-A is primarily induced by tissue hypoxia and it regulates endothelial cell survival, proliferation, permeability and migration mainly through the VEGF-receptor 2 (VEGFR2). VEGF can also be derived from the tumor-ECM. Beside the increased amount of VEGF, the receptors VEGF-R1, VEGF-R2 and VEGF-R3 are upregulated on endothelial cells in glioma in comparison to normal brain. [175- 182]

Other growth factors have also influence on angiogenesis. Epidermal growth factor (EGF), **basic fibroblast growth factor (bFGF)** and **platelet derived gfrowth factor (PDGF)** facilitates VEGF expression. The result of pathologic increased VEGF signaling in tumors is immature, highly permeable blood vessels with deteriorated blood-brain-barrier (BBB) function and subsequent parenchymal edema. In glioma, bFGF is expressed by tumor cells and endothelial cells but it can be also accumulated and stored in the extracellular matrix of glioma. [183-186]

In rapidly proliferating anaplastic gliomas oxigene supply remains constantly under the necessity, thus hypoxia remains a permanent stimuli for angiogenic factors. It seems to induce not only the secretion of growth factors, but also **interleukin-8 (Il-8)**, a chemokine released by microglia, and Il-8 is expressed in adult glioma at levels correlating to tumor grade. In glioma the interleukin-8 mediated angiogenesis is regulated by the tumor suppressor protein ING4 through the transcription factor NFκB. [187-189]

http://dx.doi.org/10.5772/50198

Interestingly, there are some molecules involved in neuronal pattering during embryogenesis that have similar functions in vascular pattern during tumor angiogenesis. One of these molecules is the **semaphorin**, that induces signal pathway through neuropilins and plexins. Neuropilins are expressed on vascular endothelial cells and function as receptors for VEGF. Their activation leads to pro-angiogenic responses even in the absent of the classical VEGF-R2 signaling and blocking neuropilin-1 can decrease tumor angiogenesis and growth. [183, 190-192]

Beside growth factors and their receptors, there are some ECM components that are overexpressed in glioma vessels in comparison to normal brain tissue, and have some stimulating effect on angiogenesis. One of the most important ECM proteins with an evident role in angiogenesis is **tenascin-C**, which is normally not expressed in the adult brain, but in glioma it can be found at the invading tumor border in the region of angiogenesis. Tenascin-C facilitates endothelial cell migration and induces VEGF expression and focal adhesion kinase phosphorylation, which are both important for angiogenesis. Another ECM protein involved in angiogenesis is **fibronectin**. The oncofetal form of fibronectin is typically only expressed during embryogenesis, but it is also produced in GBM, and it is localized to the tumor vessels. **Laminin-8** a member of the laminin family in ECM is expressed in vascular basement membrane of GBM. Its blocking in an animal model of GBM resulted in decreased tumor microvessel density and increased survival. **Versican** is also an important ECM component of the tumor angiogenesis process. The versican G3 domain facilitates endothelial cell adhesion, proliferation, and migration in vitro and blood vessel formation in nude mouse tumors. Furthermore, G3-domain expressing cells produce increased levels of fibronectin and VEGF, suggesting their common functions in angiogenesis. [193-197]

8. The possible agents for anti-angiogenic therapy

Since VEGFR play the most significant role in tumor angiogenesis, its inhibition bears the most effective possibility for decrease tumor growth. The VEGFR is a transmembrane tumor cell receptor, so blocking antibodies could close down its effect. On the other side blocking the intracellular tyrosine-kinase domain could also inhibit the activation of the signaling pathways. The latest way came into the front in past few years, when small-molecular tyrosine kinase inhibitors proved to be effective in vitro against glioma cell lines. Beside these, blocking the VEG-factor itself can also definitely decrease the stimulating effect of the receptor.

8.1. VEGF-blocking

The most known VEGF neutralizing antibody is the bevacizumab that is already a possible tool of the oncotherapy for glioblastoma. In recurrent glioma patients treated with bevacizumab combined with the chemotherapy agent irinotecan the median survival can be prolonged. As the result of a significant antitumor effect 63% radiographic response, 6-month progression-free survival in 32% of GBM patients could be achieved. Based on these favorable observations further clinical trials have been initiated to combine bevacizumab with temozolomide, the current standard of care for newly diagnosed glioblastoma patients. Another clinical trial suggests that the presence of tumor hypoxia markers predicts probable radiographic response and better survival of patients treated with combinant chemotherapy of bevacizumab and irinotecan. Gliomas treated with bevacizumab often appear as nonenhancing infiltrating laesions on MRI proving the reduced vascularity beside the ongoing invasion, so induction of anti-angiogenic therapy combined with anti-invasive therapy seems to be a possible treatment method in the future. [198-203]

8.2. VEGF-receptor blocking

Anti-angiogenic therapy with VEGF receptor inhibitor **sunitinib** normalizates tumor vasculature, so it elevates intratumoral level of temozolomide due to the improved vessel functions. **Cediranib** is a pan-VEGFR tyrosine kinase inhibitor, while **enzastaurin** is a protein kinase-C inhibitor. Both agents are already in studies. **Sorafenib** is a multikinase inhibitor, that suppresses angiogenesis by inhibiting VEGFR and PDGFR activities in endothelial cells. Sorafenib-treated mice showed significant suppression of glioblastoma cell proliferation, increased apoptosis and autophagy, and reduction of angiogenesis in vivo, phase II trials of sorafenib in patients with malignant gliomas were inducted. **Imatinib** is a kinase inhibitor of PDGFR, c-kit, and bcr-abl. In vitro studies of imatinib on glioma cell proliferation describe, that it is cytostatic agent at low concentration whereas at high concentrations it has cytotoxic effect. Imatinib monotherapy against malignant gliomas has failed to show any significant clinical benefits probable because of the moderate drug penetration across BBB and the inhibition of PDGFR alone can be insufficient to inhibit growth of malignant gliomas. In spite of these its use in combination therapy is still an interesting theme. [204-211]

8.3. Other target molecules for anti-angiogenic therapy

Tenascin-C is mainly expressed in hyperplastic vessels and it promotes migration of endothelial cells in astrocytic tumors. Therefore, blocking tenascin with an antibody to inhibit angiogenesis seems biologically reasonable, so a tenascin-specific antibody radiolabeled with I-131 was tested in patients with high-grade gliomas. The phase II studies with tenascin-blocking antibody in malignant glioma reported about a slight increase in survival time. [101, 195, 212-214]

Another ECM protein that has anti-angiogenic effect in glioma is secreted protein acidic and rich in cysteine (SPARC), also known as **osteonectin** or BM-40. Osteonectin takes part in a number of basic biologic functions, including migration, proliferation, and survival. Expression of SPARC in the nervous system is restricted normally to the angiogenic microvasculature, such as in the region of locus coeruleus and retinal astrocytes, but is not expressed in the cerebral cortex. In contrast, osteonectin is present in both tumor cells and endothelial cells in gliomas of all grades, and it is also expressed by endothelial cells and astrocytes in the adjacent tissue. Osteonectin suppresses tumor angiogenesis via inhibition of VEGF expression and secretion. [215-221]

http://dx.doi.org/10.5772/50198

8.4. Endogenous anti-angiogenic factors

A number of endogenous anti-angiogenic factors have been described that play pivotal role in tumor angiogenesis. Identifying these factors could offer some anti-cancer agent for neuro-oncological therapies. One of the best known endogenous anti-angiogenic proteins is **angiostatin.** It is mainly derived from degradation of plasminogen by proteases cathepsin-D and MMPs. In vivo studies in mice proved that angiostatin inhibits glioma angiogenesis and growth. The **thrombospondins (TSPs)** are another family of proteins that serves as an anti-angiogenic factor. In normal tissue TSP1 is produced by platelets, endothelial cells, and smooth muscle cells. Similar to angiostatin, **endostatin** is also an anti-angiogenic molecule created in glioblastoma basement membrane by proteolytic cleavage of collagen-18 by elastase, cathepsin-L, and specific MMPs. The endostatin-mediated signaling has more angiogenic inhibitory mechanism by binding to a5b1 integrin, inhibition of VEGF-R2, reduction of focal adhesion kinase-mediated endothelial cell migration, and suppression of pro-angiogenic MMP-2. A further factor is the angiogenesis inhibitor-1 (BAI1), also known as **vasculostatin,** that is produced only in glial cells and neurons of normal brain but not in blood vessels. Since vasculostatin is defnietly reduced in glioblastomas, its role in suppressing angiogenesis is glioma is strongly supposed. [222-231]

9. Conclusion

There are no simple and evidently succesful protocols for therapy of primary brain tumors. The intensive proliferation activity, the significant peritumoral infiltration and increased angiogenesis altogether are responsible for the extremely high recurrence rate of gliomas. The failure of recently administered chemotherapy arises the requirement of combination therapy. Thus besides searching a highly specific tumor marker, establishing the molecular spectrum of these tumors can be suggested. Supporting this theory, the mRNA expression pattern of the invasion-related molecules was found to be highly specific for various different histological tumor groups. So determination of the genetic signature of invasion of a glioma is thought to help in screening exact molecules as targets for individual chemotherapy. [89] Furthermore, complexity of oncotherapy with combination of antiproliferation, anti-invasive and antiangiogenic drugs could bring benefits in treatment effectiveness against brain tumors in the future.

Author details

Almos Klekner

Department of Neurosurgery, University of Debrecen, Medical and Health Science Centre, Hungary

References

[1] Burger PC, Scheithauer BW. Tumors of the central nervous system. Atlas of Tumor Pathology, third series, fascicle 1994; 10: 349-369

[2] Louis DN, Ohgaki H, Wiestler OD, Cavenee WK, Burger PC, Jouvet A, Scheithauer BW, Kleihues P. The 2007 WHO Classification of Tumours of the Central Nervous System. Acta Neuropathol 2007; 114: 197-109

[3] Miliaras G, Tsitsopoulos PP, Markoula S, Kyritsis A, Polyzoidis KS, Malamou-Mitsi V. Multifocal glioblastoma with remote cutaneous metastasis: a case report and review of the literature. Cen Eur Neurosurg 2009; 70: 39-42

[4] Czirok A, Zamir EA, Filla MB, Little CD, Rongish BJ.Extracellular matrix macroassembly dynamics in early vertebrate embryos. Curr Top Dev Biol 2006; 73: 237-258

[5] Hirose J, Kawashima H, Yoshie O,Tashiro K, Miyasaka M. Versican interacts with chemokines and modulates cellular responses. J Biol Chem 2001; 276: 5228-5234

[6] Jung S, Moon KS, Kim ST, Ryu HH, Lee YH, Jeong YI, Jung TY, Kim IY, Kim KK, Kang SS. Increased expression of intracystic matrix metalloproteinases in brain tumors: relationship to the pathogenesis of brain tumor-associated cysts and peritumoral edema. J Clin Neurosci 2007; 14:1192-1198

[7] Leivonen M, Lundin J, Nordling S, von Boguslawski K, Haglund C.Prognostic Value of Syndecan-1 Expression in Breast Cancer. Oncology 2004; 67: 11-18

[8] Pakula R, Melchior A, Denys A, Vanpouille C, Mazurier J, Allain F. Syndecan- / CD147 association is essential for cyclophilin B-induced activation of p44/42 mitogen-activated protein kinases and promotion of cell adhesion and chemotaxis. Glycobiology 2007; 17:492-503

[9] Shibata Sh, Fukada K, Suzuki Sh, Ogawa T, Yamashita Y. Histochemical localisation of versican, aggrecan and hyaluronan in the developing condylar cartilage of the fetal rat mandible. J Anat 2001; 198: 129-135

[10] Bellail AC, Hunter SB, Brat DJ, Tan C, Van Meir EG. Microregional extracellular matrix heterogeneity in brain modulates glioma cell invasion. Int J Biochem Cell Biol 2004; 36:1046–1069

[11] Gladson CL. The extracellular matrix of gliomas: modulation of cell function. J Neuropathol Exp Neurol 1999; 58:1029–1040

[12] Goldbrunner RH, Bernstein JJ, Tonn JC. Cell-extracellular matrix interaction in glioma invasion. Acta Neurochir (Wien) 1999; 141:295–305

[13] Nicholson C, Sykova. Extracellular space structure revealed by diffusion analysis. Trends Neurosci 1998; 21:207–215

[14] Novak U, Kaye AH. Extracellular matrix and the brain: components and function. J Clin Neurosci 2000; 7:280–290

[15] Paulus W. Brain extracellular matrix, adhesion molecules and glioma invasion. In: Mikkelsen T, Bjerkvig R, Laerum OD, Rosenblum ML (eds) Brain tumor invasion: biological, clinical and therapeutic considerations. Wiley-Liss, New York, 1998; pp 301–322

[16] Zamecnik J, Vargova L, Homola A, Kodet R, Sykova E. Extracellular matrix and diffusion barriers in human astrocytic tumors. Neuropathol Appl Neurobiol 2004; 30:338–350

[17] Langley RR, Fidler IJ. The seed and soil hypothesis revisited - the role of tumor–stroma interactions in metastasis to different organs. Int J Cancer 2011; 128: 2527–2535.

[18] Kalluri R. Basement membranes: structure, assembly and role in tumour angiogenesis. Nature Rev Cancer 2003; 3: 422–433.

[19] Rougon G, Hobert O. New insights into the diversity and function of neuronal immunoglobulin superfamily molecules. Annu Rev Neurosci 2003; 26: 207–238.

[20] Robinson EE, Zazzali KM, Corbett SA, et al . Alpha5beta1 integrin mediates strong tissue cohesion. J Cell Sci 2003; 116: 377–386.

[21] Humphries JD, Byron A, Humphries MJ. Integrin ligands at a glance. J Cell Sci 2006; 119: 3901–3903.

[22] Schmidt S, Friedl P. Interstitial cell migration: integrin-dependent and alternative adhesion mechanisms. Cell Tissue Res 2010; 339:83–92.

[23] Anthis NJ, Campbell ID. The tail of integrin activation. Trends Biochem Sci 2011; 36: 191–198.

[24] Schweitzer T, Vince GH, Herbold C, et al . Extraneural metastases of primary brain tumors. J Neurooncol 2001; 53: 107–114.

[25] Shapiro L, Love J, Colman DR. Adhesion molecules in the nervous system: structural insights into function and diversity. Annu Rev Neurosci 2007; 30: 451–474.

[26] Gingras MC, Roussel E, Bruner JM, et al . Comparison of cell adhesion molecule expression between glioblastoma multiforme and autologous normal brain tissue. J Neuroimmunol 1995; 57:143–153.

[27] Calogero A, Pavoni E, Gramaglia T, et al . Altered expression of alpha-dystroglycan subunit in human gliomas. Cancer Biol Ther 2006; 5: 441–448.

[28] Paulus W, Baur I, Schuppan D, et al . Characterization of integrin receptors in normal and neoplastic human brain. Am J Pathol 1993; 143: 154–163.

[29] Kawataki T, Yamane T, Naganuma H, et al . Laminin isoforms and their integrin receptors in glioma cell migration and invasiveness: evidence for a role of alpha5-laminin(s) and alpha3beta1 integrin. Exp Cell Res 2007; 313: 3819–3831.

[30] Jahn O, Tenzer S, Werner HB. Myelin proteomics: molecular anatomy of an insulating sheath. Mol Neurobiol 2009; 40: 55–72.

[31] Nakada M, Kita D, Futami K, et al . Roles of membrane type 1 matrix metalloproteinase and tissue inhibitor of metalloproteinases 2 in invasion and dissemination of human malignant glioma. J Neurosurg 2001; 94: 464–473.

[32] Leavesley DI, Ferguson GD, Wayner EA et al. Requirement of the integrin beta 3 subunit for carcinoma cell spreading or migration on vitronectin and fibrinogen. J Cell Biol 1992; 117:1101–1107

[33] Platten M, Wick W, Wild-Bode C et al. Transforming growth factors beta(1) (TGF-beta(1)) and TGF-beta(2) promote glioma cell migration via up-regulation of alpha(V)beta(3) integrin expression. Biochem Biophys Res Commun 2000; 268:607–611

[34] Guan JL, Shalloway D: Regulation of focal adhesionassociated protein tyrosine kinase by both cellular adhesion and oncogenic transformation. Nature 358: 690–692, 1992

[35] Owens LV, Xu L, Craven RJ, Dent GA, Weiner TM, Kornberg L, Liu E T, Cance W G: Overexpression of the focal adhesion inase (p125FAK) in invasive human tumors. Cancer Res 55: 2752–2755, 1995

[36] Jones G, Machado J Jr, Merlo A: Loss of focal adhesion kinase (FAK) inhibits epidermal growth factor receptordependent migration and induces aggregation of nh(2)-terminal FAK in the nuclei of apoptotic glioblastoma cells. Cancer Res, 61: 4978–4981, 2001

[37] Zagzag D, Friedlander DR, Margolis B, Grumet M, Semenza GL, Zhong H, Simons JW, Holash. J, Wiegand, SJ, Yancopoulos GD: Molecular events implicated in brain tumor angiogenesis and invasion. Pediatr Neurosurg 33: 49–55, 2000

[38] Cary LA, Guan JL: Focal adhesion kinase in integrinmediated signaling. Front: Biosci, 4: D102–113, 1999

[39] Hauck CR, Hsia DA, Schlaepfer DD: The focal adhesion kinase – a regulator of cell migration and invasion. IUBMB Life 53: 115–119, 2002

[40] Frisch SM, Vuori K, Ruoslahti E, Chan-Hui PY: Control of adhesion-dependent cell survival by focal adhesion kinase. J Cell Biol 134: 793–799, 1996

[41] Xiong W, Parsons JT: Induction of apoptosis after expression of PYK2, a tyrosine kinase structurally relatedto focal adhesion kinase. J Cell Biol 139: 529–539, 1997

[42] Graham CH, Connelly I, MacDougall JR, Kerbel RS, Stetler-Stevenson WG, Lala PK: Resistance of malignant trophoblast cells to both the anti-proliferative and antiinvasive effects of transforming growth factor-beta. Exp Cell Res 214: 93–99, 1994

[43] Merzak A, Koocheckpour S, Pilkington GJ: CD44 mediates human glioma cell adhesion and invasion in vitro. Cancer Res 54: 3988–3992, 1994

[44] Prag S, Lepekhin EA, Kolkova K, Hartmann-Petersen R, Kawa A, Walmod PS, Belman V, Gallagher H, C, Berezin V, Bock E, Pedersen N: NCAM regulates cell motility. J Cell Sci 115: 283–292, 2002

[45] Hikawa T, Mori T, Abe T, Hori S: The ability in adhesion and invasion of drug-resistant human glioma cells. J Exp Clin Cancer Res 19: 357–362, 2000

[46] Varga I, Hutóczki G, Petrás M, Kenyeres A, Scholtz B, Mikó E, Hanzély Z, Tóth J, Bognár L, Zahuczky G, Klekner A: Expression of invasion-related extracellular matrix molecules in human glioblastoma versus intracerebral lung adenocarcinoma metastasis. Cen Eur Neurosurg, 2010 Nov;71(4):173-80

[47] Naor D, Wallach-Dayan SB, Zahalka MA, et al . Involvement of CD44, a molecule with a thousand faces, in cancer dissemination. Semin Cancer Biol 2008; 18: 260–267.

[48] Ponta H, Sherman L, Herrlich PA. CD44: from adhesion molecules to signalling regulators. Nature RevMol Cell Biol 2003; 4: 33–45.

[49] Toole BP. Hyaluronan: from extracellular glue to pericellular cue. Nature reviews. Cancer.2004;4:528–539.

[50] Toole BP. Hyaluronan promotes the malignant phenotype. Glycobiology. 2002;12:37–42.

[51] Day AJ, Prestwich GD. Hyaluronan-binding proteins: tying up the giant. J Biol Chem.2002;277:4585–4588.

[52] Tsukita S, Oishi K, Sato N, Sagara J, Kawai A. ERM family members as molecular linkers between the cell surface glycoprotein CD44 and actin-based cytoskeletons. J Cell Biol. 1994;126:391–401.

[53] Lokeshwar VB, Fregien N, Bourguignon LY. Ankyrin-binding domain of CD44 (GP85) is required for the expression of hyaluronic acid-mediated adhesion function. J Cell Biol. 1994;126:1099–1109.

[54] Li H, Guo L, Li JW, Liu N, Qi R, Liu J. Expression of hyaluronan receptors CD44 and RHAMM in stomach cancers: relevance with tumor progression. Int J Oncol. 2000;17:927–932.

[55] Toole BP. Hyaluronan: from extracellular glue to pericellular cue. Nature reviews. Cancer.2004;4:528–539.

[56] Ponta H, Sherman L, Herrlich P. CD44: from adhesion molecules to signalling regulators. Nature Rev Mol Cell Biol. 2003;4:33–45.

[57] Fieber C, Plug R, Sleeman J, Dall P, Ponta H, Hofmann M. Characterisation of the murine gene encoding the intracellular hyaluronan receptor IHABP (RHAMM) Gene. 1999;226:41.

[58] Thorne RF, Legg JW, Isacke CM. The role of the CD44 transmembrane and cytoplasmic domains in coordinating adhesive and signaling events. J Cell Sci. 2004;117:373–380.

[59] Morgan MR, Humphries MJ, Bass MD. Synergistic control of cell adhesion by integrins and syndecans. Nature Rev Mol Cell Biol 2007; 8: 957–969.

[60] Xian X, Gopal S, Couchman JR. Syndecans as receptors and organizers of the extracellular matrix. Cell Tissue Res 2010; 339: 31–46.

[61] Kim C W et al., "Members of the syndecan family of heparan sulfate proteoglycans are expressed in distinct cell-, tissue-, and development-specific patterns. Molecular Biology of the Cell 5, no. 7 (July 1994): 797–805.

[62] Anttonen A et al., "Syndecan-1 expression has prognostic significance in head and neck carcinoma. British Journal of Cancer 79, no. 3-4 (February 1999): 558–564.

[63] Maret D, Gruzglin E, Sadr MS, Siu V, Shan W, Koch AW, Seidah NG, Del Maestro RF, Colman DR. Surface expression of precursor N-cadherin promotes tumor cell invasion. Neoplasia. 2010 Dec;12(12):1066-80.

[64] Kohutek ZA, diPierro CG, Redpath GT, Hussaini IM. ADAM-10-mediated N-cadherin cleavage is protein kinase C-alpha dependent and promotes glioblastoma cell migration. J Neurosci. 2009 Apr 8;29(14):4605-15.

[65] Nollet F, Kools P, van Roy F: Phylogenetic analysis of the cadherin superfamily allows identification of six major subfamilies besides several solitary members. J Mol Biol 299: 551–572, 2000

[66] Shapiro L, Weis WI. Structure and biochemistry of cadherins and catenins. Cold Spring Harbor Perspect Biol 2009; 1: a003053.

[67] Shapiro L, Love J, Colman DR. Adhesion molecules in the nervous system: structural insights into function and diversity. Annu Rev Neurosci 2007; 30: 451–474.

[68] Nollet F, Kools P, van Roy F. Phylogenetic analysis of the cadherin superfamily allows identification of six major subfamilies besides several solitary members. JMol Biol 2000; 299: 551–572.

[69] Bozzi M, Morlacchi S, Bigotti MG, et al . Functional diversity of dystroglycan. Matrix Biol 2009; 28: 179–187.

[70] Calogero A, Pavoni E, Gramaglia T, D'Amati G, Ragona G, Brancaccio A, Petrucci TC. Altered expression of alpha-dystroglycan subunit in human gliomas. Cancer Biol Ther. 2006 Apr;5(4):441-8.

[71] Gee SH, Montanaro F, Lindenbaum MH, Carbonetto S. Dystroglycan-alpha, a dystrophin-associated glycoprotein, is a functional agrin receptor. Cell 1994; 77 (5): 675–86.

[72] Pankov R, Yamada KM. Fibronectin at a glance. J Cell Sci 2002; 115 (Pt 20): 3861–3

[73] Hu B., Kong L. L., Matthews R. T., Viapiano M. S. The proteoglycan brevican binds to fibronectin after proteolytic cleavage and promotes glioma cell motility. J. Biol. Chem. 2008; 283(36):24848-59

[74] Yamagata M, Yamada KM, Yoneda M, Suzuki S, Kimata K: Chondroitin sulfate proteoglycan (PG-M-like proteoglycan) is involved in the binding of hyaluronic acid to cellular fibronectin. J Biol Chem 1986, 261(29):13526-13535.

[75] Timpl R et al. Laminin – a glycoprotein from basement membranes. J Biol Chem 1979; 254 (19): 21. 9933

[76] Guo P, Imanishi Y, Cackowski FC, et al. Up-regulation of angiopoietin- 2, matrix metalloprotease-2, membrane type 1 metalloprotease, and laminin 5 gamma 2 correlates with the invasiveness of human glioma. Am J Pathol 2005; 166:877– 890

[77] Aguiar CB, Lobão-Soares B, Alvarez-Silva M, Trentin AG.Glycosaminoglycans modulate C6 glioma cell adhesion to extracellular matrix components and alter cell proliferation and cell migration. BMC Cell Biol. 2005 Aug 19;6:31.

[78] Sanes JR, Lichtmann JW: Induction, assembly, maturation and maintenance of a postsynaptic apparatus. Nat Rev Neurosci 2001; 2(11): 791-805

[79] Delpech B, Maingonnat C, Girard N, Chauzy C, Maunoury R, Olivier A, Tayot J, Creissard P. Hyaluronan and hyaluronectin in the extracellular matrix of human brain tumour stroma. Eur J Cancer 1993; 29A:1012–1017

[80] Sadeghi N, Camby I, Goldman S, Gabius HJ, Baleriaux D, Salmon I, Decaesteckere C, Kiss R, Metens T. Effect of hydrophilic components of the extracellular matrix on quantifiable diffusion-weighted imaging of human gliomas: preliminary results of correlating apparent diffusion coefficient values and hyaluronan expression level. AJR Am J Roentgenol 2003; 181:235–241

[81] Itano N. Simple primary structure, complex turnover regulation and multiple roles of hyaluronan. J Biochem 2008; 144: 131–137.

[82] Fidler IJ. The role of the organ microenvironment in brain metastasis. Semin Cancer Biol 2011; 21: 107–112.

[83] Toole BP. Hyaluronan: from extracellular glue to pericellular cue. Nature Reviews. Cancer.2004;4:528–539.

[84] Kim MS, Park MJ, Moon EJ, Kim SJ, Lee CH, Yoo H, Shin SH, Song ES, Lee SH. Hyaluronic acid induces osteopontin via the phosphatidylinositol 3-kinase/AKT pathway to enhance the motility of human glioma cells. Cancer Res. 2005;65:686–691.

[85] Viapiano MS, Matthews RT. From barriers to bridges: chondroitin sulfate proteoglycans in Neuropathology. Trends Mol Med 2006; 12: 488–496.

[86] Yamaguchi Y. Lecticans: organizers of the brain extracellular matrix. Cell Mol Life Sci 2000; 57: 276–289.

[87] Nutt CL, Matthews RT, Hockfield S. Glial tumor invasion: a role for the upregulation and cleavage of BEHAB/brevican. Neuroscientist 2001; 7: 113-122

[88] Viapiano MS, Bi WL, Piepmeier J, Hockfield S, Matthews RT. Novel tumor-specific isoforms of BEHAB/brevican identified in human malignant gliomas. Cancer Res 2005; 65: 6726-6733

[89] Varga, G. Hutóczki, Cs. D. Szemcsák, G. Zahuczky, J. Tóth, Zs. Adamecz, A. Kenyeres, L. Bognár, Z. Hanzély, A. Klekner: Brevican, neurocan, tenascin-C and versican are mainly responsible for the invasiveness of low-grade astrocytoma. Pathol Oncol Res, Pathol Oncol Res. 2012 Apr;18(2):413-20.

[90] Akita K., Toda M., Hosoki Y., Inoue M., Fushiki S., Oohira A., Okayama M., Yamashina I., Nakada H. Heparan sulphate proteoglycans interact with neurocan and promote neurite outgrowth from cerebellar granule cells. Biochem J. 2004; 383(Pt 1): 129-38

[91] Kim C. H., Bak K. H., Kim Y. S., Kim J. M., Ko Y., Oh S. J., Kim K. M., Hong E. K. Expression of tenascin-C in astrocytic tumors: its relevance to proliferation and angiogenesis. Surg. Neurol. 2000; 54(3):235-40

[92] Swindle C. S., Tran K. T., Johnson T. D., Banerjee P., Mayes A. M., Griffith L., Wells A. Epidermal growth factor (EGF)-like repeats of human tenascin-C as ligands for EGF receptor. J. Cell Biol. 2001; 154(2):459-68

[93] Fischer D., Brown-Lüdi M.,Schulthess T., Chiquet-Ehrismann R. Concerted action of tenascin-C domains in cell adhesion, anti-adhesion and promotion of neurite outgrowth. J. Cell Sci. 1997; 110(Pt13):1513-22

[94] Hirata E., Arakawa Y., Shirahata M., Yamaguchi M., Kishi Y., Okada T., Takahashi J. A., Matsuda M., Hashimoto N. Endogenous tenascin-C enhances glioblastoma invasion with reactive change of surrounding brain tissue. Cancer Sci. 2009; 100(8):1451-9

[95] Maris C., Rorive S., Sandras F., D'Haene N., Sadeghi N., Bièche I., Vidaud M., Decaestecker C., Salmon I. Tenascin-C expression relates to clinicopathological features in pilocytic and diffuse astrocytomas. Neuropathol. Appl. Neurobiol. 2008; 34(3):316-29

[96] Gladson CL, Cheresh DA. Glioblastoma expression of vitronectin and the alpha v beta 3 integrin. Adhesion mechanism for transformed glial cells. J Clin Invest 1991; 88:1924– 1932

[97] Joester A, Faissner A. The structure and function of tenascin in the nervous system. Matrix Biol 2001; 20:13–22

[98] Mahesparan R, Read TA, Lund-Johansen M, Skaftnesmo KO, Bjerkvig R, Engebraaten O. Expression of extracellular matrix components in a highly infiltrative in vivo glioma model. Acta Neuropathol 2003; 105:49–57

[99] Oz B, Karayel FA, Gazio NL, Ozlen F, Balci K. The distribution of extracellular matrix proteins and CD44S expression in human astrocytomas. Pathol Oncol Res 2000; 6:118–124

[100] Zamecnik J, Chanova M, Tichy M, Kodet R. Distribution of the extracellular matrix glycoproteins in ependymomas— an immunohistochemical study with follow-up analysis. Neoplasma 2004; 51:214–222

[101] Zagzag D, Friedlander DR, Dosik J, Chikramane S, Chan W, Greco MA, Allen JC, Dorovini-Zis K, Grumet M: Tenascin-C expression by angiogenic vessels in human astrocytomas and by human brain endothelial cells in vitro. Cancer Res, 56: 182–189, 1996

[102] Kostianovsky M, Greco MA, Cangiarella J, Zagzag D: Tenascin-C expression in ultrastructurally defined angiogenic and vasculogenic lesions. Ultrastruct Pathol 21: 537–544, 1997

[103] Zagzag D, Capo V: Angiogenesis in the central nervous system: a role for vascular endothelial growth factor/vascular permeability factor and tenascin-C. Common molecular effectors in cerebral neoplastic, and non-neoplastic 'angiogenic diseases'. Histol Histopathol 17: 301– 321, 2002

[104] Plopper GE, McNamee HP, Dike LE, Bojanowski K, Ingber DE: Convergence of integrin and growth factor receptor signaling pathways within the focal adhesion complex. Mol Biol Cell 6: 1349–1365, 1995

[105] Mauri P, Scarpa A, Nascimbeni AC, Benazzi L, Parmagnani E, Mafficini A, Della Peruta M, Bassi C, Miyazaki K, Sorio C: Identification of proteins released by pancreatic cancer cells by multidimensional protein identification technology: a strategy for identification of novel cancer markers. Faseb J 2005, 19(9):1125-1127.

[106] Voutilainen K, Anttila M, Sillanpaa S, Tammi R, Tammi M, Saarikoski S, Kosma VM: Versican in epithelial ovarian cancer: relation to hyaluronan, clinicopathologic factors and prognosis. Int J Cancer 2003, 107(3):359-364.

[107] Aspberg A, Binkert C, Ruoslahti E: The versican C-type lectin domain recognizes the adhesion protein tenascin-R. Proc Natl Acad Sci U S A 1995, 92(23):10590-10594.

[108] Aspberg A, Adam S, Kostka G, Timpl R, Heinegard D: Fibulin-1 is a ligand for the C-type lectin domains of aggrecan and versican. J Biol Chem 1999, 274(29):20444-20449.

[109] Isogai Z, Aspberg A, Keene DR, Ono RN, Reinhardt DP, Sakai LY: Versican interacts with fibrillin-1 and links extracellular microfibrils to other connective tissue networks. J Biol Chem 2002, 277(6):4565-4572.

[110] Kawashima H, Hirose M, Hirose J, Nagakubo D, Plaas AH, Miyasaka M: Binding of a large chondroitin sulfate/dermatan sulfate proteoglycan, versican, to L-selectin, P-selectin, and CD44. J Biol Chem 2000, 275(45):35448-35456.

[111] Perides G, Asher RA, Lark MW, Lane WS, Robinson RA, Bignami A: Glial hyaluronate-binding protein: a product of metalloproteinase digestion of versican? Biochem J 1995, 312 (Pt 2):377-384.

[112] Van Lint P, Libert C (December 2007). Chemokine and cytokine processing by matrix metalloproteinases and its effect on leukocyte migration and inflammation. J. Leukoc. Biol. 82 (6): 1375–81.

[113] Wild-Bode C, Weller M, Wick W. Molecular determinants of glioma cell migration and invasion. J Neurosurg 2001; 94:978–984

[114] Demchik LL, Sameni M, Nelson K, Mikkelsen T, Sloane BF: Cathepsin B and glioma invasion. Int J Dev Neurosci 17: 483–494, 1999

[115] Rempel SA, Rosenblum ML, Mikkelsen T, Yan. PS, Ellis KD, Golembieski WA, Sameni M, Rozhin J, Ziegler G, Sloane BF: Cathepsin B expression and localization in glioma progression and invasion. Cancer Res 54: 6027–6031, 1994

[116] Sivaparvathi M, Sawaya R, Wang SW, Rayford A, Yamamoto M, Liotta LA, Nicolson GL, Rao JS: Overexpression and localization of cathepsin B during the progression of human gliomas. Clin Exp Metastasis 13: 49–56, 1995

[117] Mohanam S, Jasti SL, Kondraganti SR, Chandrasekar N, Lakka SS, Kin Y, Fuller GN, Yung AW, Kyritsis AP, Dinh DH; Olivero WC, Gujrati M, Ali-Osman F, Rao JS: Down-regulation of cathepsin B expression impairs the invasive and tumorigenic potential of human glioblastoma cells. Oncogene 20: 3665–3673, 2001

[118] Levicar N, Dewey RA, Daley E, Bates TE, Davies D, Kos J, Pilkington GJ, and Lah TT: Selective suppression of cathepsin L by antisense cDNA impairs human braintumor cell invasion in vitro and promotes apoptosis. Cancer Gene Then 10: 141–151, 2003

[119] Manabu O, Tomotsugu I,Kazuhiko K,Isao D. Angiogenesis and invasion in glioma. Brain Tumor Pathol 2011; 28:13–24

[120] Calogero A, Pavoni E, Gramaglia T, D'Amati G, Ragona G, Brancaccio A, Petrucci TC. Altered expression of alpha-dystroglycan subunit in human gliomas. Cancer Biol Ther. 2006 Apr;5(4):441-8.

[121] Demuth T, Berens ME. Molecular mechanisms of glioma cell migration and invasion. J Neurooncol 2004; 70:217–228

[122] Goodenough DA, Goliger JA, Paul DL. Connexins, connexons, and intercellular communication. Annu Rev Biochem 1996; 65:475–502

[123] Soroceanu L, Manning TJ Jr, Sontheimer H. Reduced expression of connexin-43 and functional gap junction coupling in human gliomas. Glia 2001; 33:107–117

[124] Beadle C, Assanah MC, Monzo P, Vallee R, Rosenfeld SS, Canoll P. The role of myosin II in glioma invasion of the brain. Mol Biol Cell 2008;19:3357–3368.

[125] Tonn JC, Wunderlich S, Kerkau S, Klein CE, Roosen K: Invasive behaviour of human gliomas is mediated by interindividually different integrin patterns. AnticancerRes 18: 2599–2605, 1998

[126] Taga T, Suzuki A, Gonzalez-Gomez I, Gilles FH, Stins M, Shimada H, Barsky L, Weinberg KI, Laug WE: alpha v- Integrin antagonist EMD 121974 induces apoptosis in brain tumor cells growing on vitronectin and tenascin. Int J Cancer 98: 690–697, 2002

[127] MacDonald TJ, Taga T, Shimada H, Tabrizi, P, Zlokovic BV, Cheresh DA, Laug WE: Preferential susceptibility of brain tumors to the antiangiogenic effects of an alpha(v) integrin antagonist. Neurosurgery 48: 151–157 2001

[128] Etienne-Manneville S, Hall A: Rho GTPases in cell biology. Nature 420; 629–635, 2002

[129] Reardon DA, Fink KL, Mikkelsen T, et al. Randomized phase II study of cilengitide, an integrin-targeting arginine-glycine-aspartic acid peptide, in recurrent glioblastoma multiforme. J Clin Oncol 2008;26:5610 –5617.

[130] Arslan F, Bosserhoff AK, Nickl-Jockschat T, Doerfelt A, Bogdahn U, Hau P: The role of versican isoforms V0/V1 in glioma migration mediated by transforming growth factor-beta2. Br J Cancer 2007, 96(10):1560-1568.

[131] Syrokou A, Tzanakakis GN, Hjerpe A, Karamanos NK: Proteoglycans in human malignant mesothelioma. Stimulation of their synthesis induced by epidermal, insulin and platelet-derived growth factors involves receptors with tyrosine kinase activity. Biochimie 1999, 81(7):733-744.

[132] Du WW, Yang BB, Shatseva TA, Yang BL, Deng Z, Shan SW, Lee DY, Seth A, Yee AJ: Versican G3 promotes mouse mammary tumor cell growth, migration, and metastasis by influencing EGF receptor signaling. PLoS One, 5(11):e13828

[133] Casey RC, Koch KA, Oegema TR, Jr., Skubitz KM, Pambuccian SE, Grindle SM, Skubitz AP: Establishment of an in vitro assay to measure the invasion of ovarian carcinoma cells through mesothelial cell monolayers. Clin Exp Metastasis 2003, 20(4): 343-356

[134] Nakamura JL, Haas-Kogan DA, Pieper RO: Glioma invasiveness responds variably to irradiation in a co-culture model. Int J Radiat Oncol Biol Phys 2007, 69(3):880-886.

[135] Almholt K, Juncker-Jensen A, Laerum OD, Dano K, Johnsen M, Lund LR, Romer J: Metastasis is strongly reduced by the matrix metalloproteinase inhibitor Galardin in the MMTV-PymT transgenic breast cancer model. Mol Cancer Ther 2008, 7(9): 2758-2767.

[136] Vankemmelbeke MN, Jones GC, Fowles C, Ilic MZ, Handley CJ, Day AJ, Knight CG, Mort JS, Buttle DJ: Selective inhibition of ADAMTS-1, -4 and -5 by catechin gallate esters. Eur J Biochem 2003, 270(11):2394-2403

[137] Schonherr E, Kinsella MG, Wight TN: Genistein selectively inhibits platelet-derived growth factor-stimulated versican biosynthesis in monkey arterial smooth muscle cells. Arch Biochem Biophys 1997, 339(2):353-361.

[138] Evanko SP, Angello JC, Wight TN: Formation of hyaluronan- and versican-rich pericellular matrix is required for proliferation and migration of vascular smooth muscle cells. Arterioscler Thromb Vasc Biol 1999, 19(4):1004-1013.

[139] Ween MP, Hummitzsch K, Rodgers RJ, Oehler MK, Ricciardelli C: Versican induces a pro-metastatic ovarian cancer cell behavior which can be inhibited by small hyaluronan oligosaccharides. Clin Exp Metastasis, 28(2):113-125.

[140] Zeng C, Toole BP, Kinney SD, Kuo JW, Stamenkovic I: Inhibition of tumor growth in vivo by hyaluronan oligomers. Int J Cancer 1998, 77(3):396-401.

[141] Kim MS, Park MJ, Kim SJ, Lee CH, Yoo H, Shin SH, Song ES, Lee SH. Emodin suppresses hyaluronic acid-induced MMP-9 secretion and ivnasion of gliomas cells. Int J Oncol. 2005;27:839–846.[

[142] Arata Watanabe A, Mabuchi T, Satoh E, Furuya K, Zhang L, Maeda S, Maeda S, Naganuma H. Expression of syndecans, a heparin sulfate proteoglycan, in malignant gliomas: participation of nuclear factor-kappaB in upregulation of syndecan-1 expression. J Neurooncol. 2006;77:25–32.

[143] Levin VA, Phuphanich S, Yung WK et al. Randomized, double-blind, placebo-controlled trial of marimastat in glioblastoma multiforme patients following surgery and irradiation. J Neurooncol 2006; 78:295–302

[144] Groves MD, Puduvalli VK, Hess KR et al. Phase II trial of temozolomide plus the matrix metalloproteinase inhibitor, marimastat, in recurrent and progressive glioblastoma multiforme. J Clin Oncol 2002; 20:1383–1388

[145] Sakariassen PO, Prestegarden L, Wang J et al.Angiogenesis- independent tumor growth mediated by stem-like cancer cells. Proc Natl Acad Sci USA 2006; 103:16466–16471

[146] Wang D, Anderson JC, Gladson CL. The role of the extracellular matrix in angiogenesis in malignant glioma tumors. Brain Pathol 2005;15:318 –326.

[147] Brown JM, Wilson WR. Exploiting tumour hypoxia in cancer treatment. Nat Rev Cancer 2004;4:437– 447.

[148] Kaur B, Brat DJ, Calkins CC, Van Meir EG. Brain angiogenesis inhibitor 1 is differentially expressed in normal brain and glioblastoma independently of p53 expression. Am J Pathol 2003; 162:19 –27.

[149] Brat DJ, Bellail AC, Van Meir EG. The role of interleukin-8 and its receptors in gliomagenesis and tumoral angiogenesis. Neuro Oncol 2005;7:122–133.

[150] Desbaillets I, Diserens AC, de Tribolet N, Hamou MF, Van Meir EG. Regulation of interleukin-8 expression by reduced oxygen pressure in human glioblastoma. Oncogene 1999;18:1447–1456.

[151] Fischer I, Gagner JP, Law M, Newcomb EW, Zagzag D. Angiogenesis in gliomas: biology and molecular pathophysiology. Brain Pathol 2005;15:297–310.

[152] Kaur B, Tan C, Brat DJ, Post DE, Van Meir EG. Genetic and hypoxic regulation of angiogenesis in gliomas. J Neurooncol 2004;70:229 –243.

[153] Aghi M, Chiocca EA. Contribution of bone marrow-derived cells to blood vessels in ischemic tissues and tumors. Mol Ther 2005; 12:994 –1005.

[154] Jouanneau E. Angiogenesis and gliomas: current issues and development of surrogate markers. Neurosurgery 2008;62:31–50.

[155] Aghi M, Cohen KS, Klein RJ, Scadden DT, Chiocca EA. Tumor stromal-derived factor-1 recruits vascular progenitors to mitotic neovasculature, where microenvironment influences their differentiated phenotypes. Cancer Res 2006;66:9054 –9064.

[156] Du R, Lu KV, Petritsch C, et al. HIF1alpha induces the recruitment of bone marrow-derived vascular modulatory cells to regulate tumor angiogenesis and invasion. Cancer Cell 2008;13: 206–220.

[157] Bergers G, Song S. The role of pericytes in blood-vessel formation and maintenance. Neuro Oncol 2005;7:452– 464.

[158] Reiss Y, Machein MR, Plate KH. The role of angiopoietins during angiogenesis in gliomas. Brain Pathol 2005;15:311–317.

[159] Zagzag D, Amirnovin R, Greco MA, et al. Vascular apoptosis and involution in gliomas precede neovascularization: a novel concept for glioma growth and angiogenesis. Lab Invest 2000;80: 837–849.

[160] Stratmann A, Risau W, Plate KH. Cell type-specific expression of angiopoietin-1 and angiopoietin-2 suggests a role in glioblastoma angiogenesis. Am J Pathol 1998;153:1459 –1466.

[161] Holash J, Maisonpierre PC, Compton D, et al. Vessel cooption, regression, and growth in tumors mediated by angiopoietins and VEGF. Science 1999;284:1994 –1998.

[162] Hu B, Guo P, Fang Q, et al. Angiopoietin-2 induces human glioma invasion through the activation of matrix metalloprotease- 2. Proc Natl Acad Sci U S A 2003;100:8904–8909.

[163] Rooprai HK, McCormick D. Proteases and their inhibitors in human brain tumours: a review. Anticancer Res 1997;17:4151– 4162.

[164] Raithatha SA, Muzik H, Rewcastle NB, Johnston RN, Edwards DR, Forsyth PA. Localization of gelatinase-A and gelatinase-B mRNA and protein in human gliomas. Neuro Oncol 2000;2:145– 150.

[165] Rao JS, Yamamoto M, Mohaman S, et al. Expression and localization of 92 kDa type IV collagenase/gelatinase B (MMP-9) in human gliomas. Clin Exp Metastasis 1996;14:12–18.

[166] Lakka SS, Gondi CS, Rao JS. Proteases and glioma angiogenesis. Brain Pathol 2005;15:327–341

[167] Jouanneau E. Angiogenesis and gliomas: current issues and development of surrogate markers. Neurosurgery 2008;62:31–50.

[168] Bergers G, Song S. The role of pericytes in blood-vessel formation and maintenance. Neuro Oncol 2005;7:452– 464.

[169] Ferrara N, Kerbel RS. Angiogenesis as a therapeutic target. Nature 2005;438:967–974.

[170] Anderson JC, McFarland BC, Gladson CL. New molecular targets in angiogenic vessels of glioblastoma tumours. Expert Rev Mol Med 2008;10:e23.

[171] Jouanneau E. Angiogenesis and gliomas: current issues and development of surrogate markers. Neurosurgery 2008;62:31–50.

[172] Herold-Mende C, Mueller MM, Bonsanto MM, Schmitt HP, Kunze S, Steiner HH. Clinical impact and functional aspects of tenascin-C expression during glioma progression. Int J Cancer 2002;98:362–369.

[173] Baluk P, Morikawa S, Haskell A, Mancuso M, McDonald DM. Abnormalities of basement membrane on blood vessels and endothelial sprouts in tumors. Am J Pathol 2003;163:1801–1815.

[174] Vitolo D, Paradiso P, Uccini S, Ruco LP, Baroni CD. Expression of adhesion molecules and extracellular matrix proteins in glioblastomas: relation to angiogenesis and spread. Histopathology 1996;28:521–528.

[175] Hanahan D, Folkman J. Patterns and emerging mechanisms of the angiogenic switch during tumorigenesis. Cell 1996;86:353–364.

[176] Carmeliet P, Jain RK. Angiogenesis in cancer and other diseases. Nature 2000;407:249 –257.

[177] Dvorak HF. Vascular permeability factor/vascular endothelial growth factor: a critical cytokine in tumor angiogenesis and a potential target for diagnosis and therapy. J Clin Oncol 2002;20: 4368–4380.

[178] Ferrara N. Vascular endothelial growth factor: basic science and clinical progress. Endocr Rev 2004;25:581– 611.

[179] Machein MR, Plate KH. VEGF in brain tumors. J Neurooncol 2000;50:109 –120.

[180] Plate KH, Breier G, Weich HA, Risau W. Vascular endothelial growth factor is a potential tumour angiogenesis factor in human gliomas in vivo. Nature 1992;359:845–848.

[181] Whitelock JM, Murdoch AD, Iozzo RV, Underwood PA. The degradation of human endothelial cell-derived perlecan and release of bound basic fibroblast growth factor by stromelysin, collagenase, plasmin, and heparanases. J Biol Chem 1996;271: 10079–10086.

[182] Grau SJ, Trillsch F, Herms J, et al. Expression of VEGFR3 in glioma endothelium correlates with tumor grade. J Neurooncol 2007;82:141–150.

[183] Jain RK, di Tomaso E, Duda DG, Loeffler JS, Sorensen AG, Batchelor TT. Angiogenesis in brain tumours. Nat Rev Neurosci 2007;8:610–622.

[184] Kaur B, Brat DJ, Calkins CC, Van Meir EG. Brain angiogenesis inhibitor 1 is differentially expressed in normal brain and glioblastoma independently of p53 expression. Am J Pathol 2003; 162:19 –27.

[185] Jain RK. Molecular regulation of vessel maturation. Nat Med 2003;9:685– 693.

[186] Karcher S, Steiner HH, Ahmadi R, et al. Different angiogenic phenotypes in primary and secondary glioblastomas. Int J Cancer 2006;118:2182–2189.

[187] Brat DJ, Bellail AC, Van Meir EG. The role of interleukin-8 and its receptors in gliomagenesis and tumoral angiogenesis. Neuro Oncol 2005;7:122–133.

[188] Melder RJ, Koenig GC, Witwer BP, Safabakhsh N, Munn LL, Jain RK. During angiogenesis, vascular endothelial growth factor and basic fibroblast growth factor regulate natural killer cell adhesion to tumor endothelium. Nat Med 1996;2:992–997.

[189] Garkavtsev I, Kozin SV, Chernova O, et al. The candidate tumoursuppressor protein ING4 regulates brain tumour growth and angiogenesis. Nature 2004;428:328 –332.

[190] Mamluk R, Klagsbrun M, Detmar M, Bielenberg DR. Soluble neuropilin targeted to the skin inhibits vascular permeability. Angiogenesis 2005;8:217–227.

[191] Soker S, Takashima S, Miao HQ, Neufeld G, Klagsbrun M. Neuropilin-1 is expressed by endothelial and tumor cells as an isoform-specific receptor for vascular endothelial growth factor. Cell 1998;92:735–745.

[192] Miao HQ, Klagsbrun M. Neuropilin is a mediator of angiogenesis. Cancer Metastasis Rev 2000;19:29 –37.

[193] Wang D, Anderson JC, Gladson CL. The role of the extracellular matrix in angiogenesis in malignant glioma tumors. Brain Pathol 2005;15:318 –326.

[194] Castellani P, Viale G, Dorcaratto A, et al. The fibronectin isoform containing the ED-B oncofetal domain: a marker of angiogenesis. Int J Cancer 1994;59:612– 618.

[195] Zagzag D, Shiff B, Jallo GI, et al. Tenascin-C promotes microvascular cell migration and phosphorylation of focal adhesion kinase. Cancer Res 2002;62:2660 –2668.

[196] Mariani G, Lasku A, Balza E, et al. Tumor targeting potential of the monoclonal antibody BC-1 against oncofetal fibronectin in nude mice bearing human tumor implants. Cancer 1997;80:2378– 2384.

[197] Fujita M, Khazenzon NM, Ljubimov AV, et al. Inhibition of laminin-8 in vivo using a novel poly(malic acid)-based carrier reduces glioma angiogenesis. Angiogenesis 2006;9:183–191.

[198] Stupp R, Mason WP, van den Bent MJ et al. Radiotherapy plus concomitant and adjuvant temozolomide for glioblastoma. N Engl J Med 2005; 352:987–996

[199] Vredenburgh JJ, Desjardins A, Herndon JE, 2nd, et al. Phase II trial of bevacizumab and irinotecan in recurrent malignant glioma. Clin Cancer Res 2007;13:1253–1259.

[200] Vredenburgh JJ, Desjardins A, Herndon JE, 2nd, et al. Bevacizumab plus irinotecan in recurrent glioblastoma multiforme. J Clin Oncol 2007;25:4722– 4729.

[201] Norden AD, Young GS, Setayesh K, et al. Bevacizumab for recurrent malignant gliomas: efficacy, toxicity, and patterns of recurrence. Neurology 2008;70:779 –787.

[202] Chi A, Norden AD, Wen PY. Inhibition of angiogenesis and invasion in malignant gliomas. Expert Rev Anticancer Ther 2007; 7:1537–1560.

[203] Sathornsumetee S, Cao Y, Marcello JE et al. Tumor angiogenic and hypoxic profiles predict radiographic response and survival in malignant astrocytoma patients treated with bevacizumab and irinotecan. J Clin Oncol 2008; 26:271–278

[204] Roberts WG, Whalen PM, Soderstrom E, et al. Antiangiogenic and antitumor activity of a selective PDGFR tyrosine kinase inhibitor, CP-673,451. Cancer Res 2005;65:957–966.

[205] Batchelor TT, Sorensen AG, di Tomaso E, et al. AZD2171, a pan-VEGF receptor tyrosine kinase inhibitor, normalizes tumor vasculature and alleviates edema in glioblastoma patients. Cancer Cell 2007;11:83–95.

[206] Tabatabai G, Frank B, Wick A, et al. Synergistic antiglioma activity of radiotherapy and enzastaurin. Ann Neurol 2007;61:153–161.

[207] Zhou Q, Guo P, Gallo JM. Impact of angiogenesis inhibition by sunitinib on tumor distribution of temozolomide. Clin Cancer Res 2008;14:1540 –1549.

[208] Wong ML, Prawira A, Kaye AH et al. Tumour angiogenesis: its mechanism and therapeutic implications in malignant gliomas. J Clin Neurosci 2009; 16:1119–1130

[209] Siegelin MD, Raskett CM, Gilbert CA, Ross AH, Altieri DC (2010) Sorafenib exerts anti-glioma activity in vitro and in vivo. Neurosci Lett 478:165–170

[210] Ranza E, Mazzini G, Facoetti A, Nano R. In vitro effects of the tyrosine kinase inhibitor imatinib on glioblastoma cell proliferation. J Neurooncol 2010; 96:349–357

[211] Wen PY, Yung WK, Lamborn KR et al. Phase I/II study of imatinib mesylate for recurrent malignant gliomas: North American Brain Tumor Consortium Study 2006; 99-08. Clin Cancer Res 12:4899–4907

[212] Akabani G, Reardon DA, Coleman RE, et al. Dosimetry and radiographic analysis of 131I-labeled anti-tenascin 81C6 murine monoclonal antibody in newly diagnosed patients with malignant gliomas: a phase II study. J Nucl Med 2005;46:1042–1051.

[213] Bigner DD, Brown M, Coleman RE et al. Phase I studies of treatment of malignant gliomas and neoplastic meningitis with 131I-radiolabeled monoclonal antibodies anti-tenascin 81C6 and anti-chondroitin proteoglycan sulfate Me1-14 F(ab0)2—a preliminary report. J Neurooncol 1995; 24:109–122

[214] Reardon DA, Akabani G, Coleman RE et al. Phase II trial of murine (131)I-labeled antitenascin monoclonal antibody 81C6 administered into surgically created resection cavities of patients with newly diagnosed malignant gliomas. J Clin Oncol 2002; 20:1389–1397

[215] Yunker CK, Golembieski W, Lemke N, et al. SPARC-induced increase in glioma matrix and decrease in vascularity are associated with reduced VEGF expression and secretion. Int J Cancer 2008;122:2735–2743.

[216] Rempel SA, Golembieski WA, Ge S, et al. SPARC: a signal of astrocytic neoplastic transformation and reactive response in human primary and xenograft gliomas. J Neuropathol Exp Neurol 1998;57:1112–1121.

[217] Bornstein P, Sage EH. Matricellular proteins: extracellular modulators of cell function. Curr Opin Cell Biol 2002;14:608–616.

[218] Lane TF, Iruela-Arispe ML, Johnson RS, Sage EH. SPARC is a source of copper-binding peptides that stimulate angiogenesis. J Cell Biol 1994;125:929 –943.

[219] Yan Q, Sage EH, Hendrickson AE. SPARC is expressed by ganglion cells and astrocytes in bovine retina. J Histochem Cytochem 1998;46:3–10.

[220] Lane TF, Sage EH. The biology of SPARC, a protein that modulates cell-matrix interactions. FASEB J 1994;8:163–173.

[221] Anderson JC, McFarland BC, Gladson CL. New molecular targets in angiogenic vessels of glioblastoma tumours. Expert Rev Mol Med 2008;10:e23.

[222] Kaur B, Brat DJ, Calkins CC, Van Meir EG. Brain angiogenesis inhibitor 1 is differentially expressed in normal brain and glioblastoma independently of p53 expression. Am J Pathol 2003; 162:19 –27.

[223] Wahl ML, Kenan DJ, Gonzalez-Gronow M, Pizzo SV. Angiostatin's molecular mechanism: aspects of specificity and regulation elucidated. J Cell Biochem 2005;96:242–261.

[224] O'Reilly MS, Holmgren L, Shing Y, et al. Angiostatin: a novel angiogenesis inhibitor that mediates the suppression of metastases by a Lewis lung carcinoma. Cell 1994;79:315–328.

[225] Kirsch M, Strasser J, Allende R, Bello L, Zhang J, Black PM. Angiostatin suppresses malignant glioma growth in vivo. Cancer Res 1998;58:4654–4659.

[226] Joe YA, Hong YK, Chung DS, et al. Inhibition of human malignant glioma growth in vivo by human recombinant plasminogen kringles 1-3. Int J Cancer 1999;82:694–699.

[227] Adams JC, Lawler J. The thrombospondins. Int J Biochem Cell Biol 2004;36:961–968.

[228] Strik HM, Weller M, Frank B, et al. Heat shock protein expression in human gliomas. Anticancer Res 2000;20:4457– 4462.

[229] Folkman J. Antiangiogenesis in cancer therapy—endostatin and its mechanisms of action. Exp Cell Res 2006;312:594–607.

[230] Heljasvaara R, Nyberg P, Luostarinen J, et al. Generation of biologically active endostatin fragments from human collagen XVIII by distinct matrix metalloproteases. Exp Cell Res 2005; 307:292–304.

[231] Sudhakar A, Sugimoto H, Yang C, Lively J, Zeisberg M, Kalluri R. Human tumstatin and human endostatin exhibit distinct antiangiogenic activities mediated by alpha v beta 3 and alpha 5 beta 1 integrins. Proc Natl Acad Sci U S A 2003;100:4766–4771.

Chapter 2

Gliomas Biology: Angiogenesis and Invasion

Maria Caffo, Valeria Barresi, Gerardo Caruso,
Giuseppe La Fata, Maria Angela Pino,
Giuseppe Raudino, Concetta Alafaci and
Francesco Tomasello

Additional information is available at the end of the chapter

http://dx.doi.org/10.5772/53487

1. Introduction

Glial tumors, within neuroepitelial-derived lesions, are the most common intra-assial neoplastic histotypes. Gliomas account for about 45% of all primary central nervous system (CNS) tumors and 77% of all malignant primary CNS tumors. Gliomas can originate from neural stem cells, progenitor cells, or from de-differentiated mature neural cells transformed into cancer stem cells. Although brain tumors constitute only a small proportion of overall human malignancies, they carry high rates of morbidity and mortality. Mortality is still close to 100% and the average survival of patients with glioblastoma multiforme (GBM) is less than 1 year when classical treatment is used. Recent progresses in multimodal treatment has led to only a slight increase in average survival up to 15-18 months [1]. The effectiveness of the actual chemotherapeutic approach and multimodal targeted therapies remains modest in gliomas.

Gliomas are divided into different subtypes based on cell line from which they originate. Gliomas include astrocytomas, glioblastomas, oligodendrogliomas, ependymomas and other histological subtypes. The most common gliomas are astrocytomas, oligodendrogliomas and ependymomas. Since 1993, the 4-level grading system proposed by the World Health Organization (WHO), was the most widely accepted and widespread. It is based on histologic features: nuclear atypia, presence of mitoses, endothelial proliferation. Grade I gliomas are benign with a slow proliferation rate and include pylocitic astrocytoma most common in pediatric age. Grade II gliomas are characterized by a high degree of cellular differentiation and grow diffusely into the normal brain parenchyma and are prone to malignant progression. They include astrocytoma, oligodendroglioma and oligoastrocytoma. Grade III lesions include anaplastic astrocytoma, anaplastic oligoastrocytoma and anaplastic oligodendroglioma. These tumors show a higher cellular density and a notable presence of atypia and mitotic cells. Grade IV tumors are the most malignant and also the most frequent gliomas and include glioblastoma and gliosarcoma. These tumors presented microvascular proliferations and pseudopalisading necrosis.

Conventional brain tumor treatments include surgery, radiation therapy and chemotherapy. Surgical treatment is invasive but represents the first approach for the vast majority of brain tumors due to difficulties arising in early stage detection. However, gross total removal is not always achievable in relation to the location of the tumor, to preserve vital nervous or vascular structures. Aggressive treatment modalities have extended the median survival from 4 months to 1 year, but the survival is often associated with significant impairment in the quality of life. Radiation therapy and chemotherapy are non-invasive options often used as adjuvant therapy, but may also be effective for curing early-stage tumors. Radiotherapy seems to be related only to a prolonged progression-free survival, with better control of seizures, but with no substantial differences in overall survival. Besides, patients treated with radiotherapy, have high risk to develop some complications such as post radiation leukoencephalopathy, that is characterized by dementia, gait disturbance, incontinence, deficit in attention and executive functions. In patients with recurrent GBM, the 6-months progression-free survival is only 21% after treatment with temozolomide [2]. The effectiveness of systemic chemotherapy is limited by toxic effects on healthy cells, generally resulting in morbidity or mortality of the patient. Moreover, the presence of the blood-brain barrier (BBB) limits the passage of a wide variety of anticancer agents. The high incidence of recurrence and poor prognosis of malignant gliomas compel the development of more powerful anti-cancer treatments. Action of alkylating agents, one of the most common class of chemotherapeutic drugs employed, is limited by activation of methylguanine-methyltransferase. The compromise of the quality of remaining life as well as the limited success of current treatment options in shrinking tumors, raise increasing concerns about the adverse effects of cancer treatment on brain function.

Glioma cell invasion into normal tissue is thought to be a multi-factorial process, consisting of cell interactions with extracellular matrix (ECM) and with adjacent cells, as well as accompanying biochemical processes supportive of active cell movement. Tumor cell invasion requires four distinct steps: (1) detachment of invading cells from the primary tumor mass, (2) adhesion to ECM, (3) degradation of ECM, and (4) cell motility and contractility. However, growth of tumors necessitates, also, the recruitment of a new blood supply. Angiogenesis, represent a key event in the progression of malignant gliomas. Tumor angiogenesis involves multiple cellular processes including endothelial cell proliferation, migration, reorganization of ECM and tube formation.

The advent of molecular studies allowed a new evaluation of the biology of gliomas with, a level of precision that promises interesting advances toward the development of specific and effective therapies. The introduction of molecularly targeted agents is one of the most significant advances in cancer therapy in recent years. Targeted therapies block activation of oncogenic pathways, either at the ligand-receptor interaction level or by inhibiting down-

http://dx.doi.org/10.5772/53487

stream signal transduction pathways, thereby inhibiting growth and progression of cancer. Because of their specificity, targeted therapies should theoretically have better efficacy and safety profiles than systemic cytotoxic chemotherapy or radiotherapy.

In this chapter we evaluated the invasion and angiogenesis in the glioma progression. Moreover, new pharmacological agents on the basis of the more recent literature will be evaluated.

2. Gliomas

Approximately 50% of primary brain tumors are gliomas, arising from astrocytes, oligodendrocytes, or their precursors and ependymal cells. Gliomas are classified from I to IV according to the WHO malignancy scale. Gliomas are divided into different subtypes based on cell line from which they originate. The WHO classification of CNS tumors, now in its fourth edition, is the universal standard for classifying and grading brain neoplasms. Analysis of tumour differentiation, cellularity, cytonuclear atypia, mitotic activity, microvascular proliferation, and necrosis further enables grading of the tumour as grade 2 (diffuse infiltrating low-grade gliomas), 3 (anaplastic gliomas), or 4 (glioblastomas) with increasing aggressiveness. Unfortunately, WHO morphological classification is based on subjective criteria, lacks reproducibility, and remains imperfect in its ability to predict individual outcomes. The most recent WHO classification introduced a number of significant changes that include both additions and redefinitions or clarifications of existing entities. Three new tumor types were added to the glioma section. The first of these is angiocentric glioma. Angiocentric gliomas are slowly growing solid hemispheric tumors of children and young adults. They are strongly epileptogenic, with 95% of patients presenting with intractable seizures. These tumors are characterized histologically by elongated bipolar glial tumor cells and by their striking perivascular growth pattern. Angiocentric gliomas have a low proliferative potential (MIB-1 between 1% - 5%) and have been designated as WHO grade I neoplasms. The second, pilomyxoid astrocytoma (PMA), is now formally considered as a distinct more aggressive variant of PA. PMAs typically occur at an earlier mean age and are associated with more aggressive behavior than Pas (pilocytic astrocytomas). PMAs are composed of bipolar (piloid or hairlike) cells that lie within a distinct myxoid background matrix. PMAs are currently considered WHO grade II neoplasms. Atypical choroid plexus papilloma (CPP) is the third new tumor. Cellular atypia and increased mitotic activity are reflected in more aggressive biologic behavior, with earlier metastases and higher recurrence rates than CPP. An aCPP is designated as a WHO grade II neoplasm. The 2007 WHO version recognized, also, papillary glioneuronal tumor (PGNT), rosette-forming glioneuronal tumor (RGNT) of the fourth ventricle, and the extraventricular form of neurocytoma. PGNT is a rare relatively well-circumscribed clinically indolent tumor that is exclusively found in the cerebral hemispheres. PGNTs are biphasic tumors, with both astrocytic and neuronal elements. The histologic hallmark of PGNT is the presence of hyalinized vascular pseudopapillae. Although PGNT was not formally assigned a WHO grade in the 2007 revision, this tumor generally behaves in a benign grade I fashion. RGNTs are rare slow-growing tumors of young and middle-aged adults. RGNTs contain both neurocytic and astrocytic elements. Their histologic hallmark is the formation of neurocytic perivascular pseudorosettes. RGNTs are designated as WHO grade I neoplasms. The term "central neurocytoma" describes a neuronal tumor with preferential location in the lateral ventricle body. These tumors comprise fibrillary areas mimicking neuropil plus collections of uniform round cells that have immunohistochemical and ultrastructural evidence of neuronal differentiation. A low proliferation rate is typical. Similar neoplasms have been reported outside the ventricular system, and the WHO 2007 designated the term "EVNCT" (extraventricular neurocytoma) for these uncommon tumors. Because the only distinguishing feature is location EVNCTs are included in the same histopathologic code as central neurocytoma. Both central and extraventricular neurocytomas are designated as WHO grade II neoplasms. Two new tumors of the pineal region were codified in the WHO 2007 classification, papillary tumor of the pineal region (PTPR) and pineal parenchymal tumor of intermediate differentiation (PPTID). PTPR is a rare neuroepithelial tumor that arises from the subcommissural organ and exhibits ependymal differentiation. Macroscopically, PTPRs are indistinguishable from pineocytomas. Microscopically, the tumors are easily distinguished. PTPRs show papillary architecture with pseudostratified columnar epithelium. Ultrastructural features suggesting ependymal differentiation are present. Immunohistochemistry is positive for cytokeratins. While grading of PTPRs has yet to be defined, most neuropathologists consider these as WHO grade II or III neoplasms. PPTID is a newly recognized tumor intermediate in malignancy between pineocytoma and pineoblastoma. Mild-to-moderate nuclear atypia and low-to-moderate mitotic activity result in either WHO grade II or III. PPTIDs have a much more aggressive course than pineocytomas and may warrant adjuvant therapy. PPTIDs are more common than previously recognized, accounting for up to 20% of all pineal parenchymal neoplasms. Recent reports emphasize their large size and focal invasion of adjacent structures as features that distinguish them from pineocytoma [3].

According to WHO low grade gliomas include diffuse astrocytomas (fibrillar, gemistiocytic, protoplasmatic, mixed), grade II oligodendrogliomas and oligoastrocytomas. Diagnosis of anaplastic glioma is based on the presence of mitotic activity, while vascular proliferation and necrosis are typical features of GBM. The definition of low grade glioma does not refer perhaps to I grade astrocytomas, that differ from other gliomas in relation to their biological behaviour, prognosis and genetic profile [4]. Low grade gliomas, tend perhaps to dedifferentiate: a global therapeutic approach, related to gross total (> 90%) surgical removal, radiotherapy e chemiotherapy with temozolamide, leads only to a slight prolongation of overall survival, calculated from 3 to 7 years [5]. This variability depends from various factors: age at diagnosis, tumor volume, tumor crossing the midline, neurological deficits before treatment and tumor's histology [6]. Anyway, mortality is near to 100% and only 35% of patients with glioblastoma multiforme have a median survival of one year or more.

2.1. Genetics of malignant gliomas

Cancers originate as the result of hereditary or somatic alterations in genes that control critical biological processes. The accumulation of such genetic damage over time permits the survival and progressive transformation of abnormal cell populations that eventually lead to the formation of a tumor. Consistent with their high malignant potential, gliomas exhibit a vast array of well-documented genetic changes that likely contribute to their phenotype. Gliomagenesis is characterized by several biological events, such as activated growth factor receptor signaling pathways, downregulation of many apoptotic mechanisms and unbalance among proangiogenic and antiangiogenic factors. Several growth factor receptors, such epidermal growth factor receptor (EGFR), platelet-derived growth factor receptor (PDRGF), C-Kit, vascular endhotelial growth factor receptor (VEGFR) and others growth factors receptors, are overexpressed, amplified and/or mutated in gliomas. Features of the glioma cells are the loss of tumor suppressor genes, which are critical for the cell growth, differentiation and function.

The TP53 tumor suppressor gene was identified as the main driver of chromosome 17 alterations in glioblastoma, and further studies indicated that p53 plays a critical role in monitoring the genome for DNA damage and can control cell cycle arrest to permit DNA repair or can trigger apoptosis to eliminate the damaged cell [7]. It acts as a transcriptional activator and it repress the transcription of other genes, such as IL-6, c-fos, c-jun and other oncogenes. The levels of p53 increase in G1 and S phases of the cell cycle. Cells transfected with the normal gene p53 block their growth in G1, suppressing the passage S-phase. The expression of the p53 gene cause apoptosis (programmed cell death). The effects of its mutation are the loss of cell cycle regulation, through the inactivation of $p16^{ink\text{-}4a}$, the super expression of cycline dependent kinase 4 Cdk4 and Cdk6 and of ubiquitin ligase Mdm2 and Mdm4. A similar mechanism is created after mutation of retinoblastoma (Rb), a tumor suppressor gene. Probably, TP53 is a gene responsible for the progression from low-grade to high-grade gliomas, but its mutation is an early event. Many glioma cell lines expressing p53 mutations. The mutated form of p53 has a crucial role in the regulation of neovascularization. It induces increased levels of VEGF and FGFβ through an activation of the transcription of the corresponding genes. The deletion of NFKBIA (encoding nuclear factor of κ-light polypeptide gene enhancer in B-cells inhibitor-α), an inhibitor of the EGFR-signaling pathway, promotes tumorigenesis in glioblastomas that do not have alterations of EGFR. Bredel et al. analyzed 790 human GBMs for deletions, mutations, or expression of NFKBIA and EGFR. they studied the tumor-suppressor activity of NFKBIA in tumor-cell culture and compared the molecular results with the outcome of GBM in 570 affected persons. NFKBIA is often deleted but not mutated in GBM [8].

Epidermal growth factor receptor mutations include amplifications, point mutations and deletions, with the most common alteration being the variant III deletion of the extracellular domain (EGFR-vIII mutant) [9]. Platelet-derived growth factor receptor and its ligands PDGF-A and PDGF-B are also commonly over-expressed in some glioma cells, raising the possibility of autocrine or paracrine activation [10]. Other RTK genes, such as ERBB2, another member of the EGF receptor family, and MET, which encodes the hepatocyte growth factor receptor, have also been found to be mutated in GBMs [9]. RTKs mediate cell growth and proliferation via downstream effectors such as Ras and phosphatidylinositide-3-kinase (PI3K). Activity of these proteins is tightly regulated, especially by the tumor suppressors Nf1 and Pten. The PI3K pathway is another essential survival pathway for a variety of cancer cells. The tumor suppressor Pten (phosphatase and tensin homologue on chromosome 10) negatively regulates the PI3K pathway by dephosphorylating phosphatidylinositol-3,4,5-triphosphate (PIP3) back to phosphatidylinositol-4,5-biphosphate (PIP2) [11]. Mutations in PTEN frequently involve the phosphatase domain, and mutations in PI3K typically involve the catalytic (p110α) and regulatory (p85α) domains.

Classically, GBM has been described as result endpoint from two main gliomagenesis pathways [12-13]. Primary GBM shows amplification of the EGFR, deletion or mutation of homozygous cyclin-dependent kinase (CDK) inhibitor p16INK4A/(CDKN2A), alterations in tumor-suppressor PTEN on chromosome 10, and deletion in the INK4a gene with loss of p14 and p16 [14-15]. Progression from low-grade to high-grade astrocytomas involves inactivating mutations of tumor-suppressor gene TP53 and elevated expression of PDGF ligands and receptors, accumulation of genetic alteration of retinoblastoma-associated cell cycle regulatory pathways, including deletion or mutations of cyclin-dependent kinase inhibitor p16INK4A/(CDKN2A) or the retinoblastoma susceptibility locus 1 (pRB1), as well as amplification or overexpression of cyclin-dependent kinase 4 (CDK4) and human double minute 2 (HDM2). Evolution to secondary GBM is associated with deletion of chromosome 10, which includes tumor-suppressor phosphatase and tensin homologue (PTEN). PTEN phosphatase were identified as the tumor suppressors lost on chromosomes 19 and 10, respectively. p16 can slow down cell cycle progression, whereas PTEN is a negative regulator of the phosphoinositide 3-kinase (PI3K) pathway, [16] a major signaling pathway that stimulates cellular proliferation in response to growth factor stimulation. Interestingly, only 1 copy of the gene is mutated in the tumors, suggesting that the mutations do not result in a simple loss of function. The mutation is very specific and leads to a single amino acid change (arginine 132 usually becomes histidine) in the IDH1 active site, whereby the enzyme loses its ability to catalyze conversion of isocitrate to α-ketoglutarate. It was proposed that this might have an indirect oncogenic effect through the activation of the hypoxia-inducible factor pathway, [17] a critical step in the metabolic adaptation of tumors to anaerobic growth and for the formation of new blood vessels through the angiogenic process.

Recently, attention has been focused on the role of an enzyme, isocitrate dehydrogenase 1 (IDH1), present in cytoplasm and peroxisomes, catalyzing the oxidative decarboxylation of isocitrate to alpha-ketoglutarate, reducing NADP+ to NADPH. Studies performed with seriated biopsies from gliomas, revealed that mutation of IDH1 is always found before TP53 mutation or, in case of oligodendrogliomas, before their typical deletions of chromosomes 1p and 19q. Moreover, mutation of IDH1 is quite specific, since it is extremely rare in I grade gliomas, non glioma brain tumors and in other cancers. Yan et al. studied genetic alterations of both IDH1 and of its related gene, IDH2. Genomic analysis, showed mutation of amino acid 132 of IDH1 in over 70% of patients with both low or high grade gliomas, and many of the cases negative for IDH1 mutations, had mutation involving amino acid 172 of IDH2 [18].

Studies suggest that mutant IDH1 loses its normal enzymatic activity in tumors while gaining a new pro-oncogenic activity, leading to the production of an onco-metabolite [18-20]. Other studies characterizing the genomic make-up of human glioblastoma have provided further insight into the genetic changes, core pathways and molecular subtypes underlying this disease [20-22]. Based on their gene expression profiles, The Cancer Genome Atlas Network (TCGA) further classified GBMs into four subtypes termed: proneural, neural, classical, and mesenchymal [9]. While the status of gene expression and mutation in EGFR, NF1, PDGFA, and IDH1 were defining components of these subtypes, it was also found that response to therapies was different for each subtype, suggesting that personalized treatment based on genomic alterations could lead to a more favorable outcome for this disease [23].

3. Molecular biology of glioma invasion

The cellular and molecular events that initiate and promote malignant glioma development are not completely understood. Vasculogenesis and angiogenesis potentially play distinct roles in the etiology of primary and recurrent malignant gliomas, suggesting that patient therapy should perhaps be tailored specifically against the predominant vasculature pathway at a given specific stage of gliomagenesis [24]. Cerebral gliomas show a unique pattern of invasion and, with rare exceptions, do not metastasize outside of the brain. Invading glioma cells normally migrate to distinct anatomical structures. These structures include the basement membrane (BM) of blood vessels, the subependymal space, the glial limitans externa, and parallel and intersecting nerve fiber tracts in the white matter. Invasion of tumor cells into normal tissue is thought to be a multifactorial process, consisting of cell interactions with ECM and with adjacent cells, as well as accompanying biochemical processes supportive of active cell movement. Several cell types aim active movement during various stages of embryonal development, during wound healing, and in the course of immune responses. This innate activity is regulated in a very rigid manner, suggesting that the reappearance of a motile phenotype in cancer cells results from the loss or cessation of normal inhibitory controls [25]. Critical factors in tumor cell invasion, include the detachment of invading cells from the primary tumor mass, the synthesis and deposition of ECM components by tumor cells and mesenchymal cells, the release of ECM-degrading activities for remodeling interstitial space, and the expression of adhesion molecules on glioma cell surfaces that specifically recognize and adhere to ECM components.

The detachment of invading glioma cells from the primary tumor mass involves several events, including, destabilization and disorganization of the cadherin-mediated junctions that hold the primary mass together, loss of expression of neural cell adhesion molecule, which promotes adhesion to the primary tumor mass through homophilic binding, cleavage of CD44, which anchors the primary mass to the ECM by the metalloproteinase ADAM.

Cadherin superfamily are important adhesion molecules associated with glioma invasion. Cadherins (E-, P-, and N-cadherin) form adherent junctions and may function as suppressors of tumor growth and invasion. Desmosomal cadherins interact heterotypically and provide a linkage to the intermediate filament network through association with cytosolic proteins (desmoplakin, plakoglobin). Cadherins are linked to the actin-cytoskeleton via catenins (α-, β-catenin, plakoglobin), thereby establishing molecular lines of communication to other cell-cell junctions and to cell-substratum junctions [26]. During glioma progression decreased cadherin function is correlated with de-differentiation, metastasis and poor prognosis [27]. Due to its participation in processes such as morphological differentiation and contact inhibition of growth and motility, cadherins may function as suppressors of tumor growth and invasion [25]. Perego and co-worker, showed that only glioma cells with immature adherens junctions are capable of migrating and invading through poly-1-lysine coated filters. In the process of maturation of adhesions, the Lin-7 protein forms a complex with cadherin and β-catenin [28].

The second step is a decline in the expression of connexin 43, which leads to a reduction in gap junction formation. Connexin 43 is the most abundant gap junction protein in CNS and is expressed primarily in astrocytes [29]. Cell-cell communication is important in growth control and differentiation, and it is partly achieved using gap junctions and via second messengers [30]. Decreased gap junction formation may result in fewer inhibitory signals, facilitating uncontrolled cell division and de-differentiation [31]. Has been demonstrated that reduced gap junction formation is correlated with increased motility of glioma cells in vitro [32]. Increased malignancy of glioma specimens correlates with reduced in situ gap junction formation as well as reduced connexin 43 expression [33]. The third event is cleavage of CD44, which anchors the primary mass to ECM, by the metalloproteinase ADAM. CD44 is a transmembrane glycoprotein belonging to the immunoglobulin receptor superfamily, which interacts with hyaluronic acid as its ligand. Monoclonal antibodies directed against CD44 decrease intracerebral invasion of glioma cells in vivo and through matrigel matrices in vitro [34]. CD44 can be cleaved by ADAM 10 and 17, and both the extracellular and intracellular cleaved components of CD44 promote cell migration [35].

3.1. Integrins

Integrins are heterodimeric transmembrane cell surface receptors that play a key role in the crosstalk between the cell and its surrounding stroma. Integrins regulate cell adhesion, migration, differentiation, proliferation, and survival during physiological and pathological conditions, including inflammation and cancer. Upon ligation to extracellular ligands (matrix proteins such as collagens, laminins, vitronectins and fibronectins), integrins activate downstream signaling pathways in concert with growth factor receptors, including PDGFR, EGFR and VEGFR. Preclinical data indicate that integrins play a key role in cancer initiation and progression.

Integrins contain two distinct chains, calls subunit α (alpha) and β (beta). Have been identified about 18 α and 8 β subunits. The integrin subunits penetrate the plasma membrane and typically have very short cytoplasmic domains of about 40-70 amino acids. Outside the plasma membrane, α and β chains protrude to a length of about 23 nm, the last 5 of which - thanks to the termination of each chain formed dall'NH2 - a region used to form bonds to the ECM. The molecular mass of the subunits of the integrin may range from 90 kD to 160

http://dx.doi.org/10.5772/53487

kD. The β subunits have 4 cysteine-rich repeat sequences. Both the α subunit β both bind many divalent cations. There are many ways to classify the integrins. For example, a subclass of the chains α has a structural domain in more inserted at the network termination NH2, the so-called alpha-domain A. The integrins that possess this characteristic usually form collagen (α1β1 integrins, and α2β1), or act as adhesion molecules between cell and cell (β2 integrin family). This domain α-1 is the active site for links to various integrins. Those who do not carry this domain, however, have a domain A in their active site, but this is in the β chain. In both cases, the domains A are connected to three active sites consisting of divalent cations. One of these is permanently occupied by physiological concentrations of divalent cations, and binds to a calcium ion or magnesium. The other two sites are occupied by cations when establishing ties - at least for the bonds involving an amino acid, aspartic acid, typically - in their interaction sites. An amino acid characterized in the active site of the integrin many proteins ECM, as part of the amino acid sequence Arginine-Glycine-Aspartic acid. The two main functions of integrins are cell adhesion to ECM and signal transduction from the ECM to the cell. They interact with two large groups of ligands: a variety of ECM proteins, such as fibronectin, vitronectin, fibrinogen, and cell surface molecules, that are members of the immunoglobulin supergene family, such as intracellular adhesion molecules (ICAM-1, ICAM-2) and vascular cell adhesion molecule (VCAM-1). In particular, the integrin αvβ3, which binds to fibronectin, vitronectin, and tenascin-C in ECM, is thought to play a central role in glioma invasion [36]. Increased expression of integrin αvβ3 leads to increased motility in human glioma cells with a concomitant decrease in apoptosis sensitivity.

Integrins combine the ECM out of the cell to the cytoskeleton (in particular microfilaments) within the cell. What site can bind the ECM is usually decided by the integrin α and β subunit which is composed of the same integrin. Bonds between the integrin are fibronectin, vitronectin, collagen, and laminin. The connection between the cell and the ECM makes the cell able to withstand the forces tie rods without being thrown out of the ECM. The connections between the integrin and the links in the ECM and microfilaments inside the cell are indirect: they are connected by proteins "armor" as talin, paxillin, and alpha-actinin. These act by regulating the kinase such as FAK (focal adhesion kinase - focal adhesion kinase) and the family of Src kinases to phosphorylated substrates such as the p130CAS or recruiting signal adapters such as Crk. The connection of the cell to the extracellular matrix is a basic requirement to form a multicellular organism. Integrins link the cytoskeleton to the extracellular matrix, and are recognized to be key regulators of tissue structure. They provide adhesive, migratory, and survival cues to tumor cells and to cells of the tumor microenvironment, including angiogenic endothelial cells. The integrins αvβ3 and αvβ5, among others, are highly expressed not only on the tumor vasculature and angiogenic endothelial cells, but also on tumor cells, including gliomas. Consequently, integrins have been considered as a promising therapeutic target in cancer. Monoclonal antibodies and peptide-based integrin inhibitors are being investigated for their potential therapeutic activity in various tumor types. This strategy is in advanced stage clinical development in glioblastoma, a highly vascular primary brain tumor [37].

The malignancy of glioma is dependent on diffusive properties of tumor cells that may invade widely as single cells anywhere in the brain. Integrins are the family of adhesive receptors that promote invasiveness of glioma. These heterodimeric transcellular membrane receptors are composed of two subunits, α and β, and are the major receptors for the ECM proteins. Immunohistopathological studies revealed an upregulation of α2β1, α3β1, α5β1, α6β1, and αvβ3 integrins on GBM when compared with normal brain [38].

Glioblastoma commonly displays enhanced expression of several integrins along with their ECM ligands: αvβ3 and αvβ5 (tenascin and vitronectin receptors), α5β1 (fibronectin receptor), α2β1 (collagens receptor), and α3β1, α6β4, and α6β1 (laminins receptors). Numerous studies have focused on the αv integrin family. The integrins αvβ3 and αvβ5 are markers of glioblastoma malignancy and influence a variety of processes in glioblastoma progression in vivo, including proliferation, apoptosis, and angiogenesis. Furthermore, cilengitide, an αvβ3 and αvβ5 integrins antagonist, extends mouse survival by delaying the tumor growth and is nowadays in clinical trial for recurrent malignant glioma. Two other integrins, α5β1 and α3β1, have been shown to be implicated in glioma cell adhesion and migration in vitro. The α6 integrin subunit associates with β1 or β4 subunits to form functional heterodimers that selectively bind laminins. The α6β4 integrin is essential for the organization and maintenance of epithelial hemidesmosomes that link the intermediate filaments with the extracellular matrix. The major ligand of α6β4 is the laminin-332, while α6β1 is a well-characterized laminin-111 receptor. Overexpression of α6β1 integrin has been associated with the progression of many epithelial tumors. Several studies concerning gliomas and the α6β1 ligand laminin-111 have been reported in the literature. Using immunohistochemistry studies, Gingras et al. showed that α6 integrin was strongly expressed in glioblastoma tissue, whereas it was weakly expressed in normal brain [39]. Previtali et al. confirmed that the expression of α6 was increased in glioblastoma and in other central nervous system tumors, such as meningioma, astrocytoma, and neuroblastoma, when compared with the autologous normal tissue counterpart [40]. In glioblastoma biopsies, laminin-111 is highly expressed on tumor blood vessels, but also within the brain tumor as punctuate deposits and at the tumor invasion front. In vitro, glioma cells can both secrete laminin-111 and induce its expression in normal brain tissue. Moreover, laminin-111 is one of the most permissive substrates for adhesion and migration of glioma cells in vitro. Additionally, over laminin-111, migrating glioma cells are protected from apoptosis [41].

In malignant glioma, and in particular in GBM, overexpression of αvβ3 integrin is well documented. The integrin αvβ3, which binds to fibronectin, vitronectin, and tenascin-C in ECM, is thought to play a central role in glioma invasion [36]. Increased expression of integrin αvβ3 leads to increased motility in human glioma cells with a concomitant decrease in apoptosis sensitivity. Importantly, αvβ3 integrin is expressed both on angiogenic endothelial cells and on tumor cells. Conversely, inhibition of integrin αvβ3 decreases glioma cell motility [42]. Several factors expressed in glioma cells have been found to regulate integrin expression. Particularly, uPA secreted by glioma cells has been shown to upregulate integrin αvβ3 expression by autocrine mechanism [43]. Furthermore, decreasing the in vivo expression of the β1 subunit by an antisense strategy in the intracranial C6 glioma model leads to an inhibition of glioma associated angiogenesis at the invasive edge of the tumors [44]. Down-regulated β1 integrin protein levels in vivo probably affect interactions of glioma cells with ECM components, leading to reduced migration along vascular basement membranes. The integrin α6β1 plays an important role for the regulation of glioma-initiating cells in the perivascular niche. This integrin mediates the interaction of glioma-initiating cells to laminin, an extracellular matrix protein expressed in basement membranes, including those supporting endothelial cells. This interaction provides an anchorage for glioma-initiating cells within the perivascular niche and supports their tumorigenic potential [37].

Brown et al. evaluate the role of α9β1 integrin interaction with nerve growth factor (NGF) in glioma progression, they selected the two most malignant glioblastoma cell lines: LN229, which expresses α9β1, and LN18,in which does not. Presence of the α9 integrin subunit on LN229 and absence on LN18 cell lines were verified using several assays such as monoclonal antibody adhesion microarray, Western blot analysis of cell lysates, flow cytometry, and immunocytostaining [38]. Very high expression of the α9 integrin subunit was observed only on the LN229 cell line. Western blot analysis, using polyclonal anti-α9 antibody, showed the absence of this integrin subunit on normal astrocytes. The expression of α9β1 integrin on LN229 and lack of it on LN18 was confirmed by flow cytometry and immunocytostaining analysis. The investigation of cellular responses following binding of NGF to α9β1 integrin on LN229 and LN18 cells required evaluation of the level of two other NGF receptors, TrkA and $p75^{NTR}$. Western blot analysis of cell lysates and immunocytostaining revealed negligible expression of TrkA on both types of cells, and a stable expression of $p75^{NTR}$ in comparison with PC12 neuronal cells used as a positive control. Interestingly, the level of $p75^{NTR}$ appeared to be lower on LN18 cells, which are α9β1 integrin deficient, than on LN229 cells, which are α9β1 integrin positive. This correlation was previously observed in the mRNA level of SW480 cells transfected with α9 integrin subunit. Cells transfected with the α9 subunit showed a potent increase of $p75^{NTR}$, whereas mock-transfected cells had a significantly lower expression of this NGF receptor. The opposite situation occurred for TrkA, suggesting that this specific high affinity NGF receptor has a functional complementary association with α9β1 integrin. Several factors expressed in glioma cells have been found to regulate integrin expression. Glioma expression of focal adhesion kinase, a nonreceptor cytoplasmic tyrosine kinase, has been shown to increase phosphorylation of the enhancer of filamentation 1, which in turn stimulates PDGF-mediated stimulation of glioma integrin adhesion to ECM [45].

3.2. Proteases

Extracellular proteolytic enzymes are critical for the invasive properties of malignant neoplasms [46]. Barrier to invasion do not appear as restrictive within CNS parenchyma and matrix substrates most responsible for impeding tumor migration have not been identified [47]. Nonetheless, there is a strong evidence that the expression of specific extracellular matrix proteases promotes invasive behavior by gliomas. These include the matrix metalloproteinases (MMPs), the urokinase-dependent plasminogen activating cascade, and cathepsin

B. Wild-Bode et al. [48] found that MMP-2 and MMP-3 levels and MMP-2/MMP-9 activity correlated with glioma cell migration and invasion. NF-jB, uPA, low-density lipoprotein receptor-related protein 1, and insulin-like growth factor binding protein-2 are known to upregulate MMP expression. Induced expression of tissue inhibitor of metalloproteinases-3 (TIMP-3), a putative inhibitor of MMP activity, has been shown to suppress infiltration and also to induce apoptosis in cancer cell lines. MMPs play an important role in human brain tumor invasion, probably due to an imbalance between the production of MMPs and tissue inhibitor of metalloproteinases-1 (TIMP-1) by the tumor cells. MMP-1 is the crucial enzyme able to initiate breakdown of the interstitial collagen types; in this way, it activates the other MMPs, which allows the glioma cells to infiltrate normal brain tissue.

Matrix metalloproteinases comprise a large family of zinc-dependent endoproteinases, collectively capable of degrading all ECM components. A total of 23 families of MMPs are known and these are numbered in the sequence of their discovery [49]. Originally, MMPs were classified according to their respective substrate specificity, now they are divided into eight structural subgroups, five of which are secreted and three of which are transmembrane MMPs. A signal peptide leads them to the secretory pathway. Then, these enzymes can be secreted from the cell or anchored to the plasma membrane, thereby confining their catalytic activity to the extracellular space or to the cell surface, respectively. Their function is to degrade different protein components of the ECM and of basement membranes, therefore they are essential for the interaction of individual cells with their surrounding and for the development and function of multicellular organisms [50]. Between the various substrates of MMPs we include collagens, non collagens glicoproteins, proteoglycans and other ECM components like tenascin, fibronectin and laminin, which often show tumor specific expression are also substrates [51]. The proteolytic activities of MMPs influence essential cellular processes like cell proliferation, migration and adhesion, as well as many fundamental physiological events involving tissue remodeling, such as angiogenesis, bone development, wound healing, and uterine and mammary involution [52]. However, the increasing expression of this enzymes is associated with many pathological conditions [53-54] such as rheumatoid arthritis, cardiovascular diseases or cancer progression [55]. MMP expression and activity can be regulated at different levels including gene transcription, proenzyme activation and endogenous inhibition, which act in a coordinated manner to confine the diverse MMP proteolytic activities to those conditions and locations where they are necessary. Unfortunately, these restrictive regulatory mechanisms are frequently lost in multiple pathological conditions [56]. MMPs expression is induced by different factors like EGF, TGF-β, PDGF, and various inflammation's mediated, included TNFα and IL-1β.

MMPs or matrixins are synthesized as zymogens, inactive pro-enzymes (pro-MMPs), with the zinc ion, essential for MMP activity, hidden by a cysteine-sulphydryl residue situated near the C-terminal end of the peptide. The pro-enzyme's activations starts breaking the interaction cysteine-zinc exposing, in this way the catalytic site. The fully active enzyme is generated by proteolytic cleavage of the pro-peptide domain of the partially active intermediate enzyme [50]. Once active, MMPs are regulated by interactions with endogenous inhibitors including α2-macroglobulin, thrombospondin-2, tissue inhibitors of metalloproteinases (TIMPs) and RECK (reversion-inducing cysteine-rich protein with kazal motifs) [49]. Numerous studies have investigated the expression of selected MMPs in human GBM cell lines. As it has already been reported that there are differences in the expression patterns of MMPs in different cell-lines [57]. A number of different techniques have been used to detect protease expression patterns. This may have led to dissimilar conclusions, due to disparate sensitivities and due to comparing mRNA expression with protein expression or protein activity. Variations in MMP expression may be due to in vitro selection processes or karyotype evolution, where the transcription of either the enzyme and/or its inhibitor may be affected which ultimately leads to an imbalance in the MMP-regulatory network [57]. MMP-9's production is dependent on a regulation by extracellular signal-regulated kinase (ERK), PKCα/NF-κB and jun amino-terminal kinase (JNK) signaling cascades. Glioblastomas are highly hypoxic and hypoxia upregulates MMP-2 mRNA expression in U87, U251, U373 and LN18 glioblastoma cell-lines by activation of the HIF-1α transcription factor, thereby enhancing their invasive potential. Migration and invasion of U87 and T98G GBM cells is also facilitated by NO, which can be found in high concentrations in glioblastoma tissue. NO stimulates MMP-1 expression and activity. EGF raises MMP14 expression in U251 cells, but does not influence MMP-15, -16 or MMP-24. MMP-2 expression and secretion is induced by IL-6 in U87 cells. However, IL-6 action seems to be cell-line specific, since U343 cells were not affected [57].

The inflammatory cytokine TNF-α and the immune-suppressive cytokine TGF-β have been implicated in migration and invasion of glioma cells in vitro. In U251 and in U373 cells, TNF-α stimulated the expression of MMP-9 and MMP-19. MMP-1 mRNA expression was significantly increased in U373 cells by TNF-α, whereas its expression in U251 cells remained unaffected. This may be due to the high basal level of MMP-1 expression displayed by U251 cells, where a further increase is not possible, or else it could also be a cell- line specific effect. Such an effect has been observed for MMP-1, -2, -3 and MMP-7 regulation by TNF-α and TGF-β1, which only caused a marked induction of expression in some GBM cell-lines. TNF-α enhances the invasiveness of T98G cells through an induction of MMP-3, but has no effect on MMP-1, -2 or MMP-9. However, in U251 cells TNF-α inhibits MMP-2 and decreases invasiveness into the extracellular matrix. In A172 cells, TNF-α induces gene expression and protein secretion of MMP-9. TGF-β1 alone had no effect on MMP-9 production. However, when it was added together with TNF-α a significant dose-dependent inhibition of MMP-9 secretion was observed. TGF-β1 displayed inconsistent effects on adhesion and invasiveness, depending on the cell-line examined. The invasive potential of U138 cells was markedly reduced, whereas U373 cell invasion remained unchanged. TGF-β1 caused a significant induction of MMP-11 and MMP-24 expression in U373 cells, whereas there was no impact on MMP expression in U251 cells. In U87 and LN229 cells, TGF-β upregulates MMP-2. Thus, the transcriptional modulation of MMP genes in response to TNF-α or TGF-β is not consistent, but extremely cell-line specific [57]. Elevated levels of several MMPs were also found in malignant glioma tissue samples. MMP-1 expression was increased in surgical specimens of GBM compared to low grade astrocytomas and normal brain. This increased expression is probably due to a single nucleotide polymorphism in the MMP-1 promoter at position-1607, creating a functional binding site for members of the ETS family of transcription factors. MMP-1 was expressed throughout the tumor section, particularly in the highly cellular areas of the GBM [57]. Many studies have demonstrated an intimate association between MMP-9 and tumor invasiveness. Different analyses for MMP-9 were negative in NB tissue, showed weak signals in LGA and strong expression in GBM [57]. MMP-9 is strongly expressed in blood vessels at proliferating margins, as well as tumor cells, this suggests a role in the regulation of tumor neoangiogenesis [58]. Other proteases that could be related with the development of highly invasive glial tumor are MMP-11, MMP-12, MMO-14, MMP-15, MMP-19, MMP-24, MMP-25.

A second proteolytic system that interfaces with MMPs is the urokinase pathway of plasminogen activation. This system includes urokinase (also known as urokinase-type plasminogen activator, uPA), the urokinase receptor (uPAR), and plasminogen. Urokinase is secreted as a single chain, inactive proenzyme that is activated by cleavage upon binding to its cell surface receptor uPAR. Activated uPA then converts plasminogen into plasmin, a serine protease that promotes cellular migration by the degradation of extracellular matrix proteins, activation of other matrix proteases and activation of cell surface receptors that transduce intracellular signaling for migration. Plasmin activates protease activated receptor 1 (PAR1), which is normally expressed in human astrocytes, is activated in many malignancies including GBMs, and is associated with increased invasive properties [59]. Thus, uPA and plasminogen activation can occur in the immediate vicinity of the cell membrane or, following cleavage of the uPAR GPI anchor, at greater distance in the extracellular matrix. An important biologic regulator of this cascade is plasminogen activator–inhibitor 1 (PAI1), which promotes the internalization of uPA bound uPAR [60]. uPAR has roles in cellular migration distinct from its ability to activate plasminogen though its interactions with integrins, signaling through G-protein coupled receptors, and caveolin binding [61]. There is a convincing correlative relationship between uPAR and uPA expression and malignant progression in a variety of tumor types [62]. Both neoplastic cells and stromal cells contribute to the overall activity of these pathways. In co-cultures of malignant gliomas and reactive astrocytes, most uPA and uPAR activity was derived from reactive astrocytes, whereas plasminogen was expressed in largest amounts by glioma cells [63]. Levels of uPA mRNA and its enzymatic activity are higher in human anaplastic astrocytomas and GBMs than in low grade astrocytomas and normal human brain and uPA mRNA levels have an inverse correlation with survival periods [64]. uPAR levels are significantly higher in GBMs and anaplastic astrocytomas that normal brain and low grade gliomas, with uPAR mRNA localizing to both glioma cells and endothelial cells [65]. The finding of uPAR expression at the leading edge of neoplastic infiltration and within remodeling hyperplastic blood vessels suggested that it may be playing a role in invasion and tissue remodeling. mRNA levels of both uPA and uPAR genes are increased in high grade gliomas possibly suggesting increased gene transcription [66]. In the CNS, reactive astrocytes in the vicinity of invading gliomas appear to contribute for a substantial proportion of extracellular MMP activity, both by their secretion of pro-MMP2 and the components of the plasminogen activating system, uPA and uP-AR [63]. Reactive astrocytes have also been shown to promote the invasive capabilities of glioma cells in vitro, presumably resulting from enhanced extracellular MMP-2 activity.

The cathepsins are a family of lysosomal cysteine proteases. These proteases are synthesized as inactive pro-enzymes that are activated by autocatalytic activity initiated by low pH or by other proteases including cathepsin D, uPA, and pepsin. Natural regulators of cathepsins are the cystatins, which are critical, in their inhibitory properties. Cathepsins are secreted into the extracellular space where they degrade extracellular matrix components required for invasive properties in neoplastic disease. Best studied for their roles in glioma tumorigenesis and invasion are cathepsins B, D, H, L, and S. Each of these cathepsin subtypes have higher protein levels in high grade astrocytomas than low grade tumors or normal brain and enzymatic activities, in general, correlate with protein expression [67-68]. The role of cathepsins in tumor invasion has been supported by the finding that tumor cells at the invading edge of gliomas express high levels of cathepsins, especially cathepsin B [69]. In addition, protein and enzymatic levels of cathepsins B, D, L, H, and S were found to correlate with the ability of glioblastoma cells to migrate in vitro. Once in the extracellular compartment, cathepsin B physically interacts with a protein complex at the outer cell membrane containing annexin II, p11, tPA and plasminogen [70]. Its close proximity to both the plasminogen activating cascade and MMPs is critical for regulation of their combined proteolytic functions. Upon activation, cathepsin B has its own proteolytic activity on extracellular matrix components, but also activates the cascade to convert plasminogen to plasmin and is able to activate selected MMPs [71].

3.3. Extracellular matrix

The ECM affects numerous functions and processes within the brain. During brain development, the ECM modulates the migration of glial and neuronal precursor cells, guides axonal growth cones, synapse formation and cell proliferation. The roles played by the ECM in neoplastic transformation are complex and only now beginning to be uncovered. ECM is a complex network of different collagens, proteoglycans, hyaluronic acid, laminin, fibronectin, and many other glycoproteins, including proteolytic enzymes involved in degradation and remodelling of the ECM [72]. Extracellular matrix exists in two forms: interstitial matrix that fills in the intercellular space and the more specialized BM, which is a thin sheet of extracellular matrix underlying the epithelium. ECM provides the microenvironment for the cells and serves as a tissue scaffold, guiding cell migration during embryonic development and wound repair. Integrins are a class of adhesion molecules that have a major role in the adhesion and subsequent invasion of tumor cells. ECM proteins such as fibronectin, laminins or collagens form distinct protein networks that show tissue-specific variation in composition and architecture. Cell responses to contact with these networks depend on the cell's repertoire of ECM receptors. Connections from the matrix through these receptors determine the organization of cytoskeletal structures and the localization and activation of signaling molecules leading to unique tissue specific cell functions. Changes in these ECM components are felt to modulate brain tumor growth, proliferation and invasion, although specific interactions and exact mechanisms are unknown. Cell adhesion is the binding of the cells to each other and to the ECM through cell adhesion molecules such as integrins, selectins, cadherins, the Ig (immunoglobulin) superfamily and lymphocyte homing receptors. Cell adhesion mediates cell attachment, migration, and signalling to and from the extracellular matrix. Adhesion complexes include focal adhesions, adherens junctions, tight junctions, desmosomes, hemi-desmosomes, and gap junctions. The best characterized adhesion molecules are the integrins and the best characterized adhesion complexes are focal adhesions. The extracellular ligands that anchor these adhesions include laminin, fibronectin, vitronectin, and various collagens. Focal adhesions can be considered both as sensors of force and as sites that originate cytoskeletal forces through anchored actin-microfilament bundles. Focal adhesions have many SH2-containing components (Src kinases, PI3K, SHP-2), as well as many tyrosine-phosphorylated molecules (focal adhesion kinase paxillin, tensin, caveolin).

Syndecans are a family of transmembrane heparin sulphate proteoglycans with four members, syndecans 1 to 4. Syndecans function mainly as co-receptors by binding to their ECM ligands in conjunction with other receptors, notably integrins. Through their heparin sulphate side chains, syndecans may further engage directly in ligand binding. Dystroglycans are heterodimeric complexes consisting of non-covalently associated α and β subunits with extracellular ligand-binding and transmembrane functions, respectively. Dystroglycans are a part of the larger dystrophin-associated protein (DAP) complex that connects basement membranes to the cytoskeleton, particularly via $\alpha 2$ laminins and perlecan. Ig superfamily members consist of immunoglobulin-like and fibronectin type III domains involved in homophilic and heterophilic cell–cell adhesion. The superfamily includes a variety of cell adhesion molecules (CAMs) with distinct ligand-binding specificities, including ICAM (intercellular), NCAM (neural), Ep-CAM (epithelial), L1-CAM, VCAM (vascular), ALCAM (activated leukocyte), and JAM (junctional adhesion molecule), among others. Cadherins are transmembrane proteins consisting of several tandemly repeated cadherin domains that mediate calcium-dependent homophilic cell-cell contacts. The cadherin superfamily comprises a total of more than 100 different members, with E- (epithelial) and N-cadherin (neural) most widely expressed in epithelial and neural tissues, respectively [73].

By convention, ECM components are biochemically classified fibrillar proteins (collagens), glycoproteins (laminins, fibronectin, tenascins), and several classes of proteo- glycans (heparan sulfate-, chondroitin sulfate-, dermatan sulfate-, and keratan sulfate proteoglycans). The latter mainly consist of large glycosaminoglycan (GAG) chains, covalently linked to extra- cellular or membrane bound core proteins. In contrast to other tissues, the ECM in the CNS lacks fibrillar proteins under physiological conditions. Instead the neural ECM is rich in glycoproteins and proteoglycans. It has been estimated that the neural ECM makes up about 20% of the CNS parenchyma [74]. The brain ECM is mainly deposited by astrocytes and oligodendrocytes and comprises an estimated 20% of the brain volume in adults. The main ECM components are hyaluronic acid (HA), tenascin R, and lecticans, which interconnect with each other noncovalently and form molecular networks filling the intercellular space. HA is a non-sulphated, linear, high-molecular weight glycosaminoglycan which, due to its water-binding capacity, controls the high water content of the brain interstitium. Besides tenascins and lecticans, HA binds to cell surface receptors including CD44 and ICAM-1, which together contribute to both ECM organization and cell-matrix interaction. It represents the major component of neuropil ECM and is widely distributed in the adult and embryonic brain. Malignant gliomas contain higher amounts of HA than low-grade gliomas in situ and in vitro, while the perivascular location in glioma biopsy suggests additional production by vascular stromal cells [75].

The tenascins (TN) are a family of large multimeric ECM proteins consisting of repeated structural modules including heptad repeats, epidermal growth factor (EGF)-like repeats, fibronectin type III repeats, and a globular domain shared with the fibrinogens. The TN are presumably involved in the morphogenesis of many organs and tissues [76-77]. The original tenascin discovered was TN-C, partially because of its overexpression in tumours and, inferring from cell biological studies, it has been proposed as an adhesion-modulating protein [77]. TN-C (also called neuronectin, brachinectin, myotendinous antigen, hexabrachion, glioma-mesenchymal extracellular matrix antigen, cytotactin, J1 protein, GP250 protein) has a characteristic hexabrachion structure, with as many as six arms linked to a central knob formed by disulfide bonding of cysteines in the NH2-terminal ends of polypeptides. TN-C initially appears during embryonic neural crest cell development, and it is present during brain and spinal cord organogenesis, being correlated with developmental phenomena such as cell proliferation, migration, and ECM remodelling. In addition, TN-C is transiently present in the dense mesenchyma surrounding several developing organs and tissues, including the nervous system [76-77]. Enhanced TN-C expression was detected among tumour cells, around individual cells as a fibrillary network, and around vascular channels [78]. A direct relation between the presence of TN-C and the degree of malignancy of gliomas has been reported, being TN-C reported to be expressed 5-fold higher in GBM as compared with AA and 10-fold higher as compared with juvenile pylocitic astrocytoma [79-80]. Endothelial cells in vitro attach to TN-C substrata, where they elongate, extend, and have interconnecting process. These features are lacking when endothelial cells growth on other matrix proteins, such as fibronectin, collagen, or laminin. The attachment of endothelial cells to TN-C is mediated by annexin and integrins, including $\alpha v\beta 3$ integrin, which is required for angiogenesis [79-81]. Tenascin R, another brain-specific member of the tenascin family, is a homotrimer with both lectican and integrin binding sites forming an adhesion bridge between the ECM and cells. Lecticans comprise a family of chondroitin sulphate proteoglycans with four members (brevican, versican, neurocan, and aggrecan), whereby brevican and neurocan are brain-specific. Lecticans contain HA and tenascin R binding sites and thus act as link molecules in protein–proteoglycan–glycosaminoglycan networks. Compared with peripheral interstitial tissues, a distinctive feature of the brain ECM is the absence of fibrillar collagen networks, which results in a low stiffness of the brain parenchyma. In a restricted expression pattern, fibrillar collagens I and III are, however, deposited by leptomeningeal cells, pericytes, and smooth muscle cells in blood vessels and the brain meninges, including the pia mater.

Fibronectin (FN) is a member of a family of glycoproteins that show many biological functions, including normal cell adhesion, growth, and migration. FN is involved in many cellular processes, including tissue repair, embryogenesis, blood clotting, and cell migration/adhesion. Both decreased expression and elevated degradation of FN have been shown to be responsible for some of the morphological changes observed in tumors and tumor-derived cell lines. As a peripheral protein, FN mainly acts as a bridge to link the cell surface and

ECM. Therefore, the absence or reduction of FN in tumor cells may reduce the adhesion between tumor cells and matrix components, and decrease the matrix's control of cell differentiation, proliferation, and migration. As a major protein in blood and as component of the wound provisional matrix, plasma FN contributes to tissue repair and neuronal survival following cerebral ischemia [82]. Fibronectin structure is rod-like, composed of three different types of homologous, repeating modules, types I, II, and III. These modules comprise functional domains that mediate interactions with other ECM components, with cell surface receptors and with FN itself. Twelve type I modules make up the amino-terminal and carboxy-terminal region of the molecule, and are involved mainly in fibrin and collagen binding. Only two type II modules are found in FN. They are instrumental in binding collagen. The most abundant module in FN is type III, which contains the RGD-FN receptor recognition sequence along with binding sites for other integrins and heparin. Depending on the tissue type and/or cellular conditions, the FN molecule is made up of 15-17 type III modules. In addition, there is a module that does not fall into any of these categories, called II-ICS. This module, along with EDB and EDA is regulated through alternative splicing of FN pre-mRNA. FN is an important component in the ECM of gliomas, largely in the vessel wall [83]. Expression of FN has been characterized in human GBM and in a number of astrocytoma and glioblastoma cell lines. In a study of pediatric GBM, a marked positive staining of FN in walls of small and medium size vessels was demonstrated. FN expression was seen in perivascular sheets, where it looked like a fine irregular network [83]. Knott et al. found that when normal brain tissues were invaded by glioma, ECM components such as LN, FN, and collagen type IV may are available and that tumor cells may express specific integrins, depending on the change of the interior environment, to interact with these ECM components, and enhance tumor cell invasion [84]. In vitro experiments have proven that components of ECM, LN and FN, can strongly stimulate the migration of glioma cells, which occurs after glioma cells express the relevant surface receptors [85]. Although there are many in vitro and in vivo models for FN-promoted invasion and transmigration [85], the uniqueness of these findings may be attributed to interaction between tumor cells and vascular endothelial cells (VECs), as changes of tumoral microenvironment molecules can affect tumor status and progression. Recently it has been demonstrated that FN expression is correlated with glioma migration and glioma malignancy [86]. More recently, FN has been reported to mantain extracellular matrix rigidity to promote structural rigidity, motility, and proliferation of established glioma cell lines in vitro [87]. The inhibition of FN expression in glioma cells, using short hairpin RNA-mediated silencing of gene expression, delayed cell proliferation in vitro. This delayed growth is explained, in part, by the observed reduced expression of integrin ß1 FN receptor, which was restored by the inhibition of proteosomal activity [88].

LM are a group of adhesion structural glycoproteins found in all BM as an integral part of the glia limitans externa [89]. LM the first neurite outgrowth promoting ECM identified is an adhesion glycoprotein associated with the development and regeneration of neuroectodermal tissues [89]. LM is distributed beneath vascular endothelial cells, around vascular smooth muscle cells, in the glia limitans, and beneath choroid plexus epithelial cells and plays a role in migration, neurite outgrowth, proliferation, and differentiation [90]. LM constitute the preferred substrate for growth of astrocytes and neurons, and have been found in all BM and in hyperplastic blood vessels in gliomas, gliosarcomas, and meningiomas [89]. Reactive astrocytes in situ, glioma cells in situ, as well as glioma cells lines, have been reported to express LM. Variants of LM may be expressed by astrocytes or neurons under different situations which adds to the complexity of the function and regulation of these large molecules in the CNS [91].

Type IV collagen (C-IV), the principal collagenous constituent of most BM, is mainly present in capillaries and large blood vessels. C-IV is associated with laminin, entactin, and the heparan sulphate proteoglycans perlecan. C-IV is found in areas of the normal brain, such as, beneath vascular endothelial cells, around vascular smooth muscle cells, in the glia limitans, and beneath choroid plexus epithelial cells. GBM cells are able of synthesising C-IV in vitro [72]. Bjerkvig et al. [92], demonstrated that C-IV was strongly expressed in tumour spheroids from rat glioma cell lines BT4C. In vitro the presence of C-IV in tumour vessels has been used to demonstrate vascular abnormalities in gliomas, such as BM duplication and disruption, as well as increased vascular density [93]. Recent studies have shown that GBM cells around areas of vascular proliferation, are also able to synthesise C-IV localised to the subendothelial BM of blood vessels [72].

4. Angiogenesis

Physiological angiogenesis, the formation of new blood vessels from pre-existing ones, is a strictly regulated fine-tuned process. The local balance between inducers and inhibitors of angiogenesis is critical in determining the generation or not of new vessels. Whenever this balance is perturbed pathological, uncontrolled, excessive angiogenesis occurs. Angiogenesis is a process that plays an essential role in cancer development. Coagulation and inflammation also play an important role in tumorigenesis. Their expression is controlled by over- or under-expression of certain genes [94]. Although a plethora of molecules can act as inducers of angiogenesis such as acidic fibroblast growth factor (aFGF), basic fibroblast growth factor (bFGF), transforming growth factor alpha and beta (TGF-a and -h), tumor necrosis factor alpha (TNFα) and interleukin-8 (IL-8), the major growth factors specific for vascular endothelium include members of the vascular endothelium growth factor (VEGF) and angiopoietin families, and at least one member of the large ephrin family.

Angiogenesis is believed to be the primary method of vessel formation in gliomas. Malignant gliomas are characterized by extensive microvascular proliferation. Neovascularization in brain tumors correlates directly with their biological aggressiveness, degree of malignancy and clinical recurrence and inversely with the post-operative survival of patients affected by gliomas. Among all solid tumors, GBM has been reported to be the most angiogenic by displaying the highest degree of vascular proliferation and endothelial cell hyperplasia. Such intense vascularization might be responsible for the peritumoral edema, one of the pathological features of GBM [95]. The presence of endothelial glomeruloid-like proliferation and of positive immunoreaction at level of BM of tumor vascular channel are predictive of active tumor invasiveness [83]. Diffuse astrocytomas tend to progress from grade II to grade III tumors with a time interval of several years, whereas, progression of grade III to grade IV is more rapid, typically 2 years. Primary and secondary GBMs are morphologically indistinguishable and show their histologic hallmarks, i.e., "glomeruloid" microvascular tufts and necrosis. Glioma vasculature is structurally and functionally abnormal and it correlates and leads to vasogenic edema, increased interstitial pressure, and heterogeneous delivery of oxygen and drugs [96].

Neoangiogenesis may be quantified post-operatively in brain tumors by the evaluation on surgical samples of the so-called microvessel density (MVD), which reflects the number of vessels per mm^2 within representative histological sections. Specifically, MVD is assessed in formalin-fixed and paraffin-embedded tissue sections through standard immunohistochemistry; in detail, the vessels present in the histological sections are preliminarly highlighted with peroxidase-conjugated antibodies against endothelial markers and then they are counted at light microscopy. Antibodies against several endothelial markers, such as Factor VIII, CD31, CD34 and endoglin, may be used for the quantification of MVD, with different sensitivity and specificity. For instance, following the use of antibodies against pan-endothelial markers (Factor VIII, CD31, CD34), all the vessels present in the histological section are stained, with no distinction between pre-existing and newly-formed vessels [97]. As a consequence, pan-endothelial cannot be considered as optimal markers for the quantification of neoangiogenesis. In contrast, endoglin (CD105), a 180-kDa transmembrane homodimeric glycoprotein that belongs to the TGF receptor complex [98], appears as an endothelial marker which more specifically allows the detection of vessels related to neoangiogenic process in brain tumors [97, 99-101]. Indeed, this protein is predominantly expressed by the cycling endothelial cells in the vessels of tumors [102]; even more the antibody against endoglin prefentially binds the activated endothelial cells of peri- and intra-tumor vessels that are actually involved in tumor neoangiogenesis, while a negative/weak immunoreaction for endoglin is evidenced in the vascular endothelium of normal tissues [97, 102]. Besides, in comparative studies, antibodies against endoglin have been demonstrated to be more specific in the detection of newly formed vessels in meningiomas [97], as well as in astrocytic [100] or oligodendroglial [101] neoplasias in comparison to those binding pan-endothelial markers. In addition, when MVD was assessed by using endoglin as a marker of angiogenesis, it appeared to be significantly correlated to the growth fraction and histological grade of meningiomas, and it was shown to have a prognostic impact on the overall survival and recurrence risk of these neoplasias [97]. Thus, we suggest the use of anti-endoglin antibodies instead of that of antibodies against pan-endothelial markers for the quantification of angiogenesis in brain tumors. Besides, the demonstration of endoglin expression in tumour vessels may also open therapeutic prespectives. Indeed, it has been recently shown that monoclonal antibodies against endoglin are able to induce tumour growth regression through the inhibition of the endothelial cells proliferation and angiogenesis itself [103].

The first phase in forming new blood vessels from existing vessels is the dissolution of aspects of native vessels. Glioma cells first accumulate around the existing cerebral blood vessels and lift off the astrocytic foot processes, which leads to the disruption of the normal contact between endothelial cells and the basement membrane [104]. The affected endothelial cells express angiopoietins resulting in destabilization of the vessel wall and decreased pericyte coverage. The angiopoietins are endothelial growth factors and their signal transduction pathway passes via the Tie2 receptor tyrosine kinase expressed on endothelial cells. In particular, Ang-1 and -2, have been implicated in glioma angiogenesis [105]. Ang-1 mediated activation of Tie2 is required for stabilization, remodeling and maturation of blood vessels, promotes angiogenesis and tumor growth and is associated with an increased number of highly branched vessels. Ang-1 induces phosphorylation of Tie2 and the p85 subunit of PI3K and increases PI3K activity in a dose-dependent manner, leading to endothelial cell survival via Akt signaling. In addition, Ang-1 stimulates endothelial cell migration via a PI3K-dependent activation of focal adhesion kinase (FAK), which has a key role in regulating dynamic changes in actin cytoskeletal organisation during cell migration. The biological effect of Ang-2 may depend on VEGF level. In the presence of endogenous VEGF, Ang-2 promotes vessel dilatation, remodelling of the basal lamina, proliferation and migration of endothelial cells, and stimulates sprouting of new blood vessels. In the absence of VEGF activity, Ang-2 becomes anti-angiogenic by promoting endothelial cell death and the regression of vessels [105]. Binding of Ang-2 to the Tie2 receptor on endothelial cells antagonizes this receptor's phosphorylation, thereby disrupting contacts between endothelial and periendothelial support cells and disengaging pericytes from the tumor vessels during initiation of vessel sprouting or regression. Increased expression of Ang-2 on GBM microvasculature appears early during glioma angiogenesis. Ang-2 and Tie2 expression are absent in the normal brain vasculature but are induced in tumor endothelium of coopted tumor vessels prior to their regression. Treatment of glioma cell derived mouse xenografts with a dominant negative form of Tie2 results in a significant decrease in tumor growth [106]. Maintenance of an optimal number of pericytes is necessary for successful angiogenesis in stabilizing newly formed vessels from further sprouting and to support adequate blood flow. Ang-2 may act as an antagonist to Tie2 phosphorylation, leading to destabilization of blood vessels. Therefore, Ang-2 represents a checkpoint for Ang-1/Tie2-mediated angiogenesis [107]. In brain tumor growth it's possible observe two vascular phases. In the first, the vessels are native cerebral vessels, which are co-opted by tumor cells, while in the second phase, there is true neovascularization arising from existing vessels. During the transition period between these two phases, hypoxia driven HIF-1 expression occurs which results in VEGF secretion and in the induction of neovascularization. In stage IV, angiogenesis adjacent to the necrotic area is triggered in response to increased expression of HIF-1α and VEGF. For the newly sprouting vessel is essential the deposition of proangiogenic matrix. This involves breakdown of the vascular basement membrane and extracellular matrix through the action of cathepsin B, matrix metalloproteases and other enzymes as well as the expression of matrix proteins such as fibronectin, laminin, tenascin-C and vitronectin [108]. Degradation of the vessel basement membrane and surrounding ECM, which also facilitates the invasion of endothelial cells, is an integral part of the ongoing angiogenic process. The matrix metalloproteinase family enzymes that degrade components of ECM consist of four groups according to their substrates: collagenases, gelatinases, stromelysins, and membrane-associated MMPs. Gelatinases-A (MMP-2) and gelatinases-B (MMP-9) are highly expressed in astrocytomas, and their expression levels, especially those of MMP-9, correlate with the histological grade of tumor. MMP-2 and MMP-9 expression is strongly induced by hypoxia, and these two molecules appear to have a synergistic effect on basement membrane degradation [109]. The inhibitors of MMPs are called tissue inhibitors of metalloproteinases (TIMPs), which are comprised of TIMP-1, TIMP-2, TIMP-3, and TIMP-4. The interactions between these proteases and their inhibitors play important roles in cell morphogenesis, angiogenesis, tissue remodeling, tissue repair, tumor metastasis, cirrhosis, and arthritis. After breakdown of the basement membrane, endothelial cells proliferate and migrate toward the tumor cells expressing pro-angiogenic compounds. The activation of endothelial cells results in increased expression of cell adhesion receptors, such as integrins $\alpha v\beta 3$ and $\alpha 5\beta 1$, and in increased cell survival, proliferation, and migration responses. In addition to migration of endothelial cells, migration of pericytes is an important part of tumor vessel formation. Platelet-derived growth factor secretion by activated endothelial cells recruits pericytes to the site of newly sprouting vessels and aids in establishing a new basement membrane [110].

The discovery of hypoxia inducible factor-1 (HIF-1) and the observation that hypoxia-induced HIF-1α expression in pseudopalisading cells, in tumoral necrotic areas, was concomitant with the expression of one of its target genes, VEGF, established a biological link between hypoxia and angiogenesis [111]. The most potent activator of angiogenic mechanisms in brain tumors is tissue hypoxia. One well-studied pathway is the HIF-1/VEGF-A pathway, which leads to endothelial cell proliferation and migration. HIF is a heterodimeric DNA-binding complex composed of two basic helix-loop-helix proteins of the PAS family (PER, AHR, ARNT and SIM family): the constitutive HIF-1b and one of either hypoxia-inducible a-subunits, HIF-1a or HIF-2a. In hypoxia, the a/b heterodimer binds to a core pentanucleotide sequence (RCGTG) in the hypoxia response elements (HREs) of target genes. The hypoxic microenvironment (1–2% O_2) caused by the increased oxygen consumption of hyperplasia and/or hypertrophy and the decreased oxygen delivery due to the increase in diffusion distance was assumed to contribute to the angiogenic switch. An important link between hypoxia and angiogenesis was the discovery that the expression of the potent vascular endothelial growth factor was induced by hypoxia [112]. VEGF, which regulates tumor edema and blood vessel formation, is an example of a gene regulated by an HIF-1 though an HRE. Angiogenesis is essential for development, wound healing, tissue or organ regeneration, but it is also part of pathological processes, such as cancer and certain retinopathies. It is an intricate multistep and temporally ordered process that involves a great number of genes, modifiers and pathways. Many of these genes are directly induced by HIF-1a, such as nitric oxide synthases, angiogenic and vascular growth factors and genes regulating matrix metabolism (urokinasetype plasminogen activator receptor; uPAR) [113]. Immunohistochemical expression of HIF-1α clearly correlated with the degree of glioma malignancies and predicted survival among patients with malignant gliomas and the degree of necrosis on MRI. In a recent study, has been demonstrated that SN38, the active metabolite of CPT11, exhibited an antiangiogenic effect. SN38 inhibited HIF-1α and VEGF mRNA and protein expression of glioma cells in a dose- and time-dependent manner [114]. Metronomic CPT11 treatment of gliomas exhibited growth inhibitory effects without systemic toxicity, that is, through comparison of body weight loss that was not observed by conventional CPT11 treatment. Tumor tissues treated with metronomic CPT11 exhibited decreased expression of

http://dx.doi.org/10.5772/53487

HIF-1α protein and pimonidazole expression, which were indicative of areas of hypoxia by immunohistochemistry.

4.1. Mediators of glioma angiogenesis

Glioma angiogenesis is mediated by the release of angiogenic cytokines by the tumor cells. Numerous, different cytokines have been identified so far which are able to induce angiogenesis (Figure 1). This cytokine production is either the result of overexpressing angiogenic factors through genetic alterations or is triggered by hypoxia.

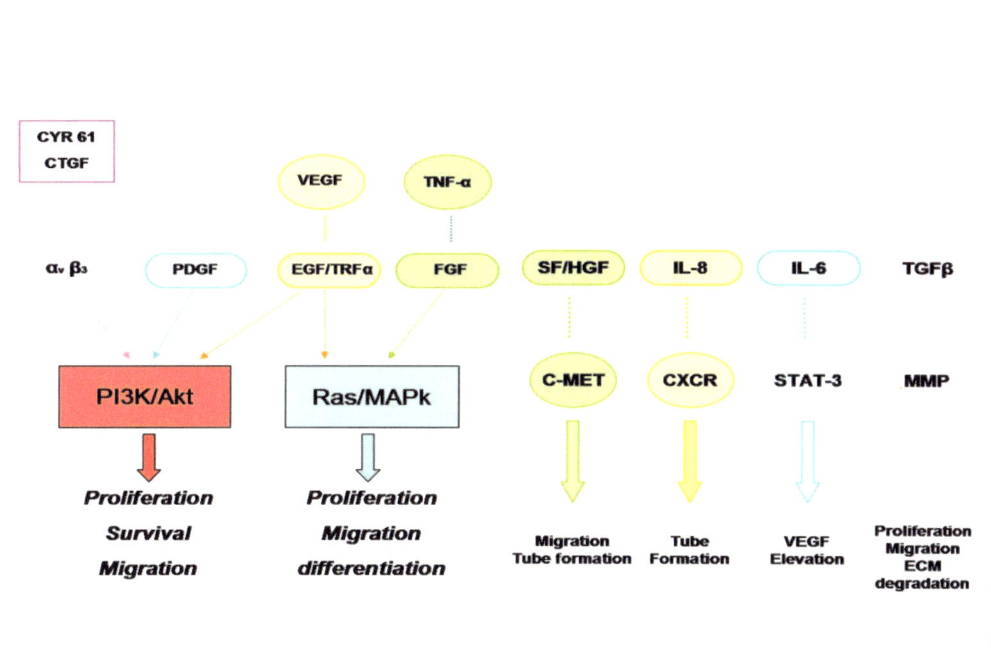

Figure 1. Representation of angiogenesis mediators in gliomas.

In the phosphatidylinositol-30 kinase (PI3K)/Akt and Ras/mitogen-activated protein kinase (MAPK) converge many angiogenic growth factors, including vascular endothelial growth factor (VEGF). These pathways modulate important cellular processes in angiogenesis, including endothelial cell proliferation, survival, migration, invasion, tube formation and extracellular matrix degradation.

CXCR = C-X-C chemokine receptor, CYR6.1 = cysteine-rich angiogenic inducer 61, CTGF = connective tissue growth factor, EGF = epidermal growth factor, FGF = fibroblast growth factor, HGF = hepatocyte growth factor, IL-6 = interleukin-6, IL-8 = interleukin-8, MMP = matrix metalloproteinases, PDGF = platelet-derived growth factor, PI3K = PI3 kinase, SF = scatter factor, TGF-a = transforming growth factor-alpha, TGF-ß = transforming growth factor-beta.

4.1.1. VEGF, VEGF-receptors and VEGF pathway

The VEGF family of growth factors and their receptors are the most important mediators of glioma angiogenesis. The VEGF family includes six glycoproteins referred to as VEGF-A, VEGF-B, VEGF-C, VEGF-D, VEGF-E, and placental growth factor. The VEGF acts as a major vascular permeability factor and as a mitogen/survival promoter for endothelial cells [115, 116]. VEGF-A and its receptors are the best characterized signaling pathway in angiogenesis and binds to two receptor tyrosine kinases (RTK) – VEGFR-1 (Flt-1) and VEGFR-2 (KDR, Flk-1) [117]. It is generally agreed that VEGFR-2 is the major receptor mediating the mitogenic, angiogenic and permeability-enhancing effects of VEGF-A. Recent evidence has suggested that VEGFR-1 participates in haematopoiesis and in the recruitment of monocytes and other bone marrow derived cells to promote tumor angiogenesis [118]. In addition, VEGFR-1 is involved in the activation of MMPs associated with matrix degradation and in the production of growth factors from endothelial cells. VEGF-A gene expression is up-regulated by hypoxia, mediated by the transcription factor HIF and the product of the von Hippel–Lindau (VHL) tumor suppressor gene. Other transcription factors capable of up-regulating VEGF transcription include the ETS-1 proto-oncogene and STAT-3. ETS proteins activate many genes involved in angiogenesis, including those that regulate VEGFR-1 and VEGFR-2, integrin b3, some MMPs and urokinase-type plasminogen activator (uPA). ETS-1 is expressed more frequently in GBM being most prominently observed in the glomeruloid tufts of GBM [119]. VEGF promotes endothelial proliferation via the activation of the MAPK pathway. VEGF also enhances vascular permeability through the MAPK signaling cascade by rearranging cadherin/catenin complexes and loosening adhering junctions between endothelial cells [120]. The VEGF-A is secreted by tumor cells as well as by stromal and inflammatory cells. VEGF-A can be linked in the extracellular matrix through the interaction with proteoglycans or glycosaminoglycans. The expression of the receptors VEGFR1 and VEGFR2 is regulated on the endothelial cells in gliomas. VEGF-A activation causes endothelial cell differentiation into a "tip" cell and a VEGF-A gradient induces "stalk" cell proliferation along an opening in the BM in forming of a new vessel sprout [121]. The ligands for VEGF3 (VEGF-C&D) are expressed by multiple cell types that surround the angiogenic vessels, suggesting the existence of a novel pro-angiogenic paracrine signaling pathways in these neoplasms. In addition to transcription factors, VEGF expression is also probably correlates with many other growth factors and their specific receptors, including transforming growth factor (TGF)-b, platelet-derived growth factor (PDGF)-B, epidermal growth factor (EGF), basic fibroblast growth factors (FGF). VEGF promotes endothelial proliferation via activation of the MAPK pathway. The activation of MAPK/ERK is associated with inhibition of the Jun-N terminal kinase (JNK) pathway in mediating the anti-apoptotic effect of VEGF. The PI3K/Akt pathway is of central importance in VEGF signaling. Activated VEGFR-2 mediates the phosphorylation of Akt, which potently inhibits endothelial cell apoptosis by interfering with various apoptosis signaling pathways. Akt also promotes endothelial cell migration, and increases the expression of HIF, leading to enhanced VEGF expression [122]. VEGF stimulates endothelial production of urokinase-type plasminogen activator (uPA), which induces conversion of plasminogen to plasmin, causing the breakdown of ECM components and leading to ECM remodeling [123]. The end result of VEGF signaling in tumors is the production of immature, highly permeable blood vessels with subsequent poor maintenance of BBB and parenchymal edema [96, 124]. Alternatively, the angiogenic effect of VEGF can be mediated through integrins, a1b1, a2b1 and avb3, which promote cell migration, proliferation and matrix remodeling.

4.1.2. FGF and FGF receptors

The FGF family of proteins and their receptors are overexpressed in various types of cancer. Binding of FGF to its receptor causes transphosphorylation and activation of intrinsic tyrosine kinase, which results in signal transduction. Both acidic FGF (aFGF) and basic FGF (bFGF) are up-regulated in GBM [125] and are responsible for resistance of endothelial cells to apoptosis. Basic fibroblast growth factor (bFGF) is expressed by vascular cells and, focally, by the tumor cells. The receptors for bFGF include FGFR1, expressed by the tumor cells and the tumor endothelial cells and the FGFR2 expressed only by the tumor cells. The anti-apoptotic effect of bFGF is mediated by increased expression of Bcl-XL and Bcl-2 via the MEK-dependent signaling pathway. In addition, bFGF stimulates the expression of VEGFR in endothelial cells.145 Similar to VEGF, aFGF and bFGF induce endothelial cell proliferation and migration. Furthermore, FGF activation leads to remodeling of ECM and degradation of the basement membrane by inducing production of plasminogen activator, collagenase and MMP in endothelial cells [127].

4.1.3. PDGF Family

PDGF-B and platelet-derived growth factor b receptor (PDGFRb) have important roles in the development and differentiation of the vessel wall [128]. PDGF is a mitogen for multiple cells of mesenchymal and neuroectodermal origin that acts through the PDGF receptors α and β. PDGF-B is required for recruitment of pericytes and maturation of the microvasculature. PDGFR-β is expressed on endothelial cells of astroglial tumors and that PDGF expression correlates with astroglial malignancy and angiogenic activity

PDGF contributes indirectly to tumor angiogenesis acting as a potent mitogenic and chemotactic stimulus for angiogenesis associated stromal cells, such as smooth muscle cells or pericytes. However, PDGF's effects on angiogenesis are mediated partly by VEGF. The angiogenic effects of PDGF are mediated through PI3K/Akt, MAPK/ERK and STAT3 signalling [129].

4.1.4. Molecules of the inflammatory cascade

Molecules of the inflammatory cascade act indirectly on angiogenesis via modulating expression of direct angiogenic factors. Interleukin-8 (IL-8) is a potent chemoattractant. But recent data suggest that it has a critical role in glial tumor angiogenesis and progression. High expression levels of PGES-1 (Prostaglandine E 1 Sinthase) and IL-8 in malignant gliomas cells and microglial cells, strongly correlated with grading tumor, are been demonstrated [130]. IL-8 expression is first observed in low grade astrocytoma in perivascular tumor areas expressing inflammatory cytokines. In malignant gliomas, IL-8 further localizes in oxygen-deprived cells surrounding necrosis. IL-8, however, stimulates angiogenesis via the interaction with the CXC chemokine receptor 1 (CXCR1), CXCR2 and Duffy antigen receptor for cytokines (DARC). DARC expression has been detected on tumour-associated endothelial cells, whereas CXCR1 and CXCR2 are found on infiltrating leukocytes near blood vessels. Macrophages are known to produce high levels of IL-8, which has a tumorigenic activity, by inducing tumor growth and angiogenesis; IL-8 is an inflammatory chemoattractant responding to the tumor microenvironment. Tumor pseudopalisading cells secrete HIF which induces IL-8 secretion. On the basis of preliminary results, the role of IL-8 as crucial angiogenesis mediator within HIF-1α pathway and crosstalk between hypoxia-induced high levels of HIF-1α and VEGF expression has been demonstrated.

The cyclooxygenase isoforms (COX-1 and COX-2) catalyze the synthesis of prostaglandins from arachidonic acid. While COX-1 is ubiquitously expressed in a wide range of tissues, COX-2 is cytokine inducible. COX-2 is expressed in human glioma cells where its expression correlates with malignancy, being highest in glioblastoma. The anti-angiogenic efficacy of COX-2 inhibitors is currently explained first by downregulation of VEGF, which results in blocking of endothelial cell proliferation and induction of endothelial cell apoptosis and second by inhibition of integrin function and signaling.

Tumor necrosis factor-α (TNF-α) is a potent proinflammatory cytokine with a quite complex role in endothelial cell survival and migration. It has impact on endothelial cell survival and migration via its TNF-receptor 1 and 2 which are both expressed on endothelial cells.

Membrane type 1-matrix metalloproteinase (MT1-MMP) expressed by the tip cell of an endothelial sprout opens up the surrounding matrix and is only later down-regulated when stalk cells come into contact with pericytes. Re-established contact between endothelial cells and pericytes induces expression of tissue inhibitor of metalloproteinases-2 (TIMP-2) in endothelial cells and TIMP-3 in pericytes in switching off the proteolytic phenotype in endothelial cells [131]. MT1-MMPs on the endothelial cell surface are also required for the subsequent step in the angiogenesis cascade of tube formation by playing a role in endothelial intracellular vacuole and lumen formation. The vessel lumen is tightly sealed by adjoining endothelial cells held together by tight and adherens junctions. A basement membrane is then produced by endothelial cells in cooperation with surrounding cells in providing structural support and maintaining endothelial cell quiescence. The BM is built up of scaffolding laminins and essential components such as collagen IV, perlecan, nidogens, and collagen XVIII [132-133]. During the maturation of new capillaries, pruning of excess or unneeded vessels for optimal perfusion is proposed to represent an adjustment to oxygen surplus while the surrounding ECM exerts mechanical strain providing traction and orientation for angiogenic microvessels [134].

Many other proangiogenic factors are upregulated in gliomas and this aspect might explain the failure of many actual antiangiogenic therapeutic strategies in gliomas management. TGF-b and its receptors are highly expressed in malignant gliomas, especially in areas of vascular hyperplasia and around necrotic regions. In glioma cells, the angiogenic effect of TGF-b is probably mediated through the enhanced expression of VEGF. TGF-b also promotes angiogenesis via the integrin signaling pathway. TGF-b upregulates expression of

$\alpha v\beta 3$ integrin that, in turn, binds to MMP-2, which leads to degradation of the ECM and enhanced endothelial cell invasion [135]. An important role has absolved by IL-1beta, IL-6, TNF-alpha and stromal-cell-derived factor (SDF)-1 alpha [46].

5. Microglia

Glioma tissues as obtained by surgical resection contain also a considerable amount of non-transformed cells. The majority of these cells are tumor-associated macrophages (TAMs) [136-137]. Resident macrophages of the brain are termed microglia. These cells invade the brain early in development and differentiate into so-called resident, ramified microglia. These tumor-associated microglia displayed an ameboid morphology similar to that described in other pathologies. Since microglia share many properties with macrophages found in non-neuronal tissues including the blood, it was possible that glioma-associated microglia could be recruited de novo from the microglial population resident in the brain, or alternatively, migrate into brain tumors from the periphery. To address this question, Badie and Schartner [138] used CD45 labeling of cells in rodent tumor models to distinguish brain microglia (CD45 low) from peripheral macrophages (CD45 high). They used CD11b/c as a general marker for macrophages and sorted the CD11b/c2 positive cells into two populations showing high and low CD45 expression. From this, they concluded that the macrophages are primarily found within tumors, while microglia was detected in all brain tissue. Thus, the precise origin of tumor microglia remains to be determined. Regardless of origin, we can define any glioma-associated monocytic cell with macrophage characteristics as a tumor-associated microglia. Candidate chemoattractants of tumor-associated microglia include monocyte chemotactic protein-3(MCP-3), colony-stimulating factor 1 (CSF-1), granulocyte-colony stimulatory factor (G-CSF), and hepathocyte growth factor/scatter factor: each of these has been shown to be released by gliomas and microglia are known to express receptors for these chemoattractant growth factors [139-140].

TAMs promote cancer progression through several mechanisms, including promotion of angiogenesis, induction of tumour growth, and enhancement of tumour cell migration and invasion. The hypoxic stress in the tumour mass leads to the expression of inflammatory molecules, which promote the recruitment of macrophages followed by conversion to the M2 phenotype. TAMs are capable to modulate and induce neovascularization and functions related to stroma formation. When TAMs are activated, in response to specific stimuli, these cells can express a repertoire of substances that promote angiogenesis. Growth factors such as acidic fibroblasts growth factor (aFGF/FGF1), basic fibroblasts growth factor (bFGF/FGF2), vascular endothelial growth factor (VEGF), granulocyte colony stimulating factor (GM-CSF), transforming growth factor-α, insulin-like growth factor-1, platelet derived growth factor (PDGF), tumour growth factor-β (TGF-β) and other monokines (e.g. tumour necrosis factor-α (TNF-α), interleukin-1, interleukin-6, interleukin-8, substance P, prostaglandins, interferons and thrombospondin which are released by tumour cells leads to the activation of macrophages and have the capability to influence the angiogenic process [141]. Therefore, macrophages recruited in situ represent an indirect pathway of amplification of angiogenesis, in concert with angiogenic molecules directly produced by tumor cells. In experimental in vitro studies, glioma cell lines seem produce high levels of a monocyte-macrophages-derived cytokine, IL-8, that induces formation of tube-like structures by human microvascular endothelial cells [142]. We previously demonstrated significant increase in IL-8 protein level in astrocytic cultures treated with PGE2. The ability of PGE2 to increase IL-8 expression in glioma cells has a significant biological impact on tumorigenesis, as shown by increased growth and reduced apoptosis in PGE2-treated cells [143]. Macrophages can exert a dual influence on blood vessel formation. On the one hand macrophages produce proangiogenic molecules on the other hand they can express anti-angiogenic molecules and damage the integrity of blood vessels. In general the pro-angiogenic functions of TAMs prevail [144].

Angiogenesis is also facilitated by TAM-derived proteases released in tumours, as extracellular proteolysis is an absolute requirement for new blood vessel formation. Macrophages can express proteases to release a number of pro-angiogenic molecules bound to heparan sulfate in proteoglycans, and fragment of fibrin and collagen, which facilitate angiogenesis. Among these, matrix metalloproteases (MMPs 1, 2, 3, 9 and 12), plasmin, urokinase plasminogen activator and receptor are the prominent ones which promotes tumour directed angiogenesis. MMPs are a family of matrix degrading enzymes including collagenase (MMP-1), gelatinase A (MMP-2), stromelysin (MMP-3), matrilysin (MMP-7), gelatinase B (MMP-9), and other MMPs. TAMs have been reported to correlate with the metastatic potential of a variety of human cancers, and they have also been shown to be a major source of MMP-9. In addition, urokinase-type plasminogen activator is a serine protease synthesized by TAMs in various human tumour types [145]. TAMs were shown to express CXCL8, which like VEGF, binds heparin in the ECM and stimulate angiogenesis [146]. Thus TAMs have the capacity to affect each phase of the angiogenic process, including degradation of the extracellular matrix, endothelial cell proliferation and endothelial cell migration. TAMs can also secrete cysteine-type lysosomal proteases and a wide variety of growth factors that can stimulate cancer growth.

New blood vessels in tumours are usually disorganized and prone to collapse, resulting in areas of inadequate perfusion and hypoxia (low oxygen tension). Additionally, rapid tumour cell proliferation in some areas may outpace the rate of new blood vessel growth, causing hypoxic areas to form [147]. The level of TAMs in tumours appears to be affected by hypoxia, a trait commonly found in these tissues. TAM numbers are generally higher in tumours containing high overall levels of hypoxia, as seen in primary human breast carcinomas and various animal tumours. Hypoxic tumours secrete higher amounts of chemoattractants and/or other factors that enhance monocyte attachment to and migration through the tumour vasculature. Once targeted to hypoxic sites, TAM functions are greatly affected by hypoxia-related factors. Because macrophages are phagocytes, they may also be attracted to hypoxic, perinecrotic areas along a trail of necrotic debris emanating from dead cells. Hypoxia also entraps TAMs by decreasing their mobility in a number of ways. One such approach involves the hypoxic up-regulation of the enzyme mitogen-activated protein kinase phosphatase (MKP-1) by macrophages. This is important because various chemoattractant receptors, including those for CCL2, VEGF, and endothelin 2, stimulate cell migration by phosphorylating the signaling enzymes MEK, ERK1/2, and p38 MAPK. Up-regulated MKP-1 rapidly dephosphorylates these molecules in TAMs, thus terminating the chemotactic response of TAMs to these chemokines [148]. Hypoxia also inhibits macrophage expression of the chemokine receptors CCR2 and CCR5 [149], further helping to immobilize TAMs. Hypoxia also induces a profound change in the phenotype of macrophages, promoting increased expression of a wide range of genes.

This is brought about by the hypoxic up-regulation of such transcription factors as hypoxia-inducible factors, HIF-1α and HIF-2α. TAMs respond to hypoxia by up-regulating a broad array of genes encoding proteins that promote the proliferation, invasion, and metastasis of tumour cells as well as tumour angiogenesis. Genes coding for M-CSF, a growth factor that promotes the survival and differentiation of macrophages, is over expressed in some human tumours, and elevated M-CSF levels correlate with high TAM numbers and poor prognosis [150]. Hypoxic macrophages are also likely to promote the invasive and/or metastatic behavior of tumour cells by releasing such pro-invasive factors as macrophage inhibitory factor [151]. Macrophage inhibitory factor is known to modulate the activities of a number of cell types in tumours, including stimulation of tumour cell motility [152]. This may involve indirect effects such as macrophage inhibitory factor-stimulated release of matrix metalloproteinase 9, which in turn degrades components of the basement membrane and extracellular matrix, thereby increasing the motility of tumour cells.

In a cultured mouse brain slice model, the invasion and growth of glioma cells was compared between normal and microglia-depleted slices. Glioma cell invasion was significantly reduced in microglia depleted slices relative to control slices [153]. The impact of microglia on glioma migration might relate to the production of membrane type 1 metalloprotease (MT1-MMP or MMP-14) that are produced by microglia in response to soluble factors released from glioma cells. Glioma cells also release metalloproteases 2 that is fully activated by MT1-MMP released from microglia. The consequent degradation of the extracellular matrix has been postulated to enhance the invasion of glioma cells into the brain parenchyma. The importance of microglia for glioma growth was further substantiated by studying animals in which microglia was depleted. The microglia-depletion in vivo was achieved by using the CD11b-HSVTK mouse model. Seven days after intracerebral glioma inoculation, ganciclovir (a specific substrate for the viral thymidine kinase HSVTK) was infused via mini-pumps into the tumor area for a further 7 days. To restrict the effect of ganciclovir on the intrinsic microglial population, the mice were irradiated before bone marrow transplanted with wild-type monocytes. The ganciclovir treatment led to a considerable depletion of microglia and to an 80% reduction in glioma volume [153].

CD68 is a monoclonal mouse antibody that labels human monocytes and macrophages. The antigen recognized by CD68 is absent from resting microglia but readily detectable in phagocytic microglia, perivascular cells and brain macrophages. In a recent study, the presence of CD68 positive cells neighboring of neoplastic cells, contiguous to necrotic and hypoxic areas within neoplastic tissue has been evidenced. The presence of TAMs that passed through vessel wall also in low-grade astrocytomas was, also, observed [154]. In anaplastic cases, neoplastic cells seem to be guided towards microglia. These data, can reinforced the hypothesis that macrophage infiltration could be closely associated with neovascularization and malignancy in human gliomas. Matrix metalloprotease activity is also regulated by the CX3CL1/CX3CR1 signaling pathway. For example, matrix metalloproteases 2, 9, and 14 are upregulated in microglia following activation of CX3CL1/CX3CR1signaling. Notably, CX3CR1 is upregulated in glioma associated microglia [155] and polymorphisms in the chemokine receptor CX3CR1 have been associated with prognosis among patients with glioma. The common CX3CR1 allele (termed V249I) was a favorable prognostic factor. Patients who had only this CX3CR1 allele had a more than 1.5 longer mean survival time. This common allele was associated with reduced microglial cell infiltration in primary tumor biopsies [155].

In a previous study has been demonstrated, in a series of GBM, the presence of laminin, fibronectin and type IV collagen in hyper-plastic vessels, in and around vascular channel, in vascular walls and at level of BM associated with endothelial glomerulus-like proliferations [83]. Laminin within the BM can bind to both endothelial cells and tumor cells and is involved in angiogenesis and tumor growth. We can hypothesized that in pilocytic astrocytoma, the ECM integrity cause a reduced macrophagic/microglial migration. In this view, an incompetent control of interactions occurs between microglial adhesive molecules and ECM substrates. In low-grade astrocytomas is achievable that low macrophage/microglial recruitment is also correlated with a lower vascular neo-angiogenesis. This relationship may influence microglial morphology, blocking microglial migration and phagocytosis [154]. To support these findings, a recent study showed an increase of CD68 positive cells which correlated with trends toward worse event-free survival [156].

6. Therapeutic strategies for malignant gliomas

The treatment of brain cancer is one of the most difficult challenge in neurosurgery and oncology. Malignant gliomas involve, in their progression, multiple aberrant signaling pathways and the blood-brain barrier (BBB) restricts the delivery of many chemotherapeutic agents. Current conventional treatments protocols include maximally safe surgical resection followed by fractionated radiation therapy of the tumor and surrounding brain parenchyma and systemic chemotherapy. However, radiation therapy is limited to a largely palliative role, and chemotherapy has provided only a modest benefit in clinical outcome. There are several factors underlying the disappointing results in brain cancer therapeutics including limited tumor cell drug uptake, intracellular drug metabolism, inherent tumor sensitivity to chemotherapy, and cellular mechanisms of resistance. The BBB protects the brain from toxins and fluctuations in systemic chemical concentrations, but it also excludes many therapeutic agents. Multimodal therapeutic approaches and molecular-based targeted therapies are modern and complex strategies potentially very efficacious and applicable to up-regulate the selectivity of therapeutic effects and down-regulate systemic toxicity and side effect toward peritumoral and safe brain tissue. Developments in molecular biology have led to a clearer understanding of the mechanisms of tumor development and resistance to therapy. As a results, new treatment strategies are emerging that target steps in the molecular pathogenesis of brain gliomas. An optimal realization of a system that overcomes the problems associated with developing effective brain tumor treatments requires the identification of neoplastic markers, and understanding their evolution over time, and the development of technology for the biomarker-targeted delivery of multiple therapeutic agents, and for the simultaneous capability of avoiding biological and biophysical barriers. In this complex phenomenon it is fundamental to improve specific selective drugs delivery systems: in this way, drugs, antisense oligonucleotides (AONs), small interference RNAs, engineered monoclonal antibodies and other therapeutic molecules may diffuse into CNS overcoming the BBB.

Glioma gene expression and its development during gliomagenesis may help to better understand the role of important molecules involved in tumor-safe brain parenchyma relationships. These molecules, such as ECM proteases, cell adhesion molecules, and their related signaling pathways, show an important role in glioma cell migration and invasion and could selectively attack to inhibit the glioma invasive rim. Various small molecule inhibitors and antibodies has been developed, and is continuing to be developed, to target key components of the signal transduction machinery, with a particular focus on growth factors and their corresponding receptors and canonical downstream signal transduction intermediates. Many of these inhibitors have potential for the treatment of glioblastoma. Testing some of these inhibitors, as well as using genetic approaches to untangling these signaling networks in well-designed model systems (including both highly representative xenograft models and mouse genetic models), is beginning to provide an emerging picture of the targetable molecular phenotype of glioblastoma.

Angiogenesis is tightly correlated with the histological grading and prognosis of gliomas. Glioma vasculature is structurally and functionally abnormal, leading to vasogenic edema, increased interstitial pressure, and heterogeneous delivery of oxygen and drugs. VEGF is the key factor implicated in the angiogenesis of gliomas. It acts as a major vascular permeability factor and as a mitogen/survival promoter for endothelial cells. VEGF expression is stimulated by hypoxia, acidosis, and many growth factors (EGFR, PDGFR, HGFR, CKit, insulin-like growth factor receptor), and their downstream signaling pathways (PI3K–Akt, Ras–MAPK) are commonly activated in gliomas. However, many other proangiogenic factors are upregulated in gliomas, and this might explain how gliomas may escape a specific antiangiogenic therapy. Antiangiogenic therapy is able to normalize the structure and function of abnormal neovasculature [96]. The normalization hypothesis states that antiangiogenic therapies may augment the effects of chemotherapy and radiotherapy by normalizing tumor vessels. Furthermore, normalizing tumor vessels might also reduce hypoxia, and thus make the tumor cells more sensitive to chemotherapy and radiation therapy [96].

6.1. Molecular targeted therapy

Elevated expression or mutation of receptors and intracellular downstream effectors has been demonstrated in gliomas. These pathways are controlled by several growth factors linked to tyrosine kinase. Specific targeting of these signaling pathways that lead to altered cellular proliferation and cell migration and invasion could provide new molecularly targeted options for glioma treatment. The introduction of molecularly targeted agents is one of the most significant advances in cancer therapy in recent years. Targeted therapies block activation of oncogenic pathways, either at the ligand–receptor interaction level or by inhibiting downstream signal transduction pathways, thereby inhibiting growth and progression of cancer. Because of their specificity, targeted therapies should theoretically have better efficacy and safety profiles than systemic cytotoxic chemotherapy or radiotherapy. The main rationale for using antiangiogenic therapies in glioblastoma is to normalize the vasculature, restoring the selective permeability of the blood-brain barrier.

6.1.1. VEGF, VEGF-receptors and VEGF pathway

VEGF-A is a member of the VEGF family that acts as a key proangiogenic factor because of its specificity to endothelial cells and the multitude of responses that it can elicit. These include ECM degradation, endothelial cell proliferation, migration and tube formation, and expression of other proangiogenic factors, such as urokinase-type plasminogen activator, plasminogen activator inhibitor-1, urokinase-type plasminogen activator receptor, and matrix metalloproteinase-1. Overexpression of VEGF-A occurs in response to hypoxia, PDGF, EGF, transforming growth factor-h, interleukin-1h, and tumor necrosis factor-a. The best-studied receptor is VEGFR-2, a potent tyrosine kinase that mediates endothelial cell signaling through the activation of Ras/Raf/MEK/MAPK, PI3K/AKT/PKB, and protein kinase C pathways. Has been suggested that blocking VEGF pathways may normalize tumor vasculature and improve chemotherapy delivery, allowing higher drug concentrations [157].

Several strategies for targeting VEGF have been proposed, such as VEGFR TKI, anti-VEGF-A and VEGFR-2 monoclonal antibodies, antisense oligonucleotides, and ribozymes. The best-studied drugs in gliomas have been vatalanib (PTK787/ZK222584), ZD6474, sorafenib (BAY 43-9006), sunitinib (SU11248), and cediranib (AZD2171). Difficulties include defining the optimal biological dose of drugs that are rarely toxic, determining the relevance of combinations with cytotoxic chemotherapy and radiotherapy, and elucidating adequate surrogate markers.

Vatalanib is a VEGFR-1 and VEGFR-2 TKI that showed activity in glioma cell lines and xenograft models [158]. A phase I study of vatalanib, and c-kit in patients with newly diagnosed GBM receiving radiation, temozolomide, and an enzyme-inducing anti-epileptic drug in order to determine the MTD of vatalanib in this patient population was evaluated. Vatalanib was well tolerated with only 2 DLTs (thrombocytopenia and elevated transaminases). Other grade 3/4 toxicities included leukopenia, lymphopenia, neutropenia, and hand-foot syndrome. Of the 13 patients evaluable for a radiographic response, 2 had a partial response and 9 had stable disease. Vatalanib significantly increased PlGF and sVEGFR1 in plasma circulation and decreased sVEGFR2 and sTie2. Vatalanib was well tolerated and this study demonstrates the safety of oral small molecule inhibitors in newly diagnosed GBM patients. Blood biomarkers may be useful as pharmacodynamic markers of response to anti-angiogenic therapies [159].

ZD6474 is a VEGFR-2 TKI with additional VEGR-3 and EGFR inhibition properties. In vivo models showed a broader spectrum of action, suggesting an antiangiogenic and anti-VEGFR preponderant effect [160]. In a glioma xenograft study, ZD6474 decreased tumor volume, lowered the tumor cell proliferation index (Ki-67), and increased tumor cell apoptosis. However, microvascular density, a typical marker of angiogenic activity, surprisingly increased, raising doubts on the antiangiogenic effects of the drug [161].

The effect of ZD6474, was also evaluated in combination with either radiotherapy or temozolomide. ZD6474 in combination with radiotherapy significantly decreased tumour area by 66% compared with controls whereas the combination with temozolomide decreased tumour area by 74% [162].

Recently, the AEE788, a reversible TK inhibitor that inhibits EGFR and VEGFR, in recurrent glioblastoma patients, was evaluated [163]. Continuous, once-daily AEE788 was associated with unacceptable toxicity and minimal activity for the treatment of recurrent glioblastoma. The study was, therefore, discontinued prematurely.

Cediranib (AZD2171) is a potent, orally available, small-molecule inhibitor of VEGF-receptor (VEGFR) tyrosine kinase activity that rapidly normalizes tumor blood vessels in patients with glioblastoma, leading to a clinical improvement in cerebral edema [164]. In a recent study, drug effects were evaluated over time through the use of magnetic resonance imaging techniques (including analysis of perfusion, permeability, and relative vessel size) and assessment of circulating progenitor cells, circulating endothelial cells, and plasma levels of several proangiogenic proteins. Results suggest that cediranib leads to a normalization of vasculature and decreased edema; however, such effects disappear overtime, which is accompanied by an increase in circulating basic fibroblast growth factor, stromal cell-derived factor-1a, and circulating endothelial cells. In mouse models, improvement in edema was associated with increased survival, despite continued tumor growth [165]. The first clinical data of the REGAL trial of cediranib plus lomustine (CCNU) to investigate whether preclinical findings will translate into improvements for patients with recurrent glioma have been negative [166].

Single-agent sunitinib, an oral small molecule inhibitor of multiple tyrosine kinase receptors, was evaluated for treatment of patients with recurrent glioblastoma and anaplastic astrocytoma (AA). For AA patients, the most common side effects were fatigue, diarrhea, hand-foot syndrome, neutropenia, thrombocytopenia, and nausea. In the GBM cohort, the most common side effects were fatigue, diarrhea, neutropenia, and thrombocytopenia. Median overall survival was 12.1 months (AA) and 12.6 months (GBM). Nonetheless, sunitinib did not demonstrate significant anti-glioma activity in patients with recurrent malignant astrocytic gliomas [167]. Recent preclinical studies suggest that treating GBM with a combination of targeted chemotherapy and radiotherapy may enhance the anti-tumor effects of both therapies. In a recent study, have been evaluated the effects of combination therapy in a mouse gliomamodel that utilizes a PDGF-IRES-Cre-expressing retrovirus to infect adult glial progenitors in mice carrying conditional deletions of Pten and p53. The addition of sunitinib to low-dose radiation caused a modest, but significant delay in tumor growth. However, no significant survival benefit was seen as tumors progressed in 100% of animals. Histological analysis revealed a reduction in vascular proliferation and a marked increase in brain invasion. The results showed that the addition of Sunitinib to radiotherapy fails to significantly alter survival in GBM despite enhancement of the effects of radiation [168].

In gliomas, despite evidence of activity in preclinical models, clinical development of bevacizumab was delayed initially because of the fear of central nervous system hemorrhage [169]. Bevacizumab is a monoclonal antibody against VEGF inhibiting angiogenesis by preventing receptor activation. Phase II clinical trials using bevacizumab in both newly diagnosed and recurrent high-grade glioma showed promising results. Bevacizumab has been shown to be safe and tolerable in malignant gliomas. In the recurrent disease setting, bevacizumab alone might be sufficient for a clinical benefit and is currently approved as a single agent for this indication. In a phase II study was evaluated the efficacy and safety of bevacizumab in Japanese patients with recurrent malignant glioma. The 6-month progression-free survival rate in the 29 patients with recurrent glioblastoma was 33.9% and the median progression-free survival was 3.3 months. The 1-year survival rate was 34.5% with a median overall survival of 10.5 months. There were eight responders (all partial responses) giving an objective response rate of 27.6%. The disease control rate was 79.3% [170].

Norden et al. [171] analyzed the pattern of recurrence in patients treated with bevacizumab and irinotecan, and their observations suggest that bevacizumab might more efficiently suppress enhancing tumor recurrence than infiltrative tumor growth. A single-institution phase II trial using the humanized monoclonal VEGF antibody bevacizumab combined with irinotecan in malignant gliomas has been reported [172]. No central nervous system hemorrhages were observed. The 6-month PFS rates were 30% and 56% in grade 4 and grade 3 gliomas, respectively, comparing favorably with historical controls. In a similar study, bevacizumab plus irinotecan in recurrent malignant gliomas improves responses, progression-free survival, and overall survival compared with historical data. Karnofsky performance status of at least 80% was a predictive factor for response and overall survival [173].

In a recent research was evaluated concurrent bevacizumab with hypofractionated stereotactic radiation therapy (HSRT) for the treatment of recurrent malignant gliomas. Despite the promising initial response seen with the addition of HSRT to bevacizumab as salvage treatment for recurrent gliomas, approximately half of patients ultimately still experience failure within the radiation field. The rate of local failure with the addition of HSRT seems to be lower than that seen with bevacizumab alone in the salvage setting [174].

Several studies of bevacizumab in combination with metronomic dosing of temozolomide or etoposide or with daily erlotinib in recurrent glioma patients are ongoing.

6.1.2. Epidermal growth factor receptor

Epidermal growth factor receptor (EGFR, ErbB1, HER1) is a tyrosine kinase receptor that is abnormally activated in 70% of solid cancers. EGFR overexpression and immunoreactivity are more common in primary tumors than in secondary glioblastomas. Activation of EGFR pathways in cancer cells has been linked to increased motility, adhesion, invasion, and proliferation of tumor cells as well as inhibition of apoptosis and induction of angiogenesis.

The EGFR transmembrane protein comprises three domains: the extracellular domain, the transmembrane domain, and the cytoplasmic domain, which harbors the tyrosine kinase activity. Ligand binding (amphiregulin, EGF, transforming growth factor TGF-β, decorin, betacellulin, epiregulin, neuroregulin) to the extracellular domain of a monomer results in its homo- or heterodimerization, inducing phosphorylation of the tyrosine kinase domain, activating several signaling pathways, in particular: phosphatidylinositol 3'-kinase/Akt/ mammalian target of rapamycin (mTOR), Ras/mitogen-activated protein kinase (MAPK), phospholipase C (PLC)/protein kinase C (PKC), and (d) c-Src [175]. These activated pathways are involved in several cell biological processes, including cell proliferation, angiogenesis, migration/adhesion, survival, and differentiation. Approximately 50% of glioblastomas overexpress EGFR and 25% express a constitutively active mutated form of EGFR. This activation occurs through several molecular mechanisms: protein overexpression, reported in ~60% of cases; gene amplification, reported in ~40% of cases; truncated transcripts encoding for a constitutionally active receptor, reported in ~20% (mainly EGFRvIII) of cases; and mutation of the extracellular domain (15%) [175]. These alterations, which are quite frequently combined in the same tumor, activate the EGFR downstream signaling pathways, promoting the oncogenic process. Therefore, several strategies have been developed in order to block the EGFR signaling pathway, including small molecule tyrosine kinase inhibitors (TKIs), monoclonal antibodies, toxin-linked conjugates, and vaccine therapies. However, caution is needed with EGFR inhibitors, because hypoxia and low glucose levels might convert the cytotoxic effects of EGFR inhibition into a cytoprotective effect.

Two main EGFR small molecule TKIs have been evaluated in gliomas: gefitinib and erlotinib. These small molecules, which are orally delivered, block the ATP pocket of the EGFR intracellular tyrosine kinase domain and thus inhibit activation of downstream signaling pathways.

Growth factor pathway expression using epidermal growth factor receptor (EGFR), mutant EGFR (EGFRvIII), platelet derived growth factor receptor (PDGFR), C-Kit and C-Abl together with phosphatase and tensin homolog (PTEN) expression and downstream activation of AKT and phosphorylated ribosomal protein S6 (P70S6K) was analysed in 26 primary glioma cultures treated with the tyrosine kinase inhibitors (TKIs) erlotinib, gefitinib and imatinib. Response for each culture was compared with the EGFR/PDGFR immunocytochemical pathway profile using hierarchical cluster analysis (HCA) and principal component analysis (PCA). Erlotinib response was not strongly associated with high expression of the growth factor pathway components. Increased EGFR expression was associated with gefitinib response; increased PDGFR-α expression was associated with imatinib response. The results of this in vitro study suggest gefitinib and imatinib may have therapeutic potential in gliomas with a corresponding growth factor receptor expression profile [176].

Gefitinib is a selective epidermal growth factor receptor tyrosine kinase inhibitor that inhibits cell growth and induces apoptosis in human glioma cells. Gefitinib also induces death of H4 cells with characteristics of the intrinsic apoptotic pathway, including Bax mitochondrial translocation, mitochondrial outer membrane permeabilization, cytochrome c cytosolic release, and caspase-9/caspase-3 activation. Gefitinib caused Bad dephosphorylation, and increased its binding preference to Bcl-2 and Bcl-xL. The dephosphorylation of Bad in gefitinib-treated cells was accompanied by reduced intracellular cyclic AMP content and protein kinase A (PKA) activity. Adenylyl cyclase activator forskolin attenuated, but PKA inhibitor H89 augmented, gefitinib-induced Bad dephosphorylation, Bax mitochondrial translocation, caspase-9/caspase-3 activation, and viability loss. Inactivation of PKA sensitized H4, T98G, and U87 cells to gefitinib cytotoxicity, Bad dephosphorylation in serine-112, and caspase-9/caspase-3 activation [177].

In a recent study, the molecular effects of the tyrosine kinase inhibitor gefitinib on the EGFR signaling pathway in human glioblastoma were investigated. Resected glioblastoma tissues exhibited high concentrations of gefitinib, 20 times higher than respective plasma. However, no significant effect on 12 pathway constituents was detected. In contrast, in vitro treatment of a glioblastoma cell line, BS-153, with endogenous EGFRwt amplification and EGFRvIII expression resulted not only in dephosphorylation of the EGFR, but also of key regulators in the pathway such as AKT. Treating established xenografts of the same cell line as an in vivo model showed dephosphorylation of the EGFR without affecting downstream signal transductors, similar to the human glioblastoma. Taken together, gefitinib reaches high concentrations in the tumor tissue and efficiently dephosphorylates its target [178]. A phase II study was designed to assess the safety and efficacy of gefitinib given with and following radiation therapy in children newly diagnosed with a poor prognosis brainstem glioma. The observation that a subset of children with this generally fatal tumor experienced long-term progression-free survival, coupled with recent observations regarding the molecular features of brainstem gliomas, raises the possibility that prospective molecular characterization may allow enrichment of treatment responders and improvement in outcome results in future studies of biologically targeted agents [179].

Comparative analysis of tissue obtained from patients before and after the start of treatment suggested that EGFR phosphorylation and downstream signaling were not markedly inhibited after treatment was started. Two main mechanisms of resistance to small molecule TKIs have been proposed. First, Stommel et al. [180] showed that several RTKs could be activated simultaneously in gliomas maintaining activation of RTKs downstream signaling pathways. Thus, inhibition of one single activated RTK is insufficient and could be easily bypassed by other activated RTKs [181]. Second, in addition to RTK activation, growth factor receptor downstream signaling pathways can be activated through a mutation of ras or PTEN or an amplification of PI3K, inducing redundant activation of the signaling pathways [182].

Haas-Kogan et al. reported that glioblastoma patients whose tumor overexpressed and amplified EGFR gene had a better tumor response to small TKIs than patients whose glioblastoma did not have these molecular abnormalities. In addition, these investigators showed that low phospho-PKB/Akt level is associated with a good tumor response to erlotinib [183].

The combination of EGFR inhibitors with inhibitors of mTOR, a distal target of the growth factor receptor signaling cascade (temsirolimus, sirolimus, everolimus), is a promising strategy. It became clear that the mechanisms of sensitivity and resistance in gliomas differ from other types of tumors, such as lung cancer, in that the sensitivity in gliomas does not seem to be linked to tyrosine kinase domain mutations. In order to achieve higher dosages than previously used in clinical trials, we conducted a phase I trial to determine the maximum tolerated dose (MTD) for the combination of erlotinib and sirolimus for the treatments of recurrent malignant gliomas. The MTD was determined to be 150 mg daily for erlotinib and

5 mg daily (after a 15 mg loading dose) for sirolimus. The dose-limiting toxicity s included rash and mucositis, hypophosphatemia, altered mental status, and neutropenia. The combination oferlotinib and sirolimus is difficult to tolerate at dosages higher than previously reported in phase II trials [184].

Ongoing trials of gefitinib, erlotinib, and other EGFR TKIs, such as lapatinib, as well as further tissue analysis of finished trials, may clarify whether selection of patients based on EGFR overexpression, EGFRvIII, pAKT, and/or PTEN expression could improve results. Other attempts to overcome resistance include trials combining EGFR TKI with cytotoxic chemotherapy and radiotherapy as well as the use of new agents that are capable of inhibiting EGFRvIII-overexpressing cell lines in vitro, such as HKI-272 (an irreversible EGFR TKI) and AEE788 [185].

A phase 2 study assessed the efficacy and safety of concurrent radiation therapy (RT) and temozolomide with pharmacodynamic dose escalation of erlotinib in patients with newly diagnosed GBM. Twenty-seven patients were treated in this study. Twenty-two (81%) patients came off study for progressive disease (18 [67%]) or adverse events (4 [15%]). Eighteen patients (67%) have died. Median progression-free survival was 2.8 months, and the median overall survival was 8.6 months. Erlotinib co-administered with RT and temozolomide was not efficacious and had an unacceptable toxicity [186].

Recently, an EGFR murine humanized monoclonal antibody, cetuximab was developed. Little is known about the efficacy of cetuximab in glioma patients. Recently, a phase I/II study combining cetuximab, radiation, and temozolomide was initiated in order to assess the safety and efficacy of this combination as first-line treatment for primary glioblastoma patients [187].

6.1.3. Platelet-derived growth factor receptor PDGFR

PDGFs are a growth factor family composed of four different polypeptide chains (PDGF-A, PDGF-B, PDGF-C, and PDGF-D) that exert their cellular effects through two types of protein tyrosine kinase receptors: PDGFR-a and PDGFR-h. Ligand binding induces receptor dimerization, activation, and autophosphorylation of the tyrosine kinase domain, which results in activation of several signal transduction pathways, including Ras-MAPK, PI3K, Src family kinase, signal transducers and activators of transcription factors (Stat), and phospholipase Cg. Overexpression of PDGF and PDGFR has been shown to play a role in the development of cancer through autocrine stimulation of cancer cells, development of angiogenesis, and control of tumor interstitial pressure. Animal gliomagenesis models have suggested that PDGFR pathways not only play a role in proliferation but also have effects on cell differentiation through dedifferentiation of mature cells, prevention of glial cell differentiation, and even promotion of cancer stem cells [188]. Inhibition of PDGFR was correlated with decreased phosphorylated extracellular signal-regulated kinase and pAKT levels, suggesting inhibition of MAPK and PI3K pathways. PDGFR and PDGF are frequently expressed in gliomas, particularly in secondary glioblastomas and seems to be associated with a poorer prognosis.

Clinical studies using the tyrosine kinase inhibitor, imatinib mesylate, in malignant gliomas, have shown no major inhibition of tumor growth or extension of survival for patients, unlike those in chronic myeloid leukemia and gastrointestinal stromal tumors. Phase I data in malignant gliomas have suggested that use of enzyme-inducing drugs significantly affects drug metabolization [189]. However, preliminary phase II results of single-agent imatinib have found only limited efficacy in unselected patients [189-190].

The effects of imatinib on the PDGFR downstream signaling pathways as well as on other cellular functions in human glioblastoma cells were studied. Western blot analysis demonstrated that imatinib was more effective in inhibiting the activated rather than the quiescent forms of the target proteins. Furthermore, the imatinib treatment induced the sustained activation of extracellular signal-regulated kinase (ERK 1/2) signaling as well as components of other downstream signaling pathways, such as PI3K/Akt, STAT3 and p38MAPK. Further analysis indicated that the activation of ERK induced by the imatinib treatment was related to the S-phase re-entry of the cell cycle in one of the three glioma cells. Imatinib significantly inhibited cell migration but not cell growth. The combination treatment of imatinib with a MEK or PI3K inhibitor resulted in significant growth inhibition but did not inhibit cell migration beyond the inhibition achieved with the imatinib treatment alone [191. In a recent study has been demonstrated that long-term culture with imatinib mesylate against PDGFR and c-Kit (stem cell factor receptor) resulted in reduced cancer stem cell ability in glioblastoma cells through cell differentiation. Derived from RG glioblastoma cells co-cultured with imatinib for 3 months, RG-IM cells showed distinct properties of cell cycle distribution and morphology in addition to significantly decreased ability to form aggregates and colonies in vitro and tumorigenicity in vivo. Furthermore, decreased expression of stem cell markers, i.e., CD133, Oct-3/4, nestin, and Bmi1, and increased terminal neural cell markers, GFAP, Tuj1, etc., were identified in RG-IM at the mRNA level [192]. Conversely, using a combination of imatinib and hydroxyurea achieved better results compared with imatinib alone or historical controls [193]. It has been hypothesized that imatinib potentializes hydroxyurea cytotoxic effects through a decrease in tumor interstitial pressure (which would increase hydroxyurea delivery to tumor cells) and a decrease in DNA repair secondary to imatinib-induced reduction of Rad 51 expression. The combination of imatinib, hydroxyurea, and vatalanib, a VEGFR inhibitor, was well tolerated in a phase I trial and has been suggested as a possible multitargeted regimen for GBM [194].

Sorafenib is an orally available antiangiogenic agent that inhibits tumor cell growth and proliferation by blocking the action of intracellular and receptor kinases, including PDGFR, RAF kinase, VEGFR2, and c-KIT. In human glioblastoma cell lines, sorafenib inhibited proliferation synergistically in combination with bortezomib, a proteosome inhibitor, and rottlerin, an experimental inhibitor of protein kinase C[195-196]. A phase II trial found that first-line TMZ and radiotherapy followed by TMZ plus sorafenib was tolerated by patients with glioblastoma, although preliminary efficacy data for this regimen were similar to data for standard therapy [197]. It has been postulated that sorafenib and protracted, daily temozolomide may provide complementary therapeutic benefit among recurrent GBM patients.

The conclusions of this study showed that sorafenib can be safely administered with daily temozolomide with a regimen with limited activity for recurrent GBM [198].

Tandutinib is an orally active inhibitor of PDGFR, FLT3, and c-KIT tyrosine kinase activity. Although no preclinical data have been reported for tandutinib in glioblastoma, 2 early-phase trials are assessing tandutinib in recurrent or progressive glioblastoma as monotherapy or combined with bevacizumab. In a novel study, targeted PDGFR-A mediated tumor growth in vitro and in vivo using the tyrosine kinase inhibitor,tandutinib (MLN-518), which strongly inhibits PDGFR-A has been evaluated. Although PDGFR-A inhibition by this agent resulted in reduced mouse tumor cell growth and increased apoptosis in vitro, and reduced tumor cell proliferation in vivo, tandutinib did reduce tumor volume at the doses tested (360 mg/kg) in vivo [199].

6.1.4. P13K and related pathways

Overactivation of the PI3K/AKT/mTOR pathway seems to play a key role in the downstream signaling pathways promoting growth and survival in several types of tumor cells, including glioma. Activation of such a pathway is triggered by stimulation of growth factor receptors (including EGFR, PDGFR, fibroblast growth factor receptor, and insulin-like growth factor-I receptor) and the Ras pathway, leading to activation of PI3K. Activated PIP3 promotes phosphorylation of AKT through translocation near the cell membrane and activation of PDK1 and PDK2. pAKT promotes phosphorylation of several downstream effectors, including MDM2, p21/p27, Bad, FKHR, nuclear factor-nB, caspase-9, glycogen synthase kinase-3h, and mTOR. mTOR plays a key role in downstream signaling of the PI3K/AKT pathway through the regulation of cellular catabolism, anabolism, proliferation, cell cycle control, autophagy, angiogenesis, and apoptosis.

In vitro studies have suggested that mTOR activity is particularly highly activated in cells with deficient PTEN function, including glioma cell lines. Alterations of PTEN expression are frequent in high-grade gliomas, with PTEN mutations being present in 15% to 40% of primary glioblastomas [200]. Preclinical studies in gliomas have suggested that PTEN-deficient tumors show enhanced sensitivity to mTOR inhibition; this provided the rationale for clinical trials of mTOR inhibitors in glioblastomas [201].

Temsirolimus (CCI-779) is a lipid soluble analog of rapamycin that inhibits mTOR by binding to FKBP-12, resulting in cell cycle arrest and decreased growth of several human cancer cell lines. In a mouse model of PDGF-B driven low-grade gliomas the use of CCI-779 demonstrated dramatic anti-proliferative effect in these tumors [202]. Again, data from other studies, demonstrated that the blockade of mTOR with CCI-779 resulted in regional apoptosis and conversion in the character of surviving tumor cells from astrocytoma to oligodendroglioma in a mouse model of Akt+KRas-induced GBMs [203]. In a recent research, a combination of perifosine and CCI-779 to inhibit Akt and mTOR respectively was adopted. In vivo, perifosine and CCI-779 showed synergy in inhibiting the PI3K/mTOR axis corresponding with decreased tumor proliferation and induction of apoptosis [204].

Recently, was reported that the combination of focal RT and mammalian target of rapamycin (mTOR) inhibition using clinically relevant concentrations of temsirolimus (CCI-779) prolongs survival in a syngeneic mouse glioma model through additive cytostatic effects. In vitro, the mTOR inhibitor CCI-779 exerted marked anti-invasive effects, irrespective of the phosphatase and tensin homolog deleted on chromosome 10 status and counteracted the proinvasive effect of sublethal irradiation. In this study, the G-protein signaling 4 (RGS4) was identified as a novel target of mTOR inhibition and a key driver of glioblastoma invasiveness, sensitive to the anti-invasive properties of CCI-779 [205]. A phase II study of temsirolimus was conducted in children and adolescents with high-grade glioma, neuroblastoma or rhabdomyosarcoma. Temsirolimus administered weekly at the dose of 75 mg/m(2) did not meet the primary objective efficacy threshold in children with high-grade glioma, neuroblastoma or rhabdomyosarcoma; however, meaningful prolonged stable disease merits further evaluation in combination therapy [206].

Prompted by in vitro evidence of synergism between mTOR inhibitors and EGFR TKI, ongoing clinical research is concentrating efforts on such combinations, including trials of temsirolimus, everolimus (RAD001), or sirolimus (rapamycin) combined with gefitinib, erlotinib, or AEE788. A phase I study combining gefitinib and sirolimus in malignant gliomas found no significant pharmacokinetic interaction between the two drugs. Preliminary results of a study using gefitinib and everolimus in unselected recurrent glioblastoma patients were recently presented. Using modified radiographic criteria, responses were found in 31% of patients, including partial and minor responses. However, median OS and PFS were not different from historical controls [207].

Enzastaurin suppress proliferation and induced apoptosis via a caspase-dependent mechanism in glioblastoma cells in vitro and inhibited growth of human glioblastoma xenografts, which was accompanied by decreased phosphorylation of downstream signaling molecules, including GSK-3b [208]. Enzastaurin is a potent a PKC/PI3K/AKT inhibitor, that reduces angiogenesis and has direct cytotoxic activity against glioma cells in preclinical studies. In a novel study, therapy was well tolerated with thrombosis, thrombocytopenia, hemorrhage, and elevated alanine aminotransferase as the most commonly observed drug-associated grade 3 or higher toxicities. The 6-month PFS was 7% for patients with glioblastoma and 16% for patients with anaplastic glioma. Enzastaurin showed, an anti-glioma activity in patients with recurrent high-grade glioma, but does not appear to have enough single-agent activity to be useful as monotherapy [209].

A recent study was conducted in patients with recurrent glioblastoma or newly diagnosed disease that was not treatable with standard (chemo)radiotherapy. In this phase 1 research, the safety and recommended dose of the oral protein kinase C-beta inhibitor (anti-angiogenic) enzastaurin in combination with single-agent temozolomide, was evaluated. The recommended dose for enzastaurin in combination with standard 4-weekly temozolomide is therefore 500 mg OD. Temozolomide did not appear to effect enzastaurin exposures at the 250 mg or 500 mg OD dose levels [210].

In vivo models showed that enzastaurin combined with radiotherapy synergistically reduced tumor volume, radiation-induced satellite tumor formation, upregulation of VEGF expression, neovascularization, and GSK-3b phosphorylation [211]. An open-label, single-arm, phase II study combined enzastaurin with temozolomide plus radiation therapy (RT) to treat glioblastoma multiforme (GBM) and gliosarcoma was reported. Progression-free survival (PFS), toxicity, and correlations between efficacy and molecular markers analyzed from tumor tissue samples were also evaluated. The treatment regimen was well tolerated. Overall survival (median, 74 weeks) and progression-free survival (median, 36 weeks) results from the current trial were comparable to those from a prior phase II study using erlotinib and were significantly better than those from 2 other previous studies that used thalidomide or cis-retinoic acid, all in combination with temozolomide plus RT [212].

In a phase II study of enzastaurin in patients with recurrent heavily pretreated glioblastoma, an interim analysis showed that objective radiographic responses occurred in ~20% of patients. The subsequent phase III trial comparing lomustine and enzastaurin at first or second recurrence was the firstphase III trial to evaluate a targeted therapy for recurrent glioblastoma. However, a planned interim analysis found that enzastaurin treatment did not significantly increase PFS, leading to enrolment being halted [213].

6.1.5. SRC and SRC-family kinases

SRC and SFKs are frequently activated in glioblastoma cell lines and patient samples. SRC and SFKs are promiscuous regulators of multiple signaling pathways regulating cell growth, proliferation, adhesion, migration, and invasion, which are important processes in tumor invasion and metastasis. In particular, SFKs mediate signaling from growth factor receptors that are commonly overexpressed in GBM. Recently, SRC and FYN (an SFK) were shown to mediate oncogenic EGFR and EGFRvIII signaling in a rodent GBM model [214].

Dasatinib is a potent inhibitor of SRC and SFK tyrosine kinase activity. Preclinical studies in a wide variety of solid tumor cell lines, including prostate, breast and glioma, have shown that dasatinib acts as a cytostatic agent, inhibiting the processes of cell proliferation, invasion and metastasis. Dasatinib also inhibits the activity of osteoclasts, which have a major role in the development of metastatic bone lesions. Dasatinib also has inhibitory activity against c-KIT and PDGFR.

In GBM cells, dasatinib inhibited migration and induced autophagic cell death, and autophagy was increased by combining dasatinib with TMZ [214-215]. In vivo, dasatinib inhibited invasion, promoted tumor regression, induced apoptosis in EGFRvIII-expressing glioblastomas, and enhanced the activity of anti-EGFR antibodies.19 Recently, it has been showed that dasatinib interacts synergistically with JSI-124, an STAT3/JAK pathway inhibitor. Depletion of Src and STAT3 by siRNA inhibits cell proliferation and migration, suggesting that Src and STA3 play a key role in these cellular responses [216].

Recently the efficacy of dasatinib, in patients with recurrent GBM after bevacizumab failure, was explored. Adult patients were treated with dasatinib 70-100 mg twice daily in combination with bevacizumab (n = 14). Of the thirteen evaluable patients, none had a complete or partial response and only one patient had stable disease after an 8 week interval. Median progression-free survival (PFS) was 28 days. Median overall survival was 78 days. The study demonstrated that Dasatinib in conjunction with bevacizumab does not appear to have activity in patients with recurrent, heavily pretreated GBM [217].

NVP-AEW541is an inhibitor of insulin-like growth factor-I receptor (IGF-IR) kinase activity on growth and signaling in a panel of glioma cell lines. NVP-AEW541 blocked phosphorylation of IGF-IR in a dose- and time-dependent manner and inhibited proliferation and clonogenicity. NVP-AEW541 also induced loss of mitochondrial membrane potential and release of cytochrome c and apoptosis-inducing factor (AIF) from mitochondria. Combined treatment with dasatinib and NVP-AEW541 induced significantly more apoptosis than either agent alone in glioma cells, but not non-neoplastic astrocytes, and synergistically inhibited clonogenic survival. Mechanistic studies indicated that combination of NVP-AEW541 and dasatinib significantly reduced pERK and pAkt and markedly increased AIF release, Bax oligomerization and loss of mitochondrial potential compared to each agent alone. These data indicate that activation of Bax plays a critical role in mediating NVP-AEW541 and dasatinib-induced apoptosis, and suggest the potential value of combining IGFR inhibition with other classes of tyrosine kinase inhibitors to potentiate therapeutic efficacy [218].

6.1.6. *Integrin inhibitors*

Integrins are transmembrane receptors for the ECM that play a role in cell adhesion and cell migration, namely, in endothelial cell migration, adhesion, and proliferation during angiogenesis. Cilengitide is a cyclic arginine– glycine–aspartic acid containing peptide that binds to and inhibits $\alpha v\beta 3$ and $\alpha v\beta 5$ integrins, which are specifically involved in angiogenesis.

Cilengitide induces apoptosis in U87 glioma cells by preventing adherence to vitronectin and tenascin, matrix protein mediators of brain tumor invasion, and growth [219]. In a phase I study (n = 51) of recurrent high grade glioma patients, cilengitide was well tolerated and was demonstrated to have some activity. An objective response was observed in five patients, with two patients demonstrating prolonged complete responses [220]. The most notable trial to date was a randomized phase II study of cilengitide, which was associated with a median survival of 10 months in recurrent glioma patients [221].

A novel study was designed to evaluate the efficacy and tumor delivery of cilengitide in patients with recurrent glioblastoma. The study accrued 30 patients with recurrent glioblastoma and, after recovery from surgery, patients were treated with cilengitide (2000 mg i.v. twice weekly, maximum of 2 years of treatment). The results confirm drug delivery and possibly retention in tumor. This study provides evidence that with established dosing, cilengitide is adequately delivered to the tumor, although as a single agent, efficacy in recurrent glioblastoma is modest [222].

In Phase I and II GBM trials, cilengitide and the combination of cilengitide with standard temozolomide and radiation demonstrate consistent antitumor activity and a favorable safety profile. Preliminary results of a phase II trial of cilengitide added to radiotherapy and temozolomide conducted in 52 patients with newly diagnosed glioblastomas suggested efficacy in a subgroup of patients, with little or no additional toxicity [223]. A multicenter, phase I/IIa study, investigated the efficacy and safety of cilengitide in combination with standard chemoradiotherapy in newly diagnosed glioblastoma. Patients were treated with cilengitide (500 mg) administered twice weekly intravenously in addition to standard radiotherapy with concomitant and adjuvant temozolomide. Treatment was continued until disease progression or for up to 35 weeks. The conclusions demonstrated that the combination of cilengitide with temozolomide and radiotherapy was well tolerated, with no additional toxicity [224]. In a recent study, the mechanisms of cilengitide-induced cytotoxicity in glioma cells was evaluated. The final data showed that cilengitide treatment induced cell detachment in glioma cells plated on vitronectin in a dose-dependent manner and decreased cell viability with increasing doses. Moreover, the authors evidenced that the treatment of glioma cells with cilengitide induced autophagy in these cells, as demonstrated by puncta LC3-GFP appearance, the increased expression of LC3II, and increased acidic vacuole formation. Some level of cell apoptosis was observed in the cilengitide-treated cells only after 48 hours of treatment, following the induction of autophagy. The pretreatment of the cells with cilengitide could increase the level of autophagy induced by γ-irradiation and significantly decreased the viability of the cells [225]. Nabors et al. examined, in a randomized phase 2 trial, the safety and efficacy of cilengitide when combined with radiation and temozolomide for patients with newly diagnosed glioblastoma multiforme. The authors showed that cilengitide was well tolerated when combined with standard chemoradiation and may improve survival for patients newly diagnosed with glioblastoma multiforme regardless of MGMT methylation status. The authors concluded that, from an efficacy and safety standpoint, future trials of this agent in this population should use the 2000 mg dose [226].

6.2. Antisense strategy

Several approaches are available to manipulate gene expression at the DNA or RNA stage of protein synthesis. In eukaryotic organism, pre-mRNA is transcribed in the nucleus, introns are spliced out and then the mature mRNA is exported from the nucleus to cytoplasm. The small subunit of the ribosome usually starts by binding to one end of the mRNA and is joined there by other eukaryotic initiation factors, forming the initiation complex. This multi-enzymatic complex scans along the mRNA strand until it reaches a start codon, and then the large subunit of ribosome attaches to the small subunit so that the translation of a protein begins. This process, by which the information of a gene is converted into protein, is referred to as "gene expression".

Several approaches are available to specifically manipulate gene expression at the DNA or RNA stage of protein synthesis. An interesting molecular targeting strategy is the introduction of single-stranded antisense oligonucleotides, specific molecules involved in cell proliferation and cell death, to modify gene expression at the translational level. Antisense oligonucleotides (AONs) are short synthetic single-stranded DNA-sequences, 13-25 nucleotides long, that bind to and induce the cleavage of homologous stretches of mRNA sequences. These result in targeted destruction of mRNA and correction of genetic aberrations. AONs thus can act as drug molecules and potentially rectify many disease conditions. RNA and DNA based oligonucleotides are the most prevalent and most practical antisense drugs.

Interactions of RNA based AONs with target mRNA inhibit gene expression by interfering with protein translation without necessarily altering mRNA stability. AONs inhibit mRNA function by several mechanisms including modulation of splicing and inhibiting protein translation by disrupting ribosome assembly.

Two different and adjunctive antisense-based approaches to modulate gene expression into cancer cells are RNA interference (RNAi) and ribozymes. RNAi is mainly responsible for the post-transcriptional regulation of gene expression but is involved in transcriptional regulation. RNAi is a process within living cells that moderates the activity of their genes. RNA interference plays a fundamental role in diverse eukaryotic functions including viral defence, chromatin remodeling, genome rearrangement, developmental timing, brain morphogenesis, and stem cell maintenance. The power of RNAi lies in the key discovery that endogenous RNAi gene silencing machinery can be hijacked to artificially regulate genes of interest. The selective effect of RNAi on gene expression makes it a valuable research tool, both in cell culture and in living organisms because synthetic double-stranded RNA (dsRNA) introduced into cells can induce suppression of specific genes of interest.

Ribozymes are small oligo-ribo-nucleotides which have a specific base sequence with natural self-splicing activity. This activity can be directed against virtually any RNA target by the inclusion of an antisense region into the ribozyme. Some ribozymes have a self-cleavage catalytic action while other ones are true catalysts and can carry out RNA slicing by transesterification (splicesome) and peptidyl transfer (in ribosomes). A major disadvantage of ribozymes at present is that, being ribonucleic acids, they are particularly sensitive to nuclease degradation. Ribozymes are not generally being considered as agents which may be exogenously administered. Whilst it should be possible to develop nuclease-resistant ribonucleotide analogues, present strategies employing ribozymes achieve their delivery by genetic means, in the form of mini-gene constructs. Ribozymes are now utilized to study gene function in HIV disease and in cancer research.

6.2.1. Antisense oligonucleotides

The choice of the target is crucial to the potential success of the therapeutic approach. The most interesting targets are involved in apoptosis, cell proliferation, neoangiogenesis and invasion.

In tumorigenic mice generated by subcutaneous injection of glioma cell lines, overexpression of antisense VEGF (C6-VEGF(-/-) mice) significantly suppressed tumor growth, decreased angiogenesis and reduced tumoral edema. Further studies by electron microscope revealed that tumor-induced hyperpermeability was mediated by formation of vesiculo-vacuolar organelles (VVO), specifically reducing the number of vesicle and caveolae in VVO, and this effect was partially blocked by antisense VEGF [227].

Recently was evaluated the suitability of folate-PAMAM dendrimer conjugates for efficient EGFR AON delivery into glioma cells, wherein they release the AON from the FA-PAMAM to knock down EGFR expression in C6 glioma cells, both in vitro and in vivo. Folic acid was coupled to the surface amino groups of G5-PAMAM dendrimer (G5D) through a 1-[3-(dimethylamino)propyl]-3-ethylcarbodiimide bond, and AONs corresponding to rat EGFR were then complexed with FA-PAMAM. The AON transfection rates mediated by FA-PAMAM and PAMAM resulting in greater suppression of EGFR expression and glioma cell growth [228]. In a previous study, was demonstrated that antisense-EGFR transfection inhibited the growth and transforming phenotype of U87MG cells. In this research, the co-transfection of U87MG cells with wild-type PTEN and antisense EGFR constructs could inhibit the cellular growth by 91.7% [229].

Inhibition of PKC-α expression by a synthetic AON inhibits proliferation of C6 glioma cells. In addition, inhibition of PKC-α expression, has also showed growth inhibition of transformed U-87 cells transfected with antisense anti-PKC-α oligonucleotide [230]. PKC- α antisense oligonucleotide treatment in GBM and in A172 GBM cells was accompanied by reduction in PKC-α levels and the induction of wild-type p53 and insulin-like growth factor-binding protein-3 (IGFBP3) 24-72 h after treatment. Increased IGFBP3 levels were accompanied by increased mRNA levels. Recombinant human IGFBP3 induced an apoptotic effect that was similar to the PKC- α antisense oligonucleotide, and its effect was blocked by IGF-I [231]. Other potential therapeutic targets are human C-raf kinase and c-Ki-RAS proteins and signal transduction kinase proteins, involved in the control of proliferation, cellular migration and differentiation, and cytoskeletal rearrangements.

In a murine model, was showed the down-regulation of proliferation rate of C6 glioma cells transfected with antisense AKT2 cDNA construct. Parental C6 cells and C6 cells, transfected with antisense construct, were implanted through lipofectamine complexes. Dominant-negative (DN-AKT2) and antisense AKT2 constructs (AS-AKT2) were transfected into rat C6 glioma cells with elevated endogenous AKT2 expression. AKT2 expression was inhibited in C6 cells transfected with AS-AKT2 but did not significantly change in cells transfected with DN-AKT2. The cell migration distance was reduced in cells transfected with DN-AKT2 or AS-AKT2 compared to the control cells and gelatin zymography showed that the production of MMP2 and MMP9 was inhibited in transfected cells [232]. Edwards et al. targeted the phosphatidylinositol 3-kinase/protein kinase B (PKB)/Akt and the Ras/MAPK pathway for their involvement in cell survival and cell proliferation. The glioblastoma cell lines U87MG, SF-188, and U251MG were transiently transfected with an antisense oligonucleotide targeting ILK (ILKAS) alone or in combination with the Raf-1 inhibitor GW5074 or with the MEK inhibitor U0126. Glioblastoma cells transfected with ILKAS exhibited reduced levels of ILK and phosphorylated PKB/Akt on Ser473. These results confirmed that combinations targeting ILK and components of the Ras/MAPK pathway result in synergy and could potentially be more effective against glioblastoma cancer than monotherapy [233].

During progression of human gliomas, the expression of capillary BM laminins containing α4 chain switches from the predominant laminin-9 into lanimin-8. Effects of antisense inhibition of laminin-8 expression in glioma therapy through an in vitro model using human GBM cell lines M059K and U-87MG co-cultured with normal human brain microvascular endothelial cells (HBMVEC) have been observed. Laminin-8 and its receptor, integrins $\alpha3\beta1$ and $\alpha6\beta1$, are important for the functioning of endothelial cell BMs, which play a role in the maintenance of the BBB. Laminin-8 plays an important role in glioma cell invasiveness, in combination with other proteins associated with glioma progression, such as tenascin-C, MMP-2 and MMP-9. In this study was demonstrated a significant reduction of invasion of co-cultures through Matrigel and through the use of morpholino oligos against $\alpha4$ and $\beta1$ chains of laminin-8 [234]. The downregulation of laminin $\alpha4$ chain using AONs inhibits the motility of human glioma cells was shown. Laminin $\alpha4$ chain appears to be an important factor in glioma migration and invasion, both in vitro and in vivo [235].

The antisense modulation of Bcl-2 expression could increase the effectiveness of conventional chemotherapeutic agent. Antisense human bcl-2 cDNA was transfected into human malignant glioma cells. The effects of bcl-2 protein down-regulation on glioma cell morphology, in vitro tumor growth, and tumorigenicity in nude mice, as well as chemosensitivity to cisplatin, were studied. Expression of antisense bcl-2 cDNA decreased bcl-2 protein by more than sixfold. Antisense bcl-2 stable transfectants (AS-bcl-2) showed profound morphological change, marked retarded cell growth in vitro and significantly increased cytotoxicity of cisplatin [236]. Phase I and II studies are also being done to test G3139 in combination with docetaxel in patients with advanced breast cancer, hormone-refractory prostate cancer, and other solid tumors. By using AONs against the first six codons of the human Bcl-2 gene transfected into malignant glioma cells (Jon52 and Roc GBM cell lines), has been demonstrated a decrease in cell growth and an increase in apoptotic death [237]. There is a link between resistance to chemotherapy in glioblastoma and expression of antiapoptotic bcl-2 family members, including bcl-XL. Anti-bcl-XL AONs (ISIS 16009, ISIS 16967) in M059K GBM cell lines have been used and demonstrated a valid correlation between reduction of bcl-XL protein expression, induction of intrinsic apoptotic pathway and enhancement of cytotoxic responses to paclitaxel treatment, resulting in a chemosensitizing effect of anti-bcl-XL therapy [238].

7. Conclusion

Cerebral gliomas remain essentially resistant to traditional cancer therapy. Radiation therapy is limited to a largely palliative role, and chemotherapy has provided only a modest benefit in the clinical outcome. Ideally we would analyze tumor tissue in order to confirm adequate concentrations of our agents; however, the difficulties of accessing brain tumor samples compared with other tumor samples in systemic cancers make this a difficult task. This also impedes our validation of biological effects in vivo, a crucial step in the assessment of new interventions and therapies.

Understanding the genetic bases of gliomas and of the invasive behavior may suggest new molecular targets to overcome the mechanisms of multi-drug-resistance of the actual therapeutic approaches and to attack at the same time different crucial biological events of gliomagenesis. In recent years, basic and preclinical studies have revealed multiple new mechanisms of gliomagenesis and corresponding targets for treatment. Glioma gene expression and its development during gliomagenesis will may help to better understand the role of important molecules involved in tumor-safe brain parenchyma relationships. These molecules, such as ECM proteases, cell adhesion molecules and their related signaling pathways show an important role in glioma cell migration and invasion and could be selectively attack to inhibit the glioma invasive rim. Targeted therapies are adopted to disrupt the function of their targets or deliver toxins to tumor cells expressing the target. However, drugs targeting single molecules show a limited efficacy, because multiple abnormalities are simultaneously present in glioma patients. It is clear that the complexity and cross-talk between signal transduction pathways limits the potential efficacy of targeting a single receptor or molecule. As a result of a tested preclinical study, clusterin, eukaryotic initiation factor-4E (eIF-4E), integrins, metalloproteinases and other key molecules (involved in invasion and angiogenesis) might be possible future interesting molecular targets in glioma therapy. Targeting of multiple signaling pathways by multitargeted kinase inhibitors or combinations of single-targeted kinase inhibitors may increase treatment efficacies. Parallel to this is the task of determining the unique molecular and genetic profiles of individual patient tumors so that the most effective therapies can be selected for those individuals. Targeted agents are likely to have the greatest potential when used in combination to increase the activity of standard chemotherapies, broadening the range of pathways inhibited by treatment and/or counteracting mechanisms of resistance. In addition, as for classic cytotoxic agents, an intact BBB may represent an important impediment limiting the efficacy of targeted therapies.

Nanotechnology provides a unique opportunity to combat cancer on the molecular scale through careful engineering of nanomedicines to specifically interact with cancer cells and inhibit cancer cell function. It is also possible to take into neoplastic tissue, novel selective contrast enhancement molecules to visualize brain tumors and to study in vivo all of their characteristics, such as cellular proliferation, angiogenesis, necrosis, tumor-safe tissue interface, and edema. There are significant opportunities to investigate the use of nuclear imaging techniques such as positron emission tomography (PET) and single-photon emission computed tomography (SPECT) for development of radiolabeled nanoparticles targeting cancer. The versatility, sensitivity and tomographic imaging capabilities of these imaging modalities will provide excellent opportunities for future development of targeted nanoparticle formulations. The surface of nanoparticles can be modified to achieve targeted delivery and improved biocompatibility. Compounds may also be encapsulated within the interior core of nanoparticles for multiple functions. Nanoparticle-based delivery systems could increase the overcoming of the BBB by the use of drugs with a targeted-cell specificity modality. This approach permits the use of a lower dose of drug, a selective drug delivery to target tumor cells, both into the central core of tumor and into the distal foci of tumor cells within areas often characterized from integrity of the BBB [239-240]. Considerable effort has been made toward the research and development of multifunctional nano-particle systems for cancer targeted imaging and therapy. Theranostic nanomedicine represent an integrated nanotherapeutic system, which can diagnose, deliver targeted therapy, and monitor the response to therapy. This integration of diagnostic imaging capability with therapeutic interventions is critical to addressing the challenges of brain tumor hetereogeneity and adaptation. As a platform technology, nanomedicine has the advantage of being able to target multiple tumor markers and deliver multiple agents simultaneously for synergy in addressing the challenges of cancer hetereogeneity and adaptative resistance. Nanoparticle drug delivery vehicles have shown the ability to encapsulate a variety of therapeutic agents such as small molecules (hydrophilic and/or hydrophobic), peptides, protein-based drugs, and nucleic acids. By encapsulating these molecules inside a nanocarrier, the solubility and stability of the drugs can be improved, providing an opportunity to reevaluate potential drugs previously ignored because of poor pharmacokinetics. Encapsulated molecules can be released from nanocarriers in a controlled manner over time to maintain a drug concentration within a therapeutic window or the release can be triggered by some stimulus unique to the delivery site [241]. The surface of the nanocarrier can be engineered to increase the blood circulation half-life and influence the bio-distribution, while attachment of targeting ligands to the surface can result in enhanced uptake by target tissues.

On the basis of the data collected and of the limits of actual standard therapeutic protocol, we think that targeted therapy represents an interesting approach to modify the biological development of gliomas, probably trying to modulate crucial pathways of gliomagenesis during precocious steps of tumor progression and more molecular targets of the same pathway or of two different pathways.

Author details

Maria Caffo[1], Valeria Barresi[2], Gerardo Caruso[1], Giuseppe La Fata[1], Maria Angela Pino[1], Giuseppe Raudino[3], Concetta Alafaci[1] and Francesco Tomasello[1]

*Address all correspondence to: mcaffo@unime.it

1 Neurosurgical Clinic, Department of Neurosciences Psychiatry and Anaesthesiology, University of Messina School of Medicine, Messina, Italy

2 Neurosurgical Clinic Department of Human Pathology, University of Messina School of Medicine, Messina, Italy

3 Neurosurgical Unit, Orthopedic Institute "Villa Salus", Augusta, Siracusa, Italy

References

[1] Caruso G., Caffo M., Raudino G., Alafaci C., Tomasello F. New Therapeutic Strategies in Gliomas Treatment. In: Abujamra A.L. (ed). Brain Tumors - Current and Emerging Therapeutic Strategies. Rijeka: Intech; 2011. p281-306.

[2] Yung WK, Albright R, Olson J, Fredericks R, Fink K, et al. A Phase II Study of Temozolamide vs. Procarbazine in Patients with Glioblastoma Multiforme at First Relapse. British Journal of Cancer 2000; 83(5) 588-593.

[3] Osborn AG, Salzman KL, Thurnher MM, Rees JH, Castillo M. The New World Health Organization Classification of Central Nervous System Tumors: What Can the Neuroradiologist Really Say? American Journal of Neuroradiology 2012; 33(5) 795-802

[4] Pouratian N, Schiff D. Management of Low-Grade Glioma. Current Neurology and Neuroscience Reports 2010; 10(3) 224-231.

[5] Pignatti F., van den Bent M, Curran D, Debruyne C, Sylvester R, et al. Prognostic Factors for Survival in Adult Patients with Cerebral Low-Grade Glioma. Journal of Clinical Oncology 2002; 20(8) 2076-2084.

[6] Weller M. Novel Diagnostic and Therapeutic Approaches to Malignant Glioma. Swiss Medical Weekly 2011; 141 w13210.

[7] Yin S., Van Meir E.G. p53 Pathway Alterations in Brain Tumors. In: Van Meir E.G. (ed). CNS Cancer: Models, Markers, Prognostic Factors, Targets and Therapeutic Approaches. New York: Humana Press (Springer); 2009. p283-314.

[8] Bredel M, Scholtens DM, Yadav AK, Alvarez AA, Renfrow JJ, et al. NFKBIA Deletion in Glioblastomas. The New England Journal of Medicine 2011; 364(7) 627-637.

[9] TCGA. Comprehensive Genomic Characterization Defines Human Glioblastoma Genes and Core Pathways. Nature 2008; 455(7216) 1061-1068.

[10] Zhu Y, Parada LF. The Molecular and Genetic Basis of Neurological Tumours. Nature Reviews Cancer 2002; 2(8) 616-626.

[11] Cully M, You H, Levine AJ, Mak TW. Beyond PTEN Mutations: the PI3K Pathway as an Integrator of Multiple Inputs During Tumorigenesis. Nature Reviews Cancer 2006; 6(3) 184-192.

[12] Lee Y, Scheck AC, Cloughesy TF, Lai A, Dong J, et al. Gene Expression Analysis of Glioblastomas Identifies the Major Molecular Basis for the Prognostic Benefit of Younger Age. BMC Medical Genomics 2008; 1 52 doi:10.1186/1755-8794-1-52.

[13] Liang Y, Diehn M, Watson N, Bollen AW, Aldape KD, et al. Gene Expression Profiling Reveals Molecularly and Clinically Distinct Subtypes of Glioblastoma Multiforme. Proceeding of the National Academy of Sciences of the USA 2005; 102(16) 5814-5819.

[14] Hanahan D, Weinberg RA. The Hallmarks of Cancer. Cell 2000; 100 (1) 57-70.

[15] Holland EC. Gliomagenesis: Genetic Alterations and Mouse Models. Nature Reviews Genetics 2001; 2(2) 120-129.

[16] Stokoe D., Furnari F.B. The PTEN/PI3 Kinase Pathway in Human Glioma. In: Van Meir, E.G. (ed). CNS Cancer: Models, Markers, Prognostic Factors, Targets and Therapeutic Approaches. New York: Humana Press (Springer); 2009. p315-357.

[17] Zhao S, Lin Y, Xu W, Jiang W, Zha Z, et al. Glioma-Derived Mutations in IDH1 Dominantly Inhibit IDH1 Catalytic Activity and Induce HIF-1alpha. Science 2009; 324(5924) 261-265.

[18] Yan H, Parsons DW, Jin G, McLendon R, Rasheed BA, et al. IDH1 and IDH2 Mutations in Gliomas. The New England Journal of Medicine 2009; 360(8) 765-773.

[19] Dang L, White DW, Gross S, Bennett BD, Bittinger MA, et al. Cancer-Associated IDH1 Mutations Produce 2-hydroxyglutarate. Nature 2009; 462(7274) 739-744.

[20] Parsons DW, Jones S, Zhang X, Lin JC, Leary RJ, et al. An Integrated Genomic Analysis of Human Glioblastoma Multiforme. Science 2008; 321(5897) 1807-1812.

[21] Phillips HS, Kharbanda S, Chen R, Forrest WF, Soriano RH, et al. Molecular Subclasses of High-Grade Glioma Predict Prognosis, Delineate a Pattern of Disease Progression, and Resemble Stages in Neurogenesis. Cancer Cell 2006; 9(3) 157-173.

[22] Carro MS, Lim WK, Alvarez MJ, Bollo RJ, Zhao X, et al. The Transcriptional Network for Mesenchymal Transformation of Brain Tumours. Nature 2010; 463(7279) 318-325.

[23] Verhaak RG, Hoadley KA, Purdom E, Wang V, Qi Y, et al. Integrated Genomic Analysis Identifies Clinically Relevant Subtypes of Glioblastoma Characterized by Abnormalities in PDGFRA, IDH1, EGFR, and NF1. Cancer Cell 2010; 17(1) 98-110.

[24] Caruso G., Caffo M., Raudino G., Raudino F., Venza M., Tomasello F. Antisense Oligonucleotides in the Treatment of Malignant Gliomas. In: Erdmann V.A., Barciszewski J. (eds). From Nucleic Acids Sequences to Molecular Medicine, RNA Technologies. Berlin Heidelberg: Springer-Verlag; 2012. p217-246.

[25] Demuth T, Berens ME. Molecular Mechanisms of Glioma Cell Migration and Invasion. Journal of Neuro-Oncology 2004; 70(2) 217-228.

[26] Perez-Moreno M, Jamora C, Fuchs E. Stickly Business: Orchestrating Cellular Signals at Adherens Junction. Cell 2003; 112 535-548.

[27] Bremnes RM, Veve R, Hirsch FR, Franklin WA. The E-Cadherin Cell-Cell Adhesion Complex and Lung Cancer Invasion, Metastasis, and Prognosis. Lung Cancer 2002; 36 107-119.

[28] Perego C, Vanoni C, Massari S, Longhi R, Pietrini G. Mammalian Lin-7 PDZ Protein Associate with Beta-Catenin at the Cell-Cell Junctions of Epithelia and Neurons. Embo J 2000; 19 3978-3989.

[29] Dermietzel R, Spray DC. Gap Junctions in the Brain: Where, What Type, How Many and Why? Trends in Neurosciences 1993; 16(5) 186-192.

[30] Goodenough DA, Goliger JA, Paul DL. Connexins, Connexons, and Intercellular Communication. Annual Review of Biochemistry 1996; 65 475-502.

[31] Ruch RJ. The Role of Gap Junctional Intercellular Communication in Neoplasia. Annals of Clinical & Laboratory Science 1994; 24(3) 216-231.

[32] McDonough WS, Johansson A, Joffee H et al. Gap Junction Intercellular Communication in Gliomas is Inversely Related to Cell Motility. International Journal of Developmental Neuroscience 1999, 17(5-6) 601-611.

[33] Soroceanu L, Manning TJ Jr, Sontheimer H. Reduced Expression of Connexin-43 and Functional Gap Junction Coupling in Human Gliomas. Glia 2001; 33(2) 107-117.

[34] Gunia S, Hussein S, Radu DL, Putz KM, Breyer R, et al. CD44s-Targeted Treatment With Monoclonal Antibody Blocks Intracerebral Invasion and Growth of 9L Gliosarcoma. Clinical and Experimental Metastasis 1999; 17(3) 221-230.

[35] Okamoto I, Kawano Y, Matsumoto M, Suga M, Kaibuchi K, et al. Regulated CD44 Cleavage Under the Control of Protein Kinase C, Calcium Influx, and the Rho Family of Small G Proteins. The Journal of Biological Chemistry 1999; 274(36) 25525-25534.

[36] Leavesley DI, Ferguson GD, Wayner EA, Cheresh Da. Requirement of the Integrin beta 3 Subunit for Carcinoma Cell Spreading or Migration on Vitronectin and Fibrinogen. The Journal of Cell Biology 1992; 117(5) 1101-1107.

[37] Tabatabai G, Weller M, Nabors B, Picard M, Reardon D, et al. Targeting Integrins in Malignant Glioma. Targeted Oncology 2010; 5(3) 175-181.

[38] Brown MC, Staniszewska I, Lazarovici P, Tuszynski GP, Del Valle L, Marcinkiewicz C. Regulatory Effect of Nerve Growth Factor in $\alpha9\beta1$ Integrin-Dependent Progression of Glioblastoma. Neuro-Oncology 2008; 10(6) 968-980.

[39] Gingras MC, Roussel E, Bruner JM, Branch CD, Moser RP. Comparison of Cell Adhesion Molecule Expression between Glioblastoma Multiforme and Autologous Normal Brain Tissue. Journal of Neuroimmunology 1995; 57(1-2) 143-53.

[40] Previtali S, Quattrini A, Nemni R, Truci G, Ducati A, Wrabetz L, Canal N. Alpha6 Beta4 and Alpha6 Beta1 Integrins in Astrocytomas and other CNS Tumors. Journal of Neuropathology and Experimental Neurology 1996; 55(4) 456-465.

[41] Delamarre E, Taboubi T, Mathieu S, Berenguer C, Rigot V, et al. Expression of Integrin $\alpha6\beta1$ Enhances Tumorigenesis in Glioma Cells. The American Journal of Pathology 2009; 175(2) 844-855.

[42] Platten M, Wick W, Wild-Bode C, Aulwurm S, Dichgans J, Weller M. Transforming Growth Factors Beta(1) (TGF-beta(1)) and TGF-beta(2) Promote Glioma Cell Migration Via Up-Regulation of Alpha(V)beta(3) Integrin Expression. Biochemical and Biophysical Research Communications 2000; 268(2) 607-611.

[43] Adachi Y, Lakka SS, Chandrasekar N, Yanamandra N, Gondi CS, et al. Down-Regulation of Integrin alpha(v)beta(3) Expression and Integrin-Mediated Signaling in Glioma Cells by Adenovirus-Mediated Transfer of Antisense Urokinase-Type Plasminogen Activator Receptor (uPAR) and Sense p16 Genes. The Journal of Biological Chemistry 2001; 276(50) 47171-47177.

[44] Bello L, Francolini M, Marthyn P, Zhang J, Carroll RS, et al. Alpha(v)beta3 and Alpha(v)beta5 Integrin Expression in Glioma Periphery. Neurosurgery 2001; 49(2) 380-389.

[45] Natarajan M, Stewart JE, Golemis EA, Pugacheva EN, Alexandropoulos K, et al. HEF1 is a Necessary and Specific Downstream Effector of FAK that Promotes the Migration of Glioblastoma Cells. Oncogene 2006; 25(12) 1721-1732.

[46] Idbaih A, Ducray F, Sierra del Rio M, Hoang-Xuan K, Delattre JY. Therapeutic Application of Noncytotoxic Molecular Targeted Therapy in Gliomas: Growth Factor Receptors and Angiogenesis Inhibitors. Oncologist 2008; 13(9) 978-992.

[47] Bellail AC, Hunter SB, Brat DJ, Tan C, van Meir EG. Microregional Extracellular Matrix Heterogeneity in Brain Modulates Glioma Cell Invasion. The International Journal of Biochemistry & Cell Biology 2004; 36(6) 1046-1069.

[48] Wild-Bode C, Weller M, Wick W. Molecular Determinants of Glioma Cell Migration and Invasion. Journal of Neurosurgery 2001; 94(6) 978-984.

[49] Egeblad M, Werb Z. New Functions for the Matrix Metalloproteinases in Cancer Progression. Nature Reviews Cancer 2002; 2(3) 161-174.

[50] Sternlicht MD, Werb Z. How Matrix Metalloproteinases Regulate Cell Behavior. Annual Review of Cell and Developmental Biology 2001; 17 463-516.

[51] Bissell MJ, Radisky D. Putting Tumours in Context. Nature Reviews Cancer 2001; 1(1) 46-54.

[52] Page-McCaw AJ, Ewald Z. Werb. Matrix Metalloproteinases and the Regulation of Tissue Remodeling. Nature Reviews Molecular Cell Biology 2007; 8(3) 221-233.

[53] Hu J, Van den Steen PE, Sang QX, Opdenakker G. Matrix Metalloproteinase Inhibitors as Therapy for Inflammatory and Vascular Diseases. Nature Reviews Drug Discovery 2007; 6(6) 480-498.

[54] López-Otín C, Matrisian LM. Emerging Roles of Proteases in Tumour Suppression. Nature Reviews Cancer 2007; 7(10) 800-808.

[55] Johnson JL, George SJ, Newby AC, Jackson CL. Divergent Effects of Matrix Metalloproteinases 3, 7, 9, and 12 on Atherosclerotic Plaque Stability in Mouse Brachiocephalic Arteries. Proceeding of the National Academy of Science of the United States of America 2005; 102(43) 15575-15580.

[56] Fanjul-Fernández M, Folgueras AR, Cabrera S, López-Otín C. Matrix Metalloproteinases: Evolution, Gene Regulation and Functional Analysis in Mouse Models. Biochimica et Biophysica Acta 2010; 1803(1) 3-19.

[57] Hagemann C, Anacker J, Ernestus RI, Vince GH. A Complete Compilation of Matrix Metalloproteinase Expression in Human Malignant Gliomas. World Journal of Clinical Oncology 2012; 3(5) 67-79.

[58] Zhao Y, Xiao A, diPierro CG, Carpenter JE, Abdel-Fattah R, et al. An Extensive Invasive Intracranial Human Glioblastoma Xenograft Model Role of High Level Matrix Metalloproteinase 9. The American Journal of Pathology 2010; 176(6) 3032-3049.

[59] Junge CE, Sugawara T, Mannaioni G, Alagarsamy S, Conn PJ, et al. The Contribution of Protease-Activated Receptor 1 to Neuronal Damage Caused by Transient Focal Cerebral Ischemia. Proceedings of the National Academy of Sciences of United States of America 2003; 100(22) 13019-13024.

[60] Loskutoff DJ, Curriden SA, Hu G, Deng G. Regulation of Cell Adhesion by PAI-1. Acta Pathologica, Microbiologica et Immunologica Scandinavica 1999; 107(1) 54-61.

[61] Resnati M, Pallavicini I, Wang JM, Oppenheim J, Serhan CN, et al. The Fibrinolytic Receptor for Urokinase Activates the G Protein-Coupled Chemotactic Receptor FPRL1/LXA4R. Proceedings of the National Academy of Sciences United States of America 2002; 99(3) 1359-1364.

[62] Bianchi E, Cohen RL, Thor III AT, Mizukami IF, Lawrence DA, et al. The Urokinase Receptor is Expressed in Invasive Breast Cancer but not in Normal Breast Tissue. Cancer Research 1994; 54(4) 861-866.

[63] Le DM, Besson A, Fogg DK, Choi KS, Waisman DM, et al. Exploitation of Astrocytes by Glioma Cells to Facilitate Invasiveness: A Mechanism Involving Matrix Metalloproteinase-2 and the Urokinase-type Plasminogen Activator-plasmin Cascade. Journal of Neuroscience 2003; 23(10) 4034-4043.

[64] Zhang X, Bu XY, Zhen HN, Fei Z, Zhang JN, Fu LA. Expression and Localisation of Urokinase-type Plasminogen Activator Gene in Gliomas. Journal of Clinical Neuroscience 2000; 7(2) 116-119.

[65] Yamamoto M, Sawaya R, Mohanam S, Bindal AK, Bruner JM, et al. Expression and Localization of Urokinase-type Plasminogen Activator in Human Astrocytomas in vivo. Cancer Research 1994; 54(14) 3656-3661.

[66] Bhattacharya A, Lakka SS, Mohanam S, Boyd D, Rao JS. Regulation of the Urokinase-type Plasminogen Activator Receptor Gene in Different Grades of Human Glioma Cell Lines. Clinical Cancer Research 2001; 7(2) 267-276.

[67] Flannery T, Gibson D, Mirakhur M, McQuaid S, Greenan C, et al. The Clinical Significance of Cathepsin S Expression in Human Astrocytomas. American Journal of Pathology 2003; 163(1) 175-182.

[68] Levicar N, Strojnik T, Kos J, Dewey RA, Pilkington GJ, Lah TT. Lysosomal Enzymes, Cathepsins in Brain Tumour Invasion. Journal of Neurooncology 2002; 58(1) 21-32.

[69] Mikkelsen T, Yan PS, Ho KL, Sameni M, Sloane BF, Rosenblum ML. Immunolocalization of Cathepsin B in Human Glioma: Implications for Tumor Invasion and Angiogenesis. Journal of Neurosurgery 1995; 83(2) 285-290.

[70] Rao JS. Molecular Mechanisms of Glioma Invasiveness: The Role of Proteases. Nature Reviews Cancer 2003; 3(7) 489-501.

[71] Kobayashi T, Honke K, Gasa S, Fujii T, Maguchi S, et al. Proteolytic Processing Sites Producing the Mature Form of Human Cathepsin D. International Journal of Biochemistry 1992; 24(9) 1487-1491.

[72] Chintala SK, Sawaya R, Gokaslan ZL, Fuller G, Rao JS. Immunohistochemical Localization of Extracellular Matrix Proteins in Human Glioma, both in Vivo and in Vitro. Cancer Letters 1996; 101(1) 107-114.

[73] Gritsenko PG, Ilina O, Friedl P. Interstitial Guidance of Cancer Invasion. Journal of Pathology 2012; 226(2) 185-199.

[74] Nicholson C, Sykova E. Extracellular Space Structure Revealed by Diffusive Analysis. Trends in Neurosciences 1998; 21(5) 207-215.

[75] Delpech B, Maingonnat C, Girard N, Chauzy C, Maunoury R, et al. Hyaluronan and Hyaluronectin in the Extracellular Matrix of Human Brain Tumor Stroma. European Journal of Cancer 1993; 29(7) 1012-1017.

[76] Bourdon MA, Ruoslahti E. Tenascin Mediates Cell Attachment through an RGD-Dependent Receptor. The Journal of Cell Biology 1989; 108(3) 1149-1155.

[77] Chiquet-Ehrismann R. Tenascins, a Growing Family of Extracellular Matrix Protein. Experientia 1995; 51(9-10) 853-862.

[78] Germanò A, Caffo M, Caruso G, La Rosa G, Galatioto S, Tomasello F. A Preliminary Study of Angiogenesis in Paediatric Glioblastoma Multiforme and its Correlation with Survival. Childs Nervous System 2001; 17(10) 577-583.

[79] Jallo GI, Friedlander DR, Kelly PJ, Wisoff JH, Grumet M, Zagzag D. Tenascin-C Expression in the Cyst Wall and Fluid of Human Brain Tumours Correlates with Angiogenesis. Neurosurgery 1997; 41(5) 1052-1059.

[80] Zagzag D, Friedlander DR, Miller DC, Dosik J, Cangiarella J, et al. Tenascin Expression in Astrocytomas Correlates with Angiogenesis. Cancer Research 1995; 55(4) 907-914.

[81] Brooks PC, Clark RA, Cheresh DA. Requirement of Vascular Integrin Alpha v Beta 3 for Angiogenesis. Science 1994; 264(5158) 569-571.

[82] Sakai T, Johnson KJ, Murozono M, Sakai K, Magnuson MA, et al. Plasma Fibronectin Supports Neuronal Survival and Reduces Brain Injury Following Transient Focal Cerebral Ischemia but is not Essential for Skin-Wound Healing and Hemostasis. Nature Medicine 2001; 7(3) 324-330.

[83] Caffo M, Germanò A, Caruso G, Meli F, Galatioto S, et al. (2004). An Immunohistochemical Study of Extracellular Matrix Proteins Laminin, Fibronectin and Type IV Collagen in Paediatric Glioblastoma Multiforme. Acta Neurochirurgica 2004; 146(10) 1113-1118.

[84] Knott JC, Mahesparan R, Garcia-Cabrera I, Bolge Tysnes B, Edvardsen K, et al. Stimulation of Extracellular Matrix Components in the Normal Brain by Invading Glioma Cells. International Journal of Cancer 1998; 75(6) 864-872.

[85] Mahesparan R, Read TA, Lund-Johansen M, Skaftnesmo KO, Bjerkvig R, Engebraaten O. Expression of Extracellular Matrix Component in a Highly Infiltrative in Vivo Glioma Model. Acta Neuropathologica 2003; 105(1) 49-57.

[86] Lin ZX, Yang LJ, Huang Q, Fu J. Activated Vascular Endothelia Regulate Invasion of Glioma Cells through Expression of Fibronectin. Chinese Medical Journal 2010; 123(13) 1754-1761.

[87] Ulrich TA, de Juan Pardo EM, Kumar S. The Mechanical Rigidity of the Extracellular Matrix Regulates the Structure, Motility, and Proliferation of Glioma Cells. Cancer Research 2009; 69(10) 4167-4174.

[88] Sengupta S, Nandi S, Hindi ES, Wainwright DA, Han Y, Lesniak MS. Short Hairpin RNA-Mediated Fibronectin Knockdown Delays Tumor Growth in a Mouse Glioma Model. Neoplasia 2010; 12(10) 837-847.

[89] Prieto AL, Edelman GM, Crossin KL. Multiple Integrins Mediate Cell Attachment to Cytotactin/Tenascin. Proceeding of the National Academy of Sciences of the United States of America 1993; 90(21) 10154-10158.

[90] Timpl R, Brown JC. The Laminins. Matrix Biology 1994; 14(4) 275-281.

[91] LeMosy EK, Lightner VA, Erickson HP. Structural Analysis of a Human Glial Variant Laminin. Experimental Cell Research 1996; 227(1) 80-88.

[92] Bjerkvig R, Laerum OD, Rucklidge GJ. Immunocytochemical Characterization of Extracellular Matrix Protein Expressed by Cultured Glioma Cells. Cancer Research 1989; 49(19) 5424-5428.

[93] Ogawa K, Oguchi M, Nakashima Y, Yamabe H. Distribution of Collagen Type IV in Brain Tumors: an Immunohistochemical Study. Journal of Neuro-Oncology 1989; 7(4) 357-366.

[94] Berindan-Neagoe I, Chiorean R, Braicu C, Florian IS, Leucuta D, et al. Quantitative mRNA Expression of Genes Involved in Angiogenesis, Coagulation and Inflammation in Multiforme Glioblastoma Tumoral Tissue versus Peritumoral Brain Tissue: Lack of Correlation with Clinical Data. European Cytokine Network 2012; 23(2) 45-55.

[95] Del Maestro RF, Megyesi JF, Farrell CL. Mechanisms of Tumor-Associated Edema: a Review. Canadian Journal of Neurological Sciences 1990; 17(2) 177-183.

[96] Jain RK, di Tomaso E, Duda DG, Loefflers LB, Sorensen AG, et al. Angiogenesis in Brain Tumours. Nature Reviews Neuroscience 2007; 8(8) 610-622.

[97] Barresi V, Cerasoli S, Vitarelli E, Tuccari G. Density of Microvessels Positive for CD105 (Endoglin) is Related to Prognosis in Meningiomas. Acta Neuropathologica 2007; 114(2) 147-156.

[98] Cheifetz S, Bellon T, Cales C, Vera S, Bernabeu C, et al. Endoglin is a Component of the Transforming Growth Factor-Beta Receptor System in Human Endothelial Cells. The Journal of Biological Chemistry 1992; 267(27) 19027-19030.

[99] Behrem S, Zarkovic K, Eskinja N, Jonjic N. Endoglin is a Better Marker than CD31 in Evaluation of Angiogenesis in Glioblastoma. Croatian Medical Journal 2005; 46(3) 417-22.

[100] Yao Y, Kubota T, Takeuchi H, Sato K. Prognostic Significance of Microvessel Density Determined by an anti-CD105/Endoglin Monoclonal Antibody in Astrocytic Tumors: Comparison with an anti-CD31 Monoclonal Antibody. Neuropathology 2005; 25(3) 201-206.

[101] Netto GC, Bleil CB, Hilbig A, Coutinho LM. Immunohistochemical Evaluation of the Microvascular Density through the Expression of TGF-Beta (CD 105/Endoglin) and CD 34 Receptors and Expression of the Vascular Endothelial Growth Factor (VEGF) in Oligodendrogliomas. Neuropathology 2008; 28(1) 17-23.

[102] Burrows FJ, Derbyshire EJ, Tazzari PL, Amlot P, Gazdar AF, et al. Up-Regulation of Endoglin on Vascular Endothelial Cells in Human Solid Tumours: Implications for Diagnosis and Therapy. Clinical Cancer Research 1995; 1(12) 1623-1634.

[103] Seon BK, Haba A, Matsuno F, Takahashi N, Tsujie M, et al. Endoglin-Targeted Cancer Therapy. Current Drug Delivery 2011; 8(1) 135-143.

[104] Zagzag D, Amirnovin R, Greco MA, Yee H, Holash J, et al. Vascular Apoptosis and Involution in Gliomas Precede Neovascularization: a Novel Concept for Glioma Growth and Angiogenesis. Laboratory Investigation 2000; 80(6) 837-849.

[105] Holash J, Maisonpierre PC, Compton D, Boland P, Alexander LR, et al. Vessel Cooption, Regression, and Growth in Tumors Mediated by Angiopoietins and VEGF. Science 1999; 284(5422) 1994-1998.

[106] Zadeh G, Qian B, Okhowat A, Sabha N, Kontos CD, Guha A. Targeting the Tie2/Tek Receptor in Astrocytomas. The American Journal of Pathology 2004; 164(2) 467-476.

[107] Mao Y, Schwarzbauer JE. Fibronectin Fibrillogenesis, a Cell-Mediated Matrix Assembly Process. Matrix Biology 2005; 24(6) 389-399.

[108] Ljubimova JY, Fujita M, Khazenzon NM, Ljubimova AV, Black KL. Changes in Laminin Isoforms Associated with Brain Tumor Invasion and Angiogenesis. Frontiers in Bioscience 2006; 11 81-88.

[109] Lakka SS, Gondi CS, Rao JS. Proteases and Glioma Angiogenesis. Brain Pathology 2005; 15(4) 327-341.

[110] Ferrara N, Kerbel RS. Angiogenesis as a Therapeutic Target. Nature 2005; 438(7070) 967-974.

[111] Semenza GL. Targeting HIF-1 for Cancer Therapy. Nature Reviews Cancer 2003; 3(10) 721-732.

[112] Shweiki D, Itin A, Soffer D, Keshet E. Vascular Endothelial Growth Factor Induced by Hypoxia May Mediate Hypoxia-Initiated Angiogenesis. Nature 1992; 359(6398) 843-845.

[113] Weidemann A, Johnson RS. Biology of HIF-1α. Cell Death & Differentiation 2008; 15(4) 621-627.

[114] Kamiyama H, Takano S, Tsuboi K, Matsumura A. Anti-Angiogenic Effects of SN38 (Active Metabolite of Irinotecan): Inhibition of Hypoxia-Inducible Factor 1 Alpha (HIF-1a)/Vascular Endothelial Growth Factor (VEGF) Expression of Glioma and Growth of Endothelial Cells. Journal of Cancer Research and Clinical Oncology 2005; 131(4) 205-213.

[115] Lee Y, Scheck AC, Cloughesy TF, Lai A, Dong J, et al. Gene Expression Analysis of Glioblastomas Identifies the Major Molecular Basis for the Prognostic Benefit of Younger Age. BMC Medical Genomics 2008; 1:52.

[116] Ito TK, Ishii G, Chiba H, Ochiai A. The VEGF Angiogenic Switch of Fibroblasts is Regulated by MMP-7 from Cancer Cells. Oncogene 2007; 26(51) 7194-7203.

[117] Ferrara N. Vascular Endothelial Growth Factor: Basic Science and Clinical Progress. Endocrine Reviews 2004; 25(4) 581-611.

[118] Gerber HP, Malik AK, Solar GP, Sherman D, Liang XH, et al. VEGF Regulates Haematopoietic Stem Cell Survival by an Internal Autocrine Loop Mechanism. Nature 2002; 417(6892) 954-958.

[119] Valter MM, Hugel A, Huang HJ, Cavenee WK, Wiestler OD, et al. Expression of the Ets-1 Transcription Factor in Human Astrocytomas is Associated with Fms-like Tyrosine Kinase-1 (Flt-1)/Vascular Endothelial growth Factor Receptor-1 Synthesis and Neoangiogenesis. Cancer Research 1999; 59(21) 5608-5614.

[120] Esser S, Lampugnani MG, Corada M, Dejana E, Risau W. Vascular Endothelial Growth Factor Induces VE-Cadherin Tyrosine Phosphorylation in Endothelial Cells. Journal of Cell Science 1998; 111(Pt 13) 1853-1865.

[121] Gerhardt H, Golding M, Fruttiger M, Ruhrberg C, Lundkvist A, et al. VEGF Guides Angiogenic Sprouting Utilizing Endothelial Tip Cell Filopodia. The Journal of Cell Biology 2003; 161(6) 1163-1177.

[122] Morales-Ruiz M, Fulton D, Sowa G, Lanquino LR, Fujio Y, et al. Vascular Endothelial Growth Factor Stimulated Actin Reorganization and Migration of Endothelial Cells is Regulated via the Serine/Threonine Kinase Akt. Circulation Research 2000; 86(8) 892-896.

[123] Wong ML, Prawira A, Kaye AH, Hovens CM. Tumour Angiogenesis: its Mechanism and Therapeutic Implications in Malignant Gliomas. Journal of Clinical Neuroscience 2009; 16(9) 1119-1130.

[124] Jain RK. Molecular Regulation of Vessel Maturation. Nature Medicine 2003; 9(6) 685-693.

[125] Schmidt NO, Westphal M, Hagel C, Ergun S, Stavrou D, et al. Levels of Vascular Endothelial Growth Factor, Hepatocyte Growth Factor/Scatter Factor and Basic Fibroblast Growth Factor in Human Gliomas and their Relation to Angiogenesis. International Journal of Cancer 1999; 84(1) 10-18.

[126] Mandriota SJ, Pepper MS. Vascular Endothelial Growth Factor-Induced in vitro Angiogenesis and Plasminogen Activator Expression are Dependent on Endogenous Basic Fibroblast Growth Factor. Journal of Cell Science 1997; 110(Pt 18) 2293-2302.

[127] Sato Y, Rifkin DB. Autocrine Activities of Basic fibroblast Growth factor: Regulation of Endothelial Cell Movement, Plasminogen Activator Synthesis, and DNA Synthesis. The Journal of Cell Biology 1988; 107(3) 1199-1205.

[128] Lindahl P, Johansson BR, Leveen P, Betsholtz C. Pericyte Loss and Microaneurysm Formation in PDGF-B-Deficient Mice. Science 1997; 277(5323) 242-245.

[129] Sun J, Wang DA, Jain RK, Carie A, Paquette S, et al. Inhibiting Angiogenesis and Tumorigenesis by a Synthetic Molecule that Blocks Binding of both VEGF and PDGF to their Receptors. Oncogene 2005; 24(29) 4701-4709.

[130] Caruso G, Caffo M, Raudino G, Alafaci C, Salpietro FM, Tomasello F. Antisense Oligonucleotides and Extracellular Matrix Proteins: Innovative Therapeutic Targets in the Treatment of High Grade Gliomas. Recent Patents on CNS Drug Discovery 2010; 5(1) 53-69.

[131] Saunders WB, Bohnsack BL, Faske SB, Anthis NJ, Bayless KJ, et al. Coregulation of Vascular Tube Stabilization by Endothelial Cell TIMP-2 and Pericyte TIMP-3. The Journal of Cell Biology 2006; 175(1) 179-191.

[132] Davis GE, Senger DR. Endothelial Extracellular Matrix: Biosynthesis, Remodeling, and Functions During Vascular Morphogenesis and neovessel Stabilization. Circulation Research 2005; 97(11) 1093-1107.

[133] Miner JH. Laminins and their Roles in Mammals. Microscopy Research Technique 2008; 71(5) 349-356.

[134] Krishnan L, Underwood CJ, Maas S, Ellis BJ, Kode TC, et al. Effect of Mechanical Boundary Conditions on Orientation of Angiogenic Microvessels. Cardiovascular Research 2008; 78(2) 324-332.

[135] Platten M, Wick W, Weller M. Malignant Glioma Biology: Role for TGF-Beta in Growth, Motility, Angiogenesis, and Immune Escape. Microscopy Research Technique 2001; 52(4) 401-410.

[136] Graeber MB, Scheithauer BW, Kreutzberg GW. Microglia in Brain Tumors. Glia 2002; 40(2) 252-259.

[137] Watters JJ, Schartner JM, Badie B. Microglia Function in Brain Tumors. Journal of Neuroscience Research 2005; 81(3) 447-455.

[138] Badie B, Schartner JM. Flow Cytometric Characterization of Tumor-Associated Macrophages in Experimental Gliomas. Neurosurgery 2000; 46(4) 957-962.

[139] Okada M, Saio M, Kito Y, Ohe N, Yano H, et al. Tumor-Associated Macrophage/Microglia Infiltration in Human Gliomas is Correlated with MCP-3, but not MCP-1. International Journal of Oncology 2009; 34(6) 1621-1627.

[140] Suzuki Y, Funakoshi H, Machide M, Matsumoto K, Nakamura T. Regulation of Cell Migration and Cytokine Production by HGF-like Protein (HLP)/Macrophage Stimulating Protein (MSP) in Primary Microglia. Biomedical Research 2008; 29(2) 77-84.

[141] Tanaka Y, Kobayashi H, Suzuki M, Kanayama N, Suzuki M, Terao T. Thymidine Phosphorylase Expression in Tumor-Infiltrating Macrophages may be Correlated with Poor Prognosis in Uterine Endometrial Cancer. Human Pathology 2002; 33(11) 1105-1113.

[142] Shono T, Ono M, Izumi H, Jimi SI, Matsushima K, et al. Involvement of the Transcription Factor NFkB in Tubular Morphogenesis of Human Microvascular Endothelial Cells by Oxidative Stress. Molecular and Cellular Biology 1996; 16(8) 4231-4239.

[143] Venza M, Visalli M, Alafaci C, Caffo M, Caruso G, et al. Interleukin-8 (IL-8) Overexpression in Astrocytomas is Induced by Prostaglandin E2 (PGE2) and is Associated to the Transcription Factors CCAAT Enhancer Binding Protein-beta (C/EPB-β) and C/EBP Homologous Protein (CHOP). Neurosurgery 2011; 69(3) 713-721.

[144] Pollard JW. Tumour-Educated Macrophages Promote Tumour Progression and Metastasis. Nature Review Cancer 2004; 4(1) 71-78.

[145] Hildenbrand R,Wolf G, Bohme B, Bleyl U, Steinborn A. Urokinase Plasminogen Activator Receptor (CD87) Expression of Tumor-Associated Macrophages in Ductal Carcinoma in situ, Breast Cancer, and Resident Macrophages of Normal Breast Tissue. Journal of Leukocyte Biology 1999; 66(1) 40-49.

[146] Hu DE, Hory Y, Fan TP. Interleukin-8 Stimulates Angiogenesis in Rats. Inflammation 1993;17:135–43.

[147] Shannon AM, Bouchier-Hayes DJ, Condron CM, Toomey D. Tumour Hypoxia, Chemotherapeutic Resistance and Hypoxia-Related Therapies. Cancer Treatment Reviews 2003; 29(4) 297-307.

[148] Murdoch C, Giannoudis A, Lewis CE. Mechanisms Regulating the Recruitment of Macrophages into Hypoxic Areas of Tumors and Other Ischemic Tissues. Blood 2004; 104(8) 2224-2234.

[149] Bosco MC, Reffo G, Puppo M, Varesio L. Hypoxia Inhibits the Expression of the CCR5 Chemokine Receptor in Macrophages. Cellular Immunology 2004; 228(1) 1-7.

[150] Sweet MJ, Hume DA. CSF-1 as a Regulator of Macrophage Activation and Immune Responses. Archivium Immunologiae et Therapiae Experimentalis 2003; 51(3) 169-177.

[151] Schmeisser A, Marquetant R, Illmer T, Graffy C, Garlichs CD, et al. The Expression of Macrophage Migration Inhibitory Factor 1alpha (MIF 1alpha) in Human Atherosclerotic plaques is Induced by Different Proatherogenic Stimuli and Associated with Plaque Instability. Atherosclerosis 2005; 178(1) 83-94.

[152] Sun B, Nishihira J, Yoshiki T, Kondo M, Sato Y, et al. Macrophage Migration Inhibitory Factor Promotes Tumor Invasion and Metastasis via the Rho-Dependent Pathway. Clinical Cancer Research 2005; 11(3) 1050-1058.

[153] Markovic DS, Glass R, Synowitz M, Rooijen N, Kettenmann H. Microglia Stimulate the Invasiveness of Glioma Cells by Increasing the Activity of Metalloprotease-2. Journal of Neuropathology & Experimental Neurology 2005; 64(9) 754-762.

[154] Caffo M, Caruso G, Barresi V, Pino MA, Venza M, et al. Immunohistochemical Study of CD68 and CR3/43 in Astrocytic Gliomas. Journal of Analytical Oncology 2012; 1(1) 42-49.

[155] Held-Feindt J, Hattermann K, Muerkoster SS, Wedderkopp H, Knerlich-Lukoschus F, et al. CX3CR1 Promotes Recruitment of Human Glioma-Infiltrating Microglia/Macrophages (GIMs). Experimental Cell Research 2010; 316(9) 1553-1566.

[156] Tibbets KM, Emnett RJ, Gao F, Perry A, Gutmann DH, Leonard JR. Histopathological Predictors of Pilocytic Astrocytoma Event-Free Survival. Acta Neuropathologica 2009; 117(6) 657-665.

[157] Jansen M, de Witt Hamer PC, Witmer AN, Troost D, van Noorden CJ. Current Perspectives on Antiangiogenesis Strategies in the Treatment of Malignant Gliomas. Brain Research Review 2004; 45(3) 143-163.

[158] Goldbrunner RH, Bendszus M, Wood J, Kiderlen M, Sasaki M, Tonn JC. PTK787/ZK222584, an Inhibitor of Vascular Endothelial Growth Factor Receptor Tyrosine Kinases, Decreases Glioma Growth and Vascularization. Neurosurgery 2004; 55(2) 426-432.

[159] Gerstner ER, Eichler AF, Plotkin SR, Drappatz J, Doyle CL, et al. Phase I Trial with Biomarker Studies of Vatalanib (PTK787) in Patients with Newly Diagnosed Glioblastoma Treated with Enzyme Inducing Anti-Epileptic Drugs and Standard Radiation and Temozolomide. Journal of Neuro-Oncology 2011; 103(2) 325-332.

[160] Ryan AJ, Wedge SR. ZD6474-a Novel Inhibitor of VEGFR and EGFR Tyrosine Kinase Activity. British Journal of Cancer 2005; 92(1) S6-13.

[161] Sandstrom M, Johansson M, Andersson U, Bergh A, Bergenheim AT, Henriksson R. The Tyrosine Kinase Inhibitor ZD6474 Inhibits Tumour Growth in an Intracerebral Rat Glioma Model. British Journal of Cancer 2004; 91(6) 1174-1180.

[162] Sandstrom M, Johansson M, Bergstrom P, Bergheneim AT, Henriksson R Effects of the VEGFR Inhibitor ZD6474 in Combination with Radiotherapy and Temozolomide in an Orthotopic Glioma Model. Journal of Neuro-Oncology 2008; 88(1) 1-9.

[163] Reardon Da, Conrad Ca, Cloughesy T, Prados MD, Friedman HS, et al. Phase I Study of AEE788, a Novel Multitarget Inhibitor of ErbB- and VEGF-Receptor-Family Tyrosine Kinases, in Recurrent Glioblastoma Patients. Cancer Chemotherapy Pharmacol 2012; 69(6) 1507-1518.

[164] Batchelor TT, Sorensen AG, di Tomaso E, Zhang WT, Duda DG, et al. AZD2171, a pan-VEGF Receptor Tyrosine Kinase Inhibitor, Normalizes Tumor Vasculature and Alleviates Edema in Glioblastoma Patients. Cancer Cell 2007; 11(1) 83-95.

[165] Kamoun WS, Ley CD, Farrar CT, Duyermaqn AM, Lahdenranta J, et al. Edema Control by Cediranib, a Vascular Endothelial Growth Factor Receptor-Targeted Kinase Inhibitor, Prolongs Survival Despite Persistent Brain Tumor Growth in Mice. Journal of Clinical Oncology 2009; 27(15) 2542-2552.

[166] Batchelor T, Mulholland P, Neyns B. A Phase III Randomized Study Comparing the Efficacy of Cediranib as Monotherapy, and in Combination with Lomustine, with Lomustine Alone in Recurrent Glioblastoma Patients. Annals of Oncology 2010; 21(8) :viii4 (LBA7).

[167] Pan E, Yu D, Yue B, Potthast L, Chowdhary S, Smith P, Chamberlain M. A Prospective Phase II Single-Institution Trial of Sunitinib for Recurrent Malignant Glioma. Journal of Neuro-Oncology 2012 Jul 26.

[168] D'Amico R, Lei L, Kennedy BC, Sisti J, Ebiana V, et al. The Addition of Sunitinib to Radiation Delays Tumor Growth in a Murine Model of Glioblastoma. Neurological Research 2012; 34(3) 252-261.

[169] Stefanik DF, Fellows WK, Rizkalla LR, Rizkalla WM, Stefanik PP, et al. Monoclonal Antibodies to Vascular Endothelial Growth Factor (VEGF) and the VEGF Receptor, FLT-1, Inhibit the Growth of C6 Glioma in a Mouse Xenograft. Journal of Neuro-Oncology 2001; 55(2) 91-100.

[170] Nagane M, Nishikawa R, Narita Y, Kobayashi H, Takano S, et al. Phase II Study of Single-agent Bevacizumab in Japanese Patients with Recurrent Malignant Glioma. Japanese Journal of Clinical Oncology 2012.

[171] Norden AD, Young GS, Setayesh K, Muzikansky A, Klufas R, et al. Bevacizumab for Recurrent Malignant Gliomas: Efficacy, Toxicity, and Patterns of Recurrence. Neurology 2008; 70(10) 779-787.

[172] Vredenburgh JJ, Desjardins A, Herndon JE II, Dowell JM, Reardon DA, et al. Phase II Trial of Bevacizumab and Irinotecan in Recurrent Malignant Gliomas. Clinical Cancer Research 2007; 13(4) 1253-1259.

[173] Gil MJ, De Las Penas R, Reynes G, Balana C, Perez-Segura P, et al. Bevacizumab Plus Irinotecan in Recurrent Malignant Glioma Shows High Overall Survival in a Multicenter Retrospective Pooled series of the Spanish Neuro-Oncology Research Group (GEINO). Anticancer Drugs 2012.

[174] Shapiro LQ, Beal K, Goenka A, Karimi S, Iwamoto FM, et al. Patterns of Failure After Concurrent Bevacizumab and Hypofractionated Stereotactic Radiation Therapy for Recurrent High-Grade Glioma. International Journal of Radiation Oncol Biol Phys 2012.

[175] Zhang H, Berezov A, Wang Q, Zhang G, Drebin J, et al. ErbB Receptors: From Oncogenes to Targeted Cancer Therapies. Journal of Clinical Investigation 2007; 117(8) 2051-2058.

[176] Kinsella P, Howley R, Doolan P, Clarke C, Madden SF, et al. Characterization and Response of Newly Developed High-Grade Glioma Cultures to the Tyrosine Kinase Inhibitors, Erlotinib, Gefitinib and Imatinib. Exp Cell Res 2012; 318(5) 641-652.

[177] Chang CY, Shen CC, Su HL, Chen CJ. Gefitinib Induces Apoptosis in Human Glioma Cells by Targeting Bad Phosphorylation. Journal of Neuro-Oncology 2011; 105(3) 507-522.

[178] Hegi ME, Diserens AC, Bady P, Kamoshima Y, Kouwenhoven MC, et al. 11. Pathway Analysis of Glioblastoma Tissue after Preoperative Treatment with the EGFR Tyrosine Kinase Inhibitor Gefitinib--a Phase II Trial. Mol Cancer Therapy 2011; 10(6) 1102-1112.

[179] Pollack IF, Stewart CF, Kocak M, Poussaint TY, Broniscer A, et al. A Phase II Study of Gefitinib and Irradiation in Children with Newly Diagnosed Brainstem Gliomas: a Report from the Pediatric Brain Tumor Consortium. Neuro Oncology 2011; 13(3) 290-297.

[180] Stommel JM, Kimmelman AC, Ying H, Nabioullin R, Ponugoti AH, et al. Coactivation of Receptor Tyrosine Kinases Affects the Response of Tumor Cells to Targeted Therapies. Science 2007; 318(5848) 287-290.

[181] Ji H, Zhao X, Yuza Y, Shimamura T, Li D, et al. Epidermal Growth Factor Receptor Variant III Mutations in Lung Tumorigenesis and Sensitivity to Tyrosine Kinase Inhibitors. Proceedings of the National Academy of Science of the United States of America 2006; 103(20) 7817-7822.

[182] Broderick DK, Di C, Parrett TJ,Samuels YR, Cummins JM, et al. Mutations of PIK3CA in Anaplastic Oligodendrogliomas, High-Grade Astrocytomas, and Medulloblastomas. Cancer Research 2004; 64(15) 5048-5050.

[183] Haas-Kogan DA, Prados MD, Tihan T, Eberhard DA, Jelluma EN, et al. Epidermal Growth Factor Receptor, Protein Kinase B/Akt, and glioma Response to Erlotinib. Journal of the National Cancer Institute 2005; 97(12) 880-887.

[184] Nghiempu PL, Lai A, Green RM, Reardon DA, Cloghesy T. A Dose Escalation Trial for the Combination of Erlotinib and Sirolimus for Recurrent Malignant Gliomas. Journal of Neuro-Oncology 2012.

[185] Traxler P, Allegrini PR, Brandt R, Brueggen J, Cozens R, et al. AEE788: a Dual Family Epidermal Growth Factor Receptor/ErbB2 and Vascular endothelial Growth Factor Receptor Tyrosine Kinase Inhibitor with Antitumor and Antiangiogenic Activity. Cancer Research 2004; 64(14) 4931-4941.

[186] Peereboom DM, Shepard DR, Ahluwalia MS, Brewer CJ, Agarwal N, et al. Phase II Trial of Erlotinib with Temozolomide and Radiation in Patients with Newly Diagnosed Glioblastoma Multiforme. Journal of Neuro-Oncology 2010; 98(1) 93-99.

[187] Combs SE, Heeger S, Haselmann R, Edler L, Debus J, Schulz-Ertner D. Treatment of Primary Glioblastoma Multiforme with Cetuximab, Radiotherapy and Temozolomide (GERT)-Phase I/II Trial: Study Protocol. BMC Cancer 2006; 6 133.

[188] Dai C, Celestino JC, Okada Y, Louis DN, Fuller GN, Holland EC. PDGF Autocrine Stimulation Dedifferentiates Cultured Astrocytes and Induces Oligodendrogliomas and Oligoastrocytomas from Neural Progenitors and Astrocytes in vivo. Genes & Development 2001; 15(15) 1913-1925.

[189] Wen PY, Yung WK, Lamborn KR, Dahia PL, Wang Y, et al. Phase I/II Study of Imatinib Mesylate for Recurrent Malignant Gliomas: North American Brain Tumor Consortium Study 99-08. Clinical Cancer Research 2006; 12(16) 4899-4907.

[190] Raymond E, Brandes AA, Dittrich C, Fumoleau P, Coudert B, et al. Phase II Study of Imatinib in Patients with Recurrent Gliomas of Various Histologies: a European Organisation for Research and Treatment of Cancer Brain Tumor Group Study. Journal of Clinical Oncology 2008; 26(28) 4659-4665.

[191] Dong Y, Jia L, Wang X, Tan X, Xu J, et al. Selective Inhibition of PDGFR by Imatinib Elicits the Sustained activation of ERK and Downstream Receptor Signaling in Malignant Glioma Cells. International Journal of Oncology 2011; 38(2) 555-569.

[192] Dong Y, Han Q, Zou Y, Deng Z, Lu X, et al. Long-term Exposure to Imatinib Reduced Cancer Stem Cell Ability through Induction of Cell Differentiation Via Activation of MAPK Signaling in Glioblastoma Cells. Molecular and Cellular Biochemistry 2012.

[193] Reardon DA, Egorin MJ, Quinn JA, Rich JN, Gururangan S, et al. Phase II Study of Imatinib Mesylate plus Hydroxyurea in Adults with Recurrent Glioblastoma Multiforme. Journal of Clinical Oncology 2005; 23(36) 9359-9368.

[194] Reardon DA, Egorin MJ, Desjardins A, Vredenburgh JJ, Beumer JH, et al. Phase I Pharmacokinetic Study of the Vascular Endothelial Growth Factor Receptor Tyrosine

Kinase Inhibitor Vatalanib (PTK787) plus Imatinib and Hydroxyurea for Malignant Glioma. Cancer 2009; 115(19) 2188-2198.

[195] Yu C, Friday BB, Lai JP, Yang L, Sarkaria J, et al. Cytotoxic Synergy between the Multikinase Inhibitor Sorafenib and the Proteasome Inhibitor Bortezomib in vitro: Induction of Apoptosis through Akt and c-Jun NH2-Terminal Kinase Pathways. Molecular Cancer Therapeutics 2006; 5(9) 2378-2387.

[196] Jane EP, Premkumar DR, Pollack IF. Coadministration of Sorafenib with Rottlerin Potently Inhibits Cell Proliferation and Migration in Human Malignant Glioma Cells. The Journal of Pharmacology and Experimental Therapeutics 2006; 319(3) 1070-1080.

[197] Hainsworth JD, Ervin T, Friedman E, Priego V, Murphy PB, et al. Concurrent Radiotherapy and Temozolomide Followed by Temozolomide and Sorafenib in the First-line Treatment of Patients with Glioblastoma Multiforme. Cancer 2010; 116(15) 3663-3669.

[198] Reardon Da, Vredenburgh JJ, Desjardins A, Peters K, Gururangan S, et al. Effect of CYP3A-Inducing anti-Epileptics on Sorafenib Exposure: Results of a Phase II Study of Sorafenib plus Daily Temozolomide in Adults with Recurrent Glioblastoma. Journal of Neuroncology 2011; 101(1) 57-66.

[199] Ohshima-Hosoyama S, Davare MA, Prajapati SI, Abraham J, Lal S, et al. Preclinical Testing of Tandutinib in a Transgenic Medulloblastoma Mouse Model. Journal of Pediatric Hematology/Oncology 2012; 34(2) 116-121.

[200] Zhou XP, Li YJ, Hoang-Xuan K, Laurent-Puig P, Mokhtari K, et al. Mutational Analysis of the PTEN Gene in Gliomas: Molecular and Pathological Correlations. International Journal of Cancer 1999; 84(2) 150-154.

[201] Neshat MS, Mellinghoff IK, Tran C, Stiles B, Thomas G, et al. Enhanced Sensitivity of PTEN-Deficient Tumors to Inhibition of FRAP/mTOR. Proceedings of the National Academy of Sciences of the United States of America 2001; 98(18) 10314-10319.

[202] Uhrbom L, Nerio E, Holland EC. Dissecting Tumor Maintenance Requirements using Bioluminescence Imaging of Cell Proliferation in a Mouse Glioma Model. Nature Medicine 2004; 10(11) 1257-1260.

[203] Hu X, Pandolfi PP, Li Y, Koutcher JA, Rosenblum M, et al. mTOR Promotes Survival and Astrocytic Characteristics Induced by Pten/AKT Signaling in Glioblastoma. Neoplasia 2005; 7(4) 356-368.

[204] Pitter KL, Galban CJ, Galban S, Saeed-Tehrani O, Li F, et al. Perifosine and CCI 779 Co-Operate to Induce Cell Death and Decrease Proliferation in Pten-Intact and Pten-Deficient PDGF-Driven Murine Glioblastoma. PLOS One 2011; 6(1) e14545.

[205] Weiler M, Pfenning PN, Thiepold AL, Blaes J, Jestaedt L, et al. Suppression of Proinvasive RGS4 by mTOR Inhibition Optimizes Glioma Treatment. Oncogene 2012.

[206] Georger B, Kieran MW, Grupp S, Perek D, Clancy J, et al. Phase II Trial of Temsirolimus in Children with High-Grade Glioma, Neuroblastoma and Rhabdomyosarcoma. European Journal of Cancer 2012; 48(2) 253-262.

[207] Kreisl TN, Lassman AB, Mischel PS, Rosen N, Scher HI, et al. A Pilot Study of Everolimus and Gefitinib in the Treatment of Recurrent Glioblastoma (GBM). Journal of Neurooncology 2009; 92(1) 99-105.

[208] Graff JR, McNulty AM, Hanna KR, Konicek BW, Lynch RL, et al. The Protein Kinase Cb-Selective Inhibitor, Enzastaurin (LY317615.HCl), Suppresses Signaling Through the AKT Pathway, induces Apoptosis, and Suppresses Growth of Human Colon Cancer and Glioblastoma Xenografts. Cancer Research 2005; 65(16) 7462-7469.

[209] Kreisl TN, Kotliarova S, Butman JA, Albert PS, Kim L, et al. A Phase I/II Trial of Enzastaurin in Patients with Recurrent High-Grade Gliomas. Neuro-Oncology 2010; 12(2) 181-189.

[210] Rampling R, Sanson M, Gorlia T, Lacombe D, Lai C, et al. A Phase I Study of LY317615 (Enzastaurin) and Temozolomide in Patients with Gliomas (EORTC trial 26054). Neuro-Oncology 2012; 14(3) 344-350.

[211] Tabatabai G, Frank B, Wick A, Lemke D, von Kurthy G, et al. Synergistic Antiglioma Activity of Radiotherapy and Enzastaurin. Annals of Neurology 2007; 61(2) 153-161.

[212] Butowski N, Chang SM, Lamborn KR, Polley MY, Pieper R, et al. Phase II and Pharmacogenomics Study of Enzastaurin plus Temozolomide During and Following Radiation Therapy in Patients with Newly Diagnosed Glioblastoma Multiforme and Gliosarcoma. Neuro-Oncology 2011; 13(12) 1331-1338.

[213] Wick W, Puduvalli VK, Chamberlain MC, van den Bent MJ, Carpentier AF, et al. Phase III Study of Enzastaurin Compared with Lomustine in the Treatment of Recurrent Intracranial Glioblastoma. Journal of Clinical Oncology 2010; 28(7) 1168-1174.

[214] Lu KV, Zhu S, Cvrljevic A, Huang TT, Sarkaria S, et al. Fyn and SRC are Effectors of Oncogenic Epidermal Growth Factor Receptor Signaling in Glioblastoma Patients. Cancer Research 2009; 69(17) 6889-6898.

[215] Milano V, Piao Y, LaFortune T, de Groot J. Dasatinib-Induced Autophagy is Enhanced in Combination with Temozolomide in Glioma. Molecular Cancer Therapeutics 2009; 8(2) 394-406.

[216] Premkumar DR, Jane EP, Agostino NR, Scialabba JL, Pollack IF. Dasatinib Synergizes with JSI-124 to Inhibit Growth and Migration and Induce Apoptosis of Malignant Human Glioma Cells. Journal of Carcinogenesis 2010; 9 7.

[217] Lu-Emerson C, Norden AD, Drappatz J, Quant EC, Beroukhim R, et al. Retrospective Study of Dasatinib for Recurrent Glioblastoma after Bevacizumab Failure. Journal of Neurooncology 2011; 104(1) 287-291.

[218] Premkumar DR, Jane EP, Pollack IF. Co-Administration of NVP-AEW541 and Dasatinib Induces Mitochondrial-Mediated Apoptosis through Bax Activation in Malignant Human Glioma Cell Lines. International Journal of Oncology 2010; 37(3) 633-643.

[219] Taga T, Suzuki A, Gonzalez-Gomez I, Gilles FH, Stins M, et al. Alpha v-Integrin Antagonist EMD 121974 Induces Apoptosis in Brain Tumor Cells Growing on Vitronectin and Tenascin. International Journal of Cancer 2002; 98(5) 690-697.

[220] Nabors LB, Mikkelsen T, Rosenfeld SS, Hochberg F, Akella NS, et al. Phase I and Correlative Biology Study of Cilengitide in Patients with Recurrent Malignant Glioma. Journal of Clinical Oncology 2007; 25(13) 1651-1657.

[221] Reardon DA, Fink KL, Mikkelsen T, Cloughesy TF, O'Neill A, et al. Randomized Phase II Study of Cilengitide, an Integrin-Targeting Arginine-Glycine-Aspartic Acid Peptide, in Recurrent Glioblastoma Multiforme. Journal of Clinical Oncology 2008; 26(34) 5610-5617.

[222] Gilbert MR, Kuhn J, Lamborn KR, Lieberman F, Wen PY, et al. Cilengitide in Patients with Recurrent Glioblastoma: the Results of NABTC 03-02, a Phase II Trial with Measures of Treatment Delivery. Journal of Neurooncology 2012; 106(1) 147-153.

[223] Stupp R, Goldbrunner R, Neyns B. Mature Results of a Phase I/IIa Trial of the Integrin Inhibitor Cilengitide (EMD121974) Added to Standard Concomitant and Adjuvant Temozolomide and Radiotherapy for Newly Diagnosed Glioblastoma. Neuro-Oncology 2007; 9 517.

[224] Stupp R, Hegi ME, Neyns B, Goldbrunner R, Schlegel U, et al. Phase I/IIa Study of Cilengitide and Temozolomide with Concomitant Radiotherapy Followed by Cilengitide and Temozolomide Maintenance Therapy in Patients with Newly Diagnosed Glioblastoma. Journal of Clinical Oncology 2010; 28(16) 2712-2718.

[225] Lomonaco SL, Finniss S, Xiang C, Lee HK, Jiang W, et al. Cilengitide Induces Autophagy-Mediated Cell Death in Glioma Cells. Neuro-Oncology 2011; 13(8) 857-865.

[226] Nabors LB, Mikkelsen T, Hegi ME, Ye X, Batchelor T, et al. A Safety Run-in and Randomized phase 2 Study of Cilengitide Combined with Chemoradiation for Newly Diagnosed Glioblastoma (NABTT 0306). Cancer 2012.

[227] Lin ZX, Yang LJ, Huang Q, Lin JH, Ren J, et al. Inhibition of Tumor-Induced Edema by Antisense VEGF is Mediated by Suppressive Vesiculo-Vacuolar Organelles (VVO) Formation. Cancer Science 2008; 99(12) 2540-2546.

[228] Kang C, Yuan X, Li F, Pu P, Yu S, et al. Evaluation of Folate-PAMAM for the Delivery of Antisense oligonucleotides to Rat C6 glioma cells in Vitro and in Vivo. Journal of Biomedical Material Research 2010; 93(2) 585-94.

[229] Tian XX, Zhang YG, Du J, Fang WG, Ng HK, Zheng J. Effects of Cotransfection of Antisense-EGFR and Wild-Type PTEN cDNA on Human Glioblastoma Cells. Neuropathology 2006; 26(3) 178-187.

[230] Pollack IF, Kawecki S, Lazo JS. Blocking of Glioma Proliferation in Vitro and in Vivo and Potentiating the Effects of BCNU and Cisplatin: UCN-01, a Selective Protein Kinase C Inhibitor. Journal of Neurosurgery 1996; 84(6) 1024-1032.

[231] Shen L, Dean NM, Glazer RI. Induction of p53-Dependent, Insulin-Like Growth Factor-Binding Protein-3-Mediated Apoptosis in Glioblastoma Multiforme Cells by a Protein Kinase C Alpha Antisense Oligonucleotide. Molecular Pharmacology 1999; 55(2) 396-402.

[232] Pu P, Kang C, Li J, Jiang H. Antisense and Dominant-Negative AKT2 cDNA Inhibits Glioma Cell Invasion. Tumour Biology 2004; 25(4) 172-178.

[233] Edwards LA, Verreault M, Thiessen B, Dragowska WH, Hu Y, et al. Combined Inhibition of the Phosphatidylinositol 3-Kinase/Akt and Ras/Mitogen-Activated Protein Kinase Pathways Results in Synergistic Effects in Glioblastoma Cells. Molecular Cancer Therapeutics 2006; 5(3) 645-654.

[234] Khazenzon NM, Ljubimov AV, Lakhter AJ, Fujita M, Fujiwara H, et al. Antisense Inhibition of Laminin-8 Expression Reduces Invasion of Human Gliomas in Vitro. Molecular Cancer Therapeutics 2003; 2(10) 985-894.

[235] Nagato S, Nakagawa K, Harada H, Kohno S, Fujiwara H, et al. Downregulation of Laminin α4 Chain Expression Inhibits Glioma Invasion in Vitro and in Vivo. International Journal of Cancer 2005; 117(1) 41-50.

[236] Zhu C, Li YB, Wong MC. Expression of Antisense bcl-2 cDNA Abolishes Tumorigenicity and Enhances Chemosensitivity of Human Malignant Glioma Cells. Journal of Neuroscience Research 2003; 74(1) 60-66.

[237] Julien T, Frankel B, Longo S, Kyle M, Gibson S. et al. Antisense-Mediated Inhibition of the bcl-2 Gene Induces Apoptosis in Human Malignant Glioma. Surgical Neurology 2000; 53(4) 360-369.

[238] Guensberg P, Wacheck V, Lucas T, Monia B, Pehamberger H, et al. Bcl-xL Antisense Oligonucleotides Chemosensitize Human Glioblastoma Cells. Cohemtherapy 2002; 48(4) 189-195.

[239] Caruso G, Raudino G, Caffo M, Alafaci C, Granata F, et al. Nanotechnology Platforms in Diagnosis and Treatments of Primary Brain Tumors. Recent Patents on Nanotechnology 2010; 4(2) 119-122.

[240] Caruso G, Caffo M, Alafaci C, Raudino G, Cafarella D, et al. Could Nanoparticles Systems Have a Role in the treatment of Cerebral Gliomas? Nanomedicine: Nanotechnology, Biology and Medicine 2011; 7(6) 744-752.

[241] Moghimi SM. Recent Developments in Polymeric Nanoparticle Engineering and their Applications in Experimental and Clinical Oncology. Anti-Cancer Agents inMedicinal Chemistry 2006; 6(6) 553-561.

Chapter 3

Hypoxia, Angiogenesis and Mechanisms for Invasion of Malignant Gliomas

Paula Province, Corinne E. Griguer, Xiaosi Han,
Nabors Louis B. and Hassan Fathallah Shaykh

Additional information is available at the end of the chapter

http://dx.doi.org/10.5772/53298

1. Introduction

Malignant gliomas are not only the most frequent primary brain tumor in the adult population, but also the most aggressive. Despite recent therapeutic advances, they remain associated with high morbidity and mortality. determinant of key biological features of these tumors, like their response, resistance, and patterns of recurrence when challenged by standard and new therapeutic options. Glioblastoma multiforme (GBM), the most aggressive of the astrocytic neoplasms, is characterized by both necrosis as well as high rates of endothelial proliferation and neo-vascularization. that generates a high consumption of oxygen and nutrients, thus leading to local hypoxia. The latter activates a cascade of signaling pathways leading to: 1) angiogenesis, 2) enhanced motility/invasion, 3) changes in metabolism, and 4) the ability to survive oxidative stress. This is a dynamic and multifactorial process whose outcome, either death or survival, is dependent on the timing and the rates of each of these processes, as well as on the molecular characteristics of the tumor. Therefore, hypoxia-induced enhancement of motility/invasion may determine the outcome and response to therapy of a particular GBM. We seek a better understanding of the molecular and phenotypic effects of local hypoxia in GBM. Here, we review the definition of hypoxia and its molecular and phenotypic effects on cancer cells in general and then turn our attention to its impact on malignant glioma cells. We also examine the interplay between anti-angiogenesis, survival, and enhanced motility, and explore potential therapeutic implications. We close with unresolved questions and potential future directions.

2. Malignant gliomas

2.1. Overview of gliomas

Central nervous system (CNS) neoplasms are a diverse group that varies widely in terms of clinical presentation, aggressiveness, and response to therapy, with distinctions in histology and cellular composition being largely responsible for these differences (Brat and Mapstone 2003). Of the many different types of brain tumors, gliomas are the most frequent primary brain tumors in adults (Ricard, Idbaih et al. 2012). Lower grade tumors, such as grades I and II, are commonly well-differentiated with limited amounts of increased cell density and other abnormalities. Grade III astrocytomas are anaplastic and have increased vessel and cell density, cellular atypia, and increased mitotic activity. GBM, grade IV, is characterized by the presence of necrosis and endothelial proliferation (Brat and Mapstone 2003; Westphal and Lamszus 2011).

2.2. Significance of malignant gliomas

The annual incidence of malignant gliomas is approximately 4 to 5 per 100 thousand and this group accounts for approximately 70% of the total number of new cases of malignant primary brain tumors diagnosed in the United States each year (Wen and Kesari 2008; Wen, Macdonald et al. 2010). The overall incidence of gliomas is higher among males as compared to females (7.2 per 100,000 persons-years in males versus 5.0 per 100,000-person years in females) and it is also highest among Caucasians, as compared to other ethnic groups (Peak and Levin 2010). Malignant gliomas can occur in any age group however the incidence increases in the fifth decade of life and peaks at about 65 years of age (Brat and Mapstone 2003). GBM is the most aggressive glioma. Stupp and colleagues reported that patients treated with concomitant and adjuvant Temozolomide and radiotherapy had overall survival (OS) rates of 27.2 and 9.8 percent at 2 and 5 years, respectively (Stupp, Mason et al. 2005; Stupp, Hegi et al. 2009).

3. Hypoxia

3.1. Definition of hypoxia

Oxygen plays a central role in cell biology and human cells require constant and adequate supply of oxygen. Oxygen functions as the terminal electron acceptor in the process of mitochondrial respiration, the process by which ATP is generated for use in most biochemical reactions (Semenza 2012; Semenza 2012). Hypoxia is a term used to describe reduced levels of oxygen and can be defined as a condition in which the oxygen pressure in the environment is less than 5 to 10 mmHg (Lu and Kang 2010). Hypoxia typically ranges from 0.1 percent to 3 percent oxygen, with exact definitions varying according to individual researchers (Wang, Jiang et al. 1995; Semenza 1998; Ke and Costa 2006; Palazon, Aragones et al. 2012). Normoxia for tissue culture experiments is considered approximately 21 percent oxygen. to meet consumption. For example, a local environment including a large number of metabolically active cancer cells may be hypoxic when the oxygen supply is not enhanced; to prevent hypoxia, supply must be increased. Factors that contribute to hypoxia include low partial pressure of oxygen in the blood, reduced ability of blood to carry oxygen, reduced tissue perfusion, increased diffusion distances, or inability of cells to use oxygen (Hockel and Vaupel 2001). Hypoxia is threatening to the normal cellular environment and a series of highly regulated and coordinated response-mechanisms are necessary in order for cells to survive in hypoxic environments (Wheaton and Chandel 2011).

3.2. Hypoxia and tumor cells

One of the characteristics of cancer cells is deregulated, high cellular proliferation that ultimately results in structurally and functionally abnormal blood vessels that are unable to provide an adequate amount of oxygen to meet the increased metabolic demands of proliferation, which ultimately results in hypoxia (Vaupel, Kallinowski et al. 1989; Harris 2002; Semenza 2012). Although indirect evidence for hypoxia in human tumors was first reported in the 1950s, Peter Vaupel and colleagues were among the first researchers to demonstrate direct evidence of hypoxia in human cancers, as well as linking hypoxia with increased metastasis and poor prognosis in patients with squamous tumors of the head and neck, cervical cancers, and breast cancers (Thomlinson and Gray 1955; Hockel, Schlenger et al. 1999; Hockel and Vaupel 2001; Harris 2002).

Tumor cells generally respond to hypoxia in 1 of 2 ways: either cellular proliferation is restricted and apoptosis and necrosis may occur or the tumor cells adapt to the stress of the hypoxic environment and become more aggressive (Vaupel 2008). This adaptation towards a more aggressive phenotype is accomplished by regulating the expression of various genes that have critical roles in cellular events, which include cellular proliferation, differentiation, tumor glycolysis, angiogenesis, and metastasis and invasion (Vaupel 2004; Lu and Kang 2010; Semenza 2012). Additionally, tumor cells not only acquire more invasive and metastatic properties in response to hypoxia, but also become more resistant to standard treatments, such as chemotherapies and radiation therapies (Semenza 2012). Hypoxia-associated resistance to radiation therapy can occur when the partial pressure of oxygen in a tumor is less than 25-30 mmHg. The mechanism of this resistance is thought to be multi-factorial, however some proposed possibilities include decreased oxygen concentrations, higher levels of heat shock proteins, and the presence of cells with decreased apoptotic potential (Hockel and Vaupel 2001). Hypoxia-induced resistance to chemotherapy is likely affected by inhibition of cellular proliferation, decreased effectiveness of some agents in the setting of hypoxia, tissue acidosis, and/or the loss of apoptotic potential of cells (Hockel and Vaupel 2001).

4. Molecular signals of hypoxia

Hypoxia-inducible factor (HIF) is a transcription factor that plays a critical a central role in mediating the ability to adapt to low-oxygen concentrations (Wang, Jiang et al. 1995; Semenza 1998). One of the primary cellular events in response to the initial exposure to hypoxia is activation of hypoxia-inducible factor 1 (HIF-1), a hetero-dimeric basic helix-loop-helix protein, composed of 2 subunits: HIF-1α, which is up-regulated in an oxygen-dependent manner, and HIF-1β, which is constitutively expressed (Semenza 2000; Lee, Bae et al. 2004; Zhu, Zhou et al. 2011). Over-expression of HIF-1α is seen in many cancer types associated with a poor prognosis, like malignancies of the brain, oropharynx, breast, cervix, ovary, and uterus (Semenza 2003; Lu and Kang 2010).

Hypoxia-inducible factor-2 alpha (HIF-2α) is another mammalian protein that appears to play a role in the cellular response to hypoxia (Hu, Wang et al. 2003; Semenza 2012). HIF-2α is structurally similar to HIF-1α, sharing 48 percent of the overall amino acid identity (Hu, Wang et al. 2003; Ke and Costa 2006). Unlike HIF-1α, which is ubiquitously expressed, HIF-2α is mainly expressed in the lung, endothelium, and carotid body (Kaur, Khwaja et al. 2005; Ke and Costa 2006). recently been discovered; its splice variants appear to play a role as negative regulators of HIF-1 (Gu, Moran et al. 1998; Makino, Cao et al. 2001; Ke and Costa 2006). Other important transcription factors that are activated by hypoxia include cyclic-AMP-response element-binding protein (CREB), nuclear factor-κB (NF-κB), activating protein-1 (AP-1), and metal-responsive transcription factor-1 (MTF-1) (Harris 2002; Vaupel 2004).

4.1. Mechanisms of hypoxia-induced signaling

Under normal oxygen conditions, HIF-1α is hydroxylated by prolyl hydroxylase (PHD). This hydroxylation leads to the recognition and binding of von Hippel-Lindau (VHL), which is part of an E3 ubiquitin ligase complex that targets HIF-1α for degradation through a proteasomal pathway (Wheaton and Chandel 2011; Semenza 2012). hypoxic conditions, the hydroxylation of the HIF-1α subunit by PHD is inhibited and, therefore, HIF-1α is stabilized, resulting in its translocation to the cell nucleus where it dimerizes with the HIF-1β subunit and forms the active HIF-1. Activation of HIF-1 subsequently results in the recruitment of transcriptional co-activators and this complex then binds to consensus hypoxia-responsive elements (HREs) within the promoter regions of target genes and initiates the transcription of a variety of hypoxia-responsive genes (Vaupel 2004). These genes can be grouped into 4 functional categories (see Figure), namely, survival/proliferation, metabolism, angiogenesis, and invasion/metastasis (Lu and Kang 2010).

4.2. Effects on cell proliferation and survival

Increased rates of cell proliferation and decreased rates of cell death are 2 of the defining differences between neoplastic cells and normal cells. HIF-1 plays an important role in cellular proliferation. Iyer *et al.* demonstrated that cells deficient in HIF-1α have reduced rates of cellular proliferation as compared to wild-type cells under both normoxic and hypoxic conditions, with the degree of reduction worsened in hypoxia (Iyer, Kotch et al. 1998; Feldser, Agani et al. 1999). Additionally, several growth factors that contribute to increased cell proliferation are also HIF-1 target genes. insulin-like growth factor-2 (IGF2) and transforming-

http://dx.doi.org/10.5772/53298

growth factor-alpha (TGF-α) (Feldser, Agani et al. 1999; Krishnamachary, Berg-Dixon et al. 2003). Binding of these factors to their receptors, namely insulin-like growth factor receptor-1 (IGFR1) and epidermal growth-factor receptor (EGFR), respectively, leads to autocrine signaling, resulting in both increased cell proliferation and survival as well as increased expression of HIF-1 (Semenza 2003; Ke and Costa 2006). These autocrine signaling pathways are necessary for cancer progression (Semenza 2003).

4.3. Effects on metabolism

The uptake of glucose by metastatic cancer cells is markedly increased as compared to non-cancer cells and under hypoxic conditions cells switch from the oxygen-dependent metabolic pathway, the tricarboxylic acid (TCA) cycle, to the oxygen-independent pathway, glycolysis (Dang and Semenza 1999; Ke and Costa 2006). HIF-1 plays an active role in this metabolic response to hypoxia by up-regulating the expression of glycolytic enzymes, such as aldolase A, phosphoglycerate kinase 1, and lactate dehydrogenase, that convert glucose to lactate (Vaupel 2004). HIF-1 also induces the over-expression of glucose transporters, namely *GLUT1* and *GLUT3*, that facilitate the uptake of glucose by the cells (Chen, Pore et al. 2001; Ke and Costa 2006; Semenza 2012). While it is well known that HIF-1 stimulates glycolysis, it has also been demonstrated that it can actively repress mitochondrial function and oxygen consumption by inducing pyruvate dehydrogenase kinase 1 (PDK1). Papandreou *et al* nicely demonstrated that HIF-1-dependent block of oxygen utilization results in increased oxygen availability and in decreased cell death when total oxygen is limiting (Papandreou, Cairns et al. 2006). In a feedback loop, this leads to a shut-down of the formation of mitochondrial acetyl-CoA and oxidative phosphorylation (OXPHOS), which in turn reduces the generation of mitochondrial Reactive Oxygen Species (ROS) and contributes to the generation of lactate that can be used to acidify the microenvironment leading to increase invasion and migration. Additionally, a very elegant study by Guzy *et al*. (2005 Cell metabolism) found that functionality of complex III of the mitochondrial electron transport chain (ETC) is required for the hypoxic stabilization of HIF-1α and HIF-2α and that an increase in ROS links this complex to HIF-alpha stabilization (Guzy, Hoyos et al. 2005). This important study linked an oxygen-dependent pathway to the stabilization of HIF-1. Thus, while HIF-1 controls glycolysis and shuts-down OXPHOS, functional mitochondria play a role in the regulation of HIF-1.

4.4. Effects on angiogenesis

Lee *et. al* demonstrated that inhibition of HIF-1 activity by either anthracycline chemotherapy or acriflavine prevents tumor vascularization in mouse models, thus lending support to the idea that HIF-1 activity is critical in tumor vascularization (Lee, Qian et al. 2009; Lee, Zhang et al. 2009; Semenza 2012). Angiogenesis is a complex process by which the vascular system is formed through growth of new capillaries from pre-existing vessels (Wang, Fei et al. 2004). In addition, although there is great diversity in the factors and signals that contribute to angiogenesis, the chemical signal that appears to play the most critical role in the process is Vascular Endothelial Growth Factor, or VEGF. VEGF is a pro-angiogenic growth factor that is secreted by many cells, including mesenchymal, stromal, and especially tumor cells. VEGF induces the migration of the endothelial precursor cells to sites of angiogenesis and is also responsible for the proliferation and differentiation of these cells (Ahluwalia and Gladson 2010). (Kaur, Khwaja et al. 2005). Interestingly, HIF-1 activates the transcription of VEGF by binding to the HRE in its promoter region (Forsythe, Jiang et al. 1996; Kaur, Khwaja et al. 2005). Hypoxia also increases VEGF production by stabilizing its mRNA; this effect is mediated by the 3′ un-translated region of the mRNA (Onesto, Berra et al. 2004; Kaur, Khwaja et al. 2005). Moreover, HIF-1 up-regulates the expression of additional key molecules that induce angiogenesis, including stromal-derived factor 1 (*SDF1*), placental growth factor (*PGF*), platelet-derived growth factor B (*PDGFB*), and angiopoietin (*ANGPT*) 1 and 2 (Rey and Semenza 2010; Semenza 2012). These pro-angiogenic genes increase vascular density, thus supplying oxygen and nutrients to metabolically demanding tumor cells (Ke and Costa 2006).

4.5. Effects of hypoxia on tumor invasion and motility

Metastasis is a complex process that consists of a series of highly regulated, rate-limiting steps in which tumor cells gain more invasive properties. Metastasis begins with a change in tumor plasticity in a process called epithelial-mesenchymal transition (EMT). During this process there is a loss of epithelial cell characteristics and a gain of mesenchymal gene expression. In short, this process is characterized by the down-regulation of epithelial (E)-cadherin, involved in adherence junctions and endothelial stabilization, and the up-regulation of mesenchymal (N)-cadherin, which allows cells to become more motile (Lu and Kang 2010; van Zijl, Krupitza et al. 2011). the repression of (E)-cadherin (Imai, Horiuchi et al. 2003; Krishnamachary, Zagzag et al. 2006; Yang, Wu et al. 2008; Lu and Kang 2010). Next, tumor cells begin to disrupt the integrity of the basement membrane. This is accomplished via a proteolytic cascade that is put into motion by HIF-1α-dependent up-regulation of enzymes such as cathepsin D (CTSD), urokinase-type plasminogen-activator receptor (uPAR), and matrix metalloproteinase-2 (MMP2) (Krishnamachary, Berg-Dixon et al. 2003; Lu and Kang 2010). Once the basement membrane is disrupted, tumor cells eventually penetrate the walls of blood vessels in order to become circulating tumor cells (CTCs) in a process known as intravasation (Lu and Kang 2010). (Gupta, Nguyen et al. 2007; Lu and Kang 2010). Hypoxia-induced expression of VEGF also increases the chance of intravasation through the effects of VEGF on increased microvascular permeability and interstitial fluid pressure (Sullivan and Graham 2007; Lu and Kang 2010).

Motility is also an important concept in the process of metastasis. Once the cell-cell junctions have been broken down by the down-regulation of (E)-cadherin, the cells are quickly able to reassemble the actin cytoskeleton into protrusive and invasive structures, such as lamellipodia and filopodia, that help them to migrate through the degraded extracellular matrix (ECM), into the blood vessels, and ultimately to their target location (Fathallah-Shaykh 2005). Actin-Related Protein 2/3 (Arp2/3), which is composed of 2 actin related proteins and 5 structural subunits, is controlled by the Scar/WAVE complex, also known as the WANP complex, and is essential to the rapid assembly of actin networks that make up lamellipodia (Machesky 2008). Additionally, the up-regulation of the capping protein increases the protrusion activity of invasive tumor cells (Yamaguchi, Wyckoff et al. 2005). The formation of filopodia is controlled by proteins such as fascin, diaphanous, and Mena/VASP (Machesky 2008).

5. Hypoxia and malignant gliomas

5.1. HIF in gliomas

In addition to decreased oxygen tension in brain and GBM tissues, the expression of HIF in gliomas can be affected by the activation of oncogenes, namely epidermal growth factor receptor (EGFR) and platelet-derived growth factor receptor (PDGFR), and/or the loss of tumor suppressor function through p53 and phosphatase and tensin homolog gene (PTEN*)* (Brat and Mapstone 2003; Kaur, Khwaja et al. 2005). EGFR affects the expression of HIF by activating a series of pathways, the first of which is the Phosphatidylinositol 3-kinases (PI(3)K) pathway, which ultimately leads to increased HIF-1α protein levels (Clarke, Smith et al. 2001; Kaur, Khwaja et al. 2005). EGFR amplification found in glioblastoma, as well as among other tumors, is also associated with a poor prognosis (Frederick, Wang et al. 2000; Kaur, Khwaja et al. 2005). Platelet-derived growth factor (PDGF) has 3 isoforms and 2 receptors and of these, the PDGFA isoform and the PDFGR-α receptor are over-expressed by glial tumor cells (Brat and Mapstone 2003). Furthermore, PDGF is thought to enhance the transcription and secretion of VEGF (Brat and Mapstone 2003). The *PTEN* gene, located on chromosome 10, is a tumor suppressor gene that is mutated in 20 to 40 percent of glioblastoma (Li, Yen et al. 1997; Cantley and Neel 1999; Brat and Mapstone 2003; Kaur, Khwaja et al. 2005). Loss of function of the *PTEN* gene in gliomas is associated with increased HIF-1α expression as well as tumor vascularization and Zundel *et al.* showed that over-expression of the gene in gliomas is associated with reduction in HIF-1α expression (Zundel, Schindler et al. 2000; Kaur, Khwaja et al. 2005). The p53 gene, mutated in approximately 50% of gliomas and believed to be the "guardian of the genome," exerts a key role in hypoxia by enhancing the degradation of HIF-1α, by promoting the interaction of the latter with MDM2, which enhances ubiquitination (Hollstein, Sidransky et al. 1991). Thus, expression of wild-type p53 down-regulates VEGF and therefore leads to inhibition of angiogenesis (Brat and Mapstone 2003; Hunter, Brat et al. 2003; Kaur, Khwaja et al. 2005). Interestingly, HIF-1α stabilizes p53 by direct physical interaction. p53 activity is lost in gliomas by multiple mechanisms; mutations of p53 are common in gliomas (Brat and Mapstone 2003; Kaur, Khwaja et al. 2005). In addition, the MDM2 protein, which enhances p53 degradation by ubiquitination, is over-expressed in gliomas (Reifenberger, Liu et al. 1993; Brat and Mapstone 2003). Furthermore, loss of $p14^{ARF}$ function in gliomas leads to MDM2-mediated enhanced degradation of p53 (Nakamura, Watanabe et al. 2001; Brat and Mapstone 2003).

5.2. Hypoxia, angiogenesis, and GBM

GBM are highly cellular astrocytic neoplasms; they are histologically characterized by an area of central necrosis surrounded by a highly cellular rim of viable tumor (Brat and Mapstone 2003; Giese, Bjerkvig et al. 2003). GBM also display areas of microvascular hyperplasia as well as areas of necrosis with the appearance of tumor cells pseudo-palisading around the necrotic centers. The areas of microvascular hyperplasia are examples of accelerated angiogenesis and are thought to influence the biological behavior of malignant gliomas by favoring aggressive neoplastic growth. angiogenesis in the surrounding hypoxic areas. In fact, the VEGF concentrations in glioblastoma are 200 to 300 times greater than serum concentrations (Takano, Yoshii et al. 1996; Brat and Mapstone 2003). The pseudo-palisading cells have also been shown to over-express HIF-1 and also to secrete other pro-angiogenic factors in addition to VEGF, such as interleukin 8 (IL-8) (Rong, Durden et al. 2006; Onishi, Ichikawa et al. 2011). It is also important to note that newly formed blood vessels in malignant gliomas generally have increased diameters, are highly permeable, have thickened basement membranes, and have highly proliferative endothelial cells (Lopes 2003; Onishi, Ichikawa et al. 2011).

5.3. Hypoxia and invasiveness of GBM

As discussed earlier, cancer cell migration and invasion consists of a series of highly coordinated steps including dissociation of cellular adhesions, remodeling of the actin cytoskeleton, proteolytic degradation of the ECM, and formation of new adhesions. Brain invasion is a characteristic feature of malignant gliomas. In vivo studies of glioblastoma have shown that tumor hypoxia results in increased cell migration (Plasswilm, Tannapfel et al. 2000). Once again, the pseudopalisading cells found around the necrotic cores in GBM, which up-regulate HIF-1, appear to be hypoxic and migrating away from the necrotic core (Elstner, Holtkamp et al. 2007; Onishi, Ichikawa et al. 2011). discovery has revealed that the protein MINK, which inactivates ADF/cofilin by phosphorylation, is up-regulated in glioma cells as compared to normal brain cells (Fathallah-Shaykh 2005). Additionally, under hypoxic conditions, glioblastoma induce the expression of c-Met, which stimulates gliomas cells to secrete urokinase plasminogen activator (uPA), which converts circulating plasminogen into plasmin. The latter helps promote invasion by degrading ECM proteins as well as by activating matrix metalloproteins, including MMP2, up-regulated in glioma cells (Fathallah-Shaykh 2005; Martens, Schmidt et al. 2006; Eckerich, Zapf et al. 2007; Onishi, Ichikawa et al. 2011).

5.4. Hypoxia and cell survival in GBM

Microarray analysis of cultured glioma cells revealed over-expression of molecules that protect them from reactive oxygen species (ROS) and endoplasmic reticulum (ER)-induced apoptosis (Fathallah-Shaykh 2005). ROS, generated by the rapid multiplication of cancer cells, cause a release of cytochrome c leading to apoptosis (Filomeni, Aquilano et al. 2003; Petrosillo, Ruggiero et al. 2003; Fathallah-Shaykh 2005). Glioma cells appear to acquire protective mechanisms against ROS-induced apoptosis. First, by up-regulating protective enzymes such as *AKR1A1* and *AKR1C1*, which belong to the aldo-keto reductase enzyme super-family (Sanli and Blaber 2001; Fathallah-Shaykh 2005). Second, by up-regulating several antioxidants, some of which include *PDG*, *TALDO1*, *AFG3L1*, *ANT2*, *GSTP1*, and *PRDX1* (Berggren, Husbeck et al. 2001; Nonn, Berggren et al. 2003; Fathallah-Shaykh 2005)., nuclear factor κB (NF- κB) has been reported to be constitutively activated in cultured glioma cells and GBM surgical samples (Bharti and Aggarwal 2002; Robe, Bentires-Alj et al. 2004; Wang, Zhang et al. 2004; Fathallah-Shaykh 2005).

The ER, one of the cells largest organelles, is responsible for folding, glysolating, and sorting proteins to their correct destinations, as well as for synthesizing lipids and cholesterol components of the cell membrane. When homeostasis is disrupted in the ER, mis-folded and un-folded proteins can accumulate with the ER lumen, resulting in *ER stress*, which shuts off protein synthesis leading to apoptosis. This response is beneficial to the cell as a safeguard against carcinogenesis because mis-folded proteins may acquire aberrant functions. On the other hand, bypassing this response is an important milestone in the development of cancer. Glioma cells appear to acquire pathways that help them recover from *ER stress* and avoid apoptosis. A normal ER stress-induced response ultimately leads to inactivation of the eukaryotic initiation factor 2 (eIF-2α), which shuts off protein synthesis. By up-regulating activating transcription factor 4 (ATF4), malignant glioma cells appear to bypass the ER stress-induced protein synthesis inhibition. ATF4 induces the growth arrest and DNA damage-inducible protein (GADD34), which dephosphorylates eIF2α, causing protein synthesis recovery (Connor, Weiser et al. 2001; Novoa, Zeng et al. 2001; Brush, Weiser et al. 2003; Fathallah-Shaykh 2005).

6. Linking hypoxia, invasion, and angiogenesis

6.1. Hypoxia, invasion, and angiogenesis in malignant gliomas

Hypoxia, invasion, and angiogenesis are interrelated through a variety of molecular pathways and feedback loops. divide and increase in number, they often out-grow their diffusion-limited oxygen supplies and hypoxia results. Once the tumor micro-environment becomes hypoxic, cellular and molecular signaling pathways are initiated in order to promote overall tumor survival. These adaptive responses include: 1) increasing cellular resistance to hypoxia, 2) favoring metabolic pathways that are optimal in hypoxia, 3) increasing motility and invasive properties in order to seek new oxygen supplies, and 4) initiating angiogenesis in order to create a new vascular supply, or a combination of these responses. (Shimizu, Eguchi et al. 1995). Therefore, there is evidence that local oxygen concentrations modulate a switch between proliferative phenotype and an invasive in GBM cells; this is called the "Go or Grow" mechanism (Giese, Kluwe et al. 1996; Giese, Loo et al. 1996; Hatzikirou, Basanta et al. 2012).

When considering angiogenesis as the adaptive mechanism in glial cells, it is necessary to evaluate the relationship between the rate of angiogenesis and the rate of cellular division. If cellular division proceeds at a rate faster than angiogenesis, then oxygen supply cannot meet metabolic demands causing not only local necrosis, but also dissemination of tumor cells by enhanced brain invasion. On the other hand, if angiogenesis proceeds at a rate faster than cellular division then oxygen supplies are sufficient to meet metabolic demands and no necrosis occurs, which is characteristic of anaplastic astrocytoma.

6.2. Anti-angiogenic agents as treatment for malignant gliomas

Both prospective and retrospective clinical trials have shown that Bevacizumab, an anti-angiogenic agent, is effective as a single-agent against recurrent glioblastoma as compared to historical controls of salvage chemotherapy (Friedman, Prados et al. 2009; Kreisl, Kim et al. 2009; Raizer, Grimm et al. 2010). The Roche-sponsored AVAglio international multicenter phase III clinical trial, comparing standard of care to standard of care plus Bevacizumab for the treatment of newly-diagnosed GBM, is completed; the results will be presented at The Society for Neuro-Oncology 2012 meeting. It is noteworthy that Bevacizumab has a positive significant impact on progression-free survival times (Norden, Drappatz et al. 2009; van den Bent, Vogelbaum et al. 2009; Keunen, Johansson et al. 2011).

Interestingly, *in vivo* GBM models have shown that anti-angiogenic agents enhance tumor cell migration/invasion. Keunen and colleagues studied a human GBM xenograft model, derived from patient tumor spheroids, in rats. The results revealed that Bevacizumab induces vascular remodeling that leads to increased tumor cell invasion into normal brain parenchyma, associated with a hypoxic tumor microenvironment and a glycolytic metabolism (Keunen, Johansson et al. 2011). Plasswilm *et al.* implanted cultured glioma cells in a chicken embryo model and showed that local hypoxia promotes tumor spread and the development of secondary tumor cell bulks (Plasswilm, Tannapfel et al. 2000).

6.3. Implications for treatment of malignant gliomas

Treatment with Bevacizumab also has important implications for how tumor progression is defined. Traditionally, tumor progression has been measured according to the MacDonald criteria which define progression by increase in contrast enhancement. However, as a result of blood-brain barrier stabilization secondary to anti-angiogenic agents, contrast enhancement is no longer a reliable measure of progression. Therefore, the Response Assessment in Neuro-Oncology (RANO) Working Group developed the RANO criteria as a means to address potential progression by non-enhancing T2/FLAIR (fluid attenuated inversion recovery) lesions as well as by increases in contrast enhancement in malignant gliomas (Province, Han et al. 2011). The use of anti-angiogenic agents, namely Bevacizumab, has also raised many questions about patterns of recurrence in malignant gliomas. Additionally, although there is some conflicting data on this subject secondary to poor study design and low study power, there is evidence that patients who are treated with Bevacizumab exhibit more diffuse or distant recurrence patterns as compared to those who do not receive Bevacizumab. Once again, the possibility of more diffuse and distant recurrence patterns may be explained by the "Go or Grow" mechanism, as explained above, with further supporting evidence derived from the glioblastoma xenograft model, also detailed above (Keunen, Johansson et al. 2011; Hatzikirou, Basanta et al. 2012).

Hypoxia-mediated enhancement of brain invasion has profound biological and clinical implications on GBM, in particular in the context of treatment with anti-angiogenic drugs. Recall that necrosis is a hallmark of GBM; thus, one can safely assume that, by the time of the initial clinical presentation, GBM cells have already invaded the surrounding brain parenchyma because of local hypoxia. This feature of GBM may limit the effectiveness of local therapeutic options, like radiation therapy and surgical resection. Furthermore, one could argue that, though anti-angiogenic drugs prolong progression free survival times, they may create a more aggressive and invasive tumor by hypoxia-mediated enhancement of motility, which delays clinical progression. These patients may experience a so-called "honeymoon period," in which they may appear stable; however, once they recur, the rate of progression of Bevacizumab-treated tumors may be very acute secondary to the large volume of invaded brain. This rationale may explain the limited effects of Bevacizumab on overall survival times.

7. Future directions

The Figure depicts the effects of HIF-1α on key cellular functions. Though some of the signaling molecules are known, we seem to be only looking at the tip of the iceberg. More research is needed to fit the pieces of the puzzle. What other molecules are activated by hypoxia to influence the 4 phenotypes shown in the Figure? How do they relate to HIF-1? Are there feedback loops between the phenotypes? That is, does motility affect metabolism and vice versa? We have presented a succinct view of the molecular basis of the four phenotypes; however, a detailed analysis is not within the scope of this chapter.

Although preclinical studies have revealed a molecular link between hypoxia, angiogenesis, and invasion, the clinical implications of these relationships are still not well known and future studies are needed. Drawing from what has already been established regarding the effects of anti-angiogenic agents on increased migration and invasion in malignant gliomas, a plausible direction for future therapeutic development would include blocking not only angiogenesis but also invasion and migration. motility agents in malignant GBM will result in significant improvement in PFS as well as overall survival times by blocking two of the primary mechanisms for their survival.

8. Conclusion

From this chapter, it is our hope that the reader has gained an understanding of the extensive role of hypoxia in brain tumors, with specific regard to its role in angiogenesis, invasion, metabolism, and overall survival of the tumor. Furthermore, although the use of anti-angiogenic agents as therapeutic options for malignant gliomas has provided some promising results, it has also revealed the need for further molecular research into the mechanisms for invasion of malignant gliomas, especially as it relates to the hypoxic environments created by anti-angiogenic drugs. Hopefully, this combination of efforts to decrease both angiogenesis and invasion will result in the development of more promising therapeutic agents to treat this disease.

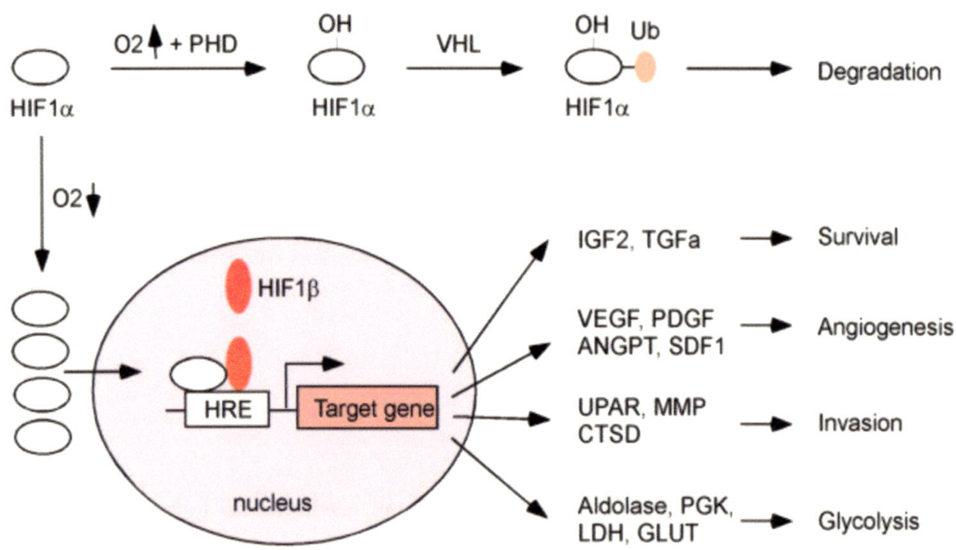

Figure 1. Cartoon illustrating signaling and degradation of HIF-1α in hypoxia. Under normal oxygen supply, one of the two proline residues (Pro-402, Pto-564) in HIF-1α is hydroxylated by prolyl hydroxylase. Once hydroxylated HIF-1α is recognized by VHL, an E3 ubiquitin (Ub) ligase, which targets HIF-1α for degradation through the proteasomal pathway. In hypoxic conditions, hydroxylation is inhibited causing the accumulation of HIF-1α, which translocates to nucleus where it associates with HIF-1β then binds to the HIF responsive Element (HRE) of target genes activating their transcription. The HIF targeting genes modulate cell survival, metabolism, angiogenesis, and tumor invasion. PGK: phosphoglycerate kinase, LDH: lactate dehydrogenase.

Author details

Paula Province, Corinne E. Griguer, Xiaosi Han, Nabors Louis B. and Hassan Fathallah Shaykh

The University of Alabama at Birmingham, Birmingham, Alabama, United States of America

http://dx.doi.org/10.5772/53298

References

[1] Ahluwalia, M. S. and C. L. Gladson (2010). "Progress on antiangiogenic therapy for patients with malignant glioma." J Oncol 2010: 689018.

[2] Berggren, M. I., B. Husbeck, et al. (2001). "Thioredoxin peroxidase-1 (peroxiredoxin-1) is increased in thioredoxin-1 transfected cells and results in enhanced protection against apoptosis caused by hydrogen peroxide but not by other agents including dexamethasone, etoposide, and doxorubicin." Arch Biochem Biophys 392(1): 103-109.

[3] Bharti, A. C. and B. B. Aggarwal (2002). "Nuclear factor-kappa B and cancer: its role in prevention and therapy." Biochem Pharmacol 64(5-6): 883-888.

[4] Brat, D. J. and T. B. Mapstone (2003). "Malignant glioma physiology: cellular response to hypoxia and its role in tumor progression." Ann Intern Med 138(8): 659-668.

[5] Brush, M. H., D. C. Weiser, et al. (2003). "Growth arrest and DNA damage-inducible protein GADD34 targets protein phosphatase 1 alpha to the endoplasmic reticulum and promotes dephosphorylation of the alpha subunit of eukaryotic translation initiation factor 2." Mol Cell Biol 23(4): 1292-1303.

[6] Cantley, L. C. and B. G. Neel (1999). "New insights into tumor suppression: PTEN suppresses tumor formation by restraining the phosphoinositide 3-kinase/AKT pathway." Proc Natl Acad Sci U S A 96(8): 4240-4245.

[7] Chen, C., N. Pore, et al. (2001). "Regulation of glut1 mRNA by hypoxia-inducible factor-1. Interaction between H-ras and hypoxia." J Biol Chem 276(12): 9519-9525.

[8] Clarke, K., K. Smith, et al. (2001). "Mutant epidermal growth factor receptor enhances induction of vascular endothelial growth factor by hypoxia and insulin-like growth factor-1 via a PI3 kinase dependent pathway." Br J Cancer 84(10): 1322-1329.

[9] Connor, J. H., D. C. Weiser, et al. (2001). "Growth arrest and DNA damage-inducible protein GADD34 assembles a novel signaling complex containing protein phosphatase 1 and inhibitor 1." Mol Cell Biol 21(20): 6841-6850.

[10] Dang, C. V. and G. L. Semenza (1999). "Oncogenic alterations of metabolism." Trends Biochem Sci 24(2): 68-72.

[11] Eckerich, C., S. Zapf, et al. (2007). "Hypoxia can induce c-Met expression in glioma cells and enhance SF/HGF-induced cell migration." Int J Cancer 121(2): 276-283.

[12] Elstner, A., N. Holtkamp, et al. (2007). "Involvement of Hif-1 in desferrioxamine-induced invasion of glioblastoma cells." Clin Exp Metastasis 24(1): 57-66.

[13] Fathallah-Shaykh, H. M. (2005). "Genomic discovery reveals a molecular system for resistance to oxidative and endoplasmic reticulum stress in cultured glioma." Arch Neurol 62(2): 233-236.

[14] Fathallah-Shaykh, H. M. (2005). "Logical networks inferred from highly specific discovery of transcriptionally regulated genes predict protein states in cultured gliomas." Biochem Biophys Res Commun 336(4): 1278-1284.

[15] Feldser, D., F. Agani, et al. (1999). "Reciprocal positive regulation of hypoxia-inducible factor 1alpha and insulin-like growth factor 2." Cancer Res 59(16): 3915-3918.

[16] Filomeni, G., K. Aquilano, et al. (2003). "Reactive oxygen species-dependent c-Jun NH2-terminal kinase/c-Jun signaling cascade mediates neuroblastoma cell death induced by diallyl disulfide." Cancer Res 63(18): 5940-5949.

[17] Forsythe, J. A., B. H. Jiang, et al. (1996). "Activation of vascular endothelial growth factor gene transcription by hypoxia-inducible factor 1." Mol Cell Biol 16(9): 4604-4613.

[18] Frederick, L., X. Y. Wang, et al. (2000). "Diversity and frequency of epidermal growth factor receptor mutations in human glioblastomas." Cancer Res 60(5): 1383-1387.

[19] Friedman, H. S., M. D. Prados, et al. (2009). "Bevacizumab alone and in combination with irinotecan in recurrent glioblastoma." J Clin Oncol 27(28): 4733-4740.

[20] Giese, A., R. Bjerkvig, et al. (2003). "Cost of migration: invasion of malignant gliomas and implications for treatment." J Clin Oncol 21(8): 1624-1636.

[21] Giese, A., L. Kluwe, et al. (1996). "Migration of human glioma cells on myelin." Neurosurgery 38(4): 755-764.

[22] Giese, A., M. A. Loo, et al. (1996). "Dichotomy of astrocytoma migration and proliferation." Int J Cancer 67(2): 275-282.

[23] Gu, Y. Z., S. M. Moran, et al. (1998). "Molecular characterization and chromosomal localization of a third alpha-class hypoxia inducible factor subunit, HIF3alpha." Gene Expr 7(3): 205-213.

[24] Gupta, G. P., D. X. Nguyen, et al. (2007). "Mediators of vascular remodelling co-opted for sequential steps in lung metastasis." Nature 446(7137): 765-770.

[25] Guzy, R. D., B. Hoyos, et al. (2005). "Mitochondrial complex III is required for hypoxia-induced ROS production and cellular oxygen sensing." Cell Metab 1(6): 401-408.

[26] Harris, A. L. (2002). "Hypoxia--a key regulatory factor in tumour growth." Nat Rev Cancer 2(1): 38-47.

[27] Hatzikirou, H., D. Basanta, et al. (2012). "'Go or grow': the key to the emergence of invasion in tumour progression?" Math Med Biol 29(1): 49-65.

[28] Hockel, M., K. Schlenger, et al. (1999). "Hypoxic cervical cancers with low apoptotic index are highly aggressive." Cancer Res 59(18): 4525-4528.

[29] Hockel, M. and P. Vaupel (2001). "Tumor hypoxia: definitions and current clinical, biologic, and molecular aspects." J Natl Cancer Inst 93(4): 266-276.

[30] Hollstein, M., D. Sidransky, et al. (1991). "p53 mutations in human cancers." Science 253(5015): 49-53.

[31] Hu, C. J., L. Y. Wang, et al. (2003). "Differential roles of hypoxia-inducible factor 1alpha (HIF-1alpha) and HIF-2alpha in hypoxic gene regulation." Mol Cell Biol 23(24): 9361-9374.

[32] Hunter, S. B., D. J. Brat, et al. (2003). "Alterations in molecular pathways of diffusely infiltrating glial neoplasms: application to tumor classification and anti-tumor therapy (Review)." Int J Oncol 23(4): 857-869.

[33] Imai, T., A. Horiuchi, et al. (2003). "Hypoxia attenuates the expression of E-cadherin via up-regulation of SNAIL in ovarian carcinoma cells." Am J Pathol 163(4): 1437-1447.

[34] Iyer, N. V., L. E. Kotch, et al. (1998). "Cellular and developmental control of O2 homeostasis by hypoxia-inducible factor 1 alpha." Genes Dev 12(2): 149-162.

[35] Kaur, B., F. W. Khwaja, et al. (2005). "Hypoxia and the hypoxia-inducible-factor pathway in glioma growth and angiogenesis." Neuro Oncol 7(2): 134-153.

[36] Ke, Q. and M. Costa (2006). "Hypoxia-inducible factor-1 (HIF-1)." Mol Pharmacol 70(5): 1469-1480.

[37] Keunen, O., M. Johansson, et al. (2011). "Anti-VEGF treatment reduces blood supply and increases tumor cell invasion in glioblastoma." Proc Natl Acad Sci U S A 108(9): 3749-3754.

[38] Kreisl, T. N., L. Kim, et al. (2009). "Phase II trial of single-agent bevacizumab followed by bevacizumab plus irinotecan at tumor progression in recurrent glioblastoma." J Clin Oncol 27(5): 740-745.

[39] Krishnamachary, B., S. Berg-Dixon, et al. (2003). "Regulation of colon carcinoma cell invasion by hypoxia-inducible factor 1." Cancer Res 63(5): 1138-1143.

[40] Krishnamachary, B., D. Zagzag, et al. (2006). "Hypoxia-inducible factor-1-dependent repression of E-cadherin in von Hippel-Lindau tumor suppressor-null renal cell carcinoma mediated by TCF3, ZFHX1A, and ZFHX1B." Cancer Res 66(5): 2725-2731.

[41] Lee, J. W., S. H. Bae, et al. (2004). "Hypoxia-inducible factor (HIF-1)alpha: its protein stability and biological functions." Exp Mol Med 36(1): 1-12.

[42] Lee, K., D. Z. Qian, et al. (2009). "Anthracycline chemotherapy inhibits HIF-1 transcriptional activity and tumor-induced mobilization of circulating angiogenic cells." Proc Natl Acad Sci U S A 106(7): 2353-2358.

[43] Lee, K., H. Zhang, et al. (2009). "Acriflavine inhibits HIF-1 dimerization, tumor growth, and vascularization." Proc Natl Acad Sci U S A 106(42): 17910-17915.

[44] Li, J., C. Yen, et al. (1997). "PTEN, a putative protein tyrosine phosphatase gene mutated in human brain, breast, and prostate cancer." Science 275(5308): 1943-1947.

[45] Lopes, M. B. (2003). "Angiogenesis in brain tumors." Microsc Res Tech 60(2): 225-230.

[46] Lu, X. and Y. Kang (2010). "Hypoxia and hypoxia-inducible factors: master regulators of metastasis." Clin Cancer Res 16(24): 5928-5935.

[47] Machesky, L. M. (2008). "Lamellipodia and filopodia in metastasis and invasion." FEBS Lett 582(14): 2102-2111.

[48] Makino, Y., R. Cao, et al. (2001). "Inhibitory PAS domain protein is a negative regulator of hypoxia-inducible gene expression." Nature 414(6863): 550-554.

[49] Martens, T., N. O. Schmidt, et al. (2006). "A novel one-armed anti-c-Met antibody inhibits glioblastoma growth in vivo." Clin Cancer Res 12(20 Pt 1): 6144-6152.

[50] Nakamura, M., T. Watanabe, et al. (2001). "p14ARF deletion and methylation in genetic pathways to glioblastomas." Brain Pathol 11(2): 159-168.

[51] Nonn, L., M. Berggren, et al. (2003). "Increased expression of mitochondrial peroxiredoxin-3 (thioredoxin peroxidase-2) protects cancer cells against hypoxia and drug-induced hydrogen peroxide-dependent apoptosis." Mol Cancer Res 1(9): 682-689.

[52] Norden, A. D., J. Drappatz, et al. (2009). "An exploratory survival analysis of anti-angiogenic therapy for recurrent malignant glioma." J Neurooncol 92(2): 149-155.

[53] Novoa, I., H. Zeng, et al. (2001). "Feedback inhibition of the unfolded protein response by GADD34-mediated dephosphorylation of eIF2alpha." J Cell Biol 153(5): 1011-1022.

[54] Onesto, C., E. Berra, et al. (2004). "Poly(A)-binding protein-interacting protein 2, a strong regulator of vascular endothelial growth factor mRNA." J Biol Chem 279(33): 34217-34226.

[55] Onishi, M., T. Ichikawa, et al. (2011). "Angiogenesis and invasion in glioma." Brain Tumor Pathol 28(1): 13-24.

[56] Palazon, A., J. Aragones, et al. (2012). "Molecular pathways: hypoxia response in immune cells fighting or promoting cancer." Clin Cancer Res 18(5): 1207-1213.

[57] Papandreou, I., R. A. Cairns, et al. (2006). "HIF-1 mediates adaptation to hypoxia by actively downregulating mitochondrial oxygen consumption." Cell Metab 3(3): 187-197.

[58] Peak, S. J. and V. A. Levin (2010). "Role of bevacizumab therapy in the management of glioblastoma." Cancer Manag Res 2: 97-104.

[59] Petrosillo, G., F. M. Ruggiero, et al. (2003). "Role of reactive oxygen species and cardiolipin in the release of cytochrome c from mitochondria." FASEB J 17(15): 2202-2208.

[60] Plasswilm, L., A. Tannapfel, et al. (2000). "Hypoxia-induced tumour cell migration in an in vivo chicken model." Pathobiology 68(3): 99-105.

[61] Province, P., X. Han, et al. (2011). Anti-Angiogenic Therapy for Malignant Glioma: Insights and Future Directions. Management of CNS Tumors. D. M. Garami, InTech.

[62] Raizer, J. J., S. Grimm, et al. (2010). "A phase 2 trial of single-agent bevacizumab given in an every-3-week schedule for patients with recurrent high-grade gliomas." Cancer 116(22): 5297-5305.

[63] Reifenberger, G., L. Liu, et al. (1993). "Amplification and overexpression of the MDM2 gene in a subset of human malignant gliomas without p53 mutations." Cancer Res 53(12): 2736-2739.

[64] Rey, S. and G. L. Semenza (2010). "Hypoxia-inducible factor-1-dependent mechanisms of vascularization and vascular remodelling." Cardiovasc Res 86(2): 236-242.

[65] Ricard, D., A. Idbaih, et al. (2012). "Primary brain tumours in adults." Lancet 379(9830): 1984-1996.

[66] Robe, P. A., M. Bentires-Alj, et al. (2004). "In vitro and in vivo activity of the nuclear factor-kappaB inhibitor sulfasalazine in human glioblastomas." Clin Cancer Res 10(16): 5595-5603.

[67] Rong, Y., D. L. Durden, et al. (2006). "'Pseudopalisading' necrosis in glioblastoma: a familiar morphologic feature that links vascular pathology, hypoxia, and angiogenesis." J Neuropathol Exp Neurol 65(6): 529-539.

[68] Sanli, G. and M. Blaber (2001). "Structural assembly of the active site in an aldo-keto reductase by NADPH cofactor." J Mol Biol 309(5): 1209-1218.

[69] Semenza, G. L. (1998). "Hypoxia-inducible factor 1 and the molecular physiology of oxygen homeostasis." J Lab Clin Med 131(3): 207-214.

[70] Semenza, G. L. (2000). "HIF-1: mediator of physiological and pathophysiological responses to hypoxia." J Appl Physiol 88(4): 1474-1480.

[71] Semenza, G. L. (2003). "Targeting HIF-1 for cancer therapy." Nat Rev Cancer 3(10): 721-732.

[72] Semenza, G. L. (2012). "Hypoxia-inducible factors in physiology and medicine." Cell 148(3): 399-408.

[73] Semenza, G. L. (2012). "Hypoxia-inducible factors: mediators of cancer progression and targets for cancer therapy." Trends Pharmacol Sci 33(4): 207-214.

[74] Shimizu, S., Y. Eguchi, et al. (1995). "Prevention of hypoxia-induced cell death by Bcl-2 and Bcl-xL." Nature 374(6525): 811-813.

[75] Stupp, R., M. E. Hegi, et al. (2009). "Effects of radiotherapy with concomitant and adjuvant temozolomide versus radiotherapy alone on survival in glioblastoma in a randomised phase III study: 5-year analysis of the EORTC-NCIC trial." Lancet Oncol 10(5): 459-466.

[76] Stupp, R., W. P. Mason, et al. (2005). "Radiotherapy plus concomitant and adjuvant temozolomide for glioblastoma." N Engl J Med 352(10): 987-996.

[77] Sullivan, R. and C. H. Graham (2007). "Hypoxia-driven selection of the metastatic phenotype." Cancer Metastasis Rev 26(2): 319-331.

[78] Takano, S., Y. Yoshii, et al. (1996). "Concentration of vascular endothelial growth factor in the serum and tumor tissue of brain tumor patients." Cancer Res 56(9): 2185-2190.

[79] Thomlinson, R. H. and L. H. Gray (1955). "The histological structure of some human lung cancers and the possible implications for radiotherapy." Br J Cancer 9(4): 539-549.

[80] van den Bent, M. J., M. A. Vogelbaum, et al. (2009). "End point assessment in gliomas: novel treatments limit usefulness of classical Macdonald's Criteria." J Clin Oncol 27(18): 2905-2908.

[81] van Zijl, F., G. Krupitza, et al. (2011). "Initial steps of metastasis: cell invasion and endothelial transmigration." Mutat Res 728(1-2): 23-34.

[82] Vaupel, P. (2004). "The role of hypoxia-induced factors in tumor progression." Oncologist 9 Suppl 5: 10-17.

[83] Vaupel, P. (2008). "Hypoxia and aggressive tumor phenotype: implications for therapy and prognosis." Oncologist 13 Suppl 3: 21-26.

[84] Vaupel, P., F. Kallinowski, et al. (1989). "Blood flow, oxygen and nutrient supply, and metabolic microenvironment of human tumors: a review." Cancer Res 49(23): 6449-6465.

[85] Wang, G. L., B. H. Jiang, et al. (1995). "Hypoxia-inducible factor 1 is a basic-helix-loop-helix-PAS heterodimer regulated by cellular O2 tension." Proc Natl Acad Sci U S A 92(12): 5510-5514.

[86] Wang, H., W. Zhang, et al. (2004). "Analysis of the activation status of Akt, NFkappaB, and Stat3 in human diffuse gliomas." Lab Invest 84(8): 941-951.

[87] Wang, Y., D. Fei, et al. (2004). "Biological activity of bevacizumab, a humanized anti-VEGF antibody in vitro." Angiogenesis 7(4): 335-345.

[88] Wen, P. Y. and S. Kesari (2008). "Malignant gliomas in adults." N Engl J Med 359(5): 492-507.

[89] Wen, P. Y., D. R. Macdonald, et al. (2010). "Updated response assessment criteria for high-grade gliomas: response assessment in neuro-oncology working group." J Clin Oncol 28(11): 1963-1972.

[90] Westphal, M. and K. Lamszus (2011). "The neurobiology of gliomas: from cell biology to the development of therapeutic approaches." Nat Rev Neurosci 12(9): 495-508.

http://dx.doi.org/10.5772/53298

[91] Wheaton, W. W. and N. S. Chandel (2011). "Hypoxia. 2. Hypoxia regulates cellular metabolism." Am J Physiol Cell Physiol 300(3): C385-393.

[92] Yamaguchi, H., J. Wyckoff, et al. (2005). "Cell migration in tumors." Curr Opin Cell Biol 17(5): 559-564.

[93] Yang, M. H., M. Z. Wu, et al. (2008). "Direct regulation of TWIST by HIF-1alpha promotes metastasis." Nat Cell Biol 10(3): 295-305.

[94] Zhu, S., Y. Zhou, et al. (2011). "Transcriptional upregulation of MT2-MMP in response to hypoxia is promoted by HIF-1alpha in cancer cells." Mol Carcinog 50(10): 770-780.

[95] Zundel, W., C. Schindler, et al. (2000). "Loss of PTEN facilitates HIF-1-mediated gene expression." Genes Dev 14(4): 391-396.

Chapter 4

Brain Tumor–Induced Angiogenesis: Approaches and Bioassays

Stefan W. Hock, Zheng Fan, Michael Buchfelder,
Ilker Y. Eyüpoglu and Nic E. Savaskan

Additional information is available at the end of the chapter

http://dx.doi.org/10.5772/53182

1. Introduction

Investigation on tumor angiogenesis has taken a discontinuous path through history. Studies on blood vessels of the human body are documented for the first time in the 17th century BC by the description of a heartbeat. The Ebers Papyrus (16th century BC) reports how the heart is connected to arteries and primarily describes the high vascularization of tumors. Later, Hippocrates (460-370 BC) made a description that should have a great impact on cancer research: He interpreted the vessels around a malignant tumor as claws of a crab and therefore named the disease *'karkinos'*. From there on tumor vessels had been described with no conceptional impact on therapeutic approaches. In 1971, Judah Folkman kicked a stone with his landmark papers on tumor-induced angiogenesis, thereby promoting a completely new view on cancer biology and therapy. He showed evidence that the tumor is not able to grow beyond a certain barrier without a network of newly recruited microvessels, stating that the tumor stimulates the proliferation of host endothelial cells via secreted factors. Folkman concluded that tumor growth is an angiogenesis-dependent process and thus anti-angiogenetic approaches could be a promising new therapy. [1, 2].

Since then the field of angiogenesis developed dynamically, becoming an actual research avalanche in the past decades. Key molecules and their receptors have been identified, certain hierarchies in signaling have been unveiled and angiogenesis is named as one of the ten hallmarks of cancer development [3]. However, the therapeutic approach to brain tumors is more complicated and has been hampered for tumor heterogeneity, delivery of drugs to the central nervous system and neurotoxic side-effects still represent the main challenges. Furthermore, the role of participating cells remains to be unraveled, i.e. whether interactions between host and tumor cells are required for vessel formation [4, 5, 6].

Blood vessels deliver oxygen and nutrients and are crucially needed for cell survival, cell function and evacuating carbon dioxide and metabolic waste. All cells of the human body reside in a 100 μm-radius to a capillary blood vessel. The close connection between brain and vessels is seen during brain development and axon growth, insofar as the same guidance molecules are recruited for axon targeting and vessel growth [7]. In particular proliferating cells in a tissue depend strongly on continuous blood supply and have an immanent aptitude to foster angiogenesis. They create a microenvironment of contact-dependent (short-range) and secreted (long-range) factors which promote the generation and growth of blood vessels. Thus, it is tempting to speculate that neoplasms have to evolve angiogenic abilities to induce neovasculature in order to develop and progress in size [8, 9, 10]. Beside normal development, physiological tissue remodeling, tumor growth, metastasis and inflammation, angiogenesis is associated with a wide range of other pathologies such as cardio-vascular and ocular diseases [11].

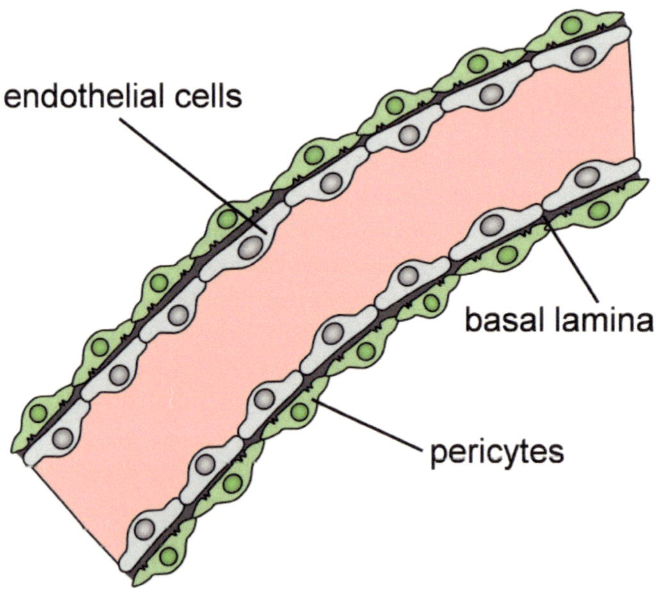

Figure 1. Vessel scheme showing the three main cellular components. The inner layer consists of endothelial cells, lining the inside (lumen) of the vessel. The tube is covered on the outer side by pericytes and smooth muscle cells. The relation of endothelial cells and pericytes is specifically in the brain with a ratio of 1:1. In between is a layer of extracellular matrix tissue known as basal lamina.

During development, two physiological processes of vessel growth can be distinguished: First angiogenesis as the sprouting of vessels and capillaries from pre-existing ones, and second vasculogenesis which describes the process of *de novo* formation of vessels from bone marrow-derived progenitor cells. In the mature state in adulthood new vessels are believed to be formed solely through angiogenesis. In contrast, tumor cell proliferation appears in an uncontrolled manner with replicative immortality and sustained angiogenesis is reinforced by vasculogenesis. While in physiological processes e.g. wound healing, angiogenesis is merely active transiently, an "angiogenic switch" is almost always turned on in tumor development. It appears plausible that the angiogenic switch is redox dependent and controlled by counterbalancing positive and negative factors, either inducing or blocking angiogenesis [12, 13]. The angiogenesis-inducing factors, such as vascular endothelial growth factor-A (VEGF-A), acidic and basic fibroblast growth factors (FGF1/2), bind to their corresponding receptors on endothelial cells. VEGF-A is one of the major players in embryonic vasculo- and angiogenesis as well as in endothelial cell survival. The expression of VEGF-A and FGF-1/-2 can be chronically upregulated by hypoxia and oncogenes. However, the blood vessels produced by chronically dominant proangiogenic factors show characteristic morphological aberrations: The tumor-induced neovasculature is marked by a high-density capillary microvessel network with extreme vessel branching, auto-looping, tortous, disorganized and enlarged vessels.

2. Identification of key angiogenic factors

Several hypotheses have been raised regarding the importance of tumor-induced angiogenesis in development and metastasis of tumors. Dr. Folkman summarized the work of insightful investigators at that time, such as Algire and Chalkley [14], Warren [15], and Greenblatt and Shubik [16], who first termed the process of 'tumor angiogenesis'. Thus, Folkman coined the concept of treating solid tumors by inhibiting angiogenesis.

Folkman's visionary hypotheses consisted of the ideas that primary tumors remain dormant in terms of angiogenesis up to a maximum size of approximately 1-2 mm in diameter. Tumor growth beyond that avascular state, switches angiogenesis on by perverting the circumvent mature host blood vessels to start sprouting towards and probably infiltrate the tumors. This process creates a network of new capillaries within and around the tumorbulk. This idea of an angiogenic switch was supported by an orphan vascular growth factor [17] produced by tumors, which has been initially termed 'tumor angiogenesis factor' (TAF) [18]. Therefore it would seem plausible to affect the tumor growth by diminishing or even preventing angiogenesis via blocking TAF or its receptors. This 'dormancy-inducing' therapeutic approach was thought not to be curative in the common sense but suggested the prevention of further tumor expansion. At best it would result in sustained regression of established tumor bulks to a size of 1-2 mm in diameter so that survival is possible through diffusion and a blood vessel supply is not necessary.

During the following decade Folkman's ideas though very logical and envisioned but still hypothetical attracted little scientific interest. The situation challenged with the identification and cloning of the first pro-angiogenic factor in the mid 1980s when Sing *et al.* isolated the **basic fibroblast growth factor** (bFGF/FGF-2) from chondrosarcoma [19]. The authors showed that bFGF is a tumor-derived growth factor, which can induce angiogenesis in different models [20]. bFGF belongs to a group of structurally related signaling molecules, all binding fibroblast growth factor receptors (aFGF/FGF-1, FGFRs). Up to now, the FGFR-family consists of four members: FGFR1, FGFR2, FGFR3 and FGFR4. Alternate splicing of FGFR1-3 gives rise to 'b' and 'c' variants resulting in seven FGFR-subtypes that can be present on the cell surface. Beside monitoring critical functions during normal development of vertebrates and invertebrates [21, 22], FGF-1 and FGF-2 take part in the promotion of endothelial cell and fibroblast proliferation and organizes endothelial cells into tube-like structures. As FGF is quite ubiquitous in the human body it is thought to have a higher angiogenic potential than other angiogenic factors (VEGF, PDGF) [23].

The interest in the research field of angiogenesis actually started to grow in the mid and late 1970s when the group of Dvorak et al. [24, 25] published their paper on one pro-angiogenic factor originally discovered in the late 1970s as a protein secreted by tumors that could increase the permeability of the microvasculature to plasma proteins [26], thus termed **vascular permeability factor** (VPF). It is the founding member of the later termed **vascular endothelial growth factor**- (VEGF-) family, a group of closely related cytokines (VEGF, VEGF-B, VEGF-C, VEGF-D, PDGF, VEGF-F) identified by Ferrera and colleagues [27, 28]with functions in the physiological and pathological processes of vasculogenesis, angiogenesis and lymphangiogenesis. VPF/VEGF (or VEGF-A) is the most important: It is essential for developmental vasculogenesis and angiogenesis, it increases the permeability of microvasculature to plasma proteins, a characteristic especially known for tumor vasculature in the beginning of tumor stroma generation [29]. VEGF is clinically relevant due to its widespread overexpression in different human cancers and is a candidate for evaluating the prognosis of individual patients. Unlike FGF, which is nonselective for endothelium and stimulates division in many different cell types, VEGF-A is a mitogen specific for the vascular endothelium. VEGF-A is a highly conserved dimeric glycoprotein (34-45kd), constituted of two chains arranged in an antiparallel fashion and bonded via disulfides. The coding region of VEGF-A on chromosome 6 consists of eight exons. Depending on the alternate splicing three different isoforms are prominently encoded in human cells with polypeptides of 189, 165 and 121 amino acids. Despite physical differences, the three VEGF-A isoforms apparently have identical biological activity when in solution.

VEGF-A signals through two major transmembrane tyrosine kinase receptors binding the factor with high affinity. The first is termed flt-1 or VEGF receptor 1 (VEGFR1) and the second is flk-1/KDR (VEGF-receptor-2, VEGFR2). Both tyrosin kinase receptors are mainly though not exclusively expressed on vascular endothelium. Especially endothelial cells of newly formed blood vessels and the vasculature of tumors expressing VEGF-A have a highly elevated expression of both receptors [30]. VEGF-A is overexpressed by the vast majority of cancers [31] and premalignant lesions (e.g. precursor lesions of breast, cervix and colon cancer) and, furthermore, correlates positively with malignant progression [32, 33].

Previously, neuropilin-1 (NRP-1, NP-1) a semaphorine receptor involved in axon guidance during brain development [34, 35] has been shown to play a role in angiogenesis-independent malignant progression [36] by increasing the affinity of various VEGF ligands to the primary VEGF-receptors. Cariboni et al. were also able to illustrate a KDR and blood vessel independent way via VEGF-NRP-1 interactions [37]. Its isoform, neuropilin-2 receptor probably modulates the affinity of VEGF-C and -D to VEGFR-3 and is thought to be important in lymphangiogenesis [38, 39].

Although the specific biological functions mediated by the different receptors are not established precisely, it seems likely that VEGFR-2 is one of the major players in tumor-induced angiogenesis and carcinogenesis. Inasmuch as VEGFR-2 is responsible for the microvascular permeability and the subsequent proliferation and migration of endothelial cells, it is holding a unique position in tumor angiogenesis:

As tumor-derived VEGF-A binds to receptors on the tumor cells themselves, VEGF-A creates a self-perpetuating loop and induces angiogenesis and carcinogenesis in a paracrine or autocrine fashion. The possibility of a therapeutic intervention stimulated academic centers as well as the biotech and pharmaceutical industries to develop VEGF-R-blockers. *Inter alia*, Sunitinib, Imatinib or Avastin/Bevacizumab have so far been created and are used as therapeutics in various cancers.

More recently a second family of ligands and receptors specific for vascular endothelial cells has emerged: the **angiopoietin-tie-system** as non-redundant regulator of endothelial cell activation [40, 41]. Curiously, in this case was that the receptors were discovered first (tie-2/tek and tie-1) and remained orphan receptors until angiopoietin-1 (ang-1) and angiopoietin-2 (ang-2) have been found to be ligands of tie-2 by Yancopolous *et al*. Ang-1 is essentially expressed by pericytes and smooth muscle cells, whereas ang-2 is stored in the granules of endothelial cells (Weibel-Palade bodies) and secreted after stimulation. Most interestingly ang-1 and ang-2 are antagonistic ligands with a high binding affinity to tie-2. While ang-1 functions as agonist to tie-2 promoting angiogenesis, inhibiting vessel leakage and suppressing inflammatory gene expression [42, 43], ang-2 behaves oppositely, causes endothelial cell apoptosis and as a result regression of newly formed vessels [44]. The situation changes completely when ang-2 acts in combination with VEGF-A, for the two work in and promote angiogenesis [45].

After focusing the first two decades of research on pro-angiogenic growth factor stimulators and how to intervene in their pathways to exogenously block the process of angiogenesis, **endogenous inhibitors** entered the scene and a large, growing family of antiangiogenic basement membrane proteins, hormone metabolites and apoptosis modulators has been discovered. Among others thrombospondin-1, interferon α/β, arresten, canstatin, angiostatin, tissue inhibitors of matrix metalloproteinases (TIMP) and vascular endothelial growth inhibitor (VEGI) have been proven to be endogenous inhibitors (Table 1).

Today, it is accepted that endogenous inhibitors activate a cellular 'brake' mechanism. This mechanism leads to altered cell-cell-interactions, malignancy associated with induced angiogenesis and other diseases like ocular disorders or rheumatoid arthritis when turned off. In case of dominant endogenous inhibitors and deactivated angiogenic switch, launching angiogenesis is (almost) impossible.

Name	Description
Angiopoietin-2 (Ang-2)	Non-matrix derived; stored in Weibel-Palade bodies; inhibits EC proliferation an migration; antagonist of ang-1; in clinical trial [46, 47]
Angiostatin	Non-matrix derived; 38-45kDa, involves either kringle domains 1-3, or smaller kringle 5 fragments [48, 49]
Arresten	Matrix derived; 26-kDa; from type IV collagen; selectively inhibits EC tube formation, interferes with FGF-2 [50, 51]
Canstatin	Matrix derived; 24-kDa; from type IV collagen; inhibits EC migration and tube formation dose-dependently [52]
Endorepellin	Matrix derived; from perlecan; inhibits several aspects of angiogenesis [53, 54]
Endostatin	Matrix derived; 20-kDa; zinc-binding fragment of type XVIII collagen; blocks angiogenesis, primary tumor growth and metastasis; interferes with FGF-2; Phase II [55]
Interferon α/β	Non-matrix derived; anti-viral proteins; Phase III (Interferon-β) [56]
Interleukins	Leukocyte-derived; heterogeneous superfamily [57]
2-Methoxyestradiol	Estradiol metabolite; Phase II [58]
Meth-1/-2	Non-matrix derived; proteins containing metalloprotease and thrombospondin domains [59]
Platelet factor-4	Inhibits FGF-2-induced EC proliferation [60]
Prolactin fragment	Derived from prolactin; 16-kDa; blocks angiogenesis; inhibits VEGF-induced Ras-activation [61]
Thrombospondin-1/-2	Matrix derived; large extracellular matrix protein; Phase II (Thrombospondin-1) [62]
TIMP	Non-matrix derived; suppress MMP activity; pluripotent effect on EC growth, apoptosis and cell differentiation [63]
Troponin I	Cartilage-derived; inhibits EC proliferation and angiogenesis [64]
Tumstatin	Matrix derived; 28-kDa from type IV collagen; apoptosis of EC [65, 66]
VEGI	174 amino acid cytokine; TNF-superfamily; autocrine apoptosis in EC [67]
Vasostatin	Non-matrix derived; fragment of calreticulin; selectively inhibits EC proliferation and angiogenesis in response to stimulus; suppresses tumor growth [68]

Table 1. Summary chart of various endogenous inhibitors of angiogenesis

http://dx.doi.org/10.5772/53182

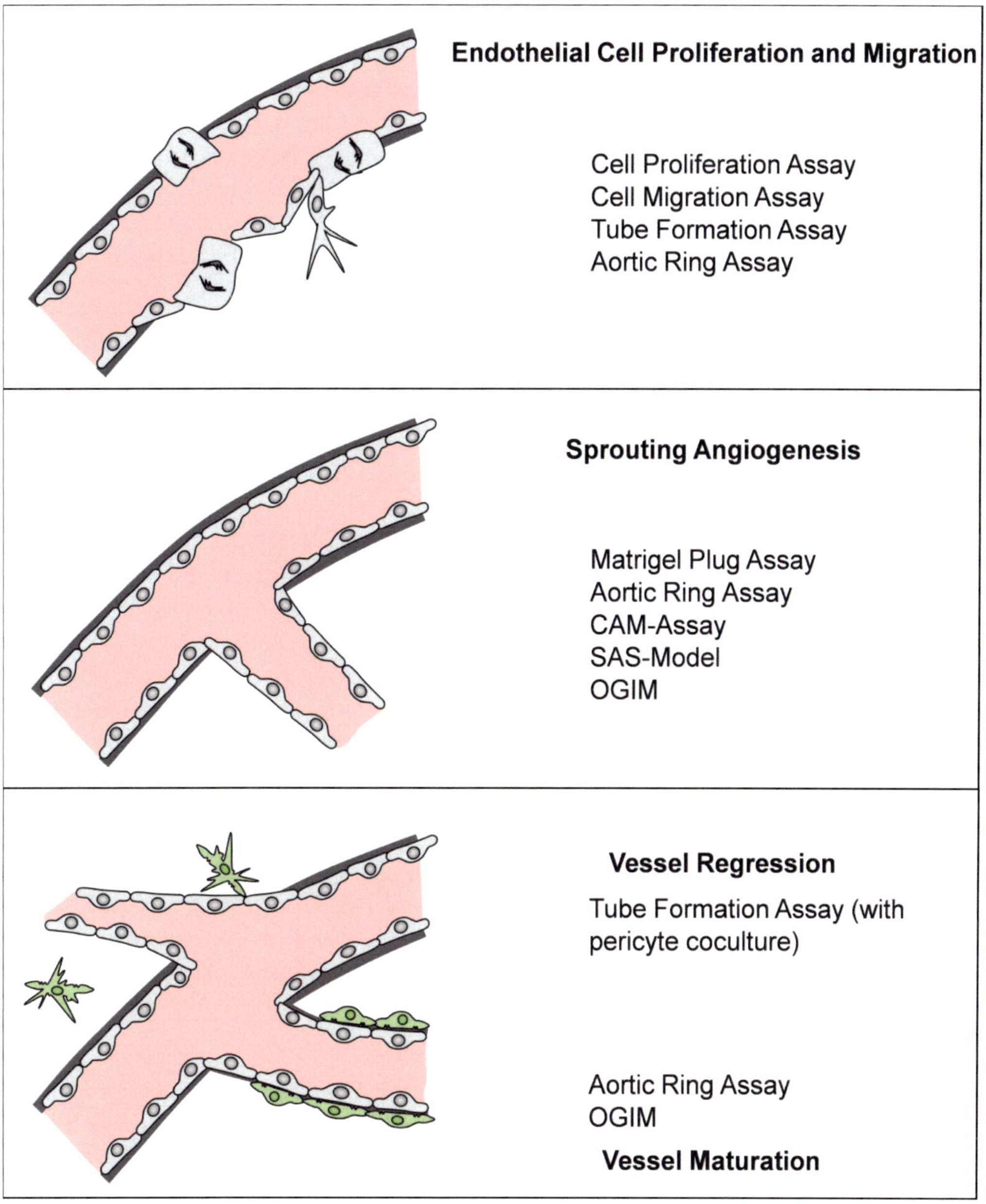

Figure 2. The key steps of angiogenesis. After binding of angiogenic factors to their receptor, endothelial cells start to proliferate and migrate towards the source of angiogenic activity (upper panel). This induces the sprouting and formation of a new branch (middle). Newly sprouted vasculature can either undergo maturation or regression (lower panel). Depending on the biological events of interest different bioassays are available with particular advantages for gauging.

3. *In vitro* assays to study brain tumor angiogenesis

The human brain is made up of various cell types of different lineages (neuroepithelial, epithelial and mesenchymal traits). Brain cells include astrocytes, oligodendrocytes, neurons, microglia, ependyma and vessels which interact with each other and form a particular environment via signaling molecules. Therefore the most important issues for *in vitro* bioassays are to reduce such complexity and to make single biological events measurable in a reasonable way. *In vitro* assays allow a high level of redundancy and permit the researcher to focus on single biological events.

Besides perictyes and the vessel-surrounding tissue, endothelial cells lining all blood vessels of the body are the prominent cells involved in neovascularization. New blood vessel formation follows in principle four cardinal steps: First step is that endothelial cells need to adhere, proliferate and permeabilize the environmental boundaries. Therefore endothelial cells undergo cell division and start to secret proteases to degrade the matrix and brake through the basal lamina, which is the second inner layer of the vessel. Second, migration and invasion towards angiogenic stimuli needs to be facilitated (VEGF, FGF, PDGF, etc.). Endothelial cells use for instance integrins to travel in tandem. This event is connected with the sprouting of newly formed vessel barbs. As a source, angiogenic stimuli can be secreted by activated lymphocytes, tumor cells, microglia and macrophages. Thirdly, endothelial vessel sprouts form new vessels and recruit cellular components to line up a fully functional vessel. The fourth key step is the modeling and reorganization process. Newly formed vessels can maturate or undergo regression. For each of the four key steps several *in vitro* assays have been developed.

3.1. Tube Formation Assay (TFA)

In the past we considered the vascular endothelium as a passive structure which acts like a filter between the blood in the vessel lumen and the vessel wall itself. In fact endothelial cells are active members of the vascular homeostasis playing a vital role in the coagulation and the fibrinolysis system as well as in adhesion and aggregation of blood platelets via secreted activators and inhibitors. These processes (among others) can be studied *in vitro* using human vascular endothelial cells isolated from umbilical veins.

Human umbilical vein endothelial cells (HUVECs) were isolated from freshly obtained human umbilical cords the first time by Eric A. Jaffe in 1973 [69]. They were able to identify the cell morphologically (Weible-Palade bodies) and immunologically (ABH antigens fitting to the donor's blood type) as human endothelial cells and demonstrated that it is possible to culture them for a period of time. Endothelial cells of all origin seem to have the ability to form three-dimensional structures (tubes, cobblestone pattern), which can be fostered by coating the plastic culture dishes with either collagen or fibrin clots. The formation of tight junctions between endothelial cells can be confirmed by electron microscopy.

The tube formation assay is a viable assay, which can be accomplished within a day. Image analysis is used generally to measure the endothelial cells ability to form tube-like structures. Further endothelial cell adhesion, migration and invasion have been reported [70]. Though

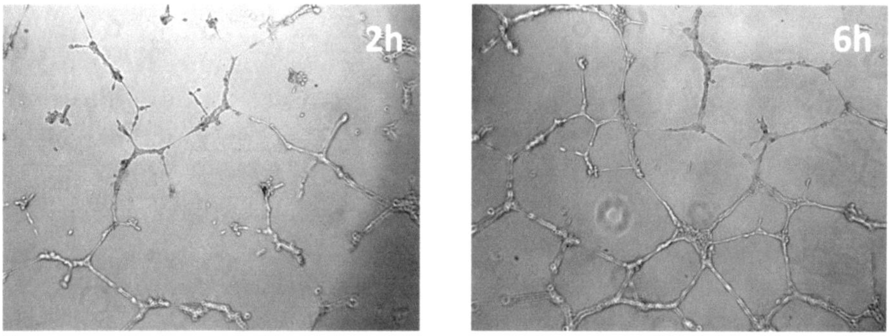

Figure 3. Tube formation assay in time lapse modus. Representative photographs of tubes formed by human umbilical vein endothelial cells (HUVECs). The left picture is taken 2 h after plating and shows beginning tube formation. The right picture is taken 6 hours after plating and shows the typical 'cobblestone' forming. Images are given as x10 magnification.

very reliable in studying the reorganization, the TFA represents only a small part of angiogenesis and allows specific predictions of the nature of different endothelial cell strains rather than testifying the angiogenic process itself.

3.2. Cell proliferation assays

There is a large variety of assays to measure cell proliferation. Well-established ones are for example the MTT-assay, in which living cells reduce 3-(4,5-Dimethylthiazol-2-yl)-2,5-diphenyltetrazolium bromide, a yellow tetrazole to purple formazan, and the thymidine incorporation assay using BrdU (5-bromo-2'-deoxyuridine), an analogue of thymidine. Both assays are performed to detect proliferating cells in living tissue, Especially the BrdU incorporation assay is most frequently used for cell proliferation studies in angiogenesis.

The cells used in proliferation assays are endothelial cells. However, it matters from which source the endothelial cells are isolated since they differ not only between large-vessel-derived endothelial cells and ones originated from microvasculature. They also seem to have distinctive characteristics when obtained from different organs and even when taken from different sites in one single organ (71, 72, 73). Another fact is the total difference between species, which cannot be ignored: One example are the pig and murine endothelial cells, which bind BSL-1 and BSL-4 (lectin from *Bandeira simplifolica*) and are therefore a target for hyper-immune destruction when implanted into patients.

The most common cell types used in this assay are either bovine aortic endothelial cells or human umbilical vein endothelial cells. During culture in the laboratory these cells are by nature in a proliferative state, while they are more in a quiescent, non-proliferative state *in vivo*. Therefore endothelial cells *in vitro* depend on the environment in which they are kept during culturing.

3.3. Cell migration assay

Cell migration is the movement of cells from one area to another induced by chemical signals. Generally cell migration plays a vital role in processes like cell differentiation, tumor metastasis and wound healing. In angiogenesis studies the focus is mainly laid on migrating endothelial cells. In terms of angiogenesis one should speak of cell invasion, for endothelial primarily degrade the basal lamina before migrating toward an angiogenic stimulus.

The assays most frequently performed are the blind-well chemotaxis chamber and the scratch-wound assay. The blind-well chemotaxis chamber is a modified Boyden chamber as used for classic neutrophil chemotaxis. Instead, endothelial cells are placed on a cell permeable filter. When an angiogenic stimulus is added into the medium below the filter, the cells start to migrate. The system is very useful in concentration-dependent effects.

In the other preferred assay, the scratch-wound assay [74, 75], HUVECs are used to be seeded into trans-wells. When the cells are 85-95% confluent a wound/scratch is set. The test is used to measure the time needed under different conditions (drug treatment, etc.) to close the wound again.

3.4. Aortic Ring Assay (ARA)

The Rat Aortic Ring Assay, originally developed by Nicosia *et al.* [76] phenocopies all the key steps in the angiogenesis process: matrix degradation, migration and proliferation of endothelial cells and structural reorganization. The basis of this assay is the excised aorta (of rats or mice) from which the connective tissue has been removed. The aortic tube will then be cut into rings or small pieces (aortic explants) and taken into culture with collagen gel. Several days after culture initiation the aortic tissue gives rise to a microvascular network of branching endothelial tubes, a process which is triggered by the dissection procedure and the growth factors produced by the rings/explants.

Since angiogenesis *in vivo* not only involves endothelial cells, but also pericytes, the basal lamina and other surrounding cells, researchers have moved to asses angiogenesis by organ culture methods. Of these, the rat aortic ring assay has become one of the most widely used ones. In particular, it has several advantages compared to "normal" *in vitro* single-cell culture: As the assay is based on explants, it does not only consist of endothelial cells which have been selected via cell passaging, but of endothelial cells and multiple other cell types which are in a non-proliferative state and therefore closer to a real-life environment. It is even possible to recapitulate all of the key steps of endothelial cell sprouting or angiogenesis: Matrix degradation, that is to say breaking through the basal lamina, which is the second layer of mature vessel enveloping the endothelial cells, migration toward a signal source, proliferation and finally reorganization or tube-forming can be analyzed. After several days in culture image analysis is used to measure length and abundance of the sprouting endothelial cells.

Although the situation in the aortic ring assay is closer to the in vivo environment than in dissociated single cell culture assays, one has to deal with the higher experimental variability due to animal strains and animal age. The main factors here are the incomplete removal of the surrounding connective tissue which can affect the sprouting and outgrowth of endothelial

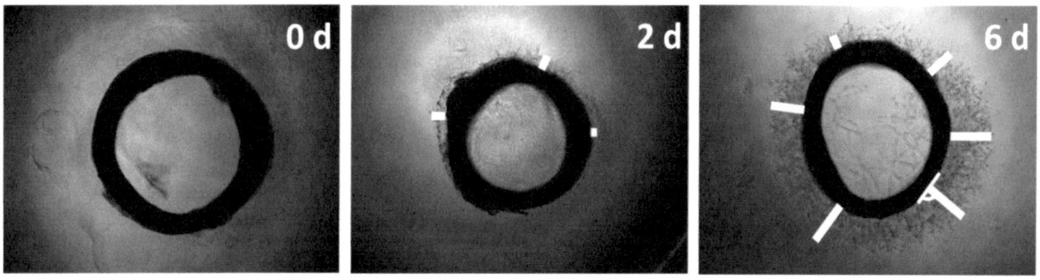

Figure 4. Aortic ring assay experiments. Phase-contrast images showing endothelial sprouting from aortic rings embedded in Matrigel and the method of quantification. To make the data comparable, we developed a tangents measure methods. Tangents are set in respect to the ring and measurements can be conducted of the sprouting distance with 90° to the tangent (white bars).

cells, the tissue from multiple animals itself which can result in an inconstant angiogenic response and last, the evaluation of the images, for the sprouting is a three-dimensional process.

The aortic ring assay is a reliable assay to test substances for their potential to positively or negatively affect angiogenesis and is able to monitor angiogenesis activity.

4. *In vivo* assays in neuro–oncology

4.1. Chronic window preparations

4.1.1. Rabbit ear chamber

In 1924 Sandison *et al.* developed the first chronic window preparation. They implanted a transparent window chamber in the ear of a rabbit [77]. The preparation allows inspection of an *in vivo* environment from outside the body, a long-term monitoring of angiogenesis is possible. Clark et al. made the first steps by studying wound-healing associated angiogenesis [78, 79]. Ide *et al.* adopted the method, transplanted tumors and were able to observe strong tumour growth associated with a newly formed vascular network [80]. Their results led to the proposal of a *'vessel growth- stimulating substance'* produced by the tumor.

4.1.2. Dorsal skinfold chamber

The dorsal skinfold chamber is an adaption of the rabbit ear chamber made by Algire *et al.* in the 1940s [81, 82]. A metal chamber with a transparent window is implanted in various animal species, in rodents it is the most widely used window preparation. The dorsal window can last 30-40 days. To study the effect of tumors on vessel formation, fluorescent tumor cells are implanted into the chamber and the angiogenic activity, infiltration by immune cells, tumor cell migration and tumor growth are then monitored by intravital microscopy (IVM) [83, 84].

The main limitation of this model is the non-organotypical environment of tumors other than skin cancer.

4.2. Chick embryo chorioallantoic membrane (CAM-) assay

A widely performed assay to test angiogenesis *in vivo* is the chorioallantoic membrane (CAM-) assay. Initially, Murphy *et al.* [85] implanted rat Jensen sarcoma cells into the CAM of chicken eggs and were able to show signs of tumor-induced angiogenesis. Highly promoted by Folkman *et al.*, the CAM-assay has been transposed to the developing field of angiogenesis [86].

Since the introduction of the CAM-assay almost a century ago multiple modifications of the original angiogenic assay were made which allow quantification of the angiogenic process. In addition chick embryos are immune-incompetent until embryonic day 17. Therefore grafting of cells of different species (e.g. human tumor cells) is possible so that the CAM-assay became a useful tool for analysis of the proangiogenic potential of test cells. The HET-CAM developed by Niels-Peter Lüpke in 1985 [87, 88] and the CAMVA (chorio allantoic membrane vascular assay) are the two modified CAM-assays mainly used in the field of angiogenesis.

The hen's egg test on the chorioallantoic membrane (HET-CAM-) assay is an organotypic model which was initially designed to replace the highly discussed Draize-test to identify irritative reactions in the eye: haemorrhage, lysis and coagulation. These three reactions of the CAM are observed on the ninth day of embryonation. Test substances are applied directly onto the CAM and the membrane is scanned after five minutes for the above named reactions. Further the test allows analysis for angiogenesis of tumor-models growing on the CAM.

The CAMVA monitors the effects of potential eye irritants, drugs or other chemicals on the blood vessels of the CAM. It was developed by Leighton *et al.* [89] in 1985 and adjusted to industrial laboratory standards by Bagley *et al.* [90, 91]. The chorioallantoic membrane vascular assay is considered suitable as an option to replace animal trials to study vascular effects. The preparation of the test starts with an egg four days after fertilization in which a small window over the CAM is cut. By sucking out approximately 3 ml of albumen, best conditions are created for optimal growth of the CAM. Thereafter, the opening is resealed and the eggs incubated for another six days. In the course of incubation, test substances are applied directly onto the CAM, followed by an examination for vascular changes in the CAM. Changes observed are hyperaemia, haemorrhaging and the occurrence of ghost vessels.

4.3. Subcutaneous Air Sac model (SAS)

The rat subcutaneous air sac (SAS-) model was promoted by Lichtenberger *et al.* [92, 93] as a straightforward method to study anti-angiogenesis *in vivo*. A sac is produced by introducing air dorsally to anesthetized rats via subcutaneous injection. So that the wall of the air sac becomes progressively thicker in time, the air sac is re-inflated every fourth day. After 10-14 days an acceptable lining of cells has been grounded and an almost transparent avascular membrane has been created. Before treated another 10 days subcutaneously with various test compounds, a sponge is implanted into the cavity. It is important to choose a good injection site which eliminates the risk of interfering and irritating the membrane. To study tumor-induced angiogenesis, tumor cells are inoculated subcutaneously on the membrane. Funahashi *et al.* modified the assay and use a tumor cell-containing chamber to determine the angiogenic effect. After the 10-day-treatment the animals are being sacrificed, the overlying skin of the air sac is removed and the transparent membrane is evaluated *in situ* for angiogenesis.

4.4. Matrigel plug assay

Most angiogenesis *in vivo* assays are very complex in both, the experimental setup and the surgical skills one needs. The matrigel plug assay is a simple *in vivo* angiogenesis assays. Derived from the engelbroth-holm-swarm (EHS) mouse sarcoma, the matrigel matrix is comparable to basement membrane proteins. It is "loaded" with either cells (mostly tumor cells) or angiogenesis-inducing substances (FGF, VEGF, etc.). Cold (and therefore liquid) matrigel is injected subcutaneously in nude mice. With increasing temperature the gel solidifies and forms a plug, which allows cell growth and vessel formation [94]. The plug is removed from the animal after 7-21 days inoculation, fixed with paraffin, stained and examined histologically.

The main benefit of the matrigel plug assay is that it is relatively easy and fast to perform, neither special experimental setup nor surgical skills are required and the test materials are available without difficulty. Nevertheless, the assay is limited to its specific organotypic location, i.e. subcutaneous. Further, matrigel is a reconstituted matrix, with a particular biochemical composition. In addition, Auerbach et al. reported considerable difficulties to maintain comparable three-dimensional plugs despite the fact that the gel volume is kept constant [95].

5. New *ex vivo* model for tumor angiogenesis

5.1. The Organotypic Glioma Invasion Model (OGIM)

The *Organotypic Glioma Invasion Model* (OGIM) is a recently developed method to study physiological angiogenesis and tumor-induced angiogenesis and allows researchers to address systematically molecular pathways of angiogenesis as well as tumor-vessel interactions [96, 97]. Furthermore, it is possible to monitor neuronal and tumor cell death, tumor proliferation and migration in time lapse with focus on specific tumor-host interactions and tumor microenvironment. The method bridges *in vitro* and *in vivo*-assays, since all cells of the brain (astrocytes, oligodendrocytes, neurons, ependymal cells microglia and vessels) are present in a natural environment.

Hippocampal brain slice cultures are acquired from postnatal rats and enhanced green fluorescent protein expressing rat glioma cells are implanted into slices in culture. After implantation cell death can be monitored in different regions of interest: The tumor bulk, the peritumoral invasion zone and the surrounding tissue. The brain slices can be kept in culture for several days after tumor implantation. Consecutively, various immunohistochemical staining for vessels can be performed. Beside the classical vessel marker, the platelet/endothelialmembrane cell adhesion molecule-1 (PECAM-1 or CD31), staining can also be performed with antibodies against laminin, factorVIII (von Willebrand - factor), and smooth muscle actin (SMA). Anti-laminin is used to stain the basal membrane, anti-vWF for endothelial cells and anti-SMA for pericytes.

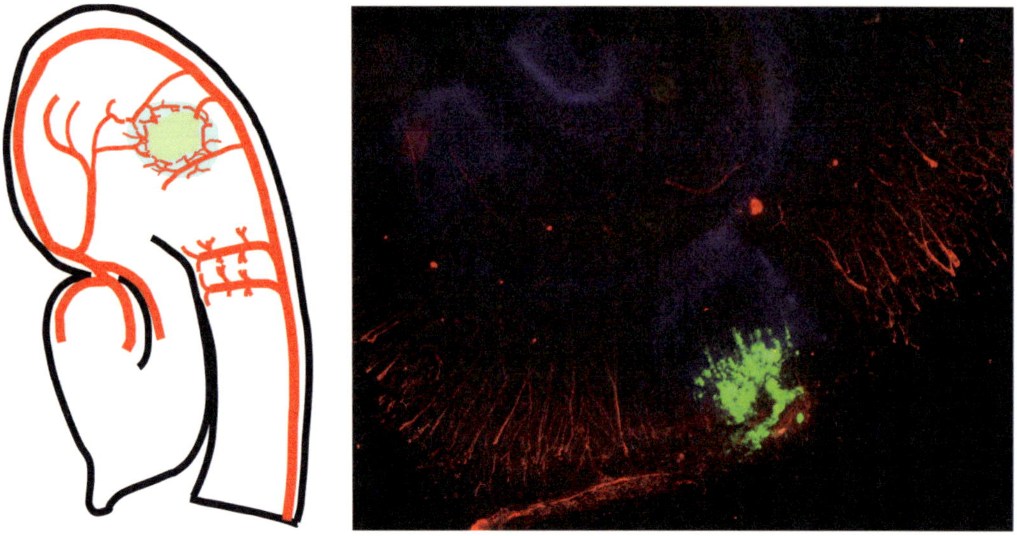

Figure 5. The Organotypic Glioma Invasion Model (OGIM) for angiogenesis studies. Left, Scheme of the brain slice and its vessels in the hippocampus and entorhinal cortex. The vessel architecture in the peritumoral invasion zone differs highly from that of the tumor zone and control area. Right, the fluorescent image shows a typical example of a GFP-tumor-implanted brain slice after immunohistochemistry performed for vessels. Green: glioma cells, blue: nuclei, red: laminin staining. The image is given as x4 magnification.

The OGIM measures vessel density (overlaying grid method), branching as well as morphological vessel aberrations such as tortuous, disorganized vessels, blind-ends and auto-loops. It is also possible to monitor and analyze vascular mimicry in a time lapse mode. In our lab we established glioma vessel features over time. The regular vessel architecture ranging from big lumen vessels down to arteriols, metarteriols and capillaries is breached and replaced by a chaotic vessel structure with probable back-and-forth blood flow and non-functional vessels with blind ends in tumors. Moreover a high-density microvessel network is produced via tumor-induction. The organotypic brain slice model represents the tumor microenvironment *in vitro* in a three-dimensional culture [98], which is biologically more relevant, but technically more challenging than migration, proliferation and cytotoxic assays being an appropriate possibility to test and optimize anti-cancer compounds.

6. Conclusion

The current development of the tumor angiogenesis field with newly identified angiogenic factors craves for robust, viable and easy to perform assays which are also assessable for analysis. Although divergent opinions exist on what are the best methods for studying angiogenesis,

http://dx.doi.org/10.5772/53182

several *in vitro* bio-assays have been established and are in worldwide use. Here we described various established *in vitro* assays commonly used in the phase of expedition and confirmation. Since at least four key steps in angiogenesis exist, i.e. proliferation, migration and invasion, sprouting and vessel formation, and vessel modeling and reorganization (maturation, regression). Thus, *in vitro* bio-assays cannot reflect all key events in one. In principle, this is also the case for *in vivo* assays. For this reason, assays make certain key vascular events assessable in a short period of time leaving others not detected. So far, established endothelial cell culture assays have a high level of redundancy and utilize endothelial cells from different origin which have been preselected for their proliferative capacity. In addition, *in vitro* tissue assays have been established which also consider the microenvironment and represent higher cellular complexity. Further, regarding the amount of data *in vitro* tests can generate, it appears also necessary to spent efforts on the precise evaluation system to be used. Some in vitro assays such as the tube formation assay allow not only for one parameter to investigate, i.e. tube formation, but open the possibility to analyze also the dynamic and morphology of such tubes. *In vivo* assays are more demanding in terms of material, time and labor. Also, these assays often require surgical skills. With all the interactions present, evaluation of certain angiogenesis processes can be hard to perform accurately. On the other hand, *in vivo* assays reflect the organotypic environment and cellular components involved. When developing antiangiogenic drugs, assays are needed that are easy to perform in a short period of time and that consider certain aspects of the *in vivo* situation to prevent artificial phenomena. We describe here a bridge technique, i.e. the o*rganotypic glioma invasion model* (OGIM), which combines the advantages of *in vitro* assays with that of the organotypic brain environment as an *in vivo* situation [98]. The OGIM is a robust *in vitro* assay enabling the investigation of key events of tumor angiogenesis within the brain. This assay allows to analyze the impact of a therapeutic within the balance of concerted factors promoting and inhibiting angiogenesis.

Acknowledgements

We thank all members of our neurooncology lab for critical suggestions and valuable comments during developing new techniques. Our work is supported in part by the German Research Foundation (DFG grant Ey 94/2-1).

Author details

Stefan W. Hock, Zheng Fan, Michael Buchfelder, Ilker Y. Eyüpoglu and Nic E. Savaskan*

*Address all correspondence to: Savaskan@gmx.net

Department of Neurosurgery, University of Erlangen-Nuremberg, Schwabachanlage, Erlangen, Germany

The authors declare no competing financial interests.

References

[1] Folkman J (1971) Tumor angiogenesis: Therapeutic implications. *N Engl J Med*285:1182–1186

[2] Cavallo T (1972) Tumor angiogenesis: Rapid induction of endothelial mitoses demonstrated by autoradiography. *J Cell Biol* 54(2):408-20

[3] Weinberg RA, Hanahan D (2011) Hallmarks of Cancer: The next Generation *Cell* 144(5): 646-74

[4] Mund JA, Case J (2011) The Role of Circulating Endothelial Progenitor Cells in Tumor Angiogenesis. *Curr. Stem. Cell Res. Ther.* 6(2):115-21

[5] Ribatti D (2011) Mast cells, angiogenesis and cancer. *Adv Exp Med Biol.* 716:270-88

[6] Ribatti D (2011) The role of pericytes in angiogenesis. *Int J Dev Biol.* 55(3):261-8.

[7] Carmeliet P, Tessier-Lavigne M (2005) Common mechanisms of nerve and blood vessel wiring. *Nature* 436(7048):193-200.

[8] Bouck N (1996) The insulin-like growth factor II/mannose 6-phosphate receptor is required for proliferin-induced angiogenesis. *Endocrinology* 137(9):3871-6.

[9] Hanahan D & Folkman J (1996) Patters and emerging mechanisms of the angiogenic switch during tumorigenesis. *Cell* 86(3):353-64.

[10] Folkman J (1997) Antiangiogenic therapy of experimental cancer does not induce acquired drug resistance. *Nature* 390(6658):404-7.

[11] Carmeliet P (2003) Angiogenesis in health and disease. *Nat. Med.* 9:653-660.

[12] Baeriswyl V, Christofori G (2009) The angiogenic switch in carcinogenesis. *Semin. Cancer Biol.* 19(5):329-37.

[13] Bergers G, Benjamin LE (2003) Tumorigenesis and the angiogenic switch. *Nat. Rev. Cancer* 3(6):401-10.

[14] Algire GH, Chalkley HW (1945) Vascular reactions of normal and malignant tissue *in vivo*. I. Vascular reactions of mice to wounds and to normal neoplastic implants. *J Natl Cancer Inst.* 6:73-85.

[15] Warren BA, Shubik P (1966) The growth of the blood vessel supply to melanoma transplants in the hamster cheek pouch. *Lab Invest.* 15:464-478.

[16] Greenblatt M, Shubik P (1968) Tumor angiogenesis: transfilter diffusion studies in the hamster by the transparent chamber technique. *J Hatl Cancer Inst.* 41:111-124.

[17] Folkman J (1971) Isolation of a tumor factor responsible for angiogenesis. *J Exp Med.* 133:275-288.

[18] Folkman J (1974) Tumor angiogenesis factor. *Cancer Res.* 34:2109-2113.

[19] Shing Y, Folkman J, Klagsbrun M (1984) Heparin affinity: purification of a tumor-derived capillary endothelial cell growth factor. *Science*. 233:1296-1299.

[20] Folkman J, Klagsbrun M (1987) Angiogenic factors. *Science*. 235:442-447.

[21] Borland CZ, Schutzman JL, Stern MJ (2001) Fibroblast growth factor signaling in Caenorhabditis elegans. *BioEssays* 23(12):1120-1130.

[22] Coumoul X, Deng CX (2003) Roles of FGF receptors in mammalian development and congenital diseases. *Birth Defects Res C Embryo Today* 69(4):286–304.

[23] Vlodavsky Cao R, Cao Y (2003) Angiogenic synergism, vascular stability and improvement of hind-limb ischemia by a combination of PDGF-BB and FGF-2. *Nature Med* 9(5): 604-13

[24] Dvorak HF, Dvorak AM, Manseau EJ (1979) Fibrin gel investment associated with line 1 and line 10 solid tumor growth, angiogenesis and fibroplasia in guinea pigs: Role of cellular immunity, myofibroblasts, microvascular damage and infaction in line 1 tumor regression. *J Natl Cancer Inst*. 62:1459-1472.

[25] Senger DR, Nagy JA, Dvorak AM, Dvorak HF (1993) Vascular permeability factor (VPF, VEGF) in tumor biology. *Cancer Metastasis Rev*. 12:303-324.

[26] Dvorak HF, Orenstein NS, Carvalho AC (1979) Induction of a fribrin-gel investment: An early event in line 10 hepatocarcinoma growth mediated by tumor-secreted products. *J Immunol*. 122:166-174.

[27] Ferrara N, Henzel WJ.(1989) Pituitary follicular cells secrete a novel heparin-binding growth factor specific for vascular endothelial cells. *Biochem Biophys Res Commun*. 161(2):851-8.

[28] Leung DW, Cachianes G, Kuang WJ, Goeddel DV, Ferrara N. (1989) Vascular endothelial growth factor is a secreted angiogenic mitogen. *Science*. 246(4935):1306-9.

[29] Brown LF, Claffey K (1997) Vascular permeability factor/vascular endothelial growth factor: A multifunctional angiogenic cytokine. *EXS*. 79:233-269.

[30] Alon T, Keshet E (1995) Vascular endothelial growth factor acts as a survival factor for newly formed retinal vessels and has implications for retinopathy of prematurity *Nature Med*. 1:1024-1028.

[31] Stiver S (2000) Vascular permeability factor/vascular endothelial growth factor (VPF/ VEGF) *J Clin Ligand Assay*. 23:193-205.

[32] Brown LF (1995) Expression of vascular permeability factor (vascular endothelial growth factor) and its receptors in breast cancer. *Hum Pathol*. 26:86-91.

[33] Wong MP (1999) Vascular endothelial growth factor is upregulated in the early pre-malignant stage of colorectal tumour progression. *Int J Cancer*. 81:845-850.

[34] Sakurai A, Doçi CL, Gutkind JS. (2012) Semaphorin signaling in angiogenesis, lymphangiogenesis and cancer. *Cell Res*. 22(1):23-32.

[35] Neufeld G, Shraga-Heled N. (2005) Semaphorins in cancer. *Front Biosci*. 10:751-60.

[36] Cao Y, Wang E, Mukhopadhyay D (2012) VEGF exerts an angiogenesis-independent function in cancer cells to promote their malignant progression. *Cancer Res*. 72(16): 3912-8.

[37] Cariboni A, Davidson K, Ruhrberg C (2011) VEGF signalling controls GnRH neuron survival via NRP1 independently of KDR and blood vessels. *Development*. 138(17): 3723-33.

[38] Susarla R, Gonzalez AM, Watkinson JC, Eggo MC. (2012) Expression of receptors for VEGFs on normal human thyroid follicular cells and their role in follicle formation. *J Cell Physiol*. 227(5):1992-2002.

[39] Xu Y, Yuan L, Mak J, Pardanaud L, Bagri A. (2010) Neuropilin-2 mediates VEGF-C-induced lymphatic sprouting together with VEGFR3. *J Cell Biol*. 188(1):115-30.

[40] Davis S, Aldrich TH, Jones PF, Acheson A, Compton DL, Jain V, Ryan TE, Bruno J, Radziejewski C, Maisonpierre PC, Yancopoulos GD (1996) Isolation of angiopoietin-1, a ligand for the TIE2 receptor, by secretion-trap expression cloning. *Cell*. 87:1161-1169.

[41] Suri C, Jones PF, Patan S, Bartunkova S, Maisonpierre PC, Davis S, Sato TN, Yancopoulos GD (1996) Requisite role of angiopoietin-1, a ligand for the TIE2 receptor, during embryonic angiogenesis. *Cell*. 87:1171-1180.

[42] Mammoto T, Parikh SM, Mammoto A, Gallagher D, Chan B, Mostoslavsky G, Ingber DE, Sukhatme VP (2007) Angiopoietin-1 requires p190 RhoGAP to protect against vascular leakage *in vivo*. *J Biol Chem*. 282:23910-23918.

[43] Witzenbichler B, Westermann D, Knueppel S, Schultheiss HP, Tschope C (2005) Protective role of angiopoietin-1 in endotoxic shock. *Circulation*. 111:97-105.

[44] Maisonpierre PC, Suri C, Jones PF, Bartunkova S, Wiegand SJ, Radziejewski C, Compton D, McClain J, Aldrich TH, Papadopoulos N, Daly TJ, Davis S, Sato TN, Yancopoulos GD (1997) Angiopoietin-2, a natural antagonist for Tie2 that disrupts *in vivo* angiogenesis. *Science*. 277(5322):55-60.

[45] Holash J, Maisonpierre PC, Compton D, Boland P, Alexander CR, Zagzag D, Yancopoulos GD, Wiegand SJ (1999) Vessel cooption, regression, and growth in tumors mediated by angiopoietins and VEGF. *Science*. 284(5422):1994-8.

[46] Davis S, Yancopoulos GD. (1999) The angiopoietins: Yin and Yang in angiogenesis. *Curr Top Microbiol Immunol*. 237:173-85

[47] Maisonpierre PC, Suri C, Jones PF, Bartunkova S, Wiegand SJ, Radziejewski C, Compton D, McClain J, Aldrich TH, Papadopoulos N, Daly TJ, Davis S, Sato TN, Yancopoulos GD. Angiopoietin-2, a natural antagonist for Tie2 that disrupts *in vivo* angiogenesis. *Science*. 277(5322):55-60.

[48] O'Reilly MS, Holmgren L, Shing Y, Sage EH, Folkman J. (1994) Angiostatin: A novel angiogenesis inhibitor that mediates the suppression of metastases by a Lewis lung carcinoma. *Cell*. 79:315-328.

[49] Cao Y, Chen A, An SS, Ji RW, Davidson D, Llinás M. (1997) Kringle 5 of plasminogen is a novel inhibitor of endothelial cell growth. *J Biol Chem*. 272(36):22924-8.

[50] Timpl R. (1996) Macromolecular organization of basement membranes. *Curr Opin Cell Biol*. 8:618–24

[51] Madri JA. (1997) Extracellular matrix modulation of vascular cell behaviour. *Transpl Immunol*. 5:179–83

[52] Kamphaus GD, Colorado PC, Panka DJ. (2000) Canstatin, a novel matrix-derived inhibitor of angiogenesis and tumor growth. *J Biol Chem*. 275:1209–15.

[53] Yurchenco PD, O'Rear JJ. (1994) Basal lamina assembly. *Curr Opin Cell Biol*. 6:674–81.

[54] Mongiat M, Sweeney SM, San Antonio JD, Fu J, Iozzo RV. (2003) Endorepellin, a novel inhibitor of angiogenesis derived from the C terminus of perlecan. *J Biol Chem*. 278:4238–49.

[55] O'Reilly MS, Boehm T, Shing Y, Fukai N, Vasios G, Lane WS, Flynn E, Birkhead JR, Olsen BR, Folkman J. (1997) Endostatin: an endogenous inhibitor of angiogenesis and tumor growth. *Cell*. 88(2):277-85.

[56] Ezekowitz RA, Mulliken JB, Folkman J. (1992) Interferon alfa-2a therapy for life-threatening hemangiomas of infancy. *N Engl J Med*. 326(22)1456-63.

[57] Strieter RM, Polverini PJ, Kunkel SL. (1995) The functional role of the ELR motif in CXC chemokine-mediated angiogenesis. *J Biol Chem*. 270:27348–57.

[58] Yue TL, Wang X, Louden CS. (1997) 2-Methoxyestradiol, an endogenous estrogen metabolite, induces apoptosis in endothelial cells and inhibits angiogenesis: possible role for stress-activated protein kinase signaling pathway and Fas expression. *Mol Pharmacol*. 51:951–62

[59] Sage EH. (1999) Pieces of eight: bioactive fragments of extracellular proteins as regulators of angiogenesis. Trends Biol Sci. 7:182

[60] Gupta SK, Hassel T, Singh JP. (1995) A potent inhibitor of endothelial cell proliferation is generated by proteolytic cleavage of the chemokine platelet factor 4. *Proc Natl Acad Sci U S A*. 92(17):7799-803.

[61] Clapp C, Martial JA, Guzman RC, Rentier-Delure F, Weiner RI. (1993) The 16-kilodalton N-terminal fragment of human prolactin is a potent inhibitor of angiogenesis. Endocrinology. 133(3):1292-9.

[62] Tolma SS, Volpert OV, Tainsky MA, Bouck N. (1994) Control of angiogenesis in fibroblasts by p53 regulation of thrombospondin-1. *Science*. 265:1582-1584

[63] Baker EA, Stephenson TJ, Reed MW, Brown NJ. (2002) Expression of proteinases and inhibitors in human breast cancer progression and survival. *Mol Pathol*. 55:300–4.

[64] Moses MA, Wiederschain D, Wu I. (1999) Troponin I is present inhuman cartilage and inhibits angiogenesis. *Proc Natl Acad Sci*. 96:2645–50.

[65] Monboisse JC, Garnotel R, Bellon G. (1994) The α3 chain of type IV collagen prevents activation of human polymorphonuclear leukocytes. *J Biol Chem*. 269:25475–82.

[66] Maeshima Y, Colorado PC, Torre A. (2000) Distinct anti-tumor properties of a type IV collagen domain derived from basement membrane. *J Biol Chem*. 275:21340–8.

[67] Zhai Y, Ni J, Jiang GW, Lu J, Xing L, Lincoln C, Carter KC, Janat F, Kozak D, Xu S, Rojas L, Aggarwal BB, Ruben S, Li LY, Gentz R, Yu GL. (1999) VEGI, a novel cytokine of the tumor necrosis factor family, is an angiogenesis inhibitor that suppresses the growth of colon carcinomas *in vivo*. *FASEB J*. 13(1):181-9.

[68] Pike SE, Yao L, Jones KD, Cherney B, Appella E, Sakaguchi K, Nakhasi H, Teruya-Feldstein J, Wirth P, Gupta G, Tosato G. (1998) Vasostatin, a calreticulin fragment, inhibits angiogenesis and suppresses tumor growth. *J Exp Med*. 188(12):2349-56.

[69] Jaffe EA (1973) Culture of Human Endothelial Cells Derived from Umbilical Veins. Identification by morphologic and immunologic criteria. *J Clin Invest* 52(11): 2745–2756.

[70] Arnaoutova I, Kleinman HK (2010) *In vitro* angiogenesis: endothelial cell tube formation on gelled basement membrane extract. *Nat Prot*.5:628-635

[71] Auerbach R (1991) Vascular endothelial cell differentiation: organ-specificity and selective affinities as the basis for developing anti-cancer strategies. *Int J Radiat Biol* 60: 1-10.

[72] Zetter BR (1990) The cellular basis of site-specific tumor metastasis. *New England J Med* 322:603-12.

[73] Arap RD, Hagbedorn M (1998) Molecular heterogeneity of the vascular endothelium revealed by *in vivo* phage display. *J Clin Invest* 102:430-7.

[74] Qin L (2006) Requirement of protein kinase D tyrosine phosphorylation for VEGF-A165-induced angiogenesis through its interaction and regulation of phospholipase Cgamma phosphorylation. *J Biol Chem* 281:32550–32558.

[75] Wang S (2008) Control of endothelial cell proliferation and migration by VEGF signaling to histone deacetylase 7. *PNAS* 22: 7738-7743.

[76] Nicosia R, Ottinetti A. (1990) Growth of microvessels in serum-free matrix culture of rat aorta: A quantitative assay of angiogenesis *in vitro*. Lab Invest 63:115-122.

[77] Sandison JC (1924) A new method for the microscopic study of living growing tissues by the introduction of a transparent chamber in the rabbit's ear. *Anat. Rec.* 28:281-287.

[78] Clark ER (1930) Recent modifications in the method of studying living cells and tissues in transparent chambers inserted in the rabbit's ear. *Anat. Rec.* 47:187-211.

[79] Clark ER, Clark EL (1932) Observations on living preformed blood vessels as seen in a transparent chamber inserted into the rabbit's ear. *Am. J. Anat.* 49:441-477.

[80] Ide AG (1939) Vascularization of the brown Pearce rabbit epithelioma transplant as seen in the transparent ear chamber. *Am. J. Roentgenol.* 42:891–899.

[81] Algire GH (1943) An adaption of the transparent-chamber technique to the mouse.*J. Nat. Cancer Inst.* 4:1-11.

[82] Algire GH, Legallais FY (1949) Recent developments in the transparent-chamber technique as adapted to the mouse. *J. Nat. Cancer Inst.* 10:225–253.

[83] Borgstrom P, Ferrara N (1996) Complete inhibition of angiogenesis and growth of microtumors by anti-vascular endothelial growth factor neutralizing antibody: novel concepts of angiostatic therapy from intravital videomicroscopy. *Cancer Res.* 56:4032–4039.

[84] Frost GI (2005) Novel syngeneic pseudo-orthotopic prostate cancer model: vascular, mitotic and apoptotic responses to castration. *Microvasc Res.* 69:1–9.

[85] Murphy JB (1913) Transplantability of tissues to the embryo of foreign species. Its bearing on questions of tissue specificity and tumor immunity. *J Exp Med* 17:482–493

[86] Knighton D, Folkman J (1977) Avascular and vascular phases of tumour growth in the chick embryo. *Br J Cancer* 35:347–356

[87] Luepke NP (1985) Hen's egg chorioallantoic membrane test for irritation potential. *Fd Chem Toxic* 23:287–91

[88] Luepke NP (1987) HET-CAM - reproducibility studies. *AM Goldberg (Ed.): Alternative methods in toxicology. Mary Ann Liebert, Inc., New York.* 5:353-363

[89] Leighton J (1985) The chick embryo in toxicology: an alternative to the rabbit eye. *Food and chemical toxicology* 23(2):293-298

[90] Bagley DM (1989) Assessing the eye irritation potential of surfactant-based materials using the chorioallantoic membrane vascular assay (CAMVA). *AM Goldberg (Ed.): Alternative methods in toxicology series - Symposium on in vitro toxicology: new directions. Mary Ann Liebert, Inc., New York.* 7:265-272

[91] Bagley DM (1991) Factors affecting use of the hens egg chorioallantoic membrane as a model for predicting eye irritation potential. *Journal of toxicology / Cutaneous and ocular toxicology.* 10:95-104

[92] Lichtenberg J (1997) The rat subcutaneous air sac model: a new and simple method for *in vivo* screening of antiangiogenesis. *Pharmacol Toxicol.* 81(6):280-4

[93] Lichtenberg J (1999) The rat Subcutaneous Air Sac model: a quantitative assay of antiangiogenesis in induced vessels. *Pharmacol Toxicol.* 84(1):34-40

[94] Akthar N (2002) The sponge/Matrigel angiogenesis assay. *Angiogenesis.* 5(1-2):75-80

[95] Auerbach R (2000) Angiogenesis assays: problems and pitfalls. *Cancer Metastasis Rev.* 19:167-172

[96] Eyüpoglu IY, Hahnen E, Heckel A, Siebzehnrübl FA, Buslei R, Fahlbusch R, Blümcke I. (2005) Malignant glioma-induced neuronal cell death in an organotypic glioma invasion model. Technical note. *J Neurosurg.* 102(4):738-44.

[97] Savaskan NE, Heckel A, Hahnen E, Engelhorn T, Doerfler A, Ganslandt O, Nimsky C, Buchfelder M, Eyüpoglu IY (2008) Small interfering RNA-mediated xCT silencing in gliomas inhibits neurodegeneration and alleviates brain edema. *Nat Med.* 14(6):629-32.

[98] Savaskan NE, Seufert S, Hauke J, Tränkle C, Eyüpoglu IY, Hahnen E. (2011) Dissection of mitogenic and neurodegenerative actions of cystine and glutamate in malignant gliomas. *Oncogene.* 6;30(1):43-53.

Section 2

Immunotherapy

Chapter 5

IGF-I Antisense and Triple-Helix Gene Therapy of Glioblastoma

Jerzy Trojan and Ignacio Briceno

Additional information is available at the end of the chapter

http://dx.doi.org/10.5772/52366

1. Introduction

1.1. General concept

There is a convergence between ontogenesis and carcinogenesis. In theory all antigens correspond to a specific stage of embryo/fetal development. These antigens – oncodevelopmental proteins - are also present in homologous neoplatic tissues during cancer growth. The first illustration of this theory is alpha-fetoprotein (AFP), a common tumor marker, which is present during the normal development of central nervous system of the rat. Immunohistochemical analysis of the localization of AFP during normal development of the central nervous system and in pathological homologous nervous tissues of teratocarcinoma, shows a remarkable parallelis [1]. A similar demonstration was demonstrated for serum albumin antigen and blood group H antigen [2]. As AFP was a specific marker for neuronal cells, a search for a specific marker of glial cells has constituted the next step in the nervous system research to distinguish glial and neuronal cells, because the known markers were not totally specific. It was demonstrated that the growth factor IGF-I (Insulin like Grow Factor I) [3-6] is present only in glial cells, and absent in neuronal cells in normal and neoplastic developmen [7]. IGF-I is, therefore, a specific marker of glioblastoma. The use of IGF-I for the study of malignant tumors, including the gliomas, became the best choice as a marker [8-10].

1.2. Anti — Gene strategies

1.2.1. Antisense

For nearly twenty years various treatments of tumors, based on the injection of antibodies directed against specific antigens and stem cells have been tested. The results were not successful because of non-selective affinity for the tumor. Moreover, direct injection of protein coupled to an isotope such as iodine-125, has also posed the problem of the limited specificity of the distribution of the protein [11]. After that, the researchers have approached the study in a radically different way, trying to stop the production of IGF-I, acting directly on the messenger RNA [7,12].

Since 1978 it is known that antisense messengers are naturally produced and destroyed in the process of DNA replicatio [13-17]. The authors successfully demonstrated that this phenomenon is possible in twenty different species. Fortunately, the researchers could produce artificial antisense messengers in a significant number [12,17-19]. Moreover, using antisense oligonucleotides associated with the photoluminescent amino-terminated poly amido amine dendrimer, they can be directly analyzed by fluorescence microscopy and flow cytometry [20]. The antisense sequences are capable of blocking the messenger RNA translation conducting to block of specific protein synthesis.

1.2.2. *Triple helix*

Since the 90s, another approach in parallel with the strategy of antisense RNA has become successful in gene therapy and clinical trials: the triple helix strategy [21-23]. The triple helix technology (HT) is the newest approach, which belongs to the antisense approach and *sensu lato* anti gene strategies. TH technology was discovered by PB Derwan and C. Helene [24,25] and its action was defined as inhibition of gene expression at the level of transcription. In short, specific oligonucleotide sequences (also called triple helix-forming oligonucleotides, TFOs) are introduced into cells by transfection using chemical carriers, such as plasmid vectors which can direct synthesis TFOs. The TFOs are linked to the genomic DNA forming the triple helix structure with the target gene and inhibiting its transcription. The TFOs usually are directed against sequences located in the promoter region of genes of interest [24]. Examples of the inhibitory activity of TFOs on target genes involved in tumorigenesis are currently available. This approach, based on the triple helix of DNA has been used for the inhibition of IGF-I, which plays a major role in tumorigenesis [26]. Triplex strategy has also been applied to the inhibition of Ras oncogenes which are the most frequently activated in human cancer. Transcription was inhibited by human Hras TFOs targeting sequences recognized by the transcription factor Sp I [27]. Moreover, synthesis of Human Tumor Necrosis Factor (TNF), which acts as an autocrine growth factor in various tumor cell lines including neuroblastoma and glioblastoma has been blocked by treatment with TFOs [28,29].

2. Experimental results

2.1. *In vitro* and *in vivo* experiments on glioma tumors

The vector of antisense type was transfected into established glioma C6 cell line. All transfected cells have changed phenotype. Morphologically these cells had an elongated appearance. Transfected glial cells have produced a large amount of antisense RNA [7,30].

Regarding *in vivo* experiment, subcutaneous injection of C6 glioma cells into DBX rats have produced a glioma tumor after ten days. When transfected glioma cells were injected (with vector carrying the cDNA antisense against IGF-I) the tumors did not develop.

The experience was reproducible in 200 rats and the results were confirmatory. It was demonstrated that if injected initially native C6 glioma cells were followed a week later by injection into another point of subcutaneously transfected glial cells, the tumor developed, but disappeared completely after 2 to 3 weeks [12].

The tumor examined histologically shortly before the death of animals, have shown an important lymphocytes / plasmocytes infiltration. Histological analysis of the tumor during its disappearance suggests that the essential mechanism is related to the presence of specifically CD8 + cytotoxic T lymphocytes. Systematic analysis of all tissues showed that these lymphocytes were of splenic origin, and were observed in very large quantities in the spleen of experimental animals (10 to15%) [12,31,32].

2.2. Mechanism of glioma tumor destruction

The cytotoxic T CD8+ cell can exert its effect, if a bridge between CD8 and the antigen of class I major histocompatibility complex (MHC) occurs [33-36]. Following transfection of glial cells with the antisense cDNA of IGF-I, the expression of MHC-I in transfected glioma cells and in vivo, is greatly enhanced (5 times). This mechanism may play a role in the cytotoxic response, although not the only one involve [37]. The bearing tumor rats receiving injections of transfected cells, have revealed a very high rate of CD8 + cells. This anti-tumor immune response has stopped the tumor development [12,31,38-40].

3. Application in clinical trial

3.1. Ethical committees

Approval for the clinical trial of gene therapy (based on the NIH clinical study No 1602, Bethesda, Maryland, 24. 11. 1993) [41] was administered by the Commission of Bioethics at the University of Medicine, Bromberg (No KB / 176/2001, 28. 06. 2002) and registered by Wiley International Gene Therapy Clinical Trial database No. 635 and 636 (J Gene Med, updated 2002), and by NATO Science program 2003/2007 - USA, France, Poland, Germany (LST 980 517).

3.2. Conditions

The NIH Committee raised a number of conditions. Initially, for all patients, tumor cells must be isolated from biopsies and cells clones to be used should be only IGF-I and GFAP positive. NIH also requires that all cells are irradiated with a dose of 5000 cGy before reinjection, to avoid the possibility of subsequent cell divisions. After irradiation, the cells must be maintained in cell culture for 24 hours.

The elimination of the plasmid in the cells before injection is ensured by the possibility of a deletion in vitro of the hygromicine for 2 to 3 weeks. (The safety of the method was guaranteed by the use of an episomal vector without the risk of integration of the DNA vector).

Gene therapy will be preceded by a lymphocyte transformation test (TTL): in vitro, the lymphocytes of patients with glioblastoma are brought into contact with their own tumor cells transfected; the increase in tritiated thymidine incorporation will allow to demonstrate the stimulation of immune cells.

The first stage is the biopsy, to harvest the cells for transfection in vitro. This step requires 4 to 6 weeks. Then, cells are frozen after verification that all cells are positive for IGF-I and GFA. In case of cellular heterogeneity after cloning, only IGF-I positive population will be frozen and preserved. The transfected cells should not produce IGF-I. The cells before injection should be irradiated. The first authorization was granted in 1994 to 12 patients [30,41].

3.3. Methodology

Primary cultures of glioma cells were etablished from biopsies of human glioblastoma patients [40]. The human glioma cell lines were transfected with plasmid vector of the "triple helix" pMT-AG TH type [26]. Clones of transfected cells, no expressing IGF-I but expressing MHC-I and B7 molecules, were selected one month after transfection. Prior to injection the transfected cells were irradiated with cGy. The first injection was performed using only cell membranes [42,43] derived from 100 000 cells, followed by two cell injection of 1 – 2 million cells, with interval of one month each (subcutaneous injection in the left arm of patients). Blood was collected before the first "membrane" vaccination, and then 3 weeks after the first and second injection. The labeling of peripheral blood lymphocytes (PBL) was performed using mouse monoclonal antibodies directed against cell surface antigens. The samples of monoclonal antibodies were used for flow cytometric analysis as follows: FITC conjugated - (a) CD45, (b) of CD4, (c) CD3, (d) CD25, (e) CD45RO, (f) CD19 (g) CD8, (h) CD8CD11b +, (i) IgG1 control antibody, and these conjugated with PE - (a) CD14, (b) CD8, (c) CD16 + CD6, (d) CD4 (CD8), e) CD4 (CD8), (f) CD5, (g) CD8CD11b-, (h) CD8CD28, (i) IgG2 (18,27) [43].

4. Clinical results

The promising results were obtained in six patients at University Hospitals of Cleveland, in two patients in Bangkok and in four patients at the University Hospital of Bromberg. Admitting that the group of glioblastoma patients treated with antisense/triple helix cell injection has given the significant results, comparatively studied two cases of colon cancer and two cases of prostate cancer patients were treated, after surgery and radiotherapy with this type of "cellular therapy (Hospital of Bromberg).

Significant changes were observed mainly after the first cell vaccination. Phenotypic changes in peripheral blood lymphocytes were as follows: an increase in the percentage of CD8 + T cells accompanied in parallel by an increase of CD8 + CD11b- and CD8CD28 + molecules, after each

http://dx.doi.org/10.5772/52366

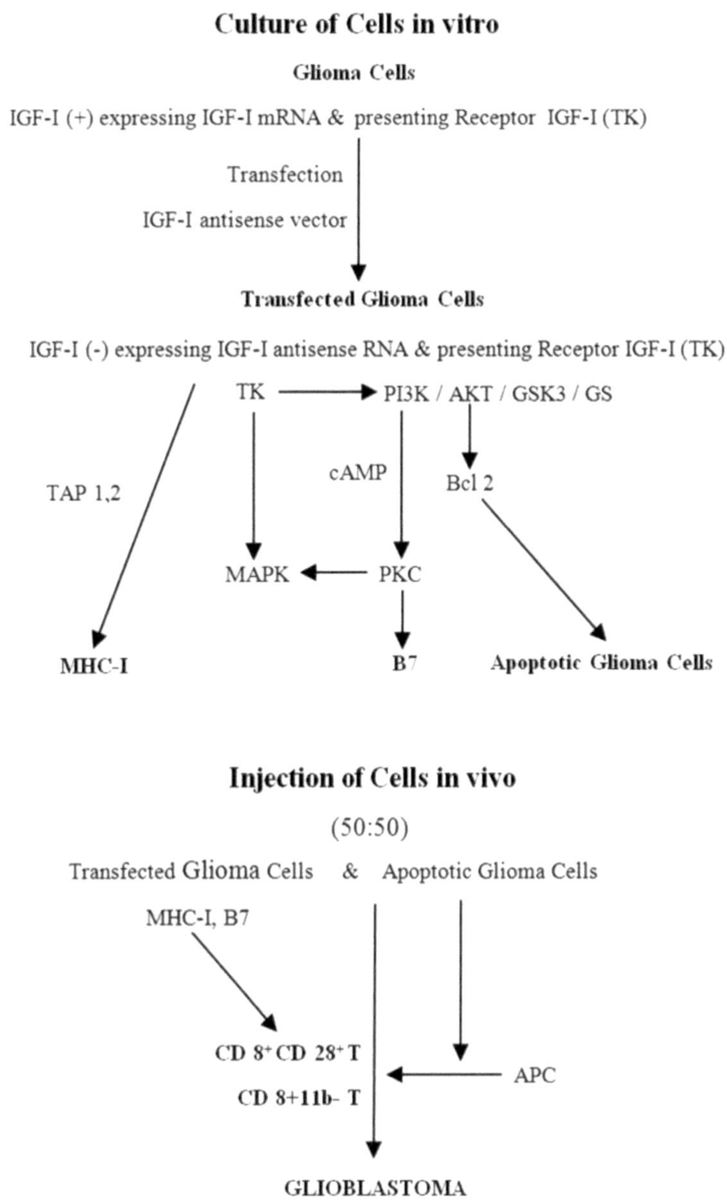

Figure 1. Antisense anti – IGF-I therapy. After *in vitro* transfection of tumor cells with a vector containing IGF-I cDNA in antisense orientation, the cells express IGF-I antisense RNA; the cells become negatively labeled with anti IGF-I antibodies, and positively with anti MHC-I and B7 antibodies. On the other hand, about half of these transfected cells become apoptotic. Both immune and apoptotic phenomena are related to signal transduction pathway. The injected transfected cells including apoptotic cells, together with induced *in vivo* APC cells, activat T lymphocytes (CTLCD8 + CD28 +). Activated CTL produce an antitumor immune response [40,44,47,61,79,80-83]. Abreviations: TAP 1,2 (transporter associated with antigen processing antigen); TK (tyrosine kinase); PI3K (phosphatidyinositol 3 kinase); PDK1 (phosphoinositide-dependent kinase 1); AKT (PKB, protein kinase B); Bcl 2 (key molecule of apoptose); GSK3 (glycogene synthetase kinase 3); GS (glycogene synthetase); MAPK (MAP kinase – mitogen activated protein kinase); PKC (protein kinaseC C).

of the three vaccinations. This alteration may reflect the increased activation of T cells cytotoxic blood (Figure 1.). Additionally, it was observed an increased percentage of lymphocytes positive for surface receptor of interleukin-2 (CD25). No changes were demonstrated in other CD molecules [44]. In our ongoing work (new protocol), 4 and 5 injections of IGF-I TH cells were introduced in patients with glioblastoma. After the fourth injection, the samples of the blood obtained from treated patients have shown a progressive increase in CD8 and NK cells, which highlights the effect of treatment on immune response. Also an increase of CD25 molecules was observed after the second and third injection. There was no difference before or after vaccination in the levels of CD3, CD16 + CD56, CD19, CD5, CD45 and CD14. The only side effect was a fever of 38°C noted after cell vaccinations. That probably corresponds to a cellular immune response (T cell induction). These changes may reflect the increased activation of cytotoxic T cells [36,45-47].

One glioblastoma patient who was treated at University Hospital of Cleveland, had lived 24 months from the time of diagnosis. Among other five glioblastoma patients treated in U.S.A. (University Hospital of Cleveland), two of the patients have survived 19 months. The treatment in U.S.A. has shown that the number of cell vaccines (between two and four) was not related to median survival of the patients. Another group of three patients treated in the U.S.A. have not responded so positively to therapy. These patients had an advanced disease with cerebral edema before gene therapy and were also treated with high doses of decadron or related steroids to reduce the effect of edema in CNS. Of course, this additional treatment has produced a negative effect on immune response and survival of patients. In two of the four patients with glioblastoma multiforme treated in Bromberg (NATO Science Program - USA / France / Poland / Germany), the average survival has ranged from 19 to 24 months, whereas the two patients in the control group survived 9.5 and 10 months respectively. Histopathological examination of removed glioblastoma tumors has shown that subjects had developed a necrosis around the tumor. Moreover the necrotic tissue surrounding the tumor has shown an infiltration of CD4 + and CD8 + T lymphocytes [32]. As to colon and prostate cancer patients the period of 19 months was also chosen as the end of clinical observations in all treated cancer patients. At 19 months, all these cancer patients were alive and the treatments were well tolerated. The PBL labelling results were similar to those obtained with glioblastoma patients (Figure 2. A,B,C) [48].

5. Discussion

The significant clinical findings were published in 2006/2012; it was demonstrated that due to the use of AS anti - IGF-I therapy following radiotherapy, the median survival of glioblastoma patients has reached 21 months. In 2010 we have reported that this survival could be explained by the immune anti-tumor response related to the increase of CD28 molecules in PBL cells analyzed after every of two "vaccinations". Moreover, this phenomenon was also observed in other tumors studied (four cases of liver cancer, colon, ovary, uterus and prostate). Phenotypic changes in peripheral blood lymphocytes (PBL) were clearly observed in all types of cancer treated with "cell therapy" - after every vaccination, an increase of CD8 + T lymphocytes,

http://dx.doi.org/10.5772/52366

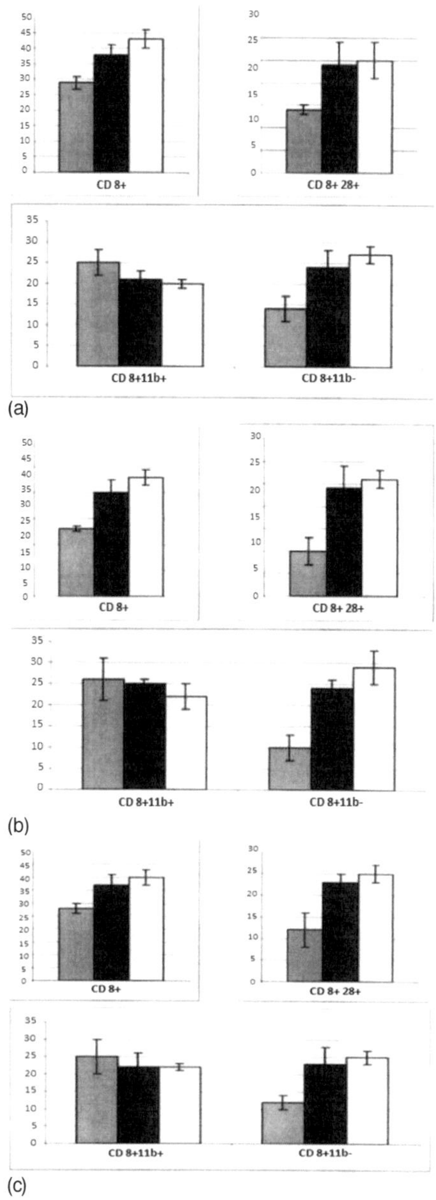

Figure 2. Flow cytometric "FACS" peripheral blood lymphocyte CD marker patterns following comparative therapies in cancers of neuroectodermal origin - glioblastoma multiforme (A), entodermal origin – colon adenocarcinoma (B), and mesodermal origin – prostate adenocaarcinoma (C). CD molecules were labelled in peripheral blood lymphocytes (PBLs) obtained from prevaccinated and "vaccinated" patients. Each of the first column corresponds to data obtained before vaccinations; each second and third column corresponds to data obtained after one and two successive cellular vaccinations (IGF-I antisense/triple helix cells). Bar graphs represent the median value of the two cases. Data are expressed as percent of positive cells when compared to the isotype control. Difference in percentage of CD8+ CD11b– and CD8+ CD28+ subpopulations from the relevant patients before and after vaccination was strongly significant with a range of *P* from 0.001 to 0.02 according to the Student's *t*-test. The *P* value for CD8+, CD8+28+, and CD8+11b– (below 0.01) is illustrated in the bar graph for statistical significance.

particularly of CD8+11b-, accompanied by a characteristic shift of CD8+11b+ to CD8+11b- (Figure 2.). This phenomenon was practically not significant in a group of patients treated only with "membrane" injections (as applied to two patients with glioblastoma) [47,48].

Glioblastoma and other malignancies were recently successfully treated with antisense therapy focused on TGF beta [49], using either antisense anti TGF beta expressing vector [50,51] or direct use of antisense oligodeoxynucleotides [52,53]. The use of phosphorothioate antisense oligonucleotides TGF beta2 (AP-12009, trabedersen) was initiated in patients with tumors that showed overexpression of TGF beta, such as high-grade gliomas - anaplastic astrocytoma (AA) or glioblastoma. Treatment was well tolerated. In 2007, the overall survival time was about 24 months, and in the control group, survival was 20 months. Recently, in three phase I/II studies and a randomized, active-controlled dose-finding phase IIb study, trabedersen treatment of high-grade glioma patients with recurrent or refractory tumor disease led to long-lasting tumor responses and so far promising survival data [52,54,55]. The results of clinical trials with other tumors that overexpress TGF beta have also been published recently [52,56]. Recently, the antisense approach, using also antisense oligonucleotides, targeting tumor neovascular trimer protein, laminin-411, was also proposed for clinical trial [57]. The innovation concerns a polymeric nanobioconjugate drug based on biodegradable, nontoxic, and nonimmunogenic polymalic acid as a universal delivery nanoplatform; this platform is applied for synthesis of nanomedicine drug which passes through the blood brain tumor barrier and tumor cell membrane. Other approach of antisense treatment, especially using antisense IGF-I-receptor has been developed [58-60]. It seems that this therapy, could be more efficient if the "cell vaccines" would be prepared after cell cloning for the expression of MHC-I. The different examples of antisense strategy in experimental and clinical trials of gliomas are showed in Table 1.

IGF-I	Antisense vector Clinical trial	Trojan et al. Biomed & Pharmacother 2010; 64(8):
TGF beta & I cell therapy	Antisense oligodeoxynucleotide Clinical trial	Dietrich et al. Curr Opin Oncol 2010; 22(6):604
Laminin-411	Antisense oligodeoxynucleotide Clinical trial	Ding et al. Proc Natl Acad Sci USA 2010; 107(42):18143.
AKT2	Antisense oligonucleotide Experimental therapy	Zhang et al. Oncol Rep 2010;24(1):65.
EGFR	Antisense oligonucleotide Experimental therapy	Li et al. Oncol Rep 2010; 23(6): 1585.
PED/PEA-15 (ERK1/2-interacting protein)	Antisense oligonucleotide Experimental therapy	Botta et al. Hum Gene Ther 2010; 21(9): 1067.
miR-21 & 5FU	Antisense oligonucleotide Experimental therapy	Ren et al. J Biomater Sci Polym Ed 2010; 21(3): 303.
miR-21	Antisense oligonucleotide	Zhou et al. Lab Invest. 2010; 90(2): 144.

IGF-I	Antisense vector Clinical trial	Trojan et al. Biomed & Pharmacother 2010; 64(8):
	Experimental therapy	
EGFR	Antisense oligonucleotide Experimental therapy	Kang et al. J Biomed Mater Res A 2010; 93(2): 585.
VEGF	Antisense (vector) Experimental therapy	Yang et al. J Neurooncol 2010; Aug 26 Epub
miR-21	Antisense oligonucleotide Experimental therapy	Zhou et al. Oncol Rep 2010; 24(1): 195.
Telomerase and tamoxifen	Antisense oligonucleotide Experimental therapy	Wang et al., Mol Med Report. 2010; 3(6): 935.
c-Met	Antisense oligonucleotide Experimental therapy	Chu et al. Oncol Rep 2010; 24(1): 189.
IGF-I	Antisense vector Clinical trial	Trojan and Anthony, Curr Signal Transd Ther. 2011; 6(3): 411.
TGF beta	Antisense oligodeoxynucleotide Clinical trial	Jashinsky et al., Curr Pharm Biotechnol. 2011; 12(12): 2203.
TGF beta	Antisense oligodeoxynucleotide Clinical trial	Hau et al., Curr Pharm Biotechnol. 2011; 12(12): 2150.
miR-10b	Antisense oligonucleotide Experimental therapy	Sun et al., Brain Res. 2011;1389: 9
micro RNA-7	Antisense oligonucleotide Experimental therapy	Lee et al., Radiother Oncol. 2011; 101(1):171.
uPAR	Antisense vector Experimental therapy	Raghu et al., Mol Cancer. 2011; 10: 130.
IGF-I	Antisense vector Clinical trial	Trojan et al., Chem Res Pract. 2012; doi:10.1155/2012/721873
miR-221/222	Antisense oligonucleotide Experimental therapy	Hao et al., Oncol Rep. 2012; 27(5): 1504.
miR-143 and miR-145	Antisense oligonucleotide Experimental therapy	Koo et al., BMC Cancer. 2012; 12: 143.
miR-1275	Antisense oligonucleotide Experimental therapy	Katsushima et al., J Biol Chem. 2012 Jun 26. [Epub]

Table 1. Examples of experimental and clinical gene therapies of gliomas using antisense technology (selection of articles of last two years).

In the strategies of anti TGF-beta and anti IGF-I and anti IGF-IR antisense techniques, the anti-tumor immune response was designated as a primary mechanism involving growth factors inhibited by antisense technology and its signaling pathway [37,51]. As PI3K/AKT/GWK3/GS pathway is considered in antisense mechanism, it was recently demonstrated that also antisense anti-glycogen synthase (GS) cells express MHC-I molecules [44,61,62]. The IGF-I, through its binding to IGF-IR, activates the PI3K/AKT transduction cascade related to the pathway of apoptosis (IRS/PI3K/AKT/Bcl or AKT / Ca2 + or GSK3 or caspases). The end result of IGF-I AS approach involves an inhibition of the pathway elements of TK/PI3K/AKT inducing an *in vivo* immune response mediated by CD8 T cells and APC cells (Figure 1.) [44].

6. Conclusions

This review draws attention to the recent studies in cancer gene therapy, particularly of glioblastoma treatment using anti - gene anti IGF-I approach. Although the number of clinical trials of "antisense" type is much lower than those of pre-clinical experimental therapies, we wish to emphasize that any experimental therapy is a potential clinical trial (Table 1.). The current clinical strategies for the treatment of gliomas are usually a combination of chemotherapy and use of different types of inhibitors (imatinib, gefitinib) including antibodies (i.e. avastin), targeting growth factors and their receptors [63-66]. The new therapies are now focusing on technology of inhibitors and antigene techniques (antisense or triple helix) used alone or combined with drug treatment [67-71]. A pharmacological strategy - the use of temozolomide introduced by R. Stupp, has offered a new hope for treatment of glioblastoma. However, although median survival has reached almost two years, we are still far from victory [72,73]. The new strategies proposing to target different growth factors, especially IGF-I, TGF-beta or VEGF, their receptors and signaling pathway elements, seem to offer a promising solution [54,73-76]. We would like to underline that the research on IGF-I which has resulted in diagnostic application – the IGF-I being considered as one of the principal precancerous markers [10,12], has conducted to experiments on suppression of IGF-I expression in tumors, following directly by immuno-gene therapy of malignant tumors. Gene therapy, particularly cellular imuno-gene therapy, and cellular immunotherapy are currently among the most promising approaches for treatment of cancer diseases [66,68,77,78].

Acknowledgements

We thank Jean-François Nicolas (Institut Pasteur, Paris) for critical review of this manuscript, Tom Thomson Philips from Scientific Lim., London, for references related to the development of the AP-12OO9 (TGF-beta2 antisense oligonucleotides phase III clinical trial of malignant tumors). We thank Dr. Pan Yuexin (CWRU, Cleveland) for the work on the logistics of antisense IGF-I vaccines and graphic presentation of CD labeling in PBL cells, and Mrs Annabelle Trojan (CURN, Cartagena) for a revision of the text. The authors were supported by the subvention of the Society ICGT Bogota.

http://dx.doi.org/10.5772/52366

Author details

Jerzy Trojan[1,2*] and Ignacio Briceno[3]

*Address all correspondence to: jerzytrojan@hotmail.com

1 INSERM U602, Paul Brousse Hospital, Paris XI University, Villejuif, France

2 INS – National Institute of Health, Department of Investigations, Bogota, Colombia

3 Faculty of Medicine, Institut of Genetics, Javeriana Pontif. University, Bogota, Colombia

No conflict of interest was signaled.

References

[1] Trojan J, Uriel J, Deugnier MA, Gaillard J. Immunocytochemical quantitative study of alphafetoprotein in normal and neoplastic neural development. Developmental Neuroscience 1984; 6: 251-259.

[2] Mollicone R, Trojan J, Oriol R. Appearance of H and B antigenes in primary sensory cells of the rat olfactory apparatus and inner ear. Developmental Brain Research 1985; 17(1): 268-279.

[3] Froesch CS, Schwander J, Zapf J. Actions of insulin-like growth factors. Annual Review of Physiology 1985; 47: 443-467.

[4] Daughaday WH, Rotwein P. Insulin-like growth factorsI and II. Peptide, messenger ribonucleic acid and gene structures, serum, and tissue concentrations. Endocrinology Review 1989; 10(1): 68-91.

[5] Le Roith D, Bondy C, Yakar S, Liu J, Butler A. The somatomedin hypothesis. Endocrinology Review 2001; 22(1): 53-74.

[6] Pollak MN, Schernhammer ES, Hankinson SE. Insulin-like growth factors and neoplasia. Nature Review Cancer 2004; 4: 505-518.

[7] Trojan J, Blossey B, Johnson T, Rudin S, Tykocinski M, Ilan J. Loss of tumorigenicity of rat glioblastoma directed by episome-based antisens cDNA transcription of insulin-like growth factor I. Proceedings of National Academy of Science USA 1992; 89: 4874-4878.

[8] Werner H, Le Roith D. New concepts in regulation and function of the insulin- like growth factors: implications for understanding normal growth and neoplasia. Cellular and Molecular Life Science 2000; 57: 932-942.

[9] Zumkeller W, Westphal M. The IGF/IGFBP system in CNS malignancy. Molecular Pathology 2001; 54: 227-229.

[10] Zumkeller W. IGFs and IGF- binding proteins as diagnostic markers and biological modulators in brain tumours. Experimental Review of Molecular Diagnostic 2002; 2: 473-477.

[11] Hajeri-Germond M, Naval J, Trojan J, Uriel J. The uptake of alphafetoprotein by C-1300 mouse neuroblastoma cells. British Journal of Cancer 1985; 51: 791-797.

[12] Trojan J, Johnson TR, Rudin SD, Ilan Ju, Tykocinski ML, Ilan J. Treatment and prevention of rat glioblastoma by immunogenic C6 cells expressing antisense insulin-like growth factor I RNA. Science 1993; 259: 94-97.

[13] Rubenstein JL, Nicolas JF, Jacob F. L'ARN non sens (nsARN) : un outil pour inactiver spécifiquement l'expression d'un gène donné in vivo [Nonsense RNA: a tool for specifically inhibiting the expression of a gene in vivo]. Copmtes Rendus Academie des Sciences Paris 1984; 299(8): 271-274.

[14] Weintraub H, Izant JG, Harland RM. Antisense RNA as a molecular tool for genetic analysis. Trends in Genetics 1985; 1(1): 23-25.

[15] Green PJ, Pines O, Inouye M. The role of antisense RNA in gene regulation. Annual Review of Biochemistry 1986; 55: 569-597.

[16] Merino E, Balbas P, Puente JL, Bolivar F. Antisense overlapping open reading frames in genes from bacteria to humans. Nucleic Acids Research 1994; 22(10): 19-77.

[17] Dias N, Stein CA. Basic concepts and antisense oligonucleotides mechanisms. Molecular Cancer Therapeutics 2002; 1: 347-355.

[18] Galderisi U, Cascino A, Giordano A. Antisense oligonucleotides as therapeutic agents. Journal of Cell Physiology 1999; 181: 251-257.

[19] Bennett CF, Butler M, Cook PD, Geary RS, Levin AA, Mehta R, Teng CL, Desmukh H, Tillman L, Hardee G. (2000). Antisense Oligonucleotides – Based Therapeutics. In: Templeton NS, Lasic DD (ed.) Gene Therapy. New York: Marcel Dekker; 2000. p305-332.

[20] Tsai YJ, Hu CC, Chu CC, Imae T. Intrinsically fluorescent PAMAM dendrimer as gene carrier and nanoprobe for nucleic acids delivery: bioimaging and transfection study. Biomacromolecules 2011; 12(12): 4283-4290.

[21] Scaggiante B, Morassutti C, Tolazzi G, Michelutti A, Baccarani M, Quadrifoglio E. Effect of unmodified triple helix-forming oligodeoxyribonucleotide targeted to human multidrug-resistance gene mdrl in MDR cancer cells. FEBS Letters 1994; 352: 380-384.

[22] Thomas T, Faaland C, Gallo M, Thomas T. Suppression of c-myc oncogene expression by a polyamine-complexed triplex forming oligonucleotide in MCF-7 breast cancer cells. Nucleic Acids Research 1995; 23: 3594-3599.

[23] Vasquez KM, Wilson IH. Triplex-directed modification of genes and gene activity. Trends in Biochemical Science 1998; 23: 4-9.

[24] Dervan P. Reagents for the site-specific cleavage of megabase DNA. Nature 1992; 359:, 87-88.

[25] Hélène C. Control of oncogene expression by antisense nucleic acids. European Journal of Cancer 1994; 30(A): 1721-1726.

[26] Shevelev A, Burfeind P, Schulze E, Rininsland F, Johnson T, Trojan J, Chernicky C, Hélène C, Ilan Ju, Ilan J. Potential triple helix-mediated inhibition of IGF-I gene expression significantly reduces tumorigenicity of glioblastoma in an animal model. Cancer Gene Therapy 1997; 4(2): 105-112.

[27] Mayfield C, Ebbinghaus S, Gee I, Jones D, Rodu B, Squibb M, Miller D. Triplex formation by the human Ha-ras promoter inhibits Spl binding and in vitro transcription. Journal of Biological Chemistry 1994; 69: 18232-18238.

[28] Aggarwal B, Schwarz L, Hogan M, Rando R. Triple helix-forming oligodeoxyribonucleotides targeted to the human tumor necrosis factor (TNF) gene inhibit TNF production and block the TNF dependent growth of human glioblastoma tumor cells. Cancer Research 1996; 56: 5156-5164.

[29] Rininsland F, Johnson TR, Chernicky CL, Schulze E, Burfeind P, Ilan J. Suppression of insulin-like growth factor type I receptor by a triple-helix strategy inhibits IGF-I transcription and tumorigenic potential of rat C6 glioblastoma cells. Proceedings of National Academy of Science USA 1997; 94:, 5854-5859.

[30] Anthony DD, Pan Y, Wu S, Shen F, Guo Y. Ex vivo and in vivo IGF-I antisense RNA strategies for treatement of cancers in humans. Advances in Experimental Medicine and Biology 1998; 45: 27-34.

[31] Trojan J, Johnson T, Rudin S, Blossey B, Kelley K, Shevelev A, Abdul-Karim F, Anthony D, Tykocinski M, Ilan Ju, Ilan J. Gene therapy of murine T eratocarcinoma: separate functions for insulin-like growth factors I and II in immunogenicity and differentiation. Proceedings of National Academy of Science USA 1994; 91: 6088-6092.

[32] Wongkajornsilp A, Ouyprasertkul M, Sangruchi T, Huabprasert S, Pan, Y, Anthony DD. The analysis of peri-tumour necrosis following the subcutaneous implantation of autologous tumor cells transfected with an episome transcribing an antisense IGF-I RNA in a glioblastoma multiforme subject. J Med Assoc Thai 2001; 4(3): 740-747.

[33] Brooks WH, Latta RB, Mahaley MS. Immunobiology of primary intracranial tumors. Journal of Neurosurgery 1981; 54: 331-337.

[34] Saji M, Moriarty J, Ban T, Singer D, Kohn L. Major Histocompatibility Complex class I gene expression in rat thyroid cells is regulated by hormones, methimazoleand io-

dide as well as interferon. Journal of Clinical Endocrinology and Metabolism 1992; 75(3): 871-878.

[35] Blanchet O, Bourge JF, Zinszner H, Israel A, Kourilsky P, Dausset J, Degos L, Paul P. Altered binding of regulatory factors to HLA class I enhancer sequence in human tumor cell lines lacking class I antigen expression. Proceedings of National Academy of Science USA 1992; 89(8): 3488-3492.

[36] Schwartz RH. Costimulation of T Iymphocytes: the role ofCD28, CTLA-4 and B7/BBI in interleukin-2 production and immunotherapy. Cell 1992; 71: 1065- 1068.

[37] Trojan J, Duc HT, Upegui-Gonzalez L, Hor F, Guo Y, Anthony DD, Ilan J. Presence of MHCI and B-7 molecules in rat and human glioma cells expressing antisense IGF-I mRNA. Neuroscience Letters 1996; 212: 9-12.

[38] Lafarge-Frayssinet C, Duc HT, Sarasin A, Frayssinet C, Anthony D, Guo Y, Trojan J. Antisense IGF-I transfer into a rat hepatoma cell line inhibits tumorigenesis by modulatig MHC-I. Cancer Gene Therapy 1997; 4(5): 276-285.

[39] Upegui-Gonzalez LC, Duc HT, Buisson Y, Arborio M, Lafarge-Frayssinet C, Jasmin C, Guo Y, Trojan J. Use of antisense strategy in the treatment of the hepatocarcinoma. Advances in Experimental Medicine and Biology 1998; 451: 35-42.

[40] Ly A, Duc HT, Kalamarides M, Trojan LA, Pan Y, Shevelev A, François J-C, Noël T, Kane A, Henin D, Anthony DD, Trojan J. Human glioma cells transformed by IGF-I triple-helix technology show immune and apoptotic characteristics determining cell selection for gene therapy of glioblastoma. Journal of Clinical Pathology (Molecular Pathology) 2001; 54(4): 230-239.

[41] Ilan J., editor. Clinical trial: Gene therapy for human brain tumors using episome based antisense cDNA transcription of Insulin like Growth Factor I. Proposal for a phase one gene therapy clilnical study. NIH no 1602. Bethesda, Maryland: NIH; 1993.

[42] Matlib MA, Kihara M, Farrell C, Dage RC. The Na+-Ca2+ exchange system in vascular smooth muscle cell membrane vesicles isolated from cultured cells and from tissue is similar. Biochimical and Biophysical Acta 1988; 939(1): 173-177.

[43] Trojan LA, Ly A, Kopinski P, Ardourel M-Y, Dufour T, Duc HT, Kasprzak H, Cloix J-F, Wei MX, Chyczewski L, Pan Y, Chatel M, Anthony DD, Trojan J. Antisense and triple helix anti IGF-I tumours vaccines - gene therapy of gliomas. International Journal of Cancer Prevention 2007; 2(4): 227-243.

[44] Trojan J, Cloix J-F, Ardourel M-Y, Chatel M, Anthony D. IGF-I biology and targeting in malignant glioma. Neuroscience 2007; 145(3): 795-812.

[45] Chen L, Ashe S, Brady WA, Hellstrom KE, Ledbetter IA, Mc Growan P, Linsley PS. Costimulation of anti-tumor immunity by the B7 counter receptor for the T lymphocyte molecules CD28 and CTLA-4. Cell 1992; 71: 1093-1102.

[46] Matthew L, Saiter B, Bhardwag N. Dendritic cells acquire antigen from apoptotic cells and induce class I restricted CTL. Nature 1998; 392: 86-89.

[47] Trojan J, Ly A, Wei MX, Kopinski P, Ardourel M-Y, Pan Y, Trojan LA, Dufour D, Shevelev A, Andres C, Chatel M, Kasprzak H, Anthony DD, Duc HT. Antisense anti-IGF-I cellular therapy of malignant tumours: immune response in cancer patients. Biomedicine & Pharmacotherapy 2010; 64(8): 576-578.

[48] Trojan J, Pan YX, Wei MX, Ly A, Shevelev A, Bierwagen M, Ardourel M-Y, Trojan LA, Alvarez A, Andres C, Noguera MC, Briceño I, Aristizabal BH, Kasprzak H, Duc HT, Anthony DD. Methodology for anti - gene anti - IGF-I therapy of malignant tumours. Chemotherapy Research and Practice 2012; doi: 10.1155/2012/721873.

[49] Kaminska B, Wesolowska A, Danilkiewicz, M. TGF beta signalling and its role in tumour pathogenesis. Acta Biochimica Polonica 2005; 52: 329-337.

[50] Fakhrai H, Dorigo O, Shawler DL, Lin H, Mercola D, Black KL, Royston Y, Sobol RE. Eradication of established intracranial rat gliomas by transforming growth factor beta antisense gene therapy. Proceedings of National Academy of Science USA 1996; 93(7): 2909-2914.

[51] Fakhrai H, Mantil JC, Liu L, Nicholson GL, Murphy-Satter CS, Ruppert J. Phase I clinical trial of a TGF-beta antisense-modified tumor cell vaccine in patients with advanced glioma. Cancer Gene Therapy 2006; 13(12): 1052-1060.

[52] Schlingensiepen KH, Schlingensiepen R, Steinbrecher A, Hau P, Bogdahn U, Fischer-Blass B, Jachimczak P. Targeted tumor therapy with the TGF-beta2 antisense compound AP 12009. Cytokine Growth Factor Review 2006; 17: 129-139.

[53] Schlingensiepen KH, Fischer-Blass B, Schmaus S, Ludwig S. Antisense therapeutics for tumor treatment: the TGF-beta2 inhibitor AP 12009 in clinical development against malignant tumors, Recent Results Cancer Research 2008; 177: 137-150.

[54] Hau P, Jachimczak P, Bogdahn U. Treatment of malignant gliomas with TGF-beta2 antisense olgonucleotides. Expert Review Anticancer Therapy 2009; 9(11): 1663-1674.

[55] Hau P, Jachimczak P, Schlaier J, Bogdahn U. TGF-β2 signaling in high-grade gliomas. Current Pharmaceutical Biotechnology 2011; 12(12): 2150-2157.

[56] Schlingensiepen KH, Jaschinski F, Lang SA, Moser C, Geissler EK, Schlitt HJ, Kielmanowicz M, Schneider A. Transforming growth factor-beta 2 gene silencing with trabedersen (AP 12009) in pancreatic cancer. Cancer Science 2011; 102(6): 1193-1200.

[57] Ding H, Inoue S, Ljubimov AV, Patil R, Portilla-Arias J, Hu J, Konda B, Wawrowsky KA, Fujita M, Karabalin N, Sasaki T, Black KL, Holler E, Ljubimova JY. Inhibition of brain tumor growth by intravenous poly (β-L-malic acid) nanobioconjugate with pH-dependent drug release [corrected]. Proceedings of National Academy of Science USA. 2010; 107(42): 18143-18148.

[58] Resnicoff M, Li W, Basak S, Herlyn D, Baserga R, Rubin R. Inhibition of rat C6 glioblastoma tumor growth by expression of insulin-like growth factor I receptor antisense mRNA. Cancer Immunology and Immunotherapy 1996; 42: 64 68.

[59] Andrews DW, Resnicoff M, Flanders AE, Kenyon L, Curtis M, Merli G, Baserga R, Iliakis G, Aiken RD. Results of a pilot study involving the use of an antisense oligodeoxynucleotide directed against the insulin like growth factor type I receptor in malignant astrocytomas. Journal of Clinical Oncology 2001; 19: 2189-2200.

[60] Baserga R. The insulin-like growth factor-I receptor as a target for cancer therapy. Expert Opinion on Therapeutic Targets 2005; 9: 753-768.

[61] Premkumar DR, Arnold B, Jane EP, Pollack IF. Synergistic interaction between 17 AAG and phosphatidylinositol 3-kinase inhibition in human malignant glioma cells. Molecular Carcinogene 2006; 45: 47-59.

[62] Ardourel M-Y, Blin M, Moret J-L, Dufour T, Duc HT, Hevor T, Trojan J, Cloix J-F. A new putative target for antisense gene therapy of glioma: glycogen synthetase. Cancer Biology and Therapy 2007; 6(5): 719-723.

[63] Stupp R, Hegi ME, van den Bent MJ, Mason WP, Weller M, Mirimanoff RO, Cairncross JG. Changing paradigms--an update on the multidisciplinary management of malignant glioma. Oncologist 2006; 11: 165-180.

[64] Reardon DA, Quinn JA, Vredenburgh JJ, Gururangan S, Friedman AH, Desjardins A, Sathornsumetee S, Herndon JE 2nd, Dowell JM, McLendon RE, Provenzale JM, Sampson JH, Smith RP, Swaisland AJ, Ochs JS, Lyons P, Tourt-Uhlig S, Bigner DD, Friedman HS, Rich JN. Phase 1 trial of gefitinib plus sirolimus in adults with recurrent malignant glioma. Clinical Cancer Research 2006; 12: 860-868.

[65] Wen PY, Yung WK, Lamborn KR, Dahia PL, Wang Y, Peng B, Abrey LE, Raizer J, Cloughesy TF, Fink K, Gilbert M, Chang S, Junck L, Schiff D, Lieberman F, Fine HA, Prados MD. Phase I/II study of imatinib mesylate for recurrent malignant gliomas: North American Brain Tumor Consortium Study 99-08. Clinical Cancer Research 2006; 12: 4899-4907.

[66] Cavazzana-Calvo M, Hacein-Bey-Abina S, Fischer A: Ten years of gene therapy: thoughts and perspectives: Medecine Science (Paris) 2010; 26(2): 115-118.

[67] Giovannangeli C, Hélène C. Progress in developments of triplex-based strategies. Antisense Nucleic Acid Drug Development 1997; 7: 413-421.

[68] Dietrich PY, Dutoit V, Tran Thang NN, Walker PR. (2010). T cell immunotherapy for malignant glioma: toward a combined approach. Current Opinion in Oncology 2010; 22(6): 604-610.

[69] Bodera P. Immunostimulatory oligonucleotides. Recent Pathology Inflammation Allergy Drug Discovery 2011; 5(1): 87-93.

[70] Piwecka M, Rolle K, Wyszko E, Żukiel R, Nowak S, Barciszewska MZ, Barciszewski J. Nucleic acid-based technologies in therapy of malignant gliomas. Current Pharmaceutical Biotechnology 2011; 12(11): 1805-1822.

[71] Catuogno S, Esposito CL, Quintavalle C, Condorelli G, de Franciscis V, Cerchia L. Nucleic acids in human glioma treatment: innovative approaches and recent results. Journal of Signal Transduction 2012; 2012:735135. Epub 2012 May 21.

[72] Hegi ME, Diserens AC, Gorlia T, Hamou MF, de Tribolet N, Weller M, Kros JM, Hainfellner JA, Mason W, Mariani L, Bromberg JE, Hau P, Mirimanoff RO, Cairncross JG, Janzer RC, Stupp R. MGMT gene silencing and benefit from temozolomide in glioblastoma. New England Journal of Medicine 2005; 352: 997-1003.

[73] Gorlia T, van den Bent MJ, Hegi ME, Mirimanoff RO, Weller M, Cairncross JG., Eisenhauer E, Belanger K, Brandes AA, Allgeier A, Lacombe D, Stupp R. Nomograms for predicting survival of patients with newly diagnosed glioblastoma: prognostic factor analysis of EORTC and NCIC trial 26981 22981/CE.3. Lancet Oncology 2008; 9(1): 29-38.

[74] Ellouk-Achard S, Djenabi S, De Oliveira GA, Dessay G, Duc HT, Zoar M, Trojan J, Claude JR, Sarasin A, Lafarge-Frayssinet C. Induction of apoptosis in rat hepatoma cells by expression of IGF-I antisense cDNA. Journal of Hepatology 1998; 29: 807-818.

[75] Goudar RK, Shi Q, Hjelmeland MD, Keir ST, McLendon RE, Wikstrand CJ, Reese ED, Conrad CA, Traxler P, Lane HA, Reardon DA, Cavenee WK, Wan XF, Bigner DD, Friedman HS, Rich JN. Combination therapy of inhibitors of epidermal growth factor receptor/vascular endothelial growth factor receptor 2 (AEE788) and the mammalian target of rapamycin (RAD001) offers improved glioblastoma tumor growth inhibition. Molecular Cancer Therapy 2005; 4: 101-112.

[76] Pan Q, Luo X, Chegini N. Blocking neuropilin-1 function has an additive effect with anti-VEGF to inhibit tumor growth. Cancer Cell 2007; 11(1): 53-67.

[77] Lemoine FM, Cherai M, Giverne C, Dimitri D, Rosenzwajg M, Trebeden-Negre H, Chaput N, Barro B, Thioun N, Gattegnio B, Selles F, Six A, Azar N, Lotz JP, Buzyn A, Sibony M, Delcourt A, Boyer O, Herson S, Klatzmann D, Lacave R. Massive expansion of regulatory T-cells following interleukin 2 treatment during a phase I-II dendritic cell-based immunotherapy of metastatic renal cancer. International Journal of Oncology 2009; 35(3): 569-581.

[78] Iwami K, Natsume A, Wakabayashi T. Gene therapy for high-grade glioma. Neurologia Medico-Chirurgica (Tokyo) 2010; 50(9): 727-736.

[79] Fonteneau JF, Larsson M, Bhardwaj N. Interactions between dead cells and dendritic in the induction of antiviral CTL responses. Current Opinion in Immunology 2002: 14: 471-477.

[80] Lebedeva IV, Stein CA. Antisense Down Regulation of the Apoptosis – Related bcl-2 and bcl-xl Proteins: a New Approach to Cancer Therapy. In: Lattime EC, Gerson SL (ed.) Gene Therapy of Cancer. New York; Academic Press. 2002. p315-330.

[81] Patel S, Doble B, Woodgett JR. Glycogen synthase kinase-3 in insulin and Wnt signalling: a double-edged sword?. Biochemical Society Transversal 2004; 32: 803-808.

[82] Beckner ME, Gobbel GT, Abounader R, Burovic F, Agostino NR, Laterra J, Pollack IF. Glycolytic glioma cells with active glycogen synthase are sensitive to PTEN and inhibitors of PI3K and gluconeogenesis. Laboratory Investigation 2005; 85: 1457-1470.

[83] Lo HW. Targeting Ras-RAF-ERK and its interactive pathways as a novel therapy for malignant gliomas. Current Cancer Drug Targets 2010; 10(8): 840–848.

Chapter 6

Using REMBRANDT to Paint in the Details of Glioma Biology: Applications for Future Immunotherapy

An Q. Dang, Neil T. Hoa, Lisheng Ge,
Gabriel Arismendi Morillo, Brian Paleo,
Esteban J. Gomez, Dayeon Judy Shon, Erin Hong,
Ahmed M. Aref and Martin R. Jadus

Additional information is available at the end of the chapter

http://dx.doi.org/10.5772/52363

1. Introduction

Microarray technology developed in the late 1990's allows one to simultaneously analyze the entire transcriptome of a given population of cells at a single time. It is essentially a microchip with each spot containing about a picogram of DNA immobilized at defined locations. This DNA captures mRNA or cDNA from defined cell populations (tissue, cell line, *etc*) in a quantitative manner. This technique allows complex patterns of global gene expressions to be quickly and easily detected between two specimens. Microarrays were initially used to describe cell cycle patterns of *Saccharomyces cerevisiae* [1]. Its powerful potential was quickly recognized and applied towards cancer. The first successful application of this technology was to show that diffuse large cell B lymphomas had two different subtypes. One subset of this cancer was easily treatable with chemotherapy; whereas, the second phenotype required a more aggressive therapy [2].

Microarray analysis of human GBM quickly revealed that this cancer could be divided into three different subtypes: neural/pro-neural, mesenchymal and classical GBM [3]. Each subset has its own unique profile of gene expression along with a unique survival pattern. The microarray data also represents a composite of the tumor and the surrounding non-cancerous cells that are involved in the microenvironment including host immune cells. Microarrays have also recently provided possible mechanisms that GBM have used to avoid the effects of anti-angiogenic therapies [4]. Thus, this *in silico* technology offers new strategies to target various cancers in still many unknown ways.

In 2005 the National Cancer Institute and the National Institute of Neurological Disorders and Stroke (NINDS) initiated the REMBRANDT (REpository for Molecular BRAin Neoplasia DaTa (http://rembrandt.nci.nih.gov/) database. This informatics venture originated from the leadership of Dr. Subhashree Madhaven (NCI Center for Bioinformatics) and Dr. Howard Fine (Glioma Molecular Diagnostic Initiative at the Center of Cancer Research). Currently this research portal molecularly characterizes a large number of primary brain tumors and correlates this gene expression, copy number data with patient survival. At this time, there are several active collaborators who are supplying information into this database: Henry Ford Institute (Detroit), Johns Hopkins University (Baltimore), National Cancer Institute-Neuro-Oncology Branch, National Institute of Neurological Disorders and Stroke (NINDS), M.D. Anderson Cancer Center (Houston), Mofitt Cancer Center (Tampa), Thomas Jefferson (Philadelphia), Univ. of California, Los Angeles, Univ. of California, San Francisco, Univ. of Pittsburgh Medical Center, and Univ. of Wisconsin Carbone Cancer Center (Madison). At the time of writing this chapter 568 brain cancer specimens are available for gene expression analysis, while 552 patients were analyzed (May-Aug 2012) for copy number studies using REMBRANDT version 1.5.5. Thus, we have a relatively large database for which we can draw good information to determine the usefulness of targeting any given gene of interest towards a given brain cancer.

Van der Bruggen, *et al.*, [5] compiled a listing of various tumor antigens that have been found within various human cancers. Tumor antigens can be defined as either being tumor-specific or tumor-associated. These tumor-associated antigens are composed of mutations, shared tumor-specific, differentiation and over-expressed antigens. Tumor specific antigens are actually quite rare. The epidermal growth factor receptor variant III (EGFRvIII) is an example of a glioma-specific tumor antigen. Most antigens used for cancer therapy are shared antigens, in which the cancers over-express these proteins. By this definition most antigens should be described as cancer-associated antigens, as opposed to cancer-specific antigens. When tumor antigens are discovered, either by molecular techniques or using immunological techniques, only a handful of tumor cases are actually evaluated to generate the initial scientific report. Hence the real scope of the true expression pattern was usually limited due to a small sampling size of the initial report. Analyzing large databases are perhaps the best way to validate the universal nature of any tumor antigen.

Traditionally, there are antibody-based or cell-mediated-based antigens. Back in the 1970's-1980's, antibody responses were viewed as the best way to treat tumors. These antibodies need to be specifically designed to bind to cancer-specific cell surface proteins. Antibodies have been detected coming from glioma patients (PHD finger proteins-3 and -20 were identified [6, 7]. When these were evaluated by REMBRANDT, there were only 1 and 5 patients who over-expressed these respective transcripts and there were no statistical significance. Many antibodies were designed against glioma cells. Antibodies targeting internal antigens will obviously not be clinically applicable, since these antibodies' binding regions can't access their targeted intracellular epitopes. Antibodies with 150,000 dalton molecular weighs can't penetrate deeply into intracellular tumor cells due to their inability to cross cell-adhesion junctions between adjacent cells. Peripherally located tumor cells usually bind the most

http://dx.doi.org/10.5772/52363

amount of antibody, leaving the more internally located ones less affected. Single chain variable antibody fragments (scFv) are being developed out of monoclonal antibody technology can penetrate deeper into tumor beds, since they have lowered molecular weights (about 15-20 kd). ScFv targeting EGFRvIII, MRP3, TRAIL and c-Met have been used in preclinical models of human gliomas [8-11]. But just like regular antibodies, the scFv will undoubtedly predominantly bind to peripheral tumor cells. The clinical efficacy of scFv still has not been firmly established.

In contrast, internal and external antigens can be processed by intracellular proteosome using a universal ubiquitization pathway. Eventually some of these antigenic peptides are presented on the cell-surface of major histocompatibility (MHC) molecules, provided they have the right affinity and the right concentration. So once the correct anti-cancer T cells are activated towards these peptides, the T cells can respond to multiple tumor cells. The caveat to this approach is that many tumor cells down-regulate their MHC expression, making themselves "invisible" to the T cells. The use of dendritic cell (DC)-based vaccines to generate endogenous T cells *in vivo* seems to show that T cell-induced therapies are a better way to treat gliomas than humoral approaches [12]. Prins, *et al*, [13] showed that DC-based therapy using the autologous tumor to prime the T cells works better against the mesenchymal type of GBM than the other two subsets. So the identification of the right tumor antigens that glioma cells possess is the Holy Grail of tumor immunotherapy.

2. Hallmarks of cancer

In 2012 Hanahan and Weinburg updated their classic "Hallmarks of Cancer" paper where they described the original six Hallmarks (resisting cell death, sustained proliferation, evading growth suppression, activating invasion and metastasis, enabling replicative immortality and inducing angiogenesis) with two more emerging Hallmarks (deregulating energetic and avoiding immune destruction), along with two enabling characteristics (genomic instability and mutation and tumor promoting inflammation) [14]. Hanahan and Weinburg pointed out that various anti-cancer therapies currently being developed actually target one of these possible ten Hallmarks of Cancer. Each of these drugs is designed to be very specific and only affect a certain cancer pathway. Hence these drugs should avoid any unwanted side effects. One obvious down-side to this way is that cancers are very resourceful and can quickly mutate to avoid the actions of this drug.

They also speculated that if you design a drug that targets two or more of these pathways, then that drug should then theoretically be more potent than a drug that targets a single "Hallmark". We think it is possible to simultaneously target multiple "Hallmarks". A whole tumor cell vaccine which targets a wide variety of possible "Hallmarks" is possible.

Figure 1 shows some representative glioma antigens that are known and can induce immune responses against seven of the "Hallmarks". So the true power of tumor vaccines using whole cells as the source of the vaccine might be that it targets multiple proposed Hallmarks of Cancer at once. So finding newer antigens that might additionally target different Hallmarks could also improve immunotherapy.

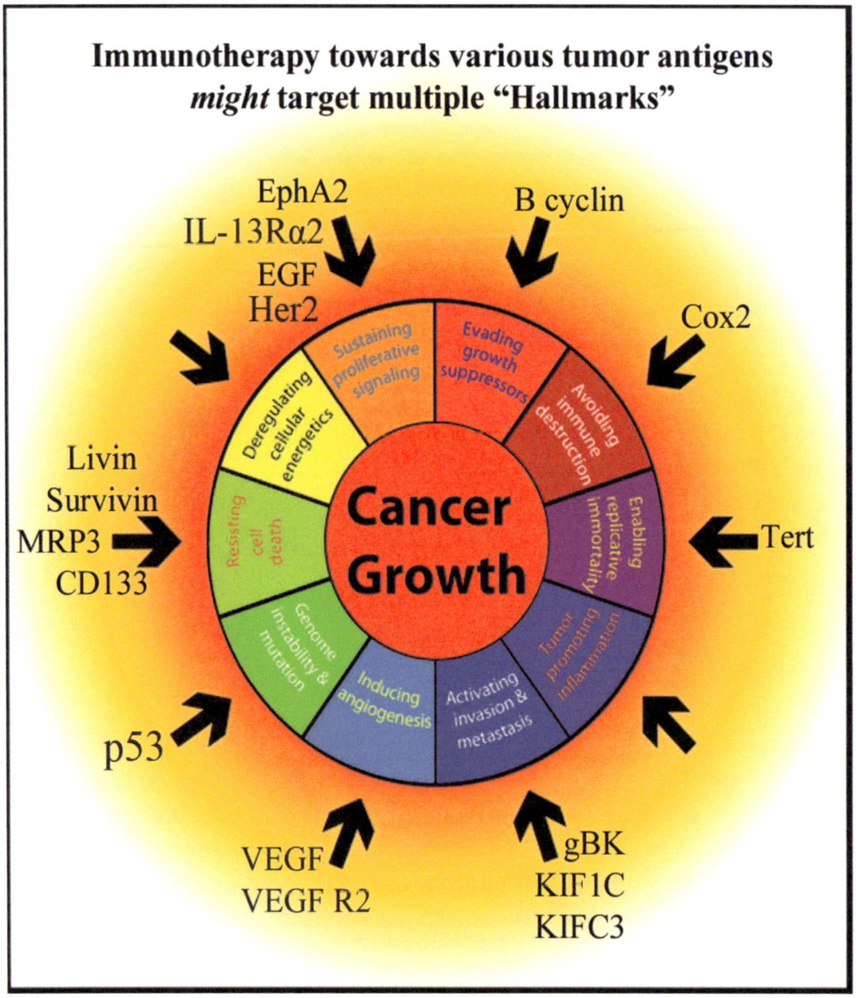

Figure 1. Whole tumor vaccines can target multiple Hallmarks of Cancer. Listed are some glioma tumor-associated antigens which can be classified under the various categories of the Hallmarks of cancer.

3. Current glioma associated tumor antigens: How well do our current tumor antigens fit the survival data of GBM?

REMBRANDT is quite easy to use. One can access the data of all glioma types or limit the selection of brain cancers to GBM, mixed gliomas, or oligodendroglioma. At the gene expression level, one can concentrate on over-expression that is 2.0-fold better than control samples,

http://dx.doi.org/10.5772/52363

or under expression < 0.5-fold expression, or an intermediate expression pattern. For this chapter we will be examining the universal nature of all glioma types. If readers want more specific brain cancer subtypes, they can easily study the various subsets of brain tumors on their own using REMBRANDT.

Previously, many tumor antigens used for glioma immunotherapy have been described [15-20]. A good tumor-associated antigen is one that is found in a large number of human glioma patients and has many different epitopes, so that many different T cell clones can respond to it, regardless of the major histocompatibility complex haplotype. The targeted antigen should also be associated with a poor prognosis. Therefore properly targeting this antigen interferes with some key glioma cell function; i.e., cell division, growth factor signaling, migration and other processes of the Hallmarks of Cancer. Improved patient survival if a successful therapy was mounted against this tumor antigen, should also eliminate those antigen-positive cells. By changing the tumor population from an antigen-positive one, to an antigen-negative one, overall survival should improve, if that antigen/protein was indeed critical to glioma biology. Even at this time, we still don't precisely know what the best glioma-specific antigens are to use for immunotherapy, except by doing expensive clinical trials. The other theoretical possibility, is that the antigen must be found on every tumor cell. In which case, every antigen-positive cell needs to be eliminated. In which case, every antigen is created equally. This question will eventually need to be answered, before immunotherapeutic cures can become a reality. Our own speculation is that not all glioma-associated antigens are equally useful.

When the currently known glioma-associated tumor antigens are subjected to REMBRANDT analysis, some of these antigens do seem to show a good inverse correlation with survival. Having more of the antigen does seem to correlate with a poorer survival in a dose-dependent manner. Figure 2 shows a representative illustration of this effect using the well-known glioma-associated antigen, IL13Rα2. There were 121 patients (red) who possessed elevated IL13Rα2 mRNA levels (21% of all glioma patients), while 115 (20% of all gliomas examined) had down-regulated IL13Rα2 expression (green). The more IL13Rα2 mRNA the patient's glioma had, the poorer the prognosis of these patients was. This data can be considered as a dose response experiment. By the Log-rank test, provided by REMBRANDT, these values were quite statistically significant from the total 568 glioma patients (blue) that were examined. Thus, this tumor antigen should be good one to target for a subset of glioma patients, since the lower the expression of IL13Rα2 lead to better patient survival. Other very good glioma-associated antigens are: EphA2, FABP7, FosL1, MRP-3, NR2E1 and podoplanin (Table 1).

Some antigens such as survivin/Birc5, CD133, her2 and Sart-2 were considered good antigens in that either their over-expression lead to poor survival or their under-expression had a better prognosis. This observation could be that some samples didn't have sufficient samples to provide a statistical significant value. WT1 also seems to be a good target. In an early clinical trial using WT-1 peptide vaccinated patients, there was some survival benefit for the first 100 weeks after the vaccination [21]. Thus, an early test of our hypothesis seems at first glance to be a viable one.

Very Good Antigens	Good Antigens	Poor Antigens
BCAN,CHI3L2, EphA2,FABP7, FosL1, IL-13Rα2, MRP3, NR2E1, PDPN, YKL-40/CHI3L1	B3GALNT/Galt3, CD133, Her2, IGF2BP3, Sart-2, Survivin, WT-1	Art-1, Art-4, ARF4L/ARL4D, CLIP2, CSPG4,EphB6, EZH2, Gnt-V, GP100, KIF1C, KIF3C, HNRPL, livin, Mage-A1, MELK, NES, NLGN4X, NRCAM, PHF-3, PHF-20, Prame, PTH-rP, PTPRZ1, Sart-1, Sart-3, SLC01C1, Sox-2, Sox-6, Sox-10, Sox-11, SSX2, TNC, Tert, Trp-2/DCT, Tyrosinase, Whsc2

Very Good Antigens: both over-expression predicts shorter patient survival and under-expression leads to longer survival rates. Statistical significance reached by REMBRANDT.

Good Antigens: one value (over expression or under-expression) achieved statistical significance.

Poor Antigens: Neither over- nor under-expression correlated with patient survival and had any statistical significance.

Table 1. Currently known Glioma-associated antigens and their predicted usefulness against all gliomas as predicted by REMBRANDT.

Unfortunately, most reported glioma-associated antigens such as Sox2, Sart3, *etc* do not seem to have any prognostic value. Their expression profile does not indicate any positive or negative effect. From this we would conclude, even though the glioma cells carry this tumor antigen, and *in vitro* experiments suggest that CTLs can kill tumor cells bearing this specific antigen, this antigen does not appear to have any selective or predictive advantage. Therefore even if a robust immune response were mounted *in vivo* by some vaccination or therapeutic process, chances are this response will not produce any demonstrable effect, unless all of those antigen-positive tumor cells were eliminated. Therefore, just because CTLs can be generated against tumor cells doesn't necessarily mean it will produce any clinical response, unless every tumor cell was eliminated. Killing every tumor within any cancer is highly doubtful.

In conclusion, some of our currently known tumor-associated antigens found in human glioma are still good ones to target by therapeutic interventions including immunological ones, while others probably will not be that much in helping eliminate this cancer. Searching out new target antigens is still a vital goal of immunotherapy and new strategies to find more appropriate antigens are required. This may be where REMBRANDT can come in quite handy in developing intelligent rationales for designing better targets for future immunotherapy (see below).

http://dx.doi.org/10.5772/52363

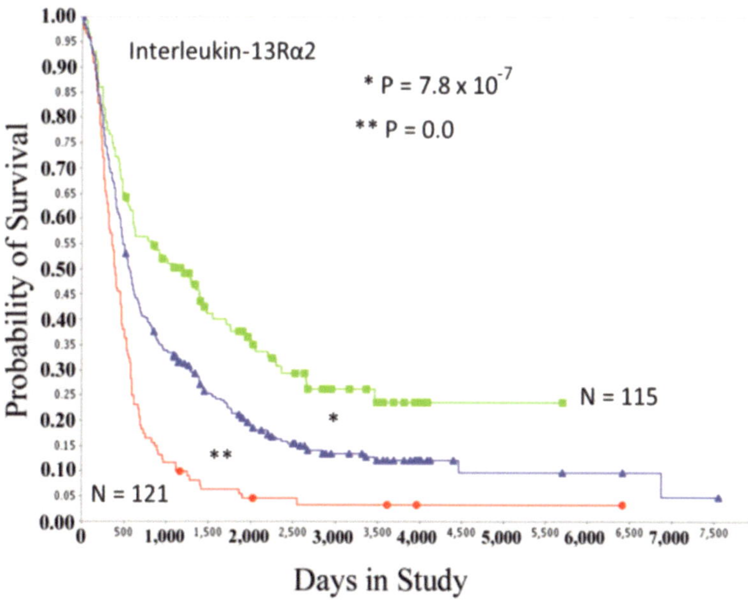

Figure 2. REMBRANDT survival of all gliomas showing differential IL13Rα2 expression. The blue symbols show the survival of all glioma patients. The red lines show the survival of IL13Rα2 over-expressing gliomas. While the green symbols show the patients that survived with a low expression of IL13Rα2. Both populations were statistically significantly different (asterisks) from the majority of all gliomas (blue).

4. Cells of the immune system involved in glioma

The immune system plays an important role in combating a wide variety of pathogens ranging from viruses, bacteria, fungi, parasites and others. Cancers can also be considered a type of pathogen that the body must rid itself of on a routine basis. In the mid-1980's, CD4+ T cell clones were classified into various subsets of T helper cells, Th1 cells produced cytokines that stimulated cell-mediated functions, while Th2 cells produced humoral immune responses [22]. New CD4 T helper subsets are still being discovered. Th9, Th17, Th22, Tfh and Treg are populations recently described in the last several years. Each subset seems to have its own niche with regards to certain immunological functions controlling certain pathogens or antigens. Besides CD4+ T cells, CD8, NK, and γδ T cells all play roles in tumor immunity.

Figure 3 shows these various subsets that are currently known along with some of their postulated effector cytokines. By REMBRANDT, we tried to analyze these different T cell subtypes. We examined their respective cytokine(s), possible effector molecules or putative transcription factors that control the transcription of these cell types.

REMBRANDT surprisingly revealed that CD4 expression had a bad prognosis for glioma patients. Over-expression of CD4 had a statistically significant poor survival prognosis, while an under-expression trended towards better survival, but this last condition was not considered significant (p=0.10). Naïve CD4+ T helper cells can give rise to numerous subtypes of CD4+ T cells: Th1, Th2, Th9, Th17, Th22, Tfh, and Treg. Thus, the sum total of all these CD4 subsets represents this poor overall survival.

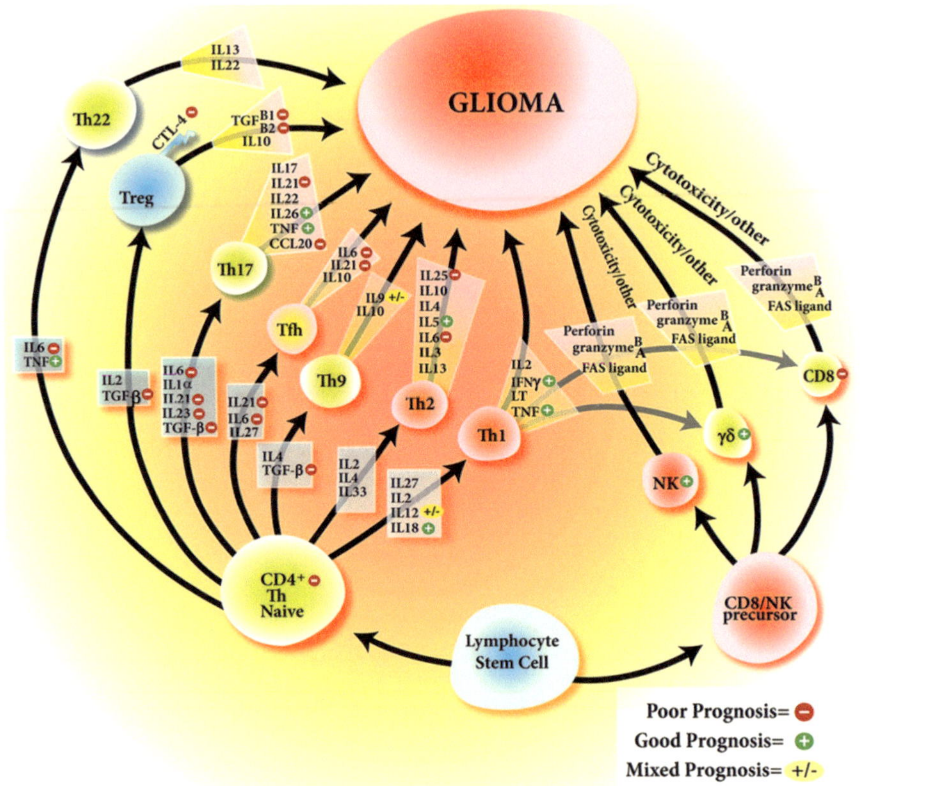

Figure 3. The cells of the Immune system and how they mediate some of their functions. Lymphocyte precursors give rise to either CD4+ or CD8/NK precursors. As a result of T cell receptor engagement along with the presence of cytokines shown in the rectangles can give rise to various T helper subsets. After the Th subsets are restimulated they can then release various cytokines as shown in the polygons. These cytokines can either affect the glioma or the cells in the local microenvironment. CD8/NK precursors can differentiate into either NK, γδ, or CD8 T cells. These cells can either kill tumor cells directly or via other undefined pathways.

In has been generally acknowledged that Th1 cells produce cell-mediated immunity that results in effective anti-tumor immune responses. Th1 cells tend to release cytokines such as IL2, IFN-γ, TNFα and LT, that either work directly on the tumor or indirectly by stimulating effector anti-tumoricidal cells, CTLs, NK, macrophages, etc. REMBRANDT suggested the expression of IL2 portrays a slightly better survival when these cytokines were elevated in patients but these were not significant. IFN-γ over-expression produced statistically significant positive outcomes while TNF down regulation lead to a worse survival. Three transcription factors, t-bet (TBX21), Signal Transducer and Activator of Transcription factor-1 and -4, Stat1 and Stat4, respectively regulate Th1 cell functions. T-bet and Stat-4 failed to show any significance. Stat1 showed a poorer survival, but we can't eliminate the possibility that glioma cells themselves directly utilize stat1 [23]. Thus, the classic Th1 cells where all Th1 associated cytokines and transcription factors that are simultaneously made, were not really displayed within human clinical gliomas.

Th2 cells are classified by their production of the cytokines IL3, IL4, IL5, IL6, IL10, IL13, and IL25. Interleukins 3, 4, 10 and 13 failed to show any significant relationship with glioma survivorship. The over-expression of IL6 and IL25 lead to poor patient survival, while over-expression of IL5 forecast better survival of glioma patients. Looking at the transcription factors that control the fate of Th2 (Gata-3, Stat6, Stat5 and MAF) also displayed a mixed effect. Stat6 was not significant, while Stat5, and MAF correlated with poorer survival. Again the secretion profiles predicted by current dogma within *in situ* Th2 cells gliomas are not consistent with current experimental conclusions about Th2 cells and their global cytokine expression pattern.

A few not so well known T helper subsets (Th9, Th22 and Tfh cells) are easily studied by microarray analyses. As a result of exposure to antigen with IL4 and TGF-β, Th9 cells can be generated. Th9 can release IL9 and IL10. As described above for these cells, IL10 didn't have any relationship with glioma survival. IL9 had a mixed expression, both under-expression and over-expression both had poor prognoses. Hence Th9 cells probably do not play an important role in glioma immunology. Th22 cells are induced after antigen exposure when IL6 and TNF are also present. These cells produce IL13 and IL22. Both cytokines appeared to be devoid of any significance, so the contributions of Th22 are probably minor. Tfh (follicular helper) cells are stimulated by IL6, IL21 and IL27. Tfh produce IL6, IL10 and IL21. Both IL6 and IL21 lead towards poor survival. Thus, Tfh cells are suspicious and may contribute to the poor response of CD4+ cells in glioma patients.

Treg cells are currently in vogue explaining poor anti-tumor immunity in many tumors including gliomas [24]. TGF-β and IL2 drive the appearance of Treg. IL2 as mentioned earlier, trends towards a favorable patient survival, however the IL2Rα (CD25) gene didn't show any significant relationship contradicting the current dogma that IL2Rα+ Treg are as predominant in GBM as previously thought [25]. The presence of TGF-β1 and TGF–β2 mRNA showed a very poor survival, glioma cells do make TGF-β1 and TGF-β2, so the initial source of stimulation of Treg may come directly from the glioma cells. Upon stimulation with TGF-β, the Treg can also release this cytokine or express the membrane form of TGF-β and thus amplifies the glioma's immunosuppressive nature. Treg use the FoxP3, Smad3 and Stat5 transcription factors. Stat5 and Smad3 showed a correlation with poor patient survival, but gliomas can also use smad3 and Stat5 [26,27], so the contribution of these transcription factors from Treg can't truly be assessed. FoxP3 is thought to be very specific for Treg, but it's presence within gliomas actually failed to show any significant correlation with patient survival. IL10 is released by Treg *in vitro*, but REMBRANDT doesn't show any survival relationship of IL10 production with gliomas, as described with Th2 and Th9 cells. The various mechanisms by which Treg can inhibit the immune system will be described in the next section (see Section 5: Immunosupression). Thus, the previously held belief that Treg are solely responsible for poor patient performance via various immunotherapies, needs a critical reassessment.

Th17 cells type also uses TGF-β to help drive their initial activation. In addition, these Th17 precursor cells require IL6, IL21, IL1α and IL1β to become polarized into the Th17 phenotype after the initial T cell receptor engagements. IL6 and IL21 over expression correlated with poor patient survival, while the expression of IL1α or IL1β subtypes didn't. Th17 cells have been identified in gliomas [28], but their precise role isn't defined. For melanomas, Th17 cells can mediate tumor destruction [29], but in colon cancer Th17 helps tumors grow [30]. REMBRANDT analysis of the transcription factors used by Th17: RORC (RORγT), RORA (RORα) and Stat3 did not show any positive or negative effects. Th17 cells release IL17A, IL17F, IL22, IL21 and IL26. The first three cytokines fail to correlate with patient survival. IL21 does show a poor patient survival prognosis, while IL26 shows a better patient survival. So the final verdict about Th17 cell's role in glioma is still undecided.

In conclusion, our current understandings of Th helper subsets seem to show multiple cytokines being expressed by cloned cells *in vitro*. However these distinct subsets can not be firmly identified *in situ*. This complexity is probably due to the complex cytokine/growth factor/environmental factors being produced within the tumor by the tumor, Treg or immune cells. One might even have to postulate subsets of these cells; e.g. Th1.1, Th1.2, Th2.1, Th2.2, Treg1.1, Treg 1.2, *etc* to explain these empirical observations. As described earlier, activated dendritic cell vaccines pulsed with autologous GBM tumors do improve GBM survival, so it will be important to describe what cytokines or subsets are correlating in those patients that are positively responding to such therapies.

CD8a is a more promiscuous marker, since it can be found on CTLs, NK, DC and other cell types. CD8b expression is exclusively found on CTLs; there were only 11 patients which over-expressed CD8b, while 89 patients down-regulated CD8b. The down-regulation of CD8b did however have a poor survival although not significant. Eosmesdermin (Eomes) is a transcription factor reported to control CTL function [31]. There was trend towards lower Eomes expression with longer patient survival occurred in 11 patients. Twenty patients over-expressed this gene, but this profile didn't alter patient survival when compared to all glioma patients. Hence, the evidence for a beneficial role of CTLs *in situ* seems to be weak.

NK cells and γδ type T cells are innate immunity-based lymphocytes. We examined a couple of NK/ γδ related genes [32]: NKG2D (KLRK1) and NKp30 (NCR3). Both of these genes when they were down-regulated lead to poor survival. Conversely, when patients presented higher expression, this produced a better survival. Both findings had statistical significance. Thus, these innate type immune cells seem to show a dose-dependent *in vivo* effectiveness. This at first glance seemed unexpected. Two targets of γδ type T cells are the MICA and MICB molecules [32]. Both of these molecules when over-expressed in glioma had poor prognoses, while low expressing gliomas had better outcomes. Hence the use of γδ type T cells to treat gliomas might be a good clinical approach [33-35]. CTLs, NK and γδ T cells use perforin (PRF1) and granzymes A and B (GRMA and GRMB) to actively lyse tumor targets *in vitro*. None of these gene expression patterns was associated with beneficial or deleterious effects. The exact mechanism by which NK/ γδ type T cells could have anti-glioma tumor effects is still unknown. This anti-tumor immunity might not actually be mediated through direct cell-mediated

http://dx.doi.org/10.5772/52363

cytotoxicity using perforin and granzymes but could be through the release of unknown cytokines or other unknown effector molecules.

One thing that can be concluded from this REMBRANDT analysis dealing with current tumor immunity is the *in situ* process is much more complicated than was previously concluded from experimental *in vitro* conditions. Hence new tools need to be developed to explore the anti-tumor mechanisms that are present within the *in situ* tumor.

5. Immunosuppression

It has been known for awhile, that advanced cancer patients, including gliomas, have abnormal and diminished immune responses [36]. This impediment undoubtedly prevents the successful application of any cellular immunotherapeutic modality and helps explain the complex T cell immune responses described above. Over the years, it has postulated that a wide range of cytokines, growth factors and micro-environmental factors (hypoxia, reactive oxygen and nitrogen) lead to diminished immunological responses [15,37,38]. Figure 4 shows these potential causes of glioma/immune suppression pathways that have been postulated over the years. Besides immunosuppressive molecules such as transforming growth factor-β subtypes 1-3 (TGF-β subtypes 1-3), interleukin-10 (IL-10), vascular endothelial cell growth factor (VEGF) or prostaglandin E (PGE), there are also suppressor cells such as T regulatory cells (Treg) and myeloid derived suppressor cells (MDSC) that contributes to the overall immunosuppressive microenvironment.

REMBRANDT data analysis does show that some cytokines/growth factors have good statistical inverse correlations with patient survival. TGF-β1 and TGF-β2 inversely correlate with patient survival in a dose-dependent manner (high expression correlated with poor survival, while low expression prognosticated a better survival). TGF-β3 doesn't appear to play much of a significant role within glioma patients. Interleukin-10 previously considered to play a major role in immunosuppression doesn't seem to have that much of an effect as seen above with the Th2 and Th9 phenotypes. VEGF inhibits immune activity via inhibitory actions upon dendritic cells [39]. Immune responses within the brain are initiated by the local dendritic cells [40].Both VEGF-A and VEGF-B over-expression significantly correlated with poor patient survival, while VEGF-C and VEGF-D failed to show any deleterious behavior. Thus, VEGF-A and VEGF-B besides promoting angiogenesis of brain cancers promotes immune suppression.

Treg and MDSC suppress the immune system through different mechanisms. Treg can release TGF-β or express cell surface TGF-β (as described above). Treg can release indoleamine-oxidase-1 (Ido-1) in various tumor models [41]. Ido-1 helps degrade the amino acid, tryptophan. T cells are very sensitive to tryptophan deprivation and become inactivated by this condition. REMBRANDT shows a significant detrimental effect when IDO-1 is over-expressed, while in those patients showing reduced expression of IDO-1 a better survival was seen. In both cases, this data was significant. Human GBM cell lines don't seem to make Ido-1, so the contribution of Ido-1 is probably from the Treg. Cytotoxic T lymphocyte antigen-4 (CTLA-4), Programmed Cell Death-1 (PCD-1), Fas Ligand (FasL), B7-H1, B7-H3 molecules which are membrane molecules and can inhibit other effector lymphocytes are possible immunosuppressive pathways of Treg. PCD1 over-expression was not associated with diminished survival, but under-expression did statistically show improved survival in a cohort of 104 patients. FasL and B7-H1 didn't show any survival effect, and are probably eliminated in their role in glioma immunology. B7-H3 was over-expressed in 203 patients and did inversely correlate with survival in a statistically significant way. There are currently thought to be two types of Treg, the natural and induced Treg subpopulations. When we examined the cell surface markers for either induced or natural Treg, nothing was immediately obvious. We postulate that *in situ* glioma Tregs are Foxp3-, FasL-, TGF-β+, Ido1+, PCD1+ and B7-H3+ based upon evaluation by REMBRANDT.

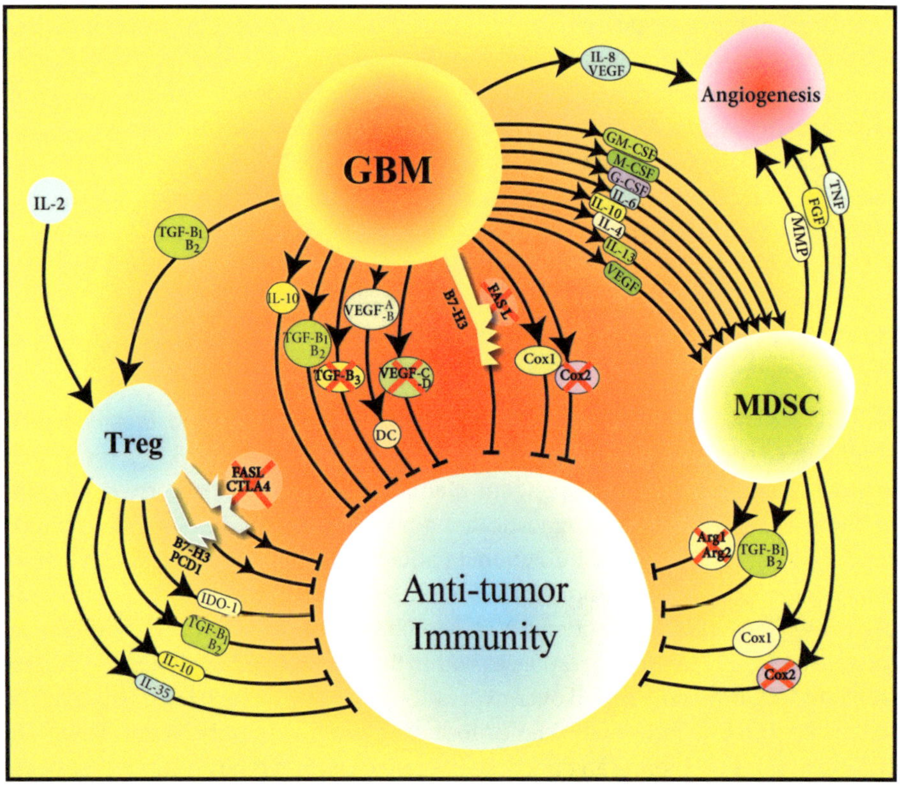

Figure 4. Mechanisms of immunosuppression found within gliomas. As a result of the glioma cell release growth factors and cytokines T regulatory (Treg) and myeloid derived suppressor cells (MDSC) are recruited. Glioma cells can express membrane proteins Fas Ligand and B7-H3. For sake of simplicity only 1 transmembrane protein is shown. Likewise Treg can express transmembrane inhibitory molecules FasL, CTLA4, B7-H3 and PCD1. A Red X indicates the pathways by REMBRANDT analysis are not likely playing a major role pathways. MDSC and gliomas can release Cox 1.

MDSC can either be composed of CD33+ cells or CD14+ cells [42]. These markers can be found on either the granulocytic or monocytic types of MDSC. MDSC are stimulated by a wide variety of cytokines and growth factors found in gliomas: GM-CSF, M-CSF, VEGF, IL1, IL4, IL6, IL13 and PGE, most of these cytokines were over-expressed by gliomas as determined by REM-

http://dx.doi.org/10.5772/52363

BRANDT. Fifty glioma patients did demonstrate an earlier demise when CD33 was determined to be over-expressed. In contrast only 8 patients down-regulated expression of CD33; this observation was not considered significant. CD14 expression was increased in 186 patients and possessed significantly shortened lives. Seventeen glioma patients were CD14 down-regulated and were approaching a significant survival advantage (p=0.058). So both types of MDSC can reside within human gliomas. MDSC can release TGF-β, arginase or prostaglandin (PGE) that prevents T cell expansion through different pathways [42]. As described above TGF-β1 and TGF-β2 are inversely correlated with glioma survival. But TGF-β can come from either Treg, the glioma itself or from MDSC. Arginase suppresses T cell function in a manner similar to IDO, in that T cells also require sufficient arginine for proper function. Two isoforms of arginase are known, Arg-1 and Arg-2. Arg-1 is a cytoplasmic enzyme; Arg-2 is a mitochondria contained enzyme. Neither form of arginase had any significant effect, eliminating this likely pathway from occurring in human gliomas. Thus, the way that MDSC mediate their actions is probably through TGF-β or PGE.

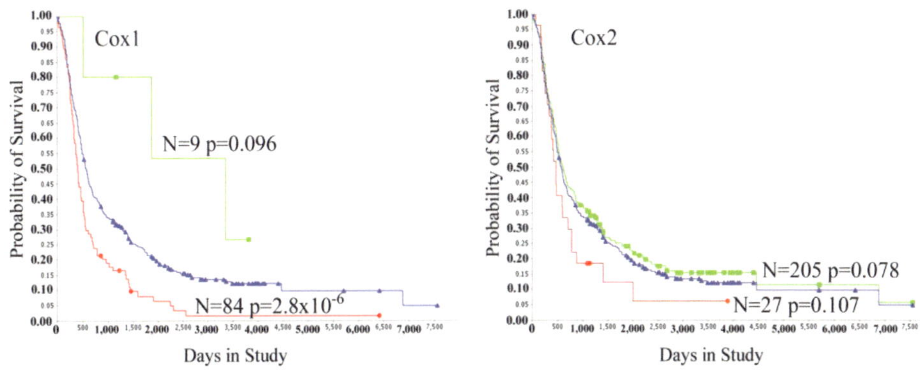

Figure 5. Survival statistics of glioma patients with Cox 1 and Cox 2 differential gene expression using REMBRANDT. The Left Panel shows the survival statistics of glioma patient analyzed for Cox 1 expression. There were 9 patient under-expressing Cox 1, which failed to achieve statistical significance. Eighty-four patients over-expressed Cox 1, which did reach a significant p value. The Right panel shows the REMBRANDT analysis of Cox 2 expression. There were 205 patients that under-expressed Cox 2, while only 27 patients over-expressed the Cox 2 transcripts. Neither phenotypes were considered significantly different from the total population of gliomas.

PGE2 is synthesized by either the cyclo-oxygenase-1 (Cox-1) or -2 (Cox-2) enzymes [43]. Cox 1 is considered by some to be a house-keeping gene and is constitutively produced and synthesizes low amounts of PGE_2. Figure 5 shows the REMBRANDT data dealing with the cyclo-oxygenases. Cox-2 is inducible and produces much more PGE_2 when cells are properly activated. Many tumors [43], including glioma cells [44,45] are reported to over-express the Cox2 enzyme. Cox2 derived epitopes have been described in human esophageal cancers that CTLs can recognize [46], so this enzyme might be a potential human glioma antigen, too. Epidemiological studies have shown that a daily dose of aspirin helps reduce PGE_2 production and lowers the incidence of a variety of cancers [47]. When Cox2 was analyzed by REMBRANDT, there was an association showing that gliomas that over-expressed Cox2 (27 patients) showed an unfavorable survival, while the under-expression of Cox 2 in 205 patients had only slightly improved patient survival. Neither of these expression patterns showed statistical significance when compared to all gliomas. Cox2 production of PGE might not therefore be a major source of PGE production as previously thought. When Cox1 expression was examined as a control, a surprisingly better correlation was found with patient survival. There were only 5 patients who under-expressed Cox 1, so statistically, this is not considered significant. Eighty-four glioma patients who over-expressed Cox1 succumbed earlier to their cancer. This later group of patients did achieve a very good statistical significance ($p = 2.8x10^{-6}$).

PGE_2 is a vasodilator and it is involved in angiogenesis so it may have multiple roles in glioma biology, besides immune suppression. Only prostaglandin receptors EP2 and EP4 were elevated within human gliomas using REMBRANDT. Based upon this REMBRANDT assessment, the role of Cox-1 needs to be investigated further in glioma biology and could be a target for therapy in some patients.

6. Growth factors, cytokines, chemokine are there targets of immunotherapy by T cells

PGE_2 receptors are coupled to G-proteins that activate adenylate cyclase, leading to an increase of intracellular cAMP which activates protein kinase A (PKA). This cellular signaling results in increased production of Vascular Endothelial Growth Factor (VEGF) and basic Fibroblast Growth Factor (bFGF) that assists new blood vessel formation (angiogenesis) (Figure 6). Glioma cells also possess growth factor and cytokine receptors, such as the interleukin-13Rα 2 (IL-13Rα2) [48], EphA2 [49], platelet derived growth factor receptor (PDGFR2) [50,51], epidermal growth factor receptor (EGFR)[52], insulin-like growth factor receptor (IGFR)[53], c-met (which binds hepatocyte growth factor/ scatter factor (HGF/SF)[54], interleukin-6 receptors (IL-6R) [55], and GM-CSF receptors [56]. Table 2 summarizes this data of growth factors/cytokines expressed within human gliomas along with their respective receptors. It can be speculated that some glioma cells use these potential autocrine growth pathways. REMBRANDT does seem to indicate that PDGF-B and PDGFR2 and the IL6/IL6R pathways are viable models of this autocrine process. The other cytokine/growth factors could be indicative of paracrine routes. Upon proper binding to their receptors, most growth factors/cytokines (EGF, IGF, PDGF, FGF, HGF/SF, Ephrin A, IL-6, IL-13 and others) use the PI3 kinase family of signal transducing docking molecules [57,58].

Upon ligation of the receptor, the Rac, Ras and Raf1 docking proteins are interacting and activate PI3K. H-ras and N-Ras have a positive correlation with poor glioma survival. Members of the Ras family, rab4,5,8,11,21,25, have been investigated with multiple aspects of signal transduction with glioma cells. But REMBRANDT showed that these rabs didn't have any significance. PI3 kinase family members do have a strong linkage with poor glioma survival by our analysis of the current data. Akt1 or Akt2 is also activated and does also show the same inverse relationship with patient survival. Thus, targeting PI3K/Akt dependent pathways are still a valid target.

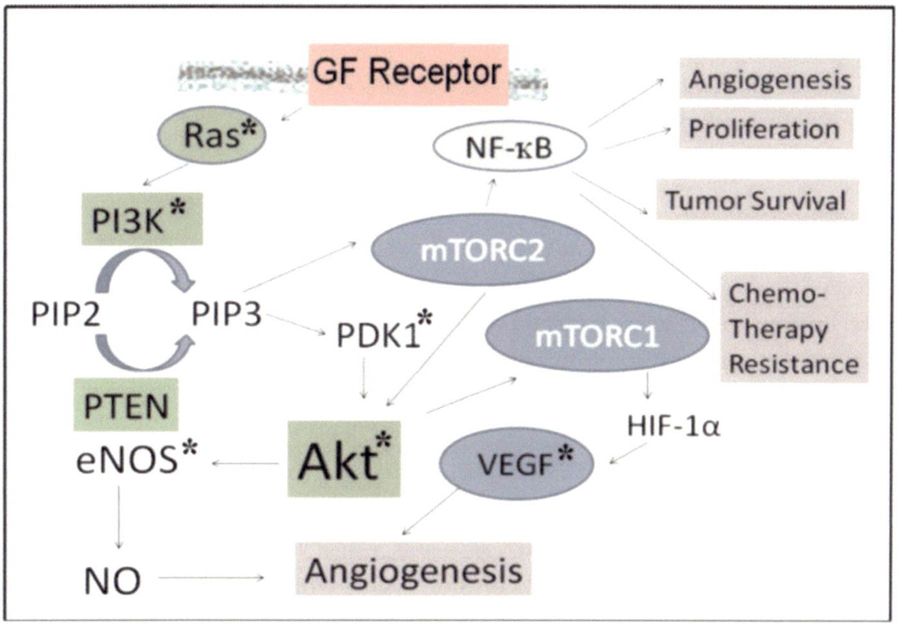

Figure 6. Generalized mechanism by which growth factor/cytokine interactions can initiate down-stream biochemical pathways. Upon binding a growth factor or cytokines, Ras/Raf/Rac signal transduction begins. PI3 kinase converts PIP2 into PIP3. PIP3 stimulates PDK1 which in turn activates Akt. eNOS is turned on by Akt. The asterisks indicate that protein is over-expressed and leads to poor patient survival by REMBRANDT.

The normal brain contains a variety of neurons, Schwann cells, glial cells, microglia and other cells. These cells are held in place and are embedded by an extracellular matrix (ECM)[59,60]. Matrix proteins besides providing cell anchorage, can also bind and sequester various soluble biological modulators. Table 3 also lists the various extracellular matrix proteins found within the brain that can bind to various glioma-related cytokines/growth factors. Several growth factors upon binding to their extracellular matrix enhance binding affinity to their receptors. Since the soluble factor is tethered to a large matrix protein, endocytosis may be slowed and allowed for increased intracellular signaling to be mediated. A prolonged signal transduction via PIP_3 can also recruits intracellular cytoskeletal elements Wave/WASP-like proteins which allows actin polymerization to be initiated at this membrane site, this can then help explain the presence of filopodia, lamellopodia, microvilli and invadopodia of gliomas [61-64]. See Section 7.2.

7. Mechanisms of invasion of gliomas

7.1. Extracellular mechanisms

It has been concluded that the reason why many human gliomas cannot be cured by conventional surgical, chemotherapeutic and radiation modalities is these tumors are very infiltrative. After the neurosurgeons and the radiation oncologists treat their patients, some remaining cancer cells have escaped these interventions. Perhaps the glioma cancer initiating cells or "stem cells" have even already migrated into new areas of the brain in searching for new sources of cytokines or other stimuli (see Section 6). There are more components that enable the glioma cells to become more invasive and can become potential targets of some therapy.

Glioma cells possess receptors/molecules than can bind to environmental components. These receptors can be either cell-adhesion integrins or CD44 [65]. The most important integrins are considered to be the $\alpha_v\beta_3$, and $\alpha_v\beta_5$ heterodimers [66]. These integrins act as receptors to bind vitronectin, fibronectin, osteopontin and cyr61 [67]. The last three ECM proteins when they were over-expressed also showed a predicted poor survival with glioma patients. Two other integrins, $\alpha_6\beta_1$ [68] and $\alpha_5\beta_1$ [69], have been reported to also play roles in glioma tumorigenesis. The $\alpha_v\beta_3$ and $\alpha_6\beta_1$ integrins are functional receptors for several heparin binding growth factors, pleiotrophin and midkine, respectively [70,71]. Midkine has been identified as a potential mediator that promotes chemoresistance within those midkine-stimulated cells [71]. As described in Table 3 some of these genes that interacted with the cytokines and growth factors were identified by REMBRANDT as significant in predicting patient outcome. REMBRANDT confirmed that CD44, α_v, α_6 and midkine lead to poorer prognoses.

Cancer cells, including gliomas do release matrix metalloproteineases (MMP) which digest the surrounding tissue and extracellular matrix allowing the cancer cells to invade surrounding tissue. By REMBRANDT we identified that MMP1, MMP2, MMP9, MMP11 and MMP14 all were associated with a bad prognosis. A natural inhibitor of the MMP, called TIMP3, associated with better patient survival when over-expressed, as current dogma predicts. So strategies that counter these MMPs or by increasing TIMP3 activity might have an important role in preventing the glioma cells from breaking its initial containment.

Gliomas might also release excess glutamate and kill surrounding normal tissue via an excitotoxic process [72]. There is speculation that gliomas can also down-regulate their glutamate receptors [73,74] so that they become impervious to the cytotoxic levels of glutamate that they release. Glutamate can be synthesized from the enzyme glutamate synthethese (GLUL) or can be scavenged via numerous catabolic pathways. Glutamate can be released via exporters that use K^+ and Na^+ cation exchangers, or SoLute Carriers (see Section 7.3 below). We found that there was no correlation with GLUL expression with patient survival or demise. So the most likely source of the released glutamate is coming via protein catabolism. The glutamate receptors GRIA1, GRIA2, GRIA3, GRIA4, GRM5 and GRM7 all correlated with a bad prognosis by a REMBRANDT analysis when they were down-regulated. The interpretation here is consistent with the initial hypothesis that this down-regulation by the glioma cells can make themselves resistant to the cytotoxic levels of glutamate found in the local microenvironment.

http://dx.doi.org/10.5772/52363

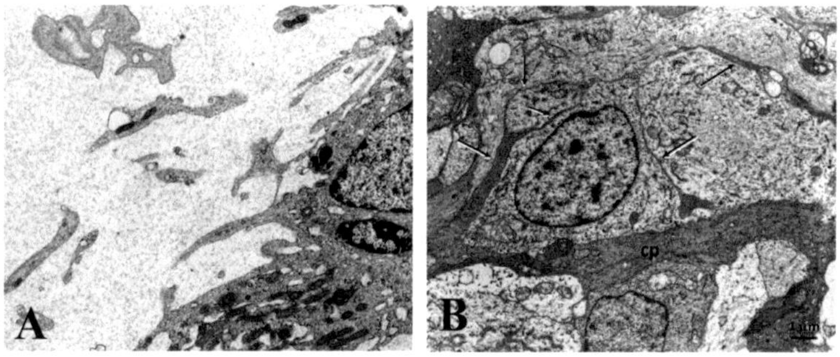

Figure 7. Electron microscopy of human GBM *in situ*. Panel A shows gliomas with microvilli invading surrounding extracellular matrix: magnified 15,000 x times. Panel B shows gliomas with filopodia invading through other cells. Magnification 5,000 x times.

7.2. Microvilli and filopodia

Cell surface superstructures including microvilli, invadopodia and filopodia have been described over the years [75-79]. These structures allow tumor cells to probe for weak spots in surrounding normal cells and then begin to invade that area as described above. Some of the gliomas found in GBM do have these microvilli structures *in situ*. Some microvilli actually had mitochondria within them (Figure 7A), and their apparent function appears linked with the ROS generation and subsequent activation of several pathways essentials for glioma invasiveness [80]. Thus, microvilli have a built in power supply to immediately supply the energy into their probing mechanisms via re-organization of microfilaments and microtubules. At some edges there were long filopodial projections that could extend past two cell- lengths. Some glioma cells possess these long filopodia and thus have the ability to probe into distant sites (Figure 7B). Glioma cells like U251 display her2/neu on their microvilli and filopodia [81]. We have also seen the receptors such as: IL13Ra2, EphA2, EGFR, PDGFR, c-Met, IGFR and IL6R on the microvilli and filopodia of U251 gliomas [unpublished data]. These microvilli also provide a novel "sea urchin" type defense that prevents various lymphocytes from mediating cytotoxicity. Thus these microvilli and filopodia can be used for multiple purposes by glioma cells and assist in their invasiveness.

We searched out the molecules that have been associated with microvilli, lamellipodia and filopodia with REMBRANT to identify pathways that are most likely being used by human gliomas. Figure 8 shows a basic schematic of how these superstructures could be composed of actin-related proteins Microfilaments, actin-binding proteins and microtubules have been reviewed in [82-84]. Microfilaments are composed of the actin family members. There are two types of actin. The monomeric, globular (G-form) represents the single unit, whereas, when these monomers polymerize, they form the filamentous, F-actin type. Actin contains both pointed and a barbed ends. The barbed end is protruding from the growing end of the F-actin polymer. Actin plays many roles in cellular processes. Actin anchors many membrane-bound proteins in place and are associated with glioma cell motility and the cytoskeleton. Surprisingly, by REMBRANDT, there was no significance of actin expression. So glioma cells probably just recycle and reuse their actin in a more efficient manner.

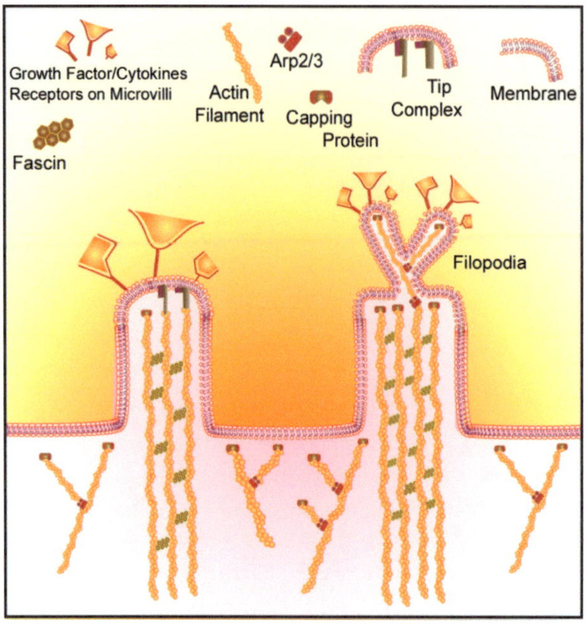

Figure 8. Schematic diagram of microvilli/filopodia. The microvilli (left) and a microvilli with a branched filopodia (right) are shown. Various growth factor/cytokine receptors and cell adhesion molecules are found on these structures. Upon binding with their ligands, the transmembrane receptors become activated and allow the nucleation of various cytoskeletal elements to begin. Hence the activated receptors can now begin a process where cell polarity is initiated.

There are molecules that crosslink the actin locking proteins together. Some proteins bundle actin polymers together making these proteins stronger, fascin is a prime example. Actin-binding proteins like Arp2/3 cause branch points within the polymerized actin strands and help explain the bending of the filopodia [85]. At least 100 proteins can associate directly or indirectly with actin some of the more important ones are listed in Table 3. It is therefore not surprising that actin-binding proteins are associated with the mobility of many cancer cells. The proteins, fascin, podoplanin, and myosin IIB, have been actively studied with regards to cancer cell motility [86-90]. These two proteins are also over-expressed in gliomas and in other cancers. The over-expression of fascin and podoplanin mRNA within gliomas is linked with a worse prognosis in those patients. Actin and fascin are important for maintaining the lamellopodia, microvilli and filopodia of various cells (Figure 8). This infiltrative nature of gliomas is believed to be the prime reason why this tumor remains such a lethal cancer, despite the best efforts to surgical remove and irradiate the surgical incision sites. So these two molecules can be considered good targets for possible molecular intervention. Table 3 summarizes as many cytoskeletal elements which have been associated with cell invasion and migration over the years and correlated them with significance by REMBRANDT.

http://dx.doi.org/10.5772/52363

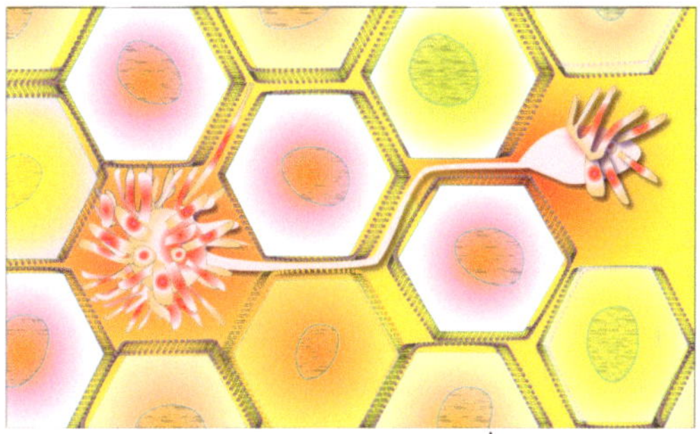
Homeostasis
High Intracellular K+
Low Intracellular Na+
Export K+
Import H2O
Import Na+
Import Cl-
Cloride Channels: CLICI
Potassium Channels: KCNMB2, KCNMB3, KCNN4, KCNQ1, KCNQ4
Sodium Channels: TRPM4, TRPM8, TRPU2, SLC9A1
Aquaporins: AQP1, AQP5, AQP9

Figure 9. Proposed model of ion channel regulation of glioma cell invasion. The main cell body (left) is in normal ionic homeostasis, where there are high intracellular K+ ion concentrations with relatively low concentrations of Na+ ions. The invading part of the cell (right) is now swelling as a result of possible activation of several ion channels listed at the bottom. K+ ions are exported while Na+ and Cl- ions along with water is imported causing the cell swell. As a result of the swelling at the leading edge the rest of the main cell body can be pulled into the new area. The bottom lines list the possible ion channels/aquaporins that were identified to be of significance by REMBRANDT.

7.3. A mechanism for glioma cells to squeeze through normal tissue

Harald Sontheimer has pioneered ion channel discovery in brain cancers. His unified hypothesis is that gliomas can shrink at the leading edge of the glioma cell [91]. In this way, the glioma cell then behaves like an amoeba and pushes itself through the normal tissue. Figure 9 shows a simplistic model of the dynamic aspects of ion-driven movements in a slightly different model 19. While at rest and in homeostasis, the glioma cell maintains its normal physiological ionic composition and has multiple filipodia projections. Some projections find an area which stimulates proper intracellular interactions and begin an invasive process. Here there is high intracellular levels of K^+, and normal concentrations of Na^+, Ca^{+2}, Cl^- and water. At the leading edge of the cell, now a disruption of normal ionic homeostasis occurs. Here K^+ channels are activated and K^+ ions are released, while Na^+ ions are allowed inside. As Na^+ ions enter, so does Cl^- anions and water, hence the cell can expand within this region of the cell. Colman et al., [92] found that one of the channels that are strongly correlated with poor survival was a CLIC1 chloride channel. REMBRANDT confirmed this ion channel expression inversely associated with poor patient survival. This chloride channel, CLIC1, also can share a subunit (BKβ as known as KCNMB2 or KCNMB3) with the big potassium (BKα, KCNMA1) ion channel channel [93]. REMBRANDT analysis showed the BKβ2 or BKβ3 chains had an inverse correlation with survival, like the CLIC1 expression. The KCNMA1/BKα ion channel failed to show any relationship with glioma patient survival. This last finding prompted us to consider whether other potassium channels could provide an alternative pathway for exporting of K^+ ions instead. The potassium channels are associated with poor glioma survival are KCNN4, KCNQ1, and KCNQ4.

For cells to maintain electroneutrality, as K^+ ions are eliminated Na+ ions must enter. REMBRANDT analysis reveals that four sodium ion channels are strongly correlated with an adverse survival rate. These sodium ion channels are TRPM8, TRPM4, TRPV2 and a sodium-hydrogen exchanger (a.k.a. NHE1, SLC9A1). As sodium ions enter the cell, so does water, so the aquaporins (water channels) are playing an active role in this dynamic swelling process, too. The aquaporins, AQP1, AQP5 and AQP9 all show dose-dependent inverse pattern of survival within glioma patients. Interestingly, AQP7 and AQP10 display an opposite pattern than the previous three aquaporins. Here over-expression of AQP7 and AQP10 lead towards better survival, while lowered expression produced a worse prognosis.

Sontheimer's lab found that a novel spliced version of the BK channel, called the glioma BK channel is found in human gliomas [94]. We created an antibody directed towards this region and confirmed that all human gliomas and many rat and mouse glioma cells lines also possessed gBK [95]. We also found that two epitopes within these gBK regions can induce human HLA-A2 restricted CTLs which lyse a variety of human cancer cells including glioma cells. Thus, ion channels have the potential to be developed into immunotherapeutic targets. So the ion channels, CLIC1, KCNMB2, KCNMB3, KCNN4, KCNQ1, KCNQ4, TRPM4, TRPM8, TRPV2 and SLC9A1 could also theoretically be targeted by immunotherapy. Dutroit and colleagues [96] have mapped a HLA-A2 derived peptidome which could stimulate possible immunotargets for CTL therapy. Some of these identified peptides did include ion and transporter channels, such as: ATP1A2, ATP2B1, CACNA1A, GRIA2, GRIA3 and SLC4A4. So immunotherapy might be directed towards these ion channels, aquaporins and transporters could be playing a role in glioma invasiveness.

7.4. "Death signatures"

Glinsky, *et al.*, [97] analyzed a wide variety of cancers by using microarray technology and discovered that a series of 11 genes (GBX2, Ki67, CCNB1, BUB1, KNTC2, USP22, HCFC1, RNF2, ANK3, FGFR2, and CES1) had a unique pattern. When this profile was expressed in those various cancers it had a high statistical probability that the patient will die of the cancer. They called this expression pattern, a "Death Signature". In theory, one would think that if an immunological intervention could be developed, these gene products might be perfect targets for immunotherapy, assuming that these genes or their synthesized proteins are actively playing a role in the cancer's aggressiveness which leads to the patient's demise. Since these genes foretold the patient death, if you could then vaccinate a patient against these antigens and prevent these genes from manifesting themselves, you should then interfere with their final outcome, death. When we examined the REMBRANDT survival data with this series of genes found in the Death Signature, there was actually very little significance; most of the gene expression patterns, when investigated individually were the opposite of what was predicted by the Death Signature concept. The only gene that correlated well with poor glioma survival was a marker for cell proliferation that pathologists regularly use as a sign of cell division, Ki67. Thus, we feel that this "Death Signature" doesn't fit too well with gliomas. In fairness to Glinsky and coworkers, they did use a large variety of cancers and they did do a multigene analysis, which REMBRANDT currently does not allow. So any multifactoral effect may have simply been masked by the complexity of their analysis.

8. Targeting the genes commonly found in human GBM

In 2010, Colman and colleagues reported a series of 31 genes that were associated with poor GBM survival [92]. When Rembrandt analysis was done using these genes, the vast majority of these genes correlated extremely well. This evaluation was much better than "Death Signature profile". Since the MD Anderson and University of California, San Francisco groups include many of their patients into REMBRANDT, it would be expected a much better correlation could be found.

One interesting finding was that a couple of these genes from the Colman, *et al.* study were also found in the glioblastoma peptidome derived from HLA-A2 alleles obtained from GBM surgical specimens [96]. These T cells-derived antigens included: CHI3L1 (YKL-40), IGFBP3 (insulin-like growth factor binding protein-3), PDPN (podoplanin) and TNC (tenascin C). We further examined these 31 genes from the Colman study and found their protein sequences. We subjected them to SYPEITHI data analysis program (http://www.syfpeithi.de/) to determine the possibility of generating nonomer peptide determinants towards their potential antigenic peptides. Table 4 summarizes this study. We limited this inquiry to those peptides that are found restricted to the HLA-0201 allele, since that is the most common HLA allele found in the US with just a little less than half the Caucasians possessing this phenotype. Some of the Colman and colleague's proteins are quite small ranging from 116 amino acids (dynein light chain) to fibronectin isoform1 that possess 2477 amino acids. For the dynein light chain there were only 12 predicted peptides that could bind to HLA-A0201 with a binding score of 16 or better. In contrast, the fibronectin isoform-1 had 236 possible peptides. In sum, these proteins provides 1,802 peptides that could theoretically be used to vaccinate patients against HLA-0201+ tumor cells. Hence this might provide a particularly rich source of very clinically relevant antigens to target glioma.

9. New targets

As we have described in Table 1, we only have 17 very good or good tumor antigens by which we can target brain cancers, thus new antigens are needed. REMBRANDT has validated *in silico* that there might be new targets that haven't been considered before. It will be important to consider targeting these molecules using a variety of mechanisms since they cause poor patient survival and their under-expression leads to better survival. This can include immunotherapy, molecular gene silencing or even knock-in strategies to take advantage of those genes which prolonged patient survival. In Table 2 we show that several growth factors, their cytokines or their extracellular matrix proteins might be potential good targets. Table 3 illustrated many intracellular cytoskeletal elements that are also good targets for either immunotherapy or potential gene knock-in. Colman's study [92] (Table 4) provided an incredible wealth of potential tumor antigens that could conceivably be targeted.

Growth factor/cytokine	Receptor	Extracellular protein capable of immobilizing
Acidic Fibroblast growth factor	FGFR*	glypican-1*
Basic Fibroblast growth factor	FGFR*	neurocan, syndecan-1*,-2*,-3, glypican-1*,-2,-3, phosphacan, nerve-glial antigen-2 (NG2) also known as chondroiten sulfate proteoglycan 4, phosphacan (PTPRZ1).
Unknown ligand	erbB2/her2*	not known
Transforming growth factor-β1**β2**β3	TGFBR1* TGFBR2** TGFBR3	syndecan-1*, decorin**, dermatan sulfate
Insulin-like growth factor-1	IGF1R	glypican-3
Hepatocyte growth factor/	c-Met*	dermatan sulfate/chondroiten sulfate B
VEGF-A**, VEGF-B**	VEGFR1 (flt1) VEGFR2 (kdr)*	glypican-1*, syndecan-2*
Platelet derived growth factor-A	PDGFR1	NG2
Platelet derived growth factor-B*	PDGFR2*	
Pleiotrophin*	nucleolin, α_v-β_3	syndecan-3
	A_6-β_1	
Midkine**	nucleolin, α_v-β_3	various heparans
	A_6-β_1	
Neuroregulin-1	erbB3 erbB4	heparan sulfated proteoglycans
Fibroblast growth factor-4	FGFR1	heparan sulfate
SDF-1 (CXCL12)	CXCR4*	syndecan-4
Epidermal growth factor*	EGFR	syndecan-2*, laminin A2**, lamininB1**, laminin A5*, laminin B3*
Interleukin-6*	IL6R*	not reported yet
Interleukin-8*	IL8RA, IL8RB*	syndecan-2*
Interleukin-13	IL13Ra1**	not reported as yet.
	IL13Ra2**	
Granulocyte-macrophage	CSF2R	syndecan-2*
Colony Stimulating Factor	c-fms	not reported as yet.

Table 2. Growth factors, cytokines and their receptors along with brain derived ECM. Single asterisk indicates either over-expression leads to poor survival or under-expression leads towards better survival. Double asterisk indicates both conditions described immediately above were true.

Thus, targeting some of these genes using DC based vaccines could encompass using whole tumor cell lysates, recombinant proteins or peptides using this information might be able to target these key proteins. One can also interfere with these vital functions of glioma invasion via molecular methods. In support of this concept, Dutroit and colleagues [96] using the peptidomics approach with HLA-A2 associated peptides has found evidence that some of these REMBRANDT validated peptides are present and could be possible targets of immunotherapy if one was to use the same starting material that they used.

Signal transduction		
Good Potential antigen	No relevance	Opposite expression
CDC42, grb2, h-ras, n-ras	c-Src, Rac1, Raf1, rab4, 5, 8, 11, 21, 25	APC, k-ras
Actin Cytoskeletal		
Actn, Arf6, basigin, caveolin1, 2, CDC42, CrkII, diaph1, erm/ moesin, filamin A, C, fascin1, grb2, gelsolin, IQGAP1, 2, 3, Mrlc2, Myh9, Nck1, paxilin, Pdpn, Ppir12a, Pfn1, Rhamm, supervillin, vimentin, Was/nWasp, Wasf2	Abi2, Actr3, Arp2, Arp3, Bcar1, caveolin 3, cofilin, c-Src, Cyfip1, diaph3, dynamin1, 2, ezrin, f-actin, fascin2, GFAP, Lmk1, Mena/Enah, MLCK, Myh2, netrin, Pak1, 3, 4, profilin 2, RhoA, Sh3pxd2a/Tks5, Ssh1, vinculin, Wasl, Wipf1	Apc, Aref/ARHGEF4, ARHGEF7, doublecortin, dynamin3, dock1, Dtnb, FAK, fascin3, Myh10, Ntn4, Pak7, Stathmin 2,3, 4, Wasf1
Tubulin cytoskeleton		
Kif2c, Kif11/eg5	Dnch2, Dynll2, Dync1l11, Dynein light chain/tctex, Kif1c, Klc2, Tubb3,5, Tubg1,2	Kif3c, /kif21b
Membrane Protein		
CD44, Itga6, Itgav, Itgb1, Itgb5, Pdpn,	Itgb3	

Table 3. Cytoskeletal proteins associated with cell migration, invasion and structure analyzed by REMBRANDT. (+) indicates significant values, opposite (+) indicates a significant value, but is opposite to what is actually predicted by current dogma.

REMBRANDT was then used to determine whether this gene is either over-expressed with a bad prognosis or under-expressed with a better survival was. When either one of those conditions was met then that antigen was considered a potentially good antigen. If both conditions were met, then it is considered a potentially very good antigen. Conversely, if neither condition was met then it was considered not good. Opposite indicates the REMBRANDT analysis contradicts the expected prediction, where over expression lead to a better survival and vice versa.

The numbers of amino acids of the translated protein are shown. This protein was then analyzed by SFYPEITHI analysis looking at possible nonamers that can theoretically bind to HLA-A*0201, as a metric for how tentatively immunogenic this protein could be. SFYPEITHI scores better than 16 were then counted. REMBRANDT was then used to determine whether

Gene	# Amino Acids	Predicted # Epitopes	Rembrandt Correl
α-actinin-1 isoform a	914	122	Very Good
Aquaporin-1, isoform1	269	66	Very Good
Chitinase-3like protein 1	383	40	Very Good
Chloride intracell. channel protein 1	241	39	Good
Collagen α2	1366	95	Very Good
Epithelial membrane protein-3	163	45	Very Good
Fatty acid binding protein-5	135	14	Very Good
Fibronectin isoform 1	2477	236	Good
Transmembrane glycoprotein NMB	572	77	Very Good
Insulin-like growth factor bind. protein-2	328	41	Very Good
Insulin-like growth factor bind. protein-3	297	33	Very Good
Lactate dehydrogenase A	332	62	Very Good
Galectin-1	135	10	Very Good
Galectin-3	250	23	Very Good
Gycoprotein (transmembrane) NMB	572	44	Very Good
Monoamine oxidase B	520	84	Very Good
Nicotinamide N-methyltransferase	264	38	Very Good
Podoplanin a	238	46	Very Good
Proteolipid protein 2	152	34	Very Good
Transmembrane protein-158 (RIS)	300	50	Very Good
Serpine A3	423	80	Very Good
Plasminogen activator inhibitor 1	402	66	Very Good
Plasma protease C1 inhibitor	500	92	Very Good
Protein S100-A10	97	15	Good
Transgelin	201	21	Very Good
Transgelin 2	199	24	Very Good
Dyncin light chain (Tctex)	116	12	No Good
Transforming growth factor-β1	390	57	Very Good
Tissue inhib. Metalloprot inhibitor 1	207	31	Very Good
Thymosin β10 (TMSB10)	44	0	Very Good
Tenascin	2201	179	No Good
VEGF-A	412	28	Very Good
Total Potential T cell epitopes: 1,802			

Table 4. SYPEITHI predicted binding epitopes for the genes restricted to HLA-A*0201 that were over-expressed in glioma and correlated with poor survival.

this gene is either over-expressed with a bad prognosis or under-expressed with a better survival. When either one of those conditions was met then that antigen was considered a potentially good antigen. If both conditions were met, then it is considered a potentially very good antigen. Conversely, if neither condition was met then it was considered not good.

http://dx.doi.org/10.5772/52363

10. Limitations and improvements for REMBRANDT

REMBRANDT type databases will be the future analyzing other types of cancer. Overall, this program is quite useful and easy to use. One must have the proper abbreviation of the gene, which can usually be found at websites like Gene Cards, Wiki Genes or the HUGO Gene Nomenclature Committee HGNC databases. Occasionally for some of the genes we searched, our analyses ran into some technical problems that won't perform the computations, obviously some glitches remain in the system that will be eventually ironed out. For the next version of REMBRANDT it will be important to allow the glioma sub-classes to be assessed: proneural, mesenchymal and classic GBM. This option will be important, since each GBM subclass has its own particular targets to be used; such as growth factor requirements proneural/neural GBM use the PDGF pathway, while classical GBM use more EGF driven pathways. YKL-40 is a marker of the mesenchymal GBM subtype and it might be a way to identify key interactions. Multivariant gene analysis, where one can analyze several genes simultaneously will also allow better analyses. So REMBRANDT version 2.0 should be enhanced with this kind of analysis.

The data we analyzed was based on gene expression measuring mRNA levels using microarrays. So the danger is that these conclusions does not necessarily mean that the corresponding proteins were synthesized. Splice variants are also not taken into account. For example gBK and BKα channels cannot be distinguished as separate isoform resulted from the current microarray platform. Nevertheless, this type of analysis will provide neuro-oncologists with some exciting concepts to think about for years to come.

11. Conclusions

After many frustrating years of attempting to use immunotherapy against cancers, tumor immunologists are starting to see successful results in melanomas, prostate cancer and in some GBM patients including high grade gliomas. The identification of better glioma-associated antigens is paramount to continue this investigative process. Many defined antigens have been discovered by serendipity and this random process has lead to developments such as using a variety of modalities: immunotoxins, chimeric antigen re-directed T cells, molecular silencing approaches, DC-based vaccines, *etc*. But there are undoubtedly many more antigens still to be discovered. Microarray analysis of tumors has already been proven to be a powerful way of classifying tumors and provide novel tumor-specific therapies. The REMBRANDT data portal allows researchers a chance to quickly assess this microarray data and quickly test potential therapies *in silico* as we have attempted to do here before doing expensive clinical trials. REMBRANDT gives one a chance to determine whether a gene has any importance in glioma biology using a large data base. In this chapter we showed that REMBRANDT offers oncologists a chance to analyze various biological pathways to see if predicted molecules seen in tissue culture cell lines are applicable with the *in situ* scenario. REMBRANDT offers immunologists a chance to now make use of the key genes involved in gliomas and then target them for immunotherapy. By targeting critical genes by therapy, one hopes to attack cancers at their strong points. REMBRANDT is pioneering this ability and its ability will undoubtedly will be copied by other medical oncologists in studying their cancer of interest. So this is the first step towards using knowledge to specifically target cancer.

Acknowledgements

We would like to thank Trina Formolo in Dr. Yetrib Hathout's lab in the Department of Integrative Systems Biology, Biochemistry & Molecular Biology at Children's National Medical Center, Washington DC, for telling us about REMBRANDT. This little suggestion blossomed into this book chapter. We also thank Susan Holsclaw of the VAMC-Long Beach for the majority of the artwork presented here. This work is sponsored by the 2012 Summer Research Fellowship Program from Southern California Institute for Research and Education, Long Beach.

Author details

An Q. Dang[1], Neil T. Hoa[1], Lisheng Ge[1], Gabriel Arismendi Morillo[2], Brian Paleo[1], Esteban J. Gomez[1], Dayeon Judy Shon[6], Erin Hong[6], Ahmed M. Aref[1,6,7] and Martin R. Jadus[1,3,4,5*]

*Address all correspondence to: martin.jadus@va.gov

1 Research Service Healthcare Group, Veterans Affairs Medical Center, Long Beach, CA, USA

2 Biological Research Institute, Faculty of Medicine, University of Zulia, Maracaibo, Venezuela

3 Diagnostic and Molecular Health Care Group, Veterans Affairs Medical Center, Long Beach, CA, USA

4 Neuro-Oncology Program, Chao Comprehensive Cancer Center, University of California, Irvine. Orange, CA, USA

5 Pathology and Laboratory Medicine, University of California Irvine, CA, USA

6 Southern California Institute for Research and Education, Veterans Affairs Medical Center, Long Beach, CA, USA

7 Modern Sciences and Arts University (MSA), Biological Science Department, Cairo, Egypt

References

[1] Spellman, P. T, Sherlock, G, Zhang, M. Q, Iyer, V. R, Anders, K, Eisen, M. B, Brown, P. O, & Botstein, D. and Bruce Futcher ((1998). Comprehensive identification of cell cycle-regulated genes of the yeast Saccharomyces cerevisiae by microarray hybridization. Mol. Biol. Cell. , 9, 3273-3297.

[2] Alizadeh, A. A, Eisen, M. B, Davis, R. E, Ma, C, Lossos, I. S, Rosenwald, A, Boldrick, J. C, Sabet, H, Tran, T, Yu, X, Powell, J. I, Yang, L, Marti, G. E, & Moore, T. Hudson J Jr, Lu L, Lewis DB, Tibshirani R, Sherlock G, Chan WC, Greiner TC, Weisenburger DD, Armitage JO, Warnke R, Levy R, Wilson W, Grever MR, Byrd JC, Botstein D, Brown PO, Staud LM ((2000). Distinct types of diffuse large B-cell lymphoma identified by gene expression profiling. Nature , 403, 503-511.

[3] Phillips, H. S, Kharbanda, S, Chen, R, Forrest, W. F, Soriano, R. H, Wu, T. D, Misra, A, Nigro, J. M, Colman, H, Soroceanu, L, Williams, P. M, Modrusan, Z, Feuerstein, B. G, & Aldape, K. (2006). Molecular subclasses of high-grade glioma predict prognosis, delineate a pattern of disease progression, and resemble stages in neurogenesis. Cancer Cell , 9, 157-173.

[4] Delay, M, Jahangiri, A, Carbonell, W. S, Hu, Y. L, Tsao, S, Tom, M. W, Paquette, J, & Tokuyasu, T. A. (2012). Microarray Analysis Verifies Two Distinct Phenotypes of Glioblastomas Resistant to Antiangiogenic Therapy. Clinical Cancer Res. , 18, 2930-42.

[5] Van Der Bruggen, P, Stroobant, V, & Vigneron, N. B. Van den Eynde. Peptide Database *Cancer Immunity,* http://www.cancerimmunity.org/peptidedatabase/Tcellepitopes.html.

[6] Struss, A. K, Romeike, B. F, Munnia, A, Nastainczyk, W, Steudel, W. I, König, J, Ohgaki, H, Feiden, W, Fischer, U, & Meese, E. (2001). PHF3-specific antibody responses in over 60% of patients with glioblastoma multiforme. Oncogene , 20, 4107-4114.

[7] Pallasch, C. P, Struss, A. K, Munnia, A, König, J, Steudel, W. I, Fischer, U, & Meese, E. (2005). Autoantibodies against GLEA2 and PHF3 in glioblastoma: Tumor-associated autoantibodies correlated with prolonged survival. International Journal of Cancer , 117, 456-459.

[8] Kuan, C. T, Wikstrand, C. J, Archer, G, Beers, R, Pastan, I, Zalutsky, M. R, & Bigner, D. D. (2000). Increased binding affinity enhances targeting of glioma xenografts by EGFRvIII-specific scFv. International Journal of Cancer , 88, 6962-6969.

[9] Kuan, C. T, Srivastava, N, Mclendon, R. E, Marasco, W. A, Zalutsky, M. R, & Bigner, D. D. (2010). Recombinant single-chain variable fragment antibodies against extracellular epitopes of human multidrug resistance protein MRP3 for targeting malignant gliomas," International Journal of Cancer. , 127, 598-611.

[10] Bremer, E, Samplonius, D, Kroesen, B. J, Van Genne, L, De Leij, L, & Helfrich, W. (2004). Exceptionally potent anti-tumor bystander activity of an scFv:sTRAIL fusion protein with specificity for EGP2 toward target antigen-negative tumor cells. Neoplasia , 6, 636-645.

[11] Solly, S. K, Nguyen, T. H, Weber, A, & Horellou, P. (2005). Targeting of c-Met and Urokinase Expressing Human Glioma Cell Lines by Retrovirus Vector Displaying Single-Chain Variable Fragment Antibody Cancer Biology & Therapy , 4, 987-992.

[12] Kim, W, & Liau, L. M. (2010). Dendritic cell vaccines for brain tumors. Neurosurgery Clinics of North America. , 21, 139-157.

[13] Prins, R. M, Soto, H, Konkankit, V, Odesa, S. K, Eskin, A, Yong, W. H, Nelson, S. F, & Liau, L. M. (2011). Gene expression profile correlates with T cell infiltration and survival in glioblastoma patients vaccinated with dendritic cell immunotherapy," Clinical Cancer Research, , 17, 1603-1615.

[14] Hanahan, D, & Weinberg, R. A. (2011). Hallmarks of Cancer: The Next Generation. Cell , 144, 646-674.

[15] Ge, L, Hoa, N, Bota, D. A, Natividad, J, Howat, A, & Jadus, M. R. (2010). Immunotherapy of brain cancers: the past, the present and future directions. Clinical and Developmental Immunology (2010:296453, 2010). doi:10.1155/2010/296453.

[16] Chow, K. H, & Gottschalk, S. (2011). Cellular immunotherapy for high-grade glioma Immunotherapy 3(3), 4 23-434 10.2217/IMT.10.110.

[17] Toda, M. (2012). Glioma Antigen. Advances in Experimental Medicine and Biology , 746, 77-84.

[18] Ge, L, Cornforth, A. N, Hoa, N. T, Delgado, C, Zhou, Y. H, & Jadus, M. R. (2012). Differential glioma-associated tumor antigen expression profiles of human glioma cells grown in hypoxia. PLOS One, in press 2012.

[19] Dietrich, P. Y, & Dutoit, V. Thang NNT, Walker PR ((2010). T-cell immunotherapy for malignant glioma: toward a combined approach. Current Opinion in Oncology , 22, 604-610.

[20] Zhang, J. G, Eguchi, J, Kruse, C. A, Gomez, G. G, Fakhrai, H, Schroter, S, Ma, W, Hoa, N, Minev, B, Delgado, C, Wepsic, H. T, Okada, H, & Jadus, M. R. (2007). Antigenic profiles of glioma cells to generate allogeneic vaccines or DC-based therapeutics. Clinical Cancer Research, , 13, 566-575.

[21] Skog, J. (2010). Glioma-specific antigens for immune therapy. Expert Review in Vaccines , 5, 793-802.

[22] Izumoto, S, Tsuboi, A, Oka, Y, Suzuki, T, Hashiba, T, Kagawa, N, Hashimoto, N, Maruno, M, Elisseeva, O. A, Shirakata, T, Kawakami, M, Oji, Y, Nishida, S, Ohno, S, Kawase, I, Hataza, J, Nakatsuka, S. I, Aozasa, K, Morita, S, Akamoto, S, Sugiyama, J,

Yoshimine, H, & Phase, T. II clinical trial of Wilms tumor 1 peptide vaccination for patients with recurrent glioblastoma multiforme. J Neurosurg , 108, 963-971.

[23] Mosmann, T. R, & Coffman, R. L. (1989). Heterogeneity of cytokine secretion patterns and functions of helper T cells Advances in Immunol, , 46, 111-147.

[24] Schaefer, L. K, Menter, D. G, & Schaefer, T. S. (2000). Activation of Stat3 and Stat1 DNA binding and transcriptional activity in human brain tumour cell lines by gp130 cytokines. Cellular Signalling , 12, 143-151.

[25] Humphries, W, Wei, J, Sampson, J. H, & Heimberger, A. B. (2010). The Role of Tregs in Glioma-Mediated Immunosuppression: Potential Target for Intervention. Neurosurg Clin N Am. , 21(1), 125-137.

[26] Andaloussi, A. E, & Lesniak, M. S. (2006). An increase in CD4+CD25+FOXP3+ regulatory T cells in tumor-infiltrating lymphocytes of human glioblastoma multiforme. Neuro. Oncol. , 8, 234-243.

[27] Rich, J. N, Zhang, M, Datto, M. B, Bigner, D. D, & Wang, X. F. (1999). Transforming growth factor-β-mediated induction and growth inhibition in astrocytes is SMAD3-dependent and a pathway prominently altered in human glioma cell lines. Journal Biological Chemistry 274: 35053- 35058., 15INK4B.

[28] Cao, S, Wang, C, Zheng, Q, Qiao, Y, Xu, K, Jiang, T, & Wu, A. (2011). STAT5 regulates glioma cell invasion by pathways dependent and independent of STAT5 DNA binding Neuroscience Letters , 487, 228-233.

[29] Wainwright, D. A, Sengupta, S, Han, Y, Ulasov, I. V, & Lesniak, M. S. (2010). The presence of IL-17A and T helper 17 cells in experimental mouse brain tumors and human glioma. PLoS ONE 5(10): e15390. doi:10.1371/journal.pone.0015390.

[30] Muranski, P, Boni, A, Antony, P. A, Cassard, L, Irvine, K. R, Kaiser, A, Paulos, C. M, Palmer, D. C, Touloukian, C. E, Ptak, K, Gattinoni, L, Wrzesinski, C, Hinrichs, C. S, Kerstann, K. W, Feigenbaum, L, Chan, C. C, & Restifo, N. P. (2008). Tumor-specific Th17-polarized cells eradicate large established melanoma. Blood , 112, 362-373.

[31] Wu, S, Rhee, K. J, Albesiano, E, Rabizadeh, S, Wu, X, Yen, H. R, Huso, D. L, Brancati, F. L, Wick, E, Mcallister, F, Housseau, F, Pardoll, D. M, & Sears, C. L. (2009). A human colonic commensal promotes colon tumorigenesis via activation of T helper type 17 T cell responses. Nature Medicine , 15, 1016-1022.

[32] Cruz-guilloty, F, Pipkin, M. E, Djuretic, I. M, Levanon, D, Lotem, J, Lichtenheld, M. G, & Groner, Y. Anjana Rao A ((2009). Runx3 and T-box proteins cooperate to establish the transcriptional program of eff ector CTLs J. Exp. Med. , 206, 51-59.

[33] Friese, M. A, Platten, M, Lutz, S. Z, Naumann, U, Aulwurm, S, Bischof, F, Bühring, H. J, Dichgans, J, Rammensee, H. G, Steinle, A, & Weller, M. (2003). MICA/NKG2D-mediated immunogene therapy of experimental gliomas. Cancer Res. , 63, 8996-9006.

[34] Bryant, N. L, Suarez-cuervo, C, Gillespie, G. Y, Markert, J. M, Nabors, L. B, Meleth, S, & Lopez, R. D. Lamb LS Jr. (2009). Characterization and immunotherapeutic potential of γδT-cells in patients with glioblastoma. Neuro. Oncol. , 11, 357-367.

[35] Lamb, L. S. (2009). T-cells as immune effectors against high-grade gliomas, Immunologic Research, , 45, 85-95.

[36] Bryant, N. L, Gillespie, G. Y, Lopez, R. D, Markert, J. M, Cloud, G. A, Langford, C. P, Arnouk, H, Su, Y, Haines, H. L, & Suarez-cuervo, C. (2011). Preclinical evaluation of ex vivo expanded/activated γδ T-cells for immunotherapy of glioblastoma multiforme, Journal of Neuro-Oncology, , 2010, 101-179.

[37] Whiteside, T. L. (2006). Immune suppression in cancer: Effects on immune cells, mechanisms and future therapeutic intervention. Seminars in Cancer , 16, 3-15.

[38] Gomez, G. G, & Kruse, C. A. (2006). Mechanisms of malignant glioma immune resistance and sources of immunosuppression, Gene Therapy & Molecular Biology, 10(A): , 133-146.

[39] Jadus, M. R, Driggers, L, & Hoa, N. Pham JTH, Natividad J, Delgado C, Jeffes EWB, Limoli C, Giedzinski E, Ge L. Mechanisms of immune evasion exhibited by different rat glioma cell lines. Chapter 4 in Neuro-Oncology and Cancer Targeted Therapy, editor: L.M. Gutierrez. Nova Science Publishers, (2010). 978-1-61668-708-3, 109-139.

[40] Gabrilovich, D. I, Chen, H. L, Girgis, K. R, Cunningham, H. T, Meny, G. M, Nadaf, S, Kavanaugh, D, & Carbone, D. P. (1996). Production of vascular endothelial growth factor by human tumors inhibits the functional maturation of dendritic cells. Nat. Med. , 2, 1096-103.

[41] Karman, J, Ling, C, Sandor, M, & Fabry, Z. (2004). Initiation of immune responses in brain is promoted by local dendritic cells. J. Immunol, , 173, 2353-2361.

[42] Munn, D. H, & Mellor, A. L. (2004). IDO and tolerance to tumors. Trends in Molecular Medicine , 10, 15-18.

[43] Gabrilovich, D. I, & Nagaraj, S. (2009). Myeloid-derived suppressor cells as regulators of the immune system Nature Reviews Immunology , 9, 162-174.

[44] Cao, Y, & Prescott, S. M. (2002). Many actions of cyclooxygenase-2 in cellular dynamics and in cancer, Journal of Cellular Physiology, , 190, 279-286.

[45] Prayson, R. A, Castilla, E. A, Vogelbaum, M. A, & Barnett, G. H. (2002). Cyclooxygenase-2 (COX-2) expression by immunohistochemistry in glioblastoma multiforme. Annals Diag Path 6:148-53 (2002).

[46] Akasaki, Y, Liu, G, Chung, H. C, Ehtesham, M, Black, K. L, & Yu, J. S. (2004). Induction of a CD4+ T regulatory type 1 response by cyclooxygenase-2-overexpressing glioma. J.Immunol. , 173, 4352-9.

[47] Gao, Y. F, Sun, Z. Q, Qi, F, Qi, Y. M, Zhai, M. X, Lou, H. P, Chen, L. X, Li, Y. X, & Wang, X. Y. (2009). Identification of a new broad-spectrum CD8+ T cell epitope from over-expressed antigen COX-2 in esophageal carcinoma. Cancer Letters , 284, 55-61.

[48] Schreinemachers, D. M, & Everson, R. B. (1994). Aspirin use and lung, colon, and breast cancer incidence in a prospective study," Epidemiology, , 5, 138-146.

[49] Debinski, W, Gibo, D. M, Slagle, B, Powers, S. K, & Gillespie, G. Y. (1999). Receptor for interleukin 13 is abundantly and specifically over-expressed in patients with glioblastoma multiforme. Int J Oncol. , 15, 481-6.

[50] Wykosky, J, Gibo, DM, Stanton, C, Debinski, W, & Eph, . 2 as a novel molecular marker and target in glioblastoma multiforme. Mol Cancer Res 3:541-551.

[51] Lokker, N. A, Sullivan, C. M, Hollenbach, S. J, Israel, M. A, & Neill, A. (2002). Platelet-derived growth factor (PDGF) autocrine signaling regulates survival and mitogenic pathways in glioblastoma cells: evidence that the novel PDGF-C and PDGF-D ligands may play a role in the development of Brain Tumors. Cancer Res , 62, 3729-3735.

[52] Fleming, T. P, Saxena, A, Clark, W. C, Robertson, J. T, Oldfield, E. H, Aaronson, S. A, & Ali, I. U. (1992). Amplification and/or overexpression of platelet-derived growth factor receptors and epidermal growth factor receptor in human glial tumors. Cancer Res. , 52, 4550-4553.

[53] Hatanpaa, K. J, Burma, S, Zhao, D, & Habib, A. A. (2010). Epidermal growth factor receptor in glioma: signal transduction, neuropathology, imaging, and radioresistance. Neoplasia , 12, 675-684.

[54] Gammeltoft, S, Ballotti, R, Kowalski, A, Westermark, B, & Van Obberghen, E. (1988). Expression of two types of receptor for insulin-like growth factors in human malignant glioma. Cancer Res. , 48, 1233-1237.

[55] Lamszus, K, Laterra, J, Westphal, M, & Rosen, E. M. (1999). Scatter factor/hepatocyte growth factor (SF/HGF) content and function in human gliomas," International Journal of Developmental Neuroscience , 17, 517-530.

[56] Weissenberger, J, Loeffler, S, Kappeler, A, Kopf, M, Lukes, A, Afanasieva, T. A, Aguzzi, A, & Weis, J. (2004). IL-6 is required for glioma development in a mouse model. Oncogene , 23, 3308-3316.

[57] Mueller, M. M, Herold-mende, C. C, Riede, D, Lange, M, Steiner, H, & Fusenig, N. E. (1999). Autocrine growth regulation by granulocyte colony stimulating factor and granulocyte-macrophage colony stimulating factor in human gliomas with tumor progression, American Journal of Pathology, , 155, 1557-1567.

[58] Joy, A. M, Beaudry, C. E, Tran, N. L, Ponce, F. A, Holz, D. R, Demuth, T, & Berens, M. E. (2003). Migrating glioma cells activate the PI3-K pathway and display decreased susceptibility to apoptosis. Journal of Cell Science , 116, 4409-4417.

[59] Cantley, L. C. (2002). The Phosphoinositide 3-Kinase Pathway Science , 296, 1655-1657.

[60] Ruoslahti, E. (1996). Brain extracellular matrix. Glycobiology , 6, 489-492.

[61] Ulrich, T. A. de Juan Pardo EM, Kumar S ((2009). The mechanical rigidity of the extracellular matrix regulates the structure, motility, and proliferation of glioma cells. Cancer Research 69: 4167.

[62] Le Clainche C Carlier MF ((2008). Regulation of actin assembly associated with protrusion and adhesion in cell migrationPhysiol Rev , 88, 489-513.

[63] Nemethova, M, Auinger, S, & Small, J. V. (2008). Building the actin cytoskeleton: filopodia contribute to the construction of contractile bundles in the lamella. Journal Cell Biol , 180, 1233-1244.

[64] Kurisu, S, & Takenawa, T. (2010). WASP and WAVE family proteins: Friends or foes in cancer invasion? Cancer Science , 101, 2093-2104.

[65] Yamazaki, D, Kurisu, S, & Takenawa, T. (2005). Regulation of cancer cell motility through actin reorganization. Cancer Science. , 96, 379-386.

[66] Isacke, C. M, & Yarwood, H. (2002). The hyaluronan receptor, CD44. International Journal of Biochemistry & Cell Biology , 34, 718-721.

[67] Abaco, D, Kaye, G. M, & Integrins, A. H. Molecular determinants of glioma invasion. Journal of Clinical Neuroscience , 11, 1041-1048.

[68] Delamarre E, Taboubi S, Mathieu S, Bérenguer C, Rigot V, Lissitzky JC, Figarella-Branger D, Ouafik LH, Luis J (2009) Expression of integrin 6β1 enhances tumorigenesis in glioma cells. American Journal of Pathology 175:844-855.

[69] Färber, K, Synowitz, M, Zahn, G, Vossmeyer, D, Stragies, R, Van Rooijen, N, & Kettenmann, H. integrin inhibitor attenuates glioma growth. Molecular and Cellular Neuroscience , 39, 579-585.

[70] Mikelis, C, Sfaelou, E, Koutsioumpa, M, & Kieffer, N. E. is a pleiotrophin receptor required for pleiotrophin-induced endothelial cell migration through receptor protein tyrosine phosphatase β/ζ. FASEB Journal , 23, 1459-1469.

[71] Kadomatsu, K, & Muramatsu, T. (2004). Midkine and pleiotrophin in neural development and cancer. Cancer Letters , 204, 127-143.

[72] Mirkin, B. L, Clark, S, Zheng, X, Chu, F, White, B. D, Greene, M, & Rebbaa, A. (2005). Identification of midkine as a mediator for intercellular transfer of drug resistance. Oncogene 24, 4965-4974.Sontheimer, H (2003) Malignant gliomas: perverting glutamate and ion homeostasis for selective advantage. Trends in Neurosciences, , 26, 543-549.

[73] Maas, S, Patt, S, Schrey, M, & Rich, A. (2001). Underediting of glutamate receptor GluR-B mRNA in malignant gliomas. Underediting of glutamate receptor GluR-B mRNA in malignant gliomas. Proc Natl Acad Sci (USA) , 98, 14687-14692.

[74] Teh, J, & Chen, S. (2012). Metabotropic glutamate receptors and cancerous growth. WIREs Membr Transp Signal , 1, 211-220.

[75] Collins, V. P, Brunk, U. T, Freddriksson, B. A, & Westermark, B. (1979). The fine structure of growing human glia and glioma cells. Acta Path. Microbiol. Scand Section , 1, 87-29.

[76] Collins, V. P, Forsby, N, Brunk, U. T, & Westermark, B. (1977). The surface morphology of cultured human glia and glioma cells. A SEM and time-lapse study at different cell densities. Cytobiologie , 16, 52-62.

[77] Spence, A. M, & Coates, P. W. (1978). Scanning electron microscopy of clones astrocytic lines derived from ethyl nitrosurea-induce rat gliomas. Virchows Arch. B Cell Path. , 28, 27-35.

[78] Höglund, A. S. (1985). The arrangement of microfilaments and microtubules in the periphery of spreading fibroblasts and glial cells. Tissue and Cell , 17, 649-666.

[79] Arismendi-morillo, G. J, & Castellano-ramirez, A. V. (2008). Ultrastructural mitochondrial pathology in human astrocytic tumors: potentials implications pro-therapeutics strategies. J. Electron Microscopy , 57, 33-39.

[80] Arismendi-morillo, G, Hoa, N. T, Ge, L, & Jadus, M. (2012). Mitochondrial network in glioma's invadopodia displays an activated state both in situ and in vitro: Potential functional implications. Ultrastructural Pathology in press.

[81] Hoa, N, Ge, L, Kuznetsov, Y, Mcpherson, A, & Cornforth, A. N. Pham JTH, Myers MP, Ahmed N, Salsman VS, Lamb, LS Jr, Bowersock JE, Hu Y, Zhou YH, Jadus MR ((2010). Glioma cells display complex cell surface topographies that resist the actions of cytolytic effector lymphocytes. Journal of Immunology , 185, 4793-4803.

[82] Bretscher, A. (1991). Microfilament Structure and Function in the Cortical Cytoskeleton. Annual Review of Cell Biology , 7, 337-374.

[83] Dos Remedios CGChhabra D, Kekic M, Dedova IV, Tsubakihara M, Berry DA ((2003). Actin binding proteins: regulation of cytoskeletal microfilaments. Physiol Rev , 83, 433-473.

[84] Cardelli, J, & Skalli, O. (2010). Divide and Conquer: the dynamic cytoskeleton of glioma. In: Glioblastoma: molecular mechanisms of pathogenesis and current therapeutic strategies S.K. Ray (ed).

[85] Winder, S. J, & Ayscough, K. R. (2004). Actin-binding proteins. J. Cell Sci , 118, 651-654.

[86] Machesky, L. M, & Li, A. (2010). Fascin: Invasive filopodia promoting metastasis. Commun Integr Biol. , 3, 263-270.

[87] Li, A, Dawson, J. C, Forero-vargas, M, Spence, H. J, Yu, X, König, I, Anderson, K, & Machesky, L. M. (2010). The actin-bundling protein fascin stabilizes actin in invadopodia and potentiates protrusive invasion. Cell Biology , 23, 339-345.

[88] Beadle, C, Assanah, M. C, Monzo, P, Vallee, R, Rosenfeld, S. S, & Canoll, P. (2008). The role of myosin II in glioma invasion of the brain. Molecular Biology of the Cell , 19, 3357-3368.

[89] Gillespie, G. Y, & Soroceanu, L. Manning TJ Jr., Gladson CL ((1999). Glioma migration can be blocked by nontoxic inhibitors of myosin II. Cancer Research 59:2076.

[90] Mishima, K, Kato, Y, Kaneko, M. K, Nishikawa, R, Hirose, T, & Matsutani, M. (2006). Increased expression of podoplanin in malignant astrocytic tumors as a novel molecular marker of malignant progression. Acta Neuropathologica , 111(5), 483-488.

[91] Sontheimer, H. (2008). An unexpected role for ion channels in brain tumor metastasis. Experimental. Biology and Medicine. , 233, 779-791.

[92] Colman, H, Zhang, L, Sulman, E. P, Mcdonald, J. M, Shooshtari, N. L, Rivera, A, Popoff, S, Nutt, C. L, Louis, D. N, Cairncross, J. G, Gilbert, M. R, Phillips, H. S, Mehta, M. P, Chakravarti, A, Pelloski, C. E, Bhat, K, Feuerstein, B. G, & Jenkins, R. B. (2010). A multigene predictor of outcome in glioblastoma. Neuro- Oncology. , 12, 49-57.

[93] Greenwood, I. A, Miller, L. J, Ohya, S, & Horowitz, B. (2002). The large conductance potassium channel-subunit can interact with and modulate the functional properties of a calcium-activated chloride channel, CLCA1. J. Biol. Chem. , 277, 22119-22122.

[94] Liu, X, Chang, Y, Reinhart, P. H, Sontheimer, H, & Chang, Y. (2002). Cloning and characterization of glioma BK, a novel BK channel isoform highly expressed in rat glioma cells. J. Neuroscience. , 22, 1840-937.

[95] Ge, L, Cornforth, A. N, Hoa, N. T, Bota, D. A, Mai, A, Kim, D. I, Chiou, S. K, & Jadus, M. R. (2012). Glioma BK channel expression in human gliomas and possible glioma specific epitopes for the immunotherapy of gliomas. J Immunol. In press.

[96] Dutoit, V, Herold-mende, C, Hilf, N, Schoor, O, Beckhove, P, Bucher, J, Dorsch, K, Flohr, S, Fritsche, J, Lewandrowski, P, Lohr, J, Rammensee, H. G, Stevanovic, S, Trautwein, C, Vass, V, Walter, S, Walker, P. R, Weinschenk, T, Singh-jasuja, H, & Dietrich, P. Y. (2012). Exploiting the glioblastoma peptidome to discover novel tumour-associated antigens for immunotherapy. Brain , 135, 1042-1054.

[97] Glinsky, G. V, Berezovska, O, & Glinskii, A. B. (2005). Microarray analysis identifies a death-from-cancer signature predicting therapy failure in patients with multiple types of cancer. Journal of Clinical Investigation , 115, 1503-1521.

Section 3

Molecular Biology of Brain Tumors and Associated Therapeutic Implications

Chapter 7

From Gliomagenesis to Multimodal Therapeutic Approaches into High-Grade Glioma Treatment

Giuseppe Raudino, Maria Caffo, Gerardo Caruso, Concetta Alafaci, Federica Raudino, Valentina Marventano, Alberto Romano, Francesco Montemagno, Massimo Belvedere, Francesco Maria Salpietro, Francesco Tomasello and Anna Schillaci

Additional information is available at the end of the chapter

http://dx.doi.org/10.5772/52782

1. Introduction

While primary malignant brain tumors account for only 2% of all adult cancers, these neoplasms cause a disproportionate rate of cancer-related disability and death. The five-year survival rates for brain tumors are the third lowest among all types of cancer, after pancreas and lung ones, respectively.

High-grade gliomas (glioblastoma multiforme [GBM] and anaplastic astrocytoma [AA]) comprise the most common types of primary central nervous system (CNS) tumors and have a combined incidence of 5-8/100,000 population. The median survival of patients with malignant gliomas treated conservatively is 14 weeks; by surgical resection alone, 20 weeks; by surgery and radiation, 36 weeks; by the addition of chemotherapy, 40-50 weeks [1].

The oncogenesis of gliomas, in particular high-grade gliomas (HGGs), the most frequent primary malignant brain tumors in adults, is driven by several biological processes and genetic alterations, involved in the transformation of a normal cell into a neoplastic one [2, 3]. Classically this step-by-step evolution from normal cells to early-stage tumors, to aggressive cancer is found in cases of "secondary" multiforme glioblastoma (GBM), derived from a lower-grade glioma, whereas some glioblastomas occur directly without previous evidence of a lower-grade tumor. This last subset of tumors are classified as "primary" or "de novo" GBM [4]. A relatively novel feature of GBM, so as of many other types of malignant tumors, is the presence inside the gross of tumors of a particular kind of tumor cells, GBM stem cells. These cells could represent the trigger and the maintenance of gliomagenesis.

The majority of GBM cases (>90%) are primary GBM, involving mainly the elderly and genetically characterized by loss of eterozygosity (LOH) 10q [70% of cases), EGFR amplification [36%), p16^{INK4a} deletion [31%) and PTEN mutations [25%). Secondary GBMs [5% of all cases of sporadic GBM) manifest in younger patients and are characterized often by TP53 mutations, the most frequent and detectable genetic alteration, already present at stage of low-grade astrocytomas, in 60% of cases. LOH 10q [10q25-qter) is the most frequent [70%) genetic alteration in both primary and secondary GBMs [5].

Gliomagenesis is driven by several biological processes and genetic alterations, involved in the transformation of a normal cell into a neoplastic one [2, 3].

One of the most fashinating and futurible therapeutic strategy against gliomas is represented by antisense therapy to block selectively glioma cells, trying to revert gliomagenetic molecular pathways towards the wild-type status. This aim could be reached through antisense molecules, delivered inside the brain and in particular inside tumoral cells, able to penetrate into glioma cells nucleus and to integrate with their genome to silence some specific genic functions. Among antisense molecules there are antisense oligonucleotides, ribozymes and RNA interference (iRNA). The specificity of hybridization makes antisense method an interesting strategy to selectively modulate the expression of genes involved in tumorigenesis. Glial tumors seem to be able to create a favorable environment for the invasion of glioma cells in cerebral parenchyma when they combine with the extracellular matrix via cell surface receptors. In this review we will focus on the different antisense approaches and on the mechanisms of action of each kind of antisense molecule and relative strategy in human gliomas therapy.

Among dysregulated molecular pathways, into brain tumor cells, there are activated growth factors signaling pathways, marked angiogenesis, downregulation of apoptotic genes and upregulation of antiapoptotic genes.

Gliomagenesis is driven by several biological events, such as activated growth factor receptor signaling pathways, downregulation of many apoptotic mechanisms and unbalance among proangiogenic and antiangiogenic factors. This last aspect is very crucial in glioma progression, because of prominent angiogenesis is a cardinal feature of malignant gliomas [2]. Several growth factor receptors, such epidermal growth factor receptor (EGFR), platelet-derived growth factor receptor (PDRGF), C-Kit, vascular endhotelial growth factor receptor (VEGFR) and other growth factors receptors, are overexpressed, amplified and/or mutaded in gliomas. Features of glioma cells are the loss of tumor suppressor genes, which are critical for cell growth, differentiation and function. These genes are TP53, the retinoblastoma (Rb) gene, the inhibitor of cyclin-dependent kinase 4a (INK4a) gene and the phosphatase and tensin homolog (PTEN) gene [6].

On the basis of this high importance of gene expression disregulation inside cancer cell genome, the modulation of gene expression at more levels, such as DNA, mRNA, proteins and transduction signal pathways, may be the most effective modality to downregulate or silence some specific genic functions pathologically upregulated or introduce genes, downregulated or deleted selectively into neoplastic cells. Therapeutic genes (Transgenes) can lead to

http://dx.doi.org/10.5772/52782

generation of anticancer drugs within the tumor (pro-drug activation), increase of selective intratumoral drug levels without increasing systemic toxicity, protection of hematopoietic cells from drug damage by inducing drug resistance and delivery of secreted fusion proteins which combine a targeting ligand and a toxin/enzyme, sensitization of tumors to radiations, that in turn can be used to induce expression of transgenes via radiation-activated promoters [7].

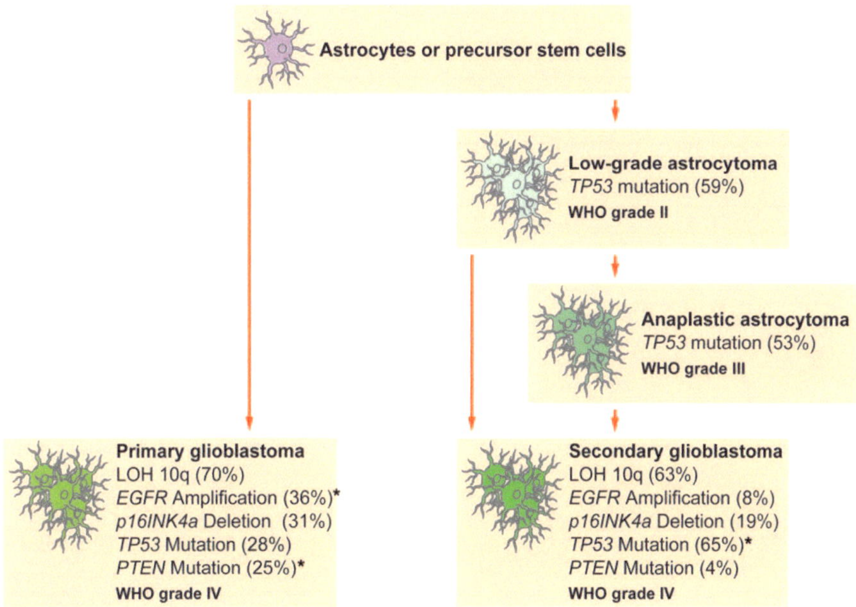

(Ohgaki and Kleihues. *AJP May 2007, Vol. 170, No. 5*)

Figure 1. De novo vs Secondary GBM genetic pathways

Progression from low-grade to high-grade astrocytomas involve inactivating mutations of tumor-suppressor gene TP53 and elevated expression of platelet-derived growth factor (PDGF) ligands and receptors, accumulation of genetic alteration of retinoblastoma-associated cell-cycle regulatory pathways, including deletion or mutations of cyclin-dependent kinase inhibitor $p16^{INK4A}$/(CDKN2A) or the retinoblastoma susceptibility locus 1 (pRB1), as well as amplification or over-expression of cyclin-dependent kinase 4 (CDK4) and human double minute 2 (HDM2). Evolution to secondary GBM is associated with deletion of chromosome 10, which includes tumor-suppressor phosphatase and tensin homolog (PTEN). The hyper-methilatyion in the promoter region and successive mutation of p16 is evident in HGGs progression. Additionally BcI2-like 12 increased expression (BcI2L12) inhibits apoptosis [8].

The astrocyte elevated gene-1 (AEG-1) is over-expressed in the majority of HGGs and stimulates cellular transformation and invasion together with the Ha-ras family of retrovirus-associated DNA sequences (RAS). Furthermore, oncogenic Ha-ras induces AEG-1 expression by modulating the phosphatidylinositol 3-kinase (PI3K)-Akt signaling pathway and contributes to the growth of HGGs. Mitogenetic signals activate a molecular cascade known as ras-mitogen activated protein kinase (Ras/MAPK). MAPK inhibits the Rb gene, activates the transcriptional factor E2F and cells enter the S phase. The INK4a gene influences the Rb pathway by activating three cyclin kinase inhibitors: p15, p16, and p19.The final result is the blockage of cyclin-dependent kinase 2, 4 and 6, triggering cell-cycle progression by inhibiting pRb. Through the new technique of genome-wide sequencing and survey of gene copy number, have been discovered novel amplicons linked to glioma progression. Table 1 summarizes the main genes involved in gliomagenesis (Tab. 1).

Gene	Chromosome	Molecular alteration	Effect of the molecular alteration	Histotype (WHO Grade)
TP53	Cr17p13.1	Mutations	Cell cycle control loss, proliferation	Astrocytoma and oligodendroglioma (Grade II) – precocious mutation in secondary GBM
PDGF-A PDGFR-α	Cr4q11-q12	Overexpressio/amplification	Proliferation/invasion	Astrocytoma and oligodendroglioma (Grade II-III)
Unknown tumor suppressor genes	1p, 19q, 4q, 9p and 11p loss	Loss of Heterozygosity	Proliferation, invasiveness, angiogenesis	Astrocytoma and oligodendroglioma (Grade II-III)
Unknown tumor suppressor genes	Cr22q	Deletion	Proliferation	Astrocytoma and oligodendroglioma (Grade II)
Rb 1	Cr13q14.2	Mutations/deletion	Cell cycle control loss, proliferation	Astrocytoma and oligodendroglioma (Grade II-III)
P16	Cr9p	CDKN2/p16 deletion	Cell cycle control loss, proliferation	Astrocytoma and oligodendroglioma (Grade II-III)
PTEN	Cr10q23	LOH	Regulation Akt/PKB signaling pathway loss; proliferation and tumor growth; invasiveness, angiogenesis	Astrocytoma and oligodendroglioma (Grade III-IV)
BAX	Cr19q24	LOH	Pro-apoptotic action loss, proliferation	Astrocytoma and oligodendroglioma (Grade II-III)
EGFR (c-erb-2)	Cr7p11-p12	Amplification/overexpression	Cell transformation and proliferation	De novo GBM
MDM2	Cr12q14.3-q15	Overexpression	Cell cycle control loss and proliferation	De novo GBM

Table 1. Main genetic alteration in human gliomas

Gliomagenesis can develop through two different ways, resulting in evolution of a cluster genic alteration directly from normal astrocyte to GBM or of a step by step different kinds of mutations of various genes passing gradually from normal astrocyte to low-grade glioma, to high-grade glioma, to GBM.

Primary GBM shows amplification of the epidermal growth factor receptor (EGFR), deletion or mutation of homozygous cyclin-dependent kinase (CDK) inhibitor $p16^{INK4A}$ /(CDKN2A), alterations in tumor suppressor PTEN on chromosome 10, and deletion in the INK4a gene with loss of p14 and p16 [6, 9]. In table 2 we, also, report the principal familial genetic syndromes associated with HGGs (Tab. 2). In the total amount of GBM, the total prevalence rate concern for the 95% cases of sporadic GBM, and only for the 5% (not more) cases of syndromic familiar cancer.

Syndrome	Involved gene	Chromosomal location	Protein function	Effect of molecular alteration	Associated tumors
Turcot [Variant form of hereditary non-polyposis colorectal cancer (HNPCC) or familial adenomatous polyposis	APC MLH1 PMS2 (mismatch repair genes) (Autosomal dominant)	5q21 3p21.3 7p22	Signal transduction, DNA mismatch repair	Hyperplasia, invasiveness and metastasis	Colorectal polyposis and primary brain tumors APC mutations are commonly associated with medulloblastoma; mismatch repair mutations are associated with glioblastoma
Gardner [Familial adenomatous polyposis, with intestinal polyposis, desmoids, osteomas, epidermoid cysts]	APC RAS DCC TP53 (Autosomal dominant)	5q21 12 18 17p13.1	Signal transduction, proliferation, cell and cell-to-matrix adhesion	Hyperplasia, invasiveness and metastasis	Colonrectal, small bowel, pancreatic, stomach, bile duct, papillary thyroid, hepatoblastoma, Brain tumors, adrenal gland cancer
Li-Fraumeny	TP53 (Autosomal dominant)	17p13.1	Transcription factor, apoptosis regulator	Abnormal protein/gain of function	Osteosarcomas, soft-tissue sarcomas, premenopausal breast, adrenal cortical, glioma, primitive neuroectodermal tumor, leukemias

Syndrome	Involved gene	Chromosomal location	Protein function	Effect of molecular alteration	Associated tumors
Von Recklinghausen Neurofibromatosis Type 1 (NF 1)	NF1 (neurofibromin) (Autosomal dominant)	17q11.2	GTPase activating protein, negative regulation of p21ras	Proliferation	Bilateral acoustic, meningioma, esp. multiple; piloid astrocytoma, mid-line glioma, diffuse glioma, intramedullary astrocytoma, spinal cord ependymoma
Neurofibromatosis Type 2 (NF 2)	NF 2	22q12.2	Cytoskeletal-cell membrane link	Proliferation	Vestibular schwannoma, peripheral schwannoma, meningioma, spinal ependymoma, astrocytoma, glial hamartoma
Tuberous sclerosis	TSC1 TSC2 (Autosomal dominant)	9q34 16p13	Not known GTPase activating protein	Cell growth and cell division control loss, proliferation	Subependymal giant cell astrocytoma, cortical tubers, cutaneous angiofibroma, peau chagrin, cardiac rhabdomyoma, adenomatous polyps of the small intestine, cysts of the lung and kidney
Retinoblastoma	RB1 (Autosomal recessive)	13q14	Regulator of transcription factors	Proliferation	Retinoblastoma, pineoblastoma, glioma, osteosarcoma
Multiple hamartoma (Cowden Disease)	APC hMLH1 hMSH2 PMS2 PTEN (Autosomal dominant)	5q21 3p21.3 2p22-21 7p22 10q23.3	Signal transduction, DNA mismatch repair	Hyperplasia; proliferation, apoptotic cell death loss, invasiveness and metastasis	Dysplastic cerebellar gangliocytoma, hamartomas (skin, breast, thyroid, colon, intestines, mouth)

http://dx.doi.org/10.5772/52782

Syndrome	Involved gene	Chromosomal location	Protein function	Effect of molecular alteration	Associated tumors
Gorlin	PTCH1 PTCH2 (Autosomal dominant)	9q22.3-q31 1p32	Transmembrane receptor	Proliferation	Medulloblastoma, meningioma, astrocytoma, multiple basal cell carcinomas, palmar and plantar pits

Table 2. Principal familial genetic syndromes associated with human gliomas

2. Glioma invasion

Glioma cells invasion consist of an active translocation of glioma cells through host cellular and extracellular matrix barriers [10].

Three steps are fundamental in the phenomenon of glioma invasion: a) adhesion of glioma cells to proteins of the surrounding extracellular matrix (ECM) mediated by cell adhesion receptors; b) degradation of ECM components by proteases secretion by glioma cells; c) migration of glioma cells into the newly created space through the ECM.

ECM is composed of proteoglycans, glycoproteins, collagens and also contains fibronectin, laminin, tenascin, hyaluronic acid, vitronectin. In recent years the glioma invasion has also been interpreted by numerous authors in terms of interaction between neoplastic cells and ECM [11].

Critical factors include the synthesis and deposition of ECM components by glioma and mesenchymal cells, the release of ECM-degrading activities for remodeling interstitial spaces, the presence of adhesion molecules (matrix receptors on glioma cell surfaces that specifically recognize and adhere to ECM components) and the effects of cell-matrix interactions on the behavior of glioma cells. ECM modification aids the loss of contact inhibition allowing tumor cells to freely migrate and invade the surrounding tissues. Changes in these ECM components are felt to modulate brain tumor growth, proliferation and invasion, although specific interactions and exact mechanisms are unknown.

Integrins, a class of adhesion molecules, play a major role in glioma cell-matrix adhesion. Integrins regulate many aspects of the cell behavior including survival, proliferation, migration and differentiation. They act with a physical trans-membrane link between the ECM and the cytoskeleton and with a bi-directional signal across the cell membrane. Integrins of the $\beta 1$ and αv classes are expressed on different cell types, including neurons, glial cells, meningeal and endothelial cells. $\beta 2$ integrins are specifically expressed by leukocytes and they are found on microglia and on infiltrating leukocytes within the CNS. Down-regulation of $\beta 1$ expression in intracerebrally transplanted glioma cells in vivo by placing $\beta 1$ antisense sequences under an inducible, tetracycline-responsive promoter markedly inhibited diffuse brain invasion [13-17].

Down-regulated β1 integrin protein levels in vivo probably affect interactions of glioma cells with ECM components, leading to reduced migration along vascular basement membranes.

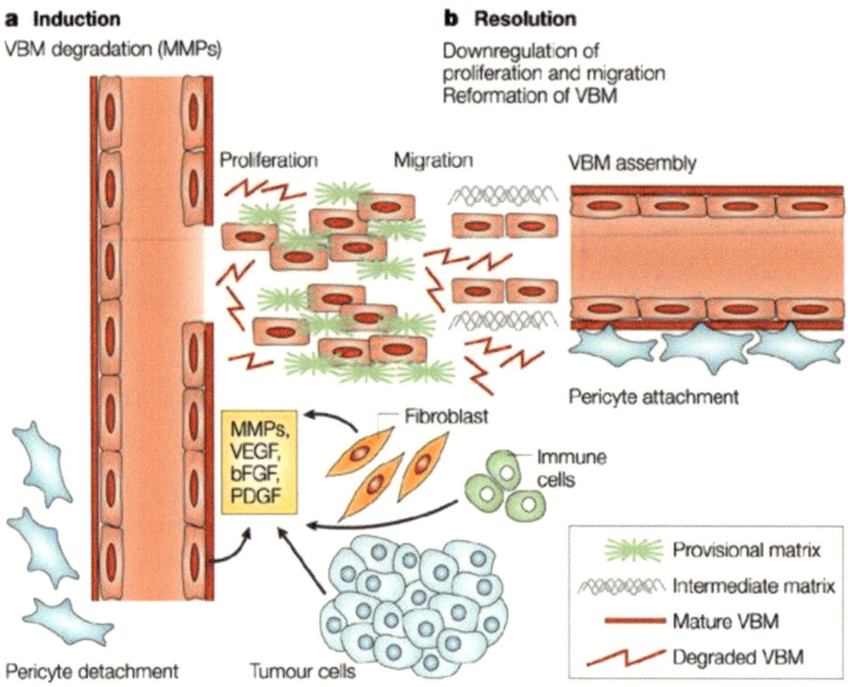

Figure 2.

The proteolytic degradation of the basement membrane (BM) is mediated by proteases, such as the matrix metalloproteases (MMPs), secreted by tumor and stromal cells [11, 12]. MMPs are secreted as proenzymes and are activated by proteolytic cleavage of their amino-terminal domain. MMPs play an important role in human brain tumor invasion, probably due to an imbalance between the production of MMPs and tissue inhibitor of metalloproteases-1 (TIMP-1) by the tumor cells. Among these molecules, MMP-1 is the crucial enzyme able to initiate breakdown of the interstitial collagens, collagen type 1, collagen type 2 and collagen type 3; in this way it activates the other MMPs which allow the glioma cells to infiltrate normal brain tissue.

3. Angiogenesis

The formation of new blood vessels from existing microvessels is angiogenesis, an histological indicator of the degree of malignancy and prognosis of patients. Of all solid tumors, malignant brain tumors show the highest degree of vascular proliferation. The WHO classification distinguishes low grade from high grade diffuse astrocytomas by the presence of microvascular proliferation as a diagnostic criterion and an independent prognostic parameter [18].

HGGs are characterized by extensive microvascular proliferation and a higher degree of vasculature. The presence of marked endothelial glomeruloid-like proliferations demonstrates active tumor invasiveness through vascular angiogenesis, disruption of pre-existing anatomical structures and neoplastic cellular migration along neoangiogenic vascular channel and through the BM, with evidence of proliferation of new fine capillaries [8, 19]. These mechanisms demonstrate a very strong and bidirectional correlation between glioma angiogenesis and invasiveness into glioma progression. The new vessel growth is stimulated through the tumor cells secretion of pro-angiogenic growth factors; these factors bind to receptors on endothelial cells thereby activating them [20].

Vascular endothelial growth factor-A (VEGF-A) is regulated in HGGs and it is secreted by tumor cells as well as by stromal and inflammatory cells. VEGF-A can be linked in the ECM through the interaction with proteoglycans or glycosaminoglycans. The expression of the receptors VEGFR1 and VEGFR2 is regulated on the endothelial cells in HGGs. The ligands for VEGF3 (VEGF-C&D) are expressed by multiple cell types that surround the angiogenic vessels, suggesting the existence of a novel pro-angiogenic paracrine signaling pathways in these neoplasms [10, 21]. Basic fibroblast growth factor (bFGF) is expressed by vascular cells and, focally, by the tumor cells too. The receptors for bFGF include FGFR1, expressed by both the tumor cells and the tumor endothelial cells; FGFR2 is expressed only by the tumor cells whereas FGFR4 is not detected in HGGs [22]. The binding of VEGF on endothelial cells activates the phosphatidylinositol-3-hydroxyl kinase (PI3K)/protein kinase B (Akt) pathway, whereas the bFGF receptors are predominantly shown through the protein kinase Cα (PKCα) pathway. The activation of endothelial cells results in increased expression of cell adhesion receptors, such as integrins $\alpha v\beta 3$ and $\alpha 5\beta 1$, and in increased cell survival, proliferation and migration responses. Other pro-angiogenic growth factors, including interleukin-8, hepatocyte growth factor, urokinase can promote or amplify angiogenesis.

Cancer angiogenesis is similar to angiogenesis seen during development except that it is less controlled and precise [23]. These blood vessels have many marked features including blind ends, erratic size and connections, and most significantly, large gaps in the endothelial lining. This last feature is important because it signifies that larger molecules can enter the tumor effectively bypassing the blood brain barrier. In fact, tumor vasculature can have intercellular gaps as large as 2 μm which is large enough for passive accumulation of 100-200nm particles into the tumor interstitium [24]. Neovascularization in brain tumors correlates directly with their biological aggressiveness, degree of malignancy and clinical recurrence and inversely with the post-operative survival of patients with gliomas. Diffuse astrocytomas tend to progress from grade II to grade III tumors with a time interval of several years, whereas, progression of grade III to grade IV is more rapid, typically 2 years. GBMs that arise from a low-grade glioma lesion are called "secondary glioblastoma".

However, in most cases, GBMs appear "de novo" and are thus termed "primary glioblastoma". Regardless of their mode of progression, primary and secondary GBMs are morphologically indistinguishable and show their histologic hallmarks, such as "glomeruloid" microvascular tufts and necrosis [25, 26].

The discovery of hypoxia inducible factor-1 (HIF-1) and the observation that hypoxia-induced HIF-1α expression in pseudopalisading cells, into intratumoral necrotic areas, was concomitant with the expression of one of its target genes, VEGF, established a biological link between hypoxia and angiogenesis [27]. The formation of new blood vessels occurs physiologically during embryogenesis. In adult life it is observed in the female reproductive system and during wound healing and in a wide range of pathologic settings, such as ischemic diseases, chronic inflammatory reactions, and neoplasia. During embryonic development, blood vessels are newly formed from endothelial precursors and hematopoietic stem cells, a process known as vasculogenesis [28]. In contrast, angiogenesis, the sprouting of new blood vessels from pre-existing ones results from an altered balance of proangiogenic factors and antiangiogenic factors [29, 10].

The sequence of events leading to the formation of new blood vessels is well characterized and involves an initial VEGF-mediated increase of vascular permeability leading to extravasation of plasma proteins associated with dilatation of native vessels and reduction in their pericyte coverage. Subsequently, endothelial cells migrate and proliferate. For this cascade to occur, deposition of a proangiogenic matrix for the newly sprouting vessel is essential. This involves breakdown of the vascular basement membrane and extracellular matrix (ECM) through the action of cathepsin B, matrix metalloproteases (MMPs) and other enzymes as well as the expression of matrix proteins such as fibronectin, laminin, tenascin-C and vitronectin. Finally, the angiogenic process culminates in the assembly of endothelial cells to form a vascular lumen followed by the elaboration of a new basement membrane and the recruitment of pericytes. In contrast to the accepted dogma that tumor development occurs in 2 phases (avascular and vascular), we observed that tumor growth in the brain follows 2 vascular phases. In the first vascular phase, the vessels are native cerebral vessels, which are coopted by tumor cells, while in the second phase, there is true neovascularization arising from existing vessels. During the transition period between these two phases, hypoxia driven HIF-1 expression occurs which results in VEGF secretion and induction of neovascularization. In Stage IV, angiogenesis adjacent to the necrotic area is triggered in response to increased expression of HIF-1α and VEGF, a process that rescues the remaining tumor cells. Thus, it is possible to suggests four sequential steps in glioma progression: i) perivascular organization, ii) proliferation, iii) vascular regression followed by necrosis, and iv) angiogenesis.

Glioma vasculature is structurally and functionally abnormal and it correlates and leads to vasogenic edema, increased interstitial pressure, and eterogeneous delivery of oxygen and drugs [23].

VEGF expression is stimulated by hypoxia and acidosis, and probably correlates with many other growth factors and their specific receptors (EGFR, HGFR, PDGFR, C-Kit, IGFR), and downstream signaling pathways (PI3K-Akt, Ras-MAPK) upregulation and activation in gliomas.

Many other proangiogenic factors are upregulated in gliomas and this aspect might explain the failure of many actual antiangiogenic therapeutic strategies in gliomas management. Among these other angiogenic factors a very important role has absolved by bFGF, IL-1beta, IL-6, IL-8, TNF-alpha and stromal-cell-derived factor (SDF)-1 alpha [2].

Another group of endothelial growth factors is represented by angiopoietins. Their signal transduction pathway passes via the Tie2 receptor tyrosine kinase expressed on endothelial cells. In particular, Ang-1 and -2, have been implicated in glioma angiogenesis. Ang-1 mediated activation of Tie2 is required for stabilization, remodelling and maturation of blood vessels, promotes angiogenesis and tumor growth and is associated with an increased number of highly branched vessels covered by pericytes. While VEGF and Ang-1 may act in concert (proliferation and maturation), Ang-2 has been implicated in further remodeling of the initial microvasculature [30, 31]. Increased expression of Ang-2 on GBM microvasculature appears early during glioma angiogenesis. However, binding of Ang-2 to the Tie2 receptor on endothelial cells antagonizes this receptor's phosphorylation, thereby disrupting contacts between endothelial and periendothelial support cells and disengaging pericytes from the tumor vessels during initiation of vessel sprouting or regression. Examination of the expression patterns of angiopoietins and their receptors suggests a role in GBM vasculature and malignant transformation. For example, increased Tie2 expression has been observed with increasing human astrocytoma grading. Ang-2 and Tie2 expression are absent in the normal brain vasculature but are induced in tumor endothelium of coopted tumor vessels prior to their regression. Of particular importance, treatment of glioma cell derived mouse xenografts with a dominant negative form of Tie2 results in a significant decrease in tumor growth [32].

A new more complex understatement of angiogenic pathways in glioma progression gives a crucial role to the Ca2+ permeable transient receptor potential (TRPC) channels in tumor angiogenesis, and in particular in endothelial permeability up-regulation, focal adhesion assembly, cell orientation and directional migration and involvement in hypoxia-induced angiogenesis and vascular remodeling. According this complex molecular pathological network, tumor angiogenesis should be not only the result of physiological adaptation to hypoxia in response to an increasing tumor mass but it should be also the result of critical genetic mutations that activate a transcriptional program for angiogenesis. Calcium (Ca2+) is an important second messenger and its entry through plasma membrane affects angiogenesis. Several reports indicate that Ca2+ permeable transient receptor potential (TRP) channels belonging to the TRPC, TRPV and TRPM represent target genes, down-stream to Notch1, PTEN, NFAT and Hif-1 transcriptional factors are activated during tumor angiogenesis. Several studies indicate that angiogenic growth factors such as vascular endothelial growth factor (VEGF) and basic firoblast growth factor (bFGF) may activate TRP channels at transcriptional and post-transcriptional levels, causing a subsequent rise in endothelial [Ca2+]i, which modulates signal transduction pathways regulating the angiogenesis. Conversely, Ca2+ influx through TRP channel activation may stimulate endothelial cells to trigger transcription, production and release of angiogenic growth factors such as VEGF and platelet-derived growth factor (PDGF) that stimulate angiogenesis.

In the field of new targeted-based molecular therapeutic approaches, TRP channels, and not only VEGF/VEGFR and HIF-1alpha, might be a promising target for new therapeutic agents to anti-angiogenic therapy [33].

4. Current treatment of glioblastoma

The efficacy of current anti-cancer multimodal therapeutic strategies in gliomas is limited by the lack of specific therapies against malignant cells, and the prognosis in patients affected by primary brain tumors is still very unfavorable. Glial tumors seem to be able to create a favorable environment for the invasion of neoplastic cells when they combine with the extracellular matrix via cell surface receptors, through the upregulation of crucial pathways such as angiogenesis and invasion. The major problem in brain drug delivery is the presence of the blood brain barrier which limits the delivery of many chemotherapeutic agents and other kinds of therapeutic molecules. This event often contributes to the failure of treatment. Current treatment of glioblastoma (GBM) is difficult and a great mysterious challenge, and, results in high recurrence rates. Upon display of symptoms of a brain tumor (seizure, chronic headache, loss of consciousness, loss of motor/sensory function) a patient will undergo MRI for detection of the tumor. This is followed by a host of treatments to remove the bulk of the tumor if possible, starting always when possible from gross total removal of tumor [34]. Patients are then monitored for recurrence. This is standard protocol for treatment of glioma regardless of grade [35]. This line of treatment can often lead to decreased quality of life. Last, if tumor recurs, there are last line treatments given after which there is no ability to treat further. The treatment of glioma is varied depending on grade, but this discussion will focus on the treatment of the most aggressive form: glioblastoma (GBM). The common treatment after detection has several components including: 1. Surgical resection of tumor from the primary site, 2. Lining of the primary site with carmustine wafers designed to kill cells in the close proximity, after gross total removal and histological confirmation of high-grade gliomas 3. Metronomic oral temozolmide chemotherapy and 4. Radiotherapy to the brain. As mentioned previously, in the case of recurrence, this treatment is coupled with anti-angiogenic therapy to prolong patients' life.

5. Surgical resection

Represents the microneurosurgical removal of the tumor from the primary site. The general procedure involves craniotomy followed by suction and gross total removal of tumor from the site. Though there are experimental imaging agents, such as optically visible fluorescent dyes coupled with intravital magnetic resonance imaging of the brain for guidance and assessment of accuracy and completion, this is not an exact science [35-37].

6. Local, intracavitary, chemotherapy

It is applied in the resection site after removal of the tumor gross in the form of Poly (lactic-co-glycolic acid)-BCNU wafers that slowly degrade and release the chemotherapeutic BCNU (Carmustine - gliadel®) into the resection site, after extemporaneous histological intraoperatory examination and confirmation of high-grade gliomas [38]. This local chemotherapeutic approach has been reported to yield a slight increase in survival times, as opposed to leaving the tumor site empty, however, it still does not allow adequate decrease in recurrence. Use of gliadel® has become less common place due to both cost-benefit analysis and preference of use by surgeons [39, 40].

7. Radiotherapy and stereotactic radiosurgery

It involves the use of gamma-irradiation in order to induce cell death through DNA damage, often inside a post-operatory adjuvant therapy. The technologic support to apply this therapeutic step does see the use of Gamma-knife, cyber-knife or conformational collimation system-based linear accelerator. This therapy is used in over 50% of all cancer patients at some point during treatment and has been in use in cancer for almost a century. In brain tumors, this treatment works by sending gamma rays through to the site of the tumor to directly damage DNA, but in longer-lasting effects, creates free radicals which can go on to cause further damage [41, 42]. Radiation therapy involves not just radiation of the tumor, as would be desirable, but irradiation of an area which can include both tumor tissue and healthy brain tissue. Radiotherapy does usually results in death of large amounts of the tumor, however, recent discoveries suggest that radiation may actually be causing side effects which can aid in recurrence. Glioma cells exposed to radiation *in vitro* show increased invasion post treatment, indicating progression and enhanced malignancy of disease [43]. Further, radiation leads to many side effects associated with cancer malignancy and disease progression, including the creation of free radical species, degradation of the extracellular matrix, inflammation and immune cells recruitment, and increased blood flow to the tumor area [44, 45].

Radiotherapy improved several clinical end points in brain tumors. Standard radiation therapy of gliomas involves the provision of 59.4 / 60 Gy, in 30/33 from 1.8 to 2 Gy daily fractions, and each should begin within 4-6 weeks after surgery. Treatment is generally given to the area of the tumor and a surrounding margin ("limited-field" method). Postoperative radiotherapy significantly prolongs median survival to approximately 12 months for glioblastoma multiforme and to 36 months for anaplastic astrocytoma [46]. A slight improvement of the results obtained with conventional radiotherapy has been achieved through the hyperfractionation daily, the use of radiosensitizers or hyperoxygenation by hyperbaric treatment [47].

Stereotactic radiotherapy is helpful for the treatment of high grade gliomas and involves the local system of radioactive sources (interstitial brachytherapy) or external targeted radiotherapy. In case of tumors of a limited volume boost stereotactic radiotherapy, administered by linear accelerator or Gamma-Knife or Cyber-knife and performed after limited-field radiotherapy, achieved a slight increase in survival in some studies [48].

The metabolic radioimmunotherapy, using radiolabeled antibodies injected systemically or intramuscularly, is still experimental because there are no phase III trials that showed a survival advantage [49].

8. Systemic chemotherapy

At present there is not a standard treatment of anaplastic oligoastrocytoma and oligodendroglioma but the common practice, based on recommendations of the National Comprehensive Cancer Network (NCCN), consists in surgery followed by radiation therapy. Adjuvant chemotherapy can also be administered and consists in PCV or TMZ.

Loss of heterozygosity (LOH) of chromosome 1p/19q (present in approximately 40-60% of oligodendroglial tumors) has been showed to be related to the sensitivity to the treatment with alkylating agents (especially TMZ and poli-chemotherapy scheme PVC) and to a more favorable prognosis. For a most appropriate therapy would therefore be necessary to look for the loss of heterozygosity 1p and 19q in all tumors with oligodendroglial component [50].

Two clinical trials are evaluating the role of chemotherapy in the treatment of anaplastic glioma correlating it to the co-deletion 1p/19q. The first, EORTC 26053-22054 is a Phase III trial on concurrent and adjuvant temozolomide chemotherapy in non-1p/19q deleted anaplastic glioma. The second is EORTC 26081-22086 a Phase III intergroup study of radiotherapy versus temozolomide alone versus radiotherapy with concomitant and adjuvant temozolomide for patients with 1p/19q codeleted anaplastic glioma.

Oligodendrogliomas and oligoastrocytomas, especially in anaplastic forms, are highly sensitive to adjuvant chemotherapy with PCV after radiation therapy, with a significant increase in progression-free survival (23 months vs. 13 months) compared to radiotherapy alone. An increase of the progression-free survival is also reflected by administering the PCV before radiotherapy. None prolongation of the median overall survival time is noted [51]. Nevertheless, there is the common practice of proposing chemotherapy as the initial therapy for pure oligodendroglioma. Further, in the case of small tumors RT remains the best therapeutic choice. Although there is no phase III clinical studies comparing PCV and TMZ in clinical practice TMZ is preferred as first line treatment for the lower toxicity and comparable efficacy to PCV. Second line chemotherapy with TMZ in recurrent oligodendroglial tumors after PCV-chemotherapy gave excellent results, and similar responses to PCV but with less toxicity [52].

Standard therapy of anaplastic astrocytoma, according to Stupp protocol, is radiotherapy with adjuvant TMZ, administered for the duration of radiotherapy (75 mg/m^2 daily) and after in six cycles (150-200 mg/m^2 for five days every 28 days). There are no randomized studies with adequate statistical power in patients with anaplastic astrocytoma that demonstrated a benefit of adjuvant or concomitant chemotherapy with nitrosoureas. In a EORTC study, comparing adjuvant dibromodulcitol and BCNU chemotherapy with radiotherapy alone in patients with anaplastic astrocytoma, no statistically significant improvement in survival was observed after BCNU/DBD adjuvant chemotherapy [53]. Temozolomide, an imidazotetrazinone acting through the formation of a reactive methyldiazonium cation and methylation of O6-guanine in DNA, induce its clinical effects through the activity of O6-alkylguanine-DNA alkyltransferase (AGT), a DNA repair protein that removes O6-alkylguanine adducts in DNA, result of translation from gene MGMT, whose grade of promoter methylation is recognized important epigenetic predictive factor to temozolomide therapeutic response. The therapeutic advantage is showed for patients with MGMT (methylguanine methyltransferase) methylated tumors. The enzyme remove alkyl groups from the O^6 position of guanine, one of the targets of alkylating agents. Epigenetic silencing of the MGMT gene in tumor tissue occurs through the methylation of the CpG islands in the promoter region. Patients whose tumors have MGMT promoter methylation are likely to benefit from the addition of TMZ chemotherapy [54]. TMZ is characterized from an excellent oral bioavailability and good penetration of the blood-brain barrier (BBB). The activity of temozolomide is highly dependent on dosing schedule, with multiple administrations being more effective than a single dose (as normally codified in Stupp protocol). Peak plasma concentration is achieved within 30-60 min of oral administration and the compound has an elimination half-life of one to two hours. Myelosuppression, which is dose limiting at 1,200 mg/m2, and nausea and vomiting are the most frequent adverse events [55].

A new promising agent, recently evaluated for the treatment of anaplastic astrocytoma, is Trabedersen, a phosphorothioate antisense oligonucleotide that act as an inhibitor of TGF- β2 (Transforming growth factor-beta 2) biosintesys. TGF- β2 levels seems to be higher in high grade gliomas. TGF-β2 is an attractive target because it regulates key mechanisms of carcinogenesis, in particular immunosuppression and metastasis. The compound was tested in phase I/II studies, in which it was administered at two doses (10 μM or 80 μM) comparing response rate, survival, and safety respect to standard chemotherapy (TMZ or PCV). Trabedersen 10 μmol/L was superior to trabedersen 80 μmol/L in both efficacy and safety for high-grade gliomas, especially in anaplastic astrocytoma. In patients with anaplastic astrocytoma, the trabedersen 10 μmol/L group had a higher overall survival rate at 24 months than the trabedersen 80 μmol/L group and the control group (83.3%, 53.3% and 41.7%, respectively). The median overall survival for patients with anaplastic astrocytoma was higher in both trabedersen groups than in the chemotherapy control group, with a survival benefit for 10 μmol/L trabedersen over chemotherapy (17.4 months). Based on the promising results of these studies, presented at the 101st annual meeting of American Association of Cancer Research, in 2010 started the pivotal Phase III study SAPPHIRE (Efficacy and Safety of AP 12009 in Adult Patients With Recurrent or Refractory Anaplastic Astrocytoma [WHO Grade 3) as Compared to Standard Treatment with Temozolomide or BCNU: A Randomized, Actively Controlled, Open label Clinical Phase 3 Study). Unfortunately, the study has been stopped prematurely in January 2012, due to slow patient recruitment [56].

Historically, the standard of care for older adult with GBM was surgical resection or biopsy, followed by involved-field radiotherapy. The new therapeutic standard is based on the results of several studies that demonstrated a significant survival benefit in GBM patients with the addition of concurrent and adjuvant TMZ to radiation. Patients treated with TMZ/RT had a median survival time of 15 months, compared with 12 months for the patients initially treated with RT alone. Further, the first group showed a 2-year survival rate of 26% compared with only 10% for the RT group. Now the standard treatment consist in surgery followed by RT with adjuvant TMZ, administered for the duration of radiotherapy and after in six cycles (Stupp protocol) [57].

A therapeutic alternative or adjunctive treatment is BCNU wafer (Gliadel®), positioned at surgery and followed by radiation therapy. Gliadel® is a biodegradable polymer wafer impregnated with BCNU. At the time of resection, up to eight wafers are implanted into the surgical cavity. Water in the interstitial fluid causes the polymer slowly to degrade. The BCNU is thus released in a controlled manner over several days to weeks and diffuses into the brain parenchyma at a high dose density. It causes a statistically significant increase in survival compared to patients treated only with surgery and radiotherapy. The SIGMA (Stupp including Gliadel for glioma) is a multi-center, spontaneous observational trial to evaluate the efficacy of Gliadel® wafers plus concomitant TMZ in patients with newly-diagnosed high grade glioma. This study is conducted at the Foundation of the Carlo Besta Neurological Institute, IRCCS, in Milan and is based on several examples in literature on this association. Samaggi et al. of the IRCCS published a study on the research and comparison of data in literature about efficacy and toxicity in patients with newly diagnosed GBM treated with the combination of Gliadel® and the Stupp protocol. Analysis of data revealed that this combination is well tolerated and it significantly improved survival without a substantial increase in toxicity [58].

Recently was demonstrated that for elderly patients with newly diagnosed glioblastoma, therapy with TMZ alone is an alternative to radiotherapy. In the study, published in the July issue of the Lancet Oncology, were recruited 412 older patients. 195 were randomly assigned to TMZ and 178 to radiotherapy. The results showed that single-agent TMZ and radiotherapy alone seem equally effective. Both treatments were well tolerated. Major side effects observed were neutropenia, (16 in the TMZ group and 2 in the RT group), lymphocytopenia (46 vs. 1), thrombocytopenia (14 vs. 4), hepatic enzyme increased (30 vs. 16), infections (35 vs. 23) and thromboembolic events (24 vs. 8). Even in older patients the MGMT methylation status of tumor is a predictive marker for the success of therapy with alkylating agents as mentioned above. So testing of tumor MGMT methylation status in elderly patients with newly diagnosed glioblastoma should be a priority to decide the best treatment [59].

9. Antiangiogenic therapy

Angiogenesis inhibition represents a new target for therapeutic intervention in malignant gliomas because GBMs are highly vascularized brain tumors and their growth seems to be angiogenesis dependent.

The inhibition of angiogenesis is achieved through the use of inhibitors of VEGF receptor (such as bevacizumab or aflibercept) or kinase or integrin inhibitors (cilengitide or erlotinib) which have been tested in several clinical trials.

The antiangiogenic effect is achieved through different mechanisms assumed on the basis of results from several studies. According to the first hypothesis (starvation hypothesis), the reduction of new blood vessels formation decreases the amount of metabolites that may reach the tumor, causing tumor cell death. According to a new hypothesis (normalization hypothesis), in the early stages (1 month) of the antiangiogenic therapy there is a normalization of the blood vessels, followed by their damage due to hypoxia, and then by the reduction of tumor growth.

http://dx.doi.org/10.5772/52782

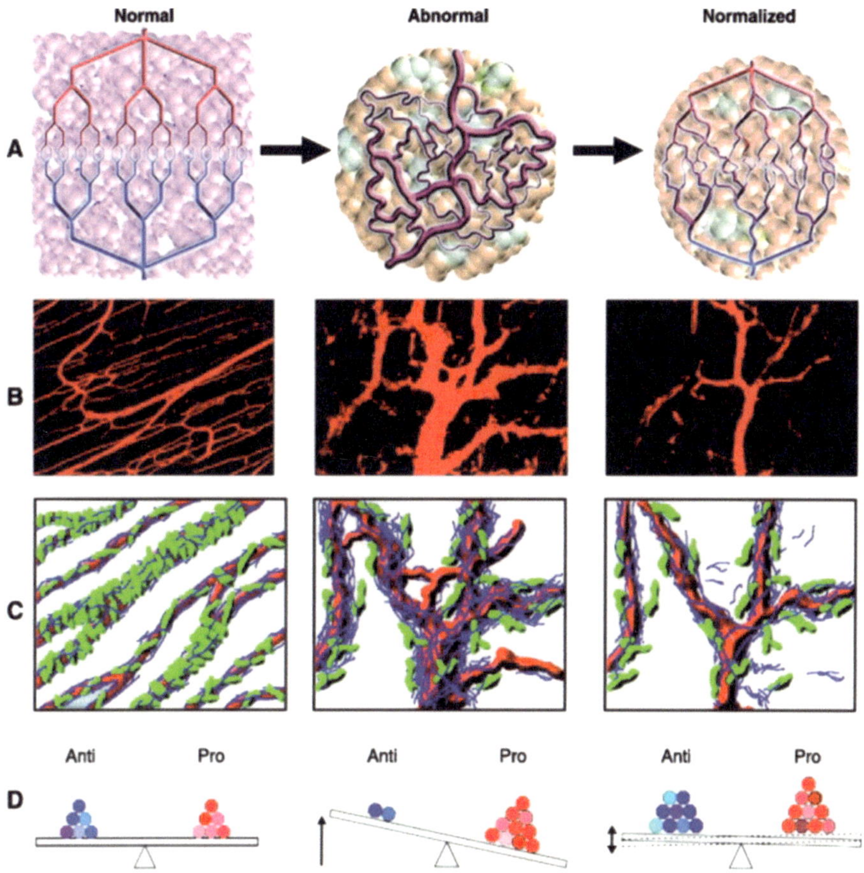

Goel S et al. Physiol Rev 2011

Figure 3.

These hypothesis have been confirmed by recent studies in which was highlighted the increase of metabolites associated with anaerobic glycolysis in the long-term therapy with anti-VEGF. This would explain the failures obtained in the treatment of solid tumors with anti-VEGF monotherapy but also the excellent results of several trials with the association anti-angiogenic agent and chemotherapy, even compared to chemotherapy alone [60].

The need to associate an antiangiogenic agent to traditional therapy is useful not only to improve the vehiculation of the anticancer drug but also to control recurrences. According to clinical experience, after surgical resection, radiotherapy and adjuvant chemotherapy with TMZ, there is a recurrence or progression within six months. This recurrence is localized in most cases where there was the resection of the primary tumor, in which are localized tumor cells infiltrated. This phenomenon has been explained assuming that the primary tumor secretes not only pro-angiogenic agents but also anti-angiogenic agents that inhibit neovascularization at the level of infiltrating tumor cells, which are located at a certain distance from the primary tumor. For this reason the use of anti-angiogenic agents is recommended not only in newly diagnosed gliomas but also in recurrences [61].

10. Anti VEGFR — Bevacizumab

Bevacizumab (Avastin®;Genentech, CA, USA) is a recombinant humanized monoclonal antibody that binds with high affinity to human VEGF preventing it from binding to its receptors VEGFR1 and VEGFR2, on the surface of endothelial cells and thereby determining the block of the cascade of events following its receptors activation. Will be therefore inhibited proliferation and increased permeability due to receptor VEGFR2 and tumor growth due to receptor VEGFR1 through the production of matrix metalloproteinases. Bevacizumab inhibits the growth of new blood vessels and reduces the blood flow to the tumor. Like other antiangiogenic agents it shows, in the initial phase of the treatment, a normalizing effect on blood vessels. This normalizing effect is important because tumor vasculature is often incomplete and tends to leak. The abnormal permeability may prevent the administration of cancer treatment such as chemotherapy. Bevacizumab can normalize the chaotic vascularization of the tumor, in order to maximize the effectiveness of the overall therapeutic strategy.

In the U.S., Avastin® is the first anti-angiogenesis therapy approved by Food and Drug Administration (FDA) to treat patients with glioblastoma multiforme (GBM) when this form of brain cancer continues to progress following standard therapy. The drug is also approved for the treatment of advanced stages of other 3 types of cancer: breast, colorectal, and non small cell lung cancer (NSCLC). Even before FDA approval, bevacizumab was widely used for this indication in the United States and in some European countries [62].

Many clinical trials evaluated efficacy of bevacizumab and irinotecan versus bevacizumab alone (and the addition of irinotecan at progression) with several results but also with many questions unanswered about the end points used, the increase in survival, the best dose and timing. Teri N. Kreisl et al. conducted a trial to evaluate single-agent activity of bevacizumab in patients with recurrent glioblastoma. The dose of bevacizumab was 10 mg/kg every 2 weeks. At tumor progression bevacizumab was associated in combination with irinotecan 340 mg/m^2 or 12 mg/m^2 every two weeks. The study found that single-agent bevacizumab has a significant antitumor effect in recurrent glioblastoma and show less overall toxicity but also a lower response rates (29% vs. 46%) compared with combination therapy. The study shows that it is not always strictly necessary the addition of irinotecan after tumor progression during the treatment with bevacizumab. It is not possible, however, exclude the contribution of irinotecan if the two agents are used together in the initial treatment. Will be necessary to conduct further studies to understand whether the addition of this drug is so useful to offset the toxic effects associated with its use [63].

Results from this trial are consistent with data presented by Vrendenburgh et al. emerged from a phase II trial testing bevacizumab plus irinotecan in recurrent GBM. They reported a response rate of 57% and a 6-month progression-free survival of 46% with this combination. The rationale of combining the two drug is based on the normalization effect of antiangiogenic agents that reduce the intratumoral pressure and increase drug delivery to tumor. But there could be also another unwanted effect, the reduction of drug penetration to the brain due to the restoring of the blood-brain barrier [64].

Avastin® is approved in Europe for the treatment of advanced stages of four types of cancer: colorectal cancer, breast cancer, lung cancer and kidney cancer. Together, these four types of cancer cause nearly 3 million deaths every year. The use of the drug in Italy for malignant gliomas is possible through the enrollment in clinical trials or the compassionate use. Compassionate use programs are intended to facilitate the availability to patients of new treatment options under development. National compassionate use programs, making medicinal products available either on a named patient basis or to cohorts of patients, are governed by individual Member States legislation. In Italy the global compassionate use is ruled by the Ministerial Decree dated 8th May 2003. Drugs under experimentation may be used outside the experimentation if there isn't a valid therapeutic alternative [65].

The neuro-oncology department of Besta Institute is conducting a study on the therapeutic use of bevacizumab and irinotecan in patients with recurrent grade III and IV glioma in the absence of therapeutic alternative since is emerged by various studies the effectiveness of this association [66]. However, not all patients respond to bevacizumab-irinotecan combination. This is probably due to the different pathways involved in tumor angiogenesis, in which VEGF is only one factor, even though prevalent. The lack of response in some patients may be related to any of the alternative routes [67].

Despite their contribution in the treatment of vascularized GBM, these agents have some serious side effects including hypertension. For this reason, this therapy is a problem for patients with underlying hypertension. In such cases is possible to associate calcium channel blockers or ACE inhibitors to cancer therapy. ACE inhibitors are often preferred because in hypertension caused by VEGF inhibitors the way of NO is involved, and it can be blocked by these antihypertensive agents. Another side effect caused by the antiangiogenic therapy is proteinuria, which can be prevented by these agents. The bevacizumab-irinotecan combination is responsible for serious side effects such as renal failure and gastric perforation, which in some cases lead to discontinuation of treatment. It is recommended that bevacizumab not be initiated for at least 28 days after surgery and until any surgical wound is fully healed and that bevacizumab be discontinued at least 28 days prior to elective surgery [62].

11. Integrin inhibitors — CILENGITIDE

Integrins are a family of transmembrane receptors whose natural ligands are represented by vibronectin, fibronectin, laminin. Their ligands are recognized by the common portion arg-gly-asp (RGD); upon binding occurs a conformational change, the formation of clusters of integrins and the activation of intracellular kinases, from which depend many intracellular signal cascades. These cascades result in the processes of proliferation, differentiation, motility, survival and cell adhesion. Some integrins are ubiquitous, others are specific for various tissues and are also expressed on the surface of different types of tumors. In such cases there will be an increase in the levels of both integrins in tumor cells than in endothelial cells in the proliferation phase during angiogenesis. Integrins most expressed are αvβ3 and αvβ5. Using these integrins as targets, will be therefore possible to obtain an antiangiogenic and anticancer effect.

There are several types of integrine inhibitors that have been evaluated in preclinical and in clinical trials: peptidomimetics (Cilengitide), antibodies (Intetumumab, Natalizumab), small organic molecules (E7820- MK0429]). The advantage of small organic molecules compared to previous compounds lies in greater stability and in oral administration instead of intravenous.

Cilengitide (developed by Merck KGaA) is a new anti-angiogenic agent for the treatment of recurrent gliomas that act as an inhibitor of integrin receptors αvβ3 and αvβ5, expressed on activated endothelial cells during angiogenesis. Integrins are proteins that facilitate the formation of new blood vessels within the tumor; blocking the receptor binding leads to the inability to invade the brain by the glioblastoma cells. This antitumoral and antiangiogenic effect of Cilengitide was demonstrated by several preclinical studies [68]. The molecule, in a phase II study presented at the American Society of Clinical Oncology (ASCO) in Chicago, was tested at two different doses (2 g or 500 mg twice a week) and provided very promising results in the group treated with the higher dose. Surprisingly, more than one third of patients in this group was still alive after one year and 22% after 2 years. 10% were still alive after 4 years [69].

Stupp et al. conducted a Phase I/IIa study of cilengitide and TMZ with concomitant radiotherapy followed by cilengitide and TMZ maintenance therapy in patients with newly diagnosed glioblastoma. Cilengitide at 500mg was administered as a 1-hour intravenous infusion twice weekly. The study highlighted how treatment with cilengitide, combined with the standard treatment, showed benefits in patients with MGMT promoter methylation. MGMT gene promoter methylation status was determined by methylation-specific polymerase chain reaction (PCR). The combination of cilengitide with TMZ and radiotherapy was well tolerated, without other side effects [70].

Merck is currently conducting two trials; the CORE study (cilengitide at a dose of 2 g twice weekly in combination with TMZ and radiotherapy) is a Phase II randomized, multicenter, open-label controlled trial investigating two regimens of intravenous cilengitide in combination with standard therapy (radiotherapy with concurrent and adjuvant TMZ) versus standard therapy alone, and is currently in progress in GBM patients with an unmethylated MGMT promoter.

The CENTRIC study is a multicenter, open-label, controlled phase III study, testing Cilengitide (at a dose of 2 g twice weekly) in combination with standard treatment (with TMZ and radiotherapy) versus standard treatment alone, in subjects with newly diagnosed glioblastoma multiforme and methylated MGMT gene promoter. Promising results in these trials probably will lead to a higher interest in integrins as targets for glioma therapy and to a bigger development of new anti-integrin agents. The results of clinical studies will be useful to explore the knowledge on the best dose of cilengitide used to obtain the desired therapeutic effect with lower side effects.

Recently the research of biomarkers predictive of patient response to anti-integrin agents has been directed toward the quantification of their expression through imaging, using radiolabeled galacto-RGD positron emission tomography, a new diagnostic technique [68].

12. Antisense approaches and mi-RNA inhibitors as anti-angiogenic agents

New antiangiogenic agents have been developed and tested in several preclinical studies with many results that encourage further research in this field. These are unconventional compounds such as siRNA and angiomirs which differently act through gene silencing. This silencing mechanism has been used to interfere with the process of angiogenesis [61].

Other treatments to halt invasion involve genetic interventions using DNA, siRNA, and microRNA delivery via a host of transfection methods [71]. These therapies are all in animal phases at the moment, largely due to the invasive nature of the interventions and the difficulties in the past twenty years with gene therapy in clinical trials. The advantage of these interventions is the ability to directly target specific genes necessary for glioma invasion without need for design of a novel drug and determination of a particular target. However, like all compounds, there are delivery issues associated with these treatments as well as possible unforeseen side effects. Another kind of new possible antisense approach is represented by long non coding RNA, different RNA-based molecules than miRNA, probably transcripted not from intronic DNA sequences. All of these antisense approaches should be reach to knockout or down-regulate pathways pathologically involved in glioma progression and invasion, trying to reverse towards normality glioma cell genome or selectively kill only glioma cells. Into this fashionable therapeutic field, our study group is improving the study of possible involvement of IL-8 and HIF-1 alpha into high-grade glioma patients to hypothesize an antisense block of both these molecules at the same time with a single approach.

13. Other potential molecular targets

Recent discoveries in molecular biology have shown further potential signaling pathways involved in the pathogenesis of malignant gliomas. Were therefore assumed new targets for novel therapeutic approaches like grow factor ligands, receptors, intracellular downstream effectors. Several studies highlighted an over-expression of EGFR in malignant gliomas, which is related with survival and proliferation of cancer cells. EGFR tyrosine kinase inhibitors (TKIs) Gefitinib (Iressa®) and Erlotinib (Tarceva®), used in combination with ionizing radiation, can increase the antitumoral effect of this therapy. The results of several phase I/II studies using Gefitinib and Erlotinib with conventional therapy in the treatment of GBM are controversial [72]. For this matter were investigated other molecular markers (besides the over-expression of EGFR) more predictive of EGFR TKIs activity. Among these there are: EGFR variant III (EGFRvIII co-expressed when there is an amplification of EGFR), phosphatase and tensin homolog (PTEN) expression, and phospho-Akt (P-Akt).

Specifically, co-expression of EGFRvIII and the tumor-suppressor protein PTEN seems to be associated with a significant clinical response to EGFR TKIs but also these results are controversial. Further studies are needed to clarify the efficacy of these agents and to select patients who may benefit from EGFR inhibitor therapy. Imatinib (Glivec®), an antagonist of PDGFR (who may be overexpressed in high grade gliomas), showed in vitro on GBM cells cytostatic or cytotoxic activity in relation to its concentration [73]. This led to clinical trials in patient with recurrent glioma. A randomized, multicenter, open-label Phase III study of imatinib in combination with hydroxyurea versus hydoxyurea alone as oral therapy in patients with progressive pretreated GBM resistant to standard dose TMZ failed to show clinically significant differences between the two treatment arms [74].

Most experimental and more traditional anti-invasive therapeutic platforms have focused on the ability of compounds to inhibit matrix metalloproteinases (MMPs) and the other extracellular matrix (ECM) components and thus limiting invasive progress of cancer cells [75].

One such compound, Marimastat, an MMP-2 inhibitor, was developed and showed promise in some clinical trials, demonstrating a possible synergic effect when used with TMZ in anaplastic astrocytoma and recurrent GBM. Despite it, actually, it isn't sure a long term therapeutic effect better than TMZ alone [76, 77]. More recently, there has been a shift in the development of novel drugs to that of more personalized therapy. In these cases, specific receptors and signaling molecules are targeted for inhibition in order to kill cancer cells. The main goal to reach the selectivity and efficacy of antitumor treatment consist on targeted therapeutic molecular-based approaches. These therapies in the field of brain tumor and in particular in case of intra-assial brain tumor, such as high-grade gliomas, represent the most fascinating challenge to achieve the killing of glioma cells into the brain and, with an adequate engineering of targeted drugs and nanoparticles systems, the population of glioma and GBM stem cells. Treatment can be modified to the individual cancer type and patient which is advantageous in reducing side effects. They work often by relying on receptor addiction of the cancer cells meaning if the receptor becomes useless through blocking, the cancer cell will almost go through withdrawal and can die [78, 79]. However, this is not known to occur with all potential targets and it is always possible that pathways will be rerouted to compensate. This type of treatment often has a side effect of halting invasion of cancer cells though more commonly treatment leads to cell death. A recent review highlights many of these compounds and their potential anti-invasive effects based on the target molecule for which they were developed. However, the exact anti-invasive effects are unknown for most of these compounds based on lack of in depth studies of invasion opting instead for survival and tumor growth measures. Most of the targets of this type of therapy are receptor tyrosine kinases (RTKs) which, upon activation by a ligand, will change conformation and phosphorylate intracellular signaling proteins leading to downstream events. In cancer, these receptors are often mutated to be constituitively active and thus require no growth factors to function. A cancer cell can actually become "addicted" to this activation and so by turning it off, the cell will die. Inhibitors of RTKs are most often antibodies due to the high specificity. The more notable RTK inhibitors are Herceptin® (against EGFR), Avastin® (against VEGF), and Tarceva® (against PDGFR). These are all used clinically for different types of cancers and have been thought to have possible anti-invasive effects due to their signaling pathways involving targets for invasion [80]. However, there is insufficient evidence to tie their effects to halting glioma invasion and as aforementioned, in vivo, Avastin causes glioma invasion. EGFR inhibition is particularly exciting due to the overexpression or mutation of EGFR in >60% of glioblastomas (de novo GBM) and alteration of glioblastoma to express EGFRvIII causes a more invasive phenotype of cells in vitro [81, 82]. However, these compounds are expensive and difficult to work with. Further, their actual role in invasion prevention is yet to be seen due to the far-reaching effects of the involved pathways.

Inhibitors of downstream proteins such as Src-kinase have shown promise in inhibiting tumor growth and progression. Based on the ability of Src to increase the invasive phenotype including cytoskeletal remodeling, MMP secretion, and adhesion disassembly, it was tested for anti-invasive activity. This treatment inhibited invasion in brain, prostate and breast cancers while also inhibiting growth, angiogenesis and proliferation [83].

Another new agent tested in clinical trials is Talampanel, a noncompetitive antagonist of the α-amino-3-hydroxy-5-methyl-4-isoxazolepropionic acid (AMPA) receptor. The receptor levels may be related with the GBM growth. This compound was tested in a multicenter Phase II study in association with standard therapy with RT and TMZ for newly diagnosed GBM. Patients showed a median survival of 20.3 months and 2 year overall survival of 41.7%. Only 29% of patients had MGMT promoter methylated [72].

14. Conclusions and future perspectives

Based on the results obtained from both the old and the most innovative therapies seems clear that a better understanding of the pathological and physiological mechanisms of brain cells can result in a more targeted therapeutic approach by designing personalized therapies. This would overcome the current limitations in the treatment and lead to a better prognosis for patients with brain tumors.

Nowday, the treatment of gliomas represents one of the most challenging areas in neurosurgery and oncology. Malignant gliomas involves multiple aberrant signaling pathways and the BBB restricts the delivery of many chemotherapeutic agents. The efficectiveness of the actual chemotherapeutic approach, multimodal targeted therapies, differently than the other malignant extracerebral tumors, remains very modest in gliomas. Considering the multitude of molecular entities and signaling pathways regulating the proliferation and cellular survival/ cell death, the inhibition of a singular target gene or transcriptional factor could not be sufficient to suppress neoplastic progression. In this intricate and complex field it seems to be very important to improve specific selective drug delivery systems to lead to diffusion of drugs, antisense oligonucleotides, small interference RNAs, engineered monoclonal antibodies and other therapeutic molecules into CNS overcoming BBB.

Considering the multitude of actually used chemotherapeutic approaches, starting from Stupp protocol (TMZ plus radiotherapy) and the results in term of recurrences and survival, the field of glioma therapy is again subject to high rate of investigation and development with the hope to postulate new possible molecular targets and therapeutic schemes to attack glioma cells. Understanding the genetic bases of gliomas and of the invasive behaviour, in particular the differentiated gene expression in distinct areas of the same tumor during glioma progression, may suggest new molecular targets to overcome the mechanisms of multi-drug-resistance of the actual therapeutic approaches to gliomas and to attack at the same time different crucial biological events of gliomagenesis.

Glioma gene expression and its development during gliomagenesis will may help to better understand the role of important molecules involved in tumor-safe brain parenchyma relationships. These molecules, such as ECM proteases, cell adhesion molecules and their related signaling pathways show an important role in glioma cell migration and invasion and could be selectively downregulated to inhibit the glioma invasive rim. It is clear that the complexity and cross-talk between signal transduction pathways limits the potential efficacy of targeting a single receptor or molecule.

We are now investigating the role of HIF (Hypoxic inducing factor) isoforms and IL-8 (Interleukine-8) in glioma progression and the possibility to block their pathways through a only antisense molecule loaded into a nonaparticle-base system, and directed against both these molecular targets. HIF-1α actively regulates downstream processes and it is also influenced by the tumor microenviroment in many different ways. Antisense inhibition of HIF may be a strong target for anti-angiogenic therapy. In fact, HIF is the crucial molecule and transcriptional factor produced in response to hypoxic conditions within HIF-1α/VEGF-regulation expression-dependent angiogenic pathway. In this molecular cascade HIF-1α up-regulated levels finally induce up-regulation of VEGF expression, and, at the same time, may stimulate gene expression of other genes involved in gliomagenesis.

Our group has recently demonstrated high expression levels of PGES-1 (Prostaglandine E 1 Sinthase) and IL-8 in HGG cells and microglial cells, strongly correlated with grading tumor. During malignancy progression, leukocyte infiltration and necrosis are two biological phenomena associated with the development of neovascularization. IL-8 expression is first observed in low grade astrocytoma in perivascular tumor areas expressing inflammatory cytokines. In HGGs, IL-8 further localizes in oxygen-deprived cells surrounding necrosis. Macrophages are known to produce high levels of IL-8, which has a tumorigenic activity, by inducing tumor growth and angiogenesis; IL-8 is an inflammatory chemoattractant responding to the tumor microenvironment. Tumor pseudopalisading cells secrete hypoxic inducing factor (HIF) which induces IL-8 secretion. On the base of our preliminary results, we hypothese an important role of IL-8 as crucial angiogenesis mediator within HIF-1α pathway and crosstalk between hypoxia-induced high levels of HIF-1α and VEGF expression. A simultaneous selective antisense strategy against two molecular targets involved at different levels in the same pathological pathway could be an attractive therapeutic mechanism aimed at enhancing an anti-angiogenic and anti-tumoral effect.

A very interesting new field of research and therapeutic application in glioma treatment is represented by studying and knowledge of differential phenotypic transcriptional profiles expressed into gliomas, and GBM in particular. Hoelzinger et al. in their study have showed two different gene expression profiles into two distinct subpopulations of glioma cells, respectively the glioma cells located inside the stationary and proliferative tumor core and the glioma cells, located inside the motile and invading tumor rim. The authors report two different pattern of gene expression, characterized respectively by high levels of IGFBP2 and vimentin into tumor core glioma cells and upregulated expression of genes involved in adhesion, extracellular signal transduction, cytoskeletal rearrangement, intracellular signal transduction and apoptosis. In particular genes upregulated in invasive cells are autotoxin (ATX), the autocrin motility factor, protein tyrosine kinase 2 beta (PYK2), ephrin B3, antiapoptotic factor B-cell lymphoma-w (BCLW) and death-associated protein 3 (DAP3). The existence of two different gene expression profiles into distinct areas of the same tumor suggests the possibility to attack different molecular pathways and steps of glioma progression at the same time, targeting selectively different subsets of glioma cells. This introduces the possibility of multiagent treatment modalities, specifically targeting invasive cells, through new molecular therapeutic approaches in conjuction with classic treatments [84].

Author details

Giuseppe Raudino[1], Maria Caffo[2], Gerardo Caruso[2], Concetta Alafaci[2], Federica Raudino[3], Valentina Marventano[3], Alberto Romano[1], Francesco Montemagno[1], Massimo Belvedere[1], Francesco Maria Salpietro[2], Francesco Tomasello[2] and Anna Schillaci[3]

1 Villa Salus Clinic, Augusta, Italy

2 Department of Neurosurgery, University of Messina, Italy

3 Department of Pharmacy, University of Catania, Italy

References

[1] N. G. Avgeropoulos, T. T. Batchelor. New Treatment Strategies for Malignant Gliomas. The Oncologist 1999;4:209-224

[2] A. Idbaih, F. Ducray et al. "Therapeutic Application of Noncytotoxic Molecular Targeted Therapy in Gliomas: Growth factor receptors and Angiogenesis Inhibitors". The Oncologist 2008;13:978-992

[3] A. El-Aneed. "Current strategies in cancer gene therapy". European Journal of Pharmacology 498 (2004) 1-8

[4] Cho-Lea Tso, W.A. Freije et al. "Distinct Transcription Profiles of Primary and Secondary Glioblastoma Subgroups". Ancer Res, January 1, 2006

[5] H. Ohgaki and P. Kleihues. "Genetic Pathways to Primary and Secondary Glioblastoma".he American Journal of Pathology, Vol. 170. No 5. 5 May 2007

[6] E.A. Maher, F.B. Furnari et al. Malignant glioma: genetics and biology of a grave matter. Genes Dev 2001; 15:1311–1333

[7] P.Y.P. Lam and X. O. Breakefield. "Potential of gene therapy for brain tumors". Human Molecular Genetics, 2001, Vol. 10, No. 7

[8] L. Bello, C. Giussani et al. Angiogenesis and invasion in gliomas. Cancer Treat Res 2004; 117:263-284

[9] D. Hanahan, R.A. Weinberg. The hallmarks of cancer. Cell 2000; 100: 57-70 – E.C. Holland Gliomagenesis: genetic alterations and mouse models. Nat Rev Genet 2001; 2: 120-129

[10] D. Hanahan, J. Folkman. Patterns and emerging mechanisms of the angiogenic switch during tumorigenesis. Cell 1996; 86:353-364

[11] J.F. Woessner. The family of matrix metalloproteinases. Ann NY Acad Sci 1994; 732:11-21

[12] J.H. Uhm, N.P. Dooley et al. Mechanisms of glioma invasion: role of matrix metalloproteinases. Can J Neurol Sci 1997; 24:3-15

[13] K. Pinkstaff, J. Detterich, G. Lynch, C. Gall. Integrin subunit gene expression is regionally differentiated in adult brain. J Neurosci 1999; 19(5): 1541-1556

[14] L.S. Jones. Integrins: Possible functions in the adult CNS. Trends Neurosci 1996; 19(2): 68-72

[15] H.K. Rooprai, T. Vanmeter et al. The role of integrins receptors in aspects of glioma invasion in vitro. Int J Dev Neurosci 1999; 17(5-6): 613-623

[16] C.L. Gladson, J.N. Wilcox et al. Cerebral microenviroment influences expression of the vitronectin gene in astrocytic tumors. J Cell Sci 1995; 108(Pt 3): 947-956

[17] L. Bello, M. Francolini et al. Alpha(v)beta3 and alpha(v)beta5 integrin expression in glioma periphery. Neurosurgery 2001; 49(2): 380-389

[18] S.I. Abdulrauf, K. Edvardsen et al. Vascular endothelial growth factor expression and vascular density as prognostic markers of survival in patients with low-grade astrocytoma. J Neurosurg 1998 88:513-520

[19] M. Caffo, A. Germanò et al. An immunohistochemical study of extracellular matrix proteins laminin, fibronectin and type IV collagen in paediatric glioblastoma multiforme. Acta Neurochir (Wien) 2004; 146(10): 1113-1118

[20] S. Liekens, E. De Clercq et al. Angiogenesis: Regulators and clinical application. Biochem Pharmacol 2001; 61(3): 253-270

[21] S.J. Grau, F. Trillsch et al. Expression of VEGFR3 in glioma endothelium correlates with tumor grade. J Neurooncol 2007; 82(2): 141-150

[22] R.S. Morrison, F. Yamaguchi et al. Basic fibroblast growth facto rand fibroblast growth factor receptor I are implicated in the growth of human astrocytomas. J Neurooncol 1994; 18: 207-216

[23] R.K. Jain et al. Angiogenesis in brain tumours. Nat Rev Neurosci, 2007. 8(8): 610-22

[24] H. Hashizume et al. Openings between defective endothelial cells explain tumor vessel leakiness. Am J Pathol, 2000. 156(4): 1363-80

[25] P. Kleihues, P.C. Burger et al. Glioblastoma. In: Pathology and Genetics of Tumours of the Nervous System, Kleihues P, Cavenee WK (eds.), 2000, pp. 29-39, IARC Press: Lyon

[26] P. Kleihues, H. Ohgaki (1999). Primary and secondary glioblastomas: from concept to clinical diagnosis. Neuro-oncology 1:44-51

[27] G.L. Semenza (2003). Targeting HIF-1 for cancer therapy. Nat Rev Cancer 3:721-732

[28] G.D. Yancopoulos, S. Davis et al. Vascular-specific growth factors and blood vessel formation. Nature, 2000, 407:242-248

[29] J. Folkman. Angiogenesis in cancer,vascular, rheumatoid and other disease. Nat Med, 1995, 1:27-31

[30] J. Holash, P.C. Maisonpierre et al. Vessel cooption, regression,and growth in tumors mediated by angiopoietins and VEGF. Science 284:1994-1998

[31] A. Stratmann, W. Risau, K.H. Plate (1998) Cell type-specific expression of angiopoietin-1 and angiopoietin-2 suggests a role in glioblastoma angiogenesis. Am J Pathol 153:1459-1466

[32] G. Zadeh, B. Qian et al. Targeting the Tie2/Tek receptor in astrocytomas. Am J Pathol 164:467-476

[33] G. Santoni, M. Beatrice et al. " New deals on the transcriptional and post-transcriptional regulation of TRP channel target genes during the angiogenesis of glioma". Journal of Experimental and Integrative Medicine 2011; 1(4):221-234

[34] R. Nishikawa. Standard therapy for glioblastoma--a review of where we are. Neurol Med Chir (Tokyo), 2010. 50(9): p. 713-9

[35] K.L. Chaichana et al., Recurrence and malignant degeneration after resection of adult hemispheric low-grade gliomas. J Neurosurg, 2010. 112(1): p. 10-7

[36] J.K. Park et al. Scale to predict survival after surgery for recurrent glioblastoma multiforme. J Clin Oncol, 2010. 28(24): p. 3838-43

[37] W. Stummer et al. Extent of resection and survival in glioblastoma multiforme:identification of and adjustment for bias. Neurosurgery, 2008. 62(3): p. 564-76

[38] F.J. Attenello et al. Use of Gliadel (BCNU) wafer in the surgical treatment of malignant glioma: a 10-year institutional experience. Ann Surg Oncol, 2008. 15(10): p. 2887-93

[39] L.R. Kleinberg et al. Clinical course and pathologic findings after Gliadel and radiotherapy for newly diagnosed malignant glioma: implications for patient management. Cancer Invest, 2004. 22(1): p. 1-9. 28

[40] M. Westphal et al. Gliadel wafer in initial surgery for malignant glioma: longterm follow-up of a multicenter controlled trial. Acta Neurochir (Wien), 2006. 148(3): p. 269-75).

[41] T. Okawa (History of radiotherapy for cancer). Gan To Kagaku Ryoho, 1999. 26 Suppl 1: p. 15-22

[42] B. Bucci et al. Fractionated ionizing radiation exposure induces apoptosis through caspase-3 activation and reactive oxygen species generation. Anticancer Res, 2006. 26(6B): p. 4549-57

[43] C. Wild-Bode et al. Sublethal irradiation promotes migration and invasiveness of glioma cells: implications for radiotherapy of human glioblastoma. Cancer Res, 2001. 61(6): p. 2744-50

[44] G.S. Bauman et al. Effects of radiation on a three-dimensional model of malignant glioma invasion. Int J Dev Neurosci, 1999. 17(5-6): p. 643-51. 45

[45] Y. Ogawa et al. Reactive oxygen species-producing site in radiation and hydrogen peroxide-induced apoptosis of human peripheral T cells: Involvement of lysosomal membrane destabilization. Int J Mol Med, 2004. 13(5): p. 655-60

[46] R.Stupp, M. E. Hegi et al.Changing Paradigms—An Update on the Multidisciplinary Management of Malignant Glioma. The Oncologist 2006;11:165–180

[47] K Ogawa, Y Yoshii et al. Phase II trial of radiotherapy after hyperbaric oxygenation with chemotherapy for high-grade gliomas, British Journal of Cancer (2006) 95, 862–868

[48] M.C. Chamberlain, P.A. Kormanik. Practical guidelines for the treatment of malignant gliomas. West J Med 1998; 168:114-120

[49] J.A. Williams, J.A. Edwards, B.W. Wessels. Targeting and therapy of human glioma xenografts in vivo using radiolabeled antibodies. Int J Radiat Oncol Biol Phys. 1990 Sep;19(3):633-42

[50] E.A. Lauren, N.L. David et al. Survey of treatment recommendations for anaplastic oligodendroglioma.Neuro Oncol. 2007 July; 9(3): 314–318

[51] M.J. van den Bent, A.F. Carpentier et al. Adjuvant procarbazine, lomustine, and vincristine improves progression-free survival but not overall survival in newly diagnosed anaplastic oligodendrogliomas and oligoastrocytomas: a randomized european organisation for research and treatment of cancer Phase I trial II. J. Clin. Oncol. 24(18), 2715–2722 (2006))

[52] M.J. van den Bent, M.J.B. Taphoorn et al. Phase II Study of First-Line Chemotherapy With Temozolomide in Recurrent Oligodendroglial Tumors: The European Organization for Research and Treatment of Cancer Brain Tumor Group Study 26971. J Clin Oncol 21:2525-2528

[53] J. Hildebrand, T. Gorlia, J.M. Kros. Adjuvant dibromodulcitol and BCNU chemotherapy in anaplastic astrocytoma: results of a randomised European Organisation for Research and Treatment of Cancer phase III study (EORTC study 26882) Eur J Cancer. 2008 Jun; 44(9): 1210-6

[54] H.S. Friedman, R.E. McLendon et al. DNA mismatch repair and O6-alkylguanine-DNA alkyltransferase analysis and response to Temodal in newly diagnosed malignant glioma. J Clin Oncol 1998;16:3851–3857

[55] N. G. Avgeropoulos, T. T. Batchelor. New Treatment Strategies for Malignant Gliomas. The Oncologist 1999;4:209-224

[56] U. Bogdahn, T. Schneider, V. Oliushine. Randomized, active-controlled phase IIb study with trabedersen (AP 12009) in recurrent or refractory high-grade glioma patients: Basis for phase III endpoints. J Clin Oncol 27:15s, 2009 (suppl; abstr 2037)

[57] Stupp R, Mason WP et al. Radiotherapy plus concomitant and adjuvant temozolomide for glioblastoma. N Engl J Med 2005;352:987–996

[58] A. Salmaggi, S. Duri et al. Loco-regional treatments in first-diagnosis glioblastoma: literature review on association between Stupp protocol and Gliadel. Neurol Sci. 2011 Nov;32 Suppl 2:S241-5

[59] W. Wick, M. Platten et al. Temozolomide chemotherapy alone versus radiotherapy alone for malignant astrocytoma in the elderly: the NOA-08 randomised, phase 3 trial. Lancet Oncol. 2012 Jul;13(7):707-715

[60] S. Goel, Dan G. Duda, Lei Xu. Normalization Of The Vasculature For Treatment Of Cancer And Other Diseases. Physiol Rev. 2011 July; 91(3): 1071–1121

[61] T. Würdinger, A. Bakhos Tannous. Special Focus: Angeogenesis in the Central Nervous System; Glioma angiogenesis ;Towards novel RNA therapeutics. Cell Adhesion & Migration 3:2, 230-235; April/May/June 2009

[62] M. G. McNamara and W. P. Mason. Antiangiogenic Therapies in Glioblastoma Multiforme. Posted: 06/13/2012; Expert Rev Anticancer Ther. 2012;12(5):643-654

[63] T. N. Kreisl, L. Kim et al. Phase II Trial of Single-Agent Bevacizumab Followed by Bevacizumab Plus Irinotecan at Tumor Progression in Recurrent Glioblastoma. J Clin Oncol 27:740-745

[64] J.J. Vredenburgh, A. Desjardins, J.E. Herndon. Bevacizumab Plus Irinotecan in Recurrent Glioblastoma Multiforme. J Clin Oncol 25:4722-4729

[65] EUROPLAN - NATIONAL CONFERENCES- Final Report of the conference in ITALY(2010)

[66] ROL – Linee Guida Terapeutiche – Tumori del Sistema Nervoso Centrale (agg. febbraio 2012)

[67] E.T. Wong, S. Brem. Taming Glioblastoma: Targeting Angiogenesis. Journal of Clinical Oncology, Vol 25, No 30 (October 20), 2007: pp 4705-4706

[68] M. C. Chamberlain, T. Cloughsey et al. A Novel Treatment for Glioblastoma-Integrin Inhibition. Posted: 04/06/2012; Expert Rev Neurother. 2012;12(4):421-435)

[69] K. Fink, T. Mikkelsen et al. Long-term effects of cilengitide, a novel integrin inhibitor, in recurrent glioblastoma: A randomized phase IIa study. J Clin Oncol 28:15s, 2010 (suppl; abstr 2010)

[70] R. Stupp, M. E. Hegi et al. Phase I/IIa Study of Cilengitide and Temozolomide With Concomitant Radiotherapy Followed by Cilengitide and Temozolomide Maintenance Therapy in Patients With Newly Diagnosed Glioblastoma. J Clin Oncol 28:2712-2718

[71] S. Takahashi et al. Downregulation of uPARP mediates cytoskeletal rearrangements and decreases invasion and migration properties in glioma cells. J Neurooncol, 2010 - 192. B. Zhang et al. Reduction of Akt2 inhibits migration and invasion of glioma cells. Int J Cancer, 2009. 125(3): p. 585-95.191, 192

[72] M. Hadziahmetovic, K. Shirai and Arnab Chakravarti. Recent Advancements in Multimodality Treatment of Gliomas: Targeted Therapy in HGG. Future Oncol. 2011;7(10):1169-1183

[73] E. Ranza, G. Mazzini et al. In vitro effects of the tyrosine kinase inhibitor imatinib on glioblastoma cell proliferation. J. Neurooncol. 96(3), 349–357 (2010)

[74] G. Dresemann, M. Weller et al. Imatinib in combination with hydroxyurea versus hydroxyurea alone as oral therapy in patients with progressive pretreated glioblastoma resistant to standard dose temozolomide. J. Neurooncol. 96(3), 393–402 (2010).

[75] J.C. Tonn et al. Effect of synthetic matrix-metalloproteinase inhibitors on invasive capacity and proliferation of human malignant gliomas in vitro. Int J Cancer, 1999. 80(5): p. 764-72

[76] M.D. Groves et al., Phase II trial of temozolomide plus marimastat for recurrent anaplastic gliomas: a relationship among efficacy, joint toxicity and anticonvulsant status. J Neurooncol, 2006. 80(1): p. 83-90

[77] M.D. Groves et al., Phase II trial of temozolomide plus the matrix metalloproteinase inhibitor, marimastat, in recurrent and progressive glioblastoma multiforme. J Clin Oncol, 2002. 20(5): p. 1383-8.

[78] I.B. Weinstein and A.K. Joe. Oncogene addiction. Cancer Res, 2008. 68(9): p.3077-80; discussion 3080

[79] I.B. Weinstein and A.K. Joe. Mechanisms of disease: Oncogene addiction—a rationale for molecular targeting in cancer therapy. Nat Clin Pract Oncol, 2006. 3(8): p. 448-57

[80] C. Di et al. Emerging therapeutic targets and agents for glioblastoma migrating cells. Anticancer Agents Med Chem, 2010. 10(7): p. 543-55

[81] J.F. De Groot et al. Tumor invasion after treatment of glioblastoma with bevacizumab: radiographic and pathologic correlation in humans and mice. Neuro Oncol, 2010. 12(3): p. 233-42

[82] P.H. Huang et al. Quantitative analysis of EGFRvIII cellular signaling networks reveals a combinatorial therapeutic strategy for glioblastoma. Proc Natl Acad Sci U S A, 2007. 104(31): p. 12867-72

[83] M.S. Ahluwalia et al. Targeting SRC in glioblastoma tumors and brain metastases: rationale and preclinical studies. Cancer Lett, 2010. 298(2): p. 139-49.

[84] D.B. Hoeltzinger, L. Mariani et al. "Gene expression profile of glioblastoma multiforme invasive phenotype points to new therapeutic targets". Neoplasia Vol 7, no 1, January 2005, 7-16

Chapter 8

Dipeptidyl Peptidase-IV and Related Proteases in Brain Tumors

Petr Busek and Aleksi Sedo

Additional information is available at the end of the chapter

http://dx.doi.org/10.5772/53888

1. Introduction

Malignant gliomas rank among the most aggressive human tumors. The hallmarks of these tumors include a highly infiltrative behavior, aberrant cell proliferation and apoptosis, increased angiogenesis and intratumoral as well as systemic immunosuppression [1, 2]. Proteases localized on the cell-surface or released extracellularly may significantly contribute to these characteristics by mediating the breakdown of the components of the extracellular matrix (ECM), liberating growth factors sequestered by binding to the ECM, regulating the activity of paracrine mediators and shedding of cell-surface proteins [3]. There is substantial evidence for the role of matrix metalloproteinases (MMP), the serine protease urokinase-type plasminogen activator (uPA) and the cysteine protease cathepsin B in glioma invasion [4], angiogenesis [5] and proliferation. In addition, expression of proteases such as cathepsin D, uPA or MMP-9 in the clinical material may predict patient prognosis [6-8]. Nevertheless, the role of several proteases including the canonical dipeptidyl peptidase-IV (DPP-IV) and related proteases in glioma progression remains largely unknown with only few studies using synthetic inhibitors or genetic manipulation to determine their function. In this chapter, we review the basic characteristics of DPP-IV and related proteases, focus on their functional role in the transformed as well as stromal cells, and discuss the implications for the biology of human gliomas.

1.1. "Dipeptidyl peptidase-IV activity and/or structure homologous" (DASH) molecules

Historically, dipeptidyl peptidase-IV (DPP-IV, EC 3.4.14.5, identical with the lymphocyte differentiation antigen CD26) was described by Hopsu-Havu and Glenner [9] in liver homogenates on the basis of its unique hydrolytic activity cleaving N-terminal dipeptides from synthetic chromogenic substrates with the proline residue in the penultimate position. The presence of similar enzymatic activity was observed in body fluids soon after that [10, 11]. At that time, DPP-IV was hypothesized to participate on the turnover of the regulatory as well as structural proteins bearing the consensus cleavage sequence. However, the speculations about its particular biological roles awaited experimental confirmation. Subsequently, multiple authors noted substantial heterogeneity of molecular forms that possessed strikingly similar enzymatic activity but differed in molecular weight, isoelectric point and subcellular localization [12]. It took several years to identify and characterize other "DPP-IV-like" molecules, individual gene products, exhibiting various degree of structural homology with the canonical DPP-IV. These comprise the intracellularly localized DPP8 and DPP9 (both still assigned under the same EC 3.4.14.5) [13, 14], the plasma membrane fibroblast activation protein-alpha/seprase (FAP, EC 3.4.21.B28) [15] as well as the DPP-IV sequentially dissimilar intracellular DPP-II (quiescent cell proline dipeptidase, DPP7, EC 3.4.14.2)[16]. Besides, highly structurally similar but hydrolytically inactive DPP6 and DPP10 were discovered later [17]. Recently, all these molecular species are by some authors referred to as the "Dipeptidyl peptidase-IV activity/and or structure homologous" (DASH) molecules [18-24]. Formerly, Glutamate carboxypeptidase II (GCPII, N-acetyl-L-aspartyl-L-glutamate peptidase I, NAALADase I, prostate specific membrane antigen, EC 3.4.17.21) and Attractin were proposed to belong to this group on the basis of the presumed DPP-IV-like enzymatic activity [24]. However, further research did not confirm the hydrolytic potential of these molecules [25, 26]. Since both of them also lack any significant structural homology with DPP-IV, they are no more included in the DASH group.

1.1.1. Dipeptidyl peptidase-IV

In humans, the canonical DPP-IV is almost ubiquitously expressed as a single-pass type II integral transmembrane glycoprotein in a variety of cell types, tissues and organs (reviewed in [11, 27]). Its soluble counterpart is detectable in body fluids, being either a product of proteolytic shedding from the cell surface or a putative specific secretory form [28]. Upregulation of the plasma membrane DPP-IV is associated with cell differentiation in e.g. T cells [29, 30], hepatocytes [31] and intestinal epithelium [32]. The expression and function of DPP-IV/CD26, a marker of a subset of activated T-cells, was intensively studied in the immune system [33]. Its crosslinking in T cells affects the synthesis and secretion of a number of cytokines and interleukins [34, 35]. DPP-IV is also identical with the adenosine daeminase binding protein and participates on the immunoregulations by influencing the pericellular concentration of free adenosine [36, 37]. The physiological relevance of the interaction of DPP-IV with plasminogen 2 [38] and several proteins of the ECM [39, 40] is still more speculated than proven.

1.1.2. Fibroblast activation protein

Possessing about 52% amino acid sequence identity with DPP-IV, FAP represents its closest homologue within the DASH group. Its gene is located on chromosome 2q23 and is believed to be a product of DPP-IV gene duplication (reviewed in [15]). FAP is typically expressed as a type II transmembrane protein and its soluble counterpart is present in blood plasma and is also known as α2-antiplasmin cleaving enzyme [41, 42]. In contrast to DPP-IV, FAP expression is substantially restricted and the majority of normal adult cells are FAP negative [27]. FAP expression is significantly induced in non-malignant states associated with tissue remodeling such as wound healing, embryogenesis, osteoarthritis as well as rheumatoid arthritis [43, 44], in liver cirhosis [45], and in cancer stroma [46]. In addition to the DPP-IV-like exopeptidase activity, FAP also possesses gelatinolytic endopeptidase activity [47, 48], and was thus suggested to participate in the degradation of structural proteins of the extracellular matrix during tissue remodeling and cancer cell invasion (reviewed in [15]). Matrix metalloproteinases (MMP), in particular MMP 2 [49], seem to be important functional partners of FAP in the modification of extracellular matrix [15]. Interestingly, heteromeric DPP-IV/FAP complexes, possessing both the DPP-IV-like exopeptidase and proline-specific endopeptidase enzymatic activity, are suspected to influence the migratory and invasive potential of fibroblasts and endothelial cells [49, 50].

1.1.3. Dipeptidyl peptidase 8 and 9

DPP8 and 9 are cytosolic dimeric proteins that are expressed in the majority of tissues including the human brain [13, 14, 51, 52], for review see [53]. The enzymatic activity of DPP 9 is thought to be important for the degradation of intracellular proline containing proteins with presentation of the peptide fragments on MHC-I molecules [54]. Some reports also suggest the involvement of both DPP8 and 9 in the processes of cell growth, migration and adhesion, probably via an indirect, enzymatic activity independent effect on the cell-extracellular matrix interactions [55]. DPP 9 may also influence the intracellular signaling cascades: DPP9 overexpression reduces the EGF mediated Akt activation by an enzyme activity dependent mechanism, and in addition DPP9 interacts with Ras [56]. Both proteases are expressed in the immune system [52, 57] and some of the effects of non-selective DPP inhibitors on immune cells may be in fact caused by the inhibition of DPP8 and 9 [53].

1.1.4. Dipeptidyl peptidase-II

DPP-II (DPP7, QPP, EC 3.4.14.2) possesses the unique DPP-IV-like enzymatic activity, but is structurally different from the canonical DPP-IV. It is a widely expressed intracellular enzyme that is typically localized in lysosomes and extralysosomal vesicles [16]. It is the only enzyme from the DASH group that has an acidic pH optimum [16]. Although the physiological function of DPP-II remains largely unknown, it is speculated to participate on the intralysosomal turnover of short peptides [58, 59]. In addition, several reports from the Huber lab argue for its role in the maintenance of quiescence in lymphocytes and fibroblasts [60, 61] and possibly also in glucose homeostasis [62]. DPP-II knockout is embryonic lethal in mice [62, 63], inhibition of DPP-II triggers apoptosis in noncycling G0 lymphocytes [64, 65] probably through deregulation of the cell cycle entry, and its absence in T cells leads to faster proliferation and differentiation into Th17 cells [63].

1.1.5. Dipeptidyl peptidase 6 and 10

DPP6 (dipeptidyl peptidase-IV like protein 1, DPPX) [66] and DPP10 (dipeptidyl peptidase-IV like protein 2)[67] are the enzymatically inactive, DPP-IV structurally related members of the DASH group [17]. Both proteins participate on the regulation of the voltage gated potassium channels [68] and may play a role in the development of the central nervous system and neurodegenerative diseases [69, 70]. There are currently no data on their role in gliomagenesis and only two studies suggested an association of mutations in DPP6 with pancreatic cancer [71, 72].

A substantial leap of interest in the DASH molecules was induced i) by the introduction of DPP-IV inhibitors in the treatment of type II diabetes [19, 244] and ii) observations of marked alterations of their expression and activity in the course of several diseases especially involving the immune system, and in cancer, where a direct pathogenetic role for DPP-IV and FAP seems to be highly probable. A significant proportion of the biologically active, mostly pro-proliferative peptides, systemic as well as local hormones, chemokines, neuropeptides, incretins and growth factors (Figure 1) contains a penultimate N-terminal proline residue as an evolutionary conserved proteolytic regulatory "check-point" [245]. Thus, the DPP-IV enzymatic activity is believed to be a functional regulator of their biological action. Limited proteolysis of these peptides by DPP-IV may lead both to quantitative and, due to the diversification of receptor subset preference, also to qualitative changes of their signaling potential [73-75].

While the systematic description of individual DASH molecules is available, including the cloning and structure resolution, the interpretations of biological studies are often equivocal because of their "moonlighting" character [76]. First, the overlap of enzymatic activities among the DASH molecules implies their sharing of similar sets of substrates (Figure 1) and thus, to some extent, DASH molecules may substitute each other. Second, DASH molecules execute more biological functions, depending on the given cell population and actual context of the biologically active substrates and the relevant receptors within the immediate environment. Third, the functional potential of DASH molecules is broadened by interactions with non-hydrolytic molecular partners (Ramirez-Montagut et al. 2004; Wang et al. 2005).

2. Expression and function of dipeptidyl peptidase-IV and related proteases in the microenvironment of human malignancies

2.1. Expression in transformed cells- tumor type specific and context dependent functions

Altered expression of DPP-IV and FAP is associated with several malignancies including brain tumors [87]. Both molecules may be expressed by the transformed as well as stromal cells and are associated with tumor promotion or suppression depending on the cancer type (for review see [88, 89, 27]). The mechanisms by which these molecules contribute to cancer pathogenesis and progression remain largely unknown, but several reports indicate that DASH molecules may serve as diagnostic and prognostic markers as well as therapeutic targets.

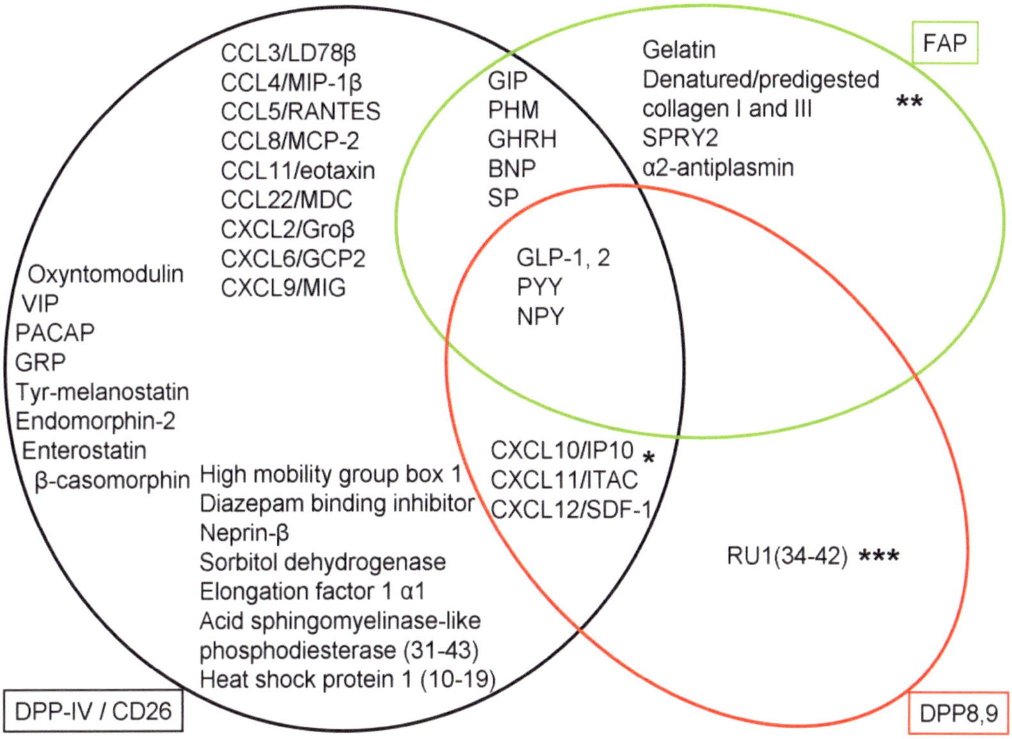

Figure 1. Potential overlaps of DPP-IV and related proteases in the processing of biologically active peptides. The pathophysiological importance of the cleavage is established e.g. for GLP-1, GIP, CXCL12 and NP Y, some of the in vitro cleaved substrates are unlikely to be of significance in vivo (e.g. Heat shock protein 1 for DPP-IV, SPRY2 for FAP). Not all identified DPP-IV substrates were tested with DPP8, 9 and FAP, the cleavage by these proteases is usually slower compared to DPP-IV. * cleavage has only been established for DPP-IV and DPP8; ** substrates of the endopeptidase activity of FAP; *** only tested for DPP8 and DPP9; VIP= Vasoactive intestinal peptide, PACAP= Pituitary adenylate cyclase-activating peptide, GRP= Gastrin-releasing peptide, GIP= Gastric inhibitory polypeptide/ glucose-dependent insulinotropic peptide, PHM= Peptide Histidine-Methionine, GHRH= Growth hormone releasing hormone, BNP= Brain natriuretic peptide, SP= Substance P, GLP-1, 2= Glucagon-like peptide-1, 2, PYY= Peptide YY, NP Y= Neuropeptide Y, SPRY2= sprouty (Drosophila) homolog 2, RU1(34-42)= antigenic peptide VPYGSFKHV. Compiled based on [15, 54, 73, 77-86].

DPP-IV expression is typical for a subset of aggressive T cell malignancies, which may be related to its function in T cell activation [90, 91]. The presence of DPP-IV is also associated with a more malignant behavior in B-cell chronic lymphocytic leukaemia [92], thyroid cancer [93], gastrointestinal stromal tumors [94], and was recently linked to a subpopulation of cancer stem cells responsible for the metastatic spread of colorectal cancer [95].

Recent studies aimed at examining the functional role of DPP-IV in malignant cells. In mesothelioma, DPP-IV is expressed in tumors in situ and in mesothelioma cell lines [96]. By binding fibronectin and collagen I, DPP-IV likely contributes to the interaction of these cells with the ECM [97]. A different mechanism may operate in Ewing sarcoma: DPP-IV (and likely also the intracellular proteases DPP8 and 9) proteolytically cleaves NP Y1-36 to NP Y3-36 and thus abolishes its cell death inducing activity in the cancer cells and switches it to an angiogenesis promoting mediator [98].

Contrary to the above cited reports, some malignancies exhibit decreased DPP-IV expression. This is typical for melanoma and melanoma derived cell lines [99-102], cancer cell lines derived from neuroblastoma [103] and prostate [104] as well as non-small-cell lung cancer [105]. It should be however noted that on the tissue level, the data on DPP-IV expression are equivocal at least for prostate and lung cancer [106-109]. DPP-IV was shown to act as a tumor suppressor in melanoma [99, 102], neuroblastoma [103], prostate [104] and non-small-lung cancer [105] cells: its reexpression in the transformed cells led do decreased growth, increased apoptosis and sensitivity to growth factor withdrawal, decreased invasiveness and slower xenotransplant growth in immunodeficient animals.

The mechanisms that account for these diverse effects of DPP-IV on tumor cells are rather poorly understood. The currently best characterized physiological function of DPP-IV is proteolytic inactivation of incretins and possibly other biologically active peptides [73, 110]. The biological relevance of this phenomenon is confirmed by the clinically exploited DPP-IV inhibitors resulting in systemic elevation of DPP-IV substrates such as GLP-1 [111]. In addition, a variety of growth factors, chemokines and neuropeptides implicated in the progression of human tumors are potential DPP-IV substrates (reviewed in [74]) and DPP-IV may therefore act as a "gate-keeper" regulating their biological function on the systemic and/or local level. The decreased clearance of biologically active substrates due to the absence of DPP-IV may lead to sustained pro-proliferative signaling and promote tumor growth and metastasis. Masur et al. [112] showed that the growth promoting and promigratory activity of GLP-2 in colon cancer cells in vitro is increased in the presence of a DPP-IV inhibitor. Similarly, the inhibition of the DPP-IV enzymatic activity facilitated metastatic spread of prostate cancer cells by preventing the cleavage of the chemokine CXCL12 (SDF-1, stromal cell derived factor -1) [113].

On the other hand, DPP-IV also triggers changes in signaling cascades and expression of molecules mediating interaction with the ECM that are harder to reconcile with the cleavage of biologically active substrates in the pericellular space. In ovarian carcinoma, DPP-IV expression led to suppression of MAPK signaling, enhanced E-cadherin expression and the downregulation of MMP-2 and MT-MMP-1, which was associated with decreased invasiveness, tumor progression and enhanced chemosensitivity [114-116]. In prostate cancer cells, re-expression of DPP-IV interfered with the signaling of a non-DPP-IV substrate bFGF and inhibited their malignant phenotype in the study by Wesley et al. [104]. Yet, Goznalez-Gronow et al. [117] identified DPP-IV as a receptor for plasminogen 2 epsilon that promoted the invasiveness of the prostate cancer cell line 1-LN.

To test the relevance of the hypothesized non-proteolytic functions of DPP-IV, several groups including ours engineered an enzymatically inactive form of DPP-IV with a single amino acid substitution in the active site ($Ser^{630} \rightarrow Ala^{630}$). Reintroduction of this mutant form of DPP-IV frequently results in similar tumor suppressing effects as observed with the enzymatically active DPP-IV [99, 102, 105, 118].

The proteolytic and non-proteolytic mechanisms may also combine and thus extend the portfolio of the biological functions of DPP-IV. Arscott et al. [103] showed that DPP-IV reexpression in neuroblastoma cells induced differentiation, increased their sensitivity to serum withdrawal and reduced their migration, invasion and pro-angiogenic capacity in vitro as well as in vivo. This was most likely caused by the downmodulation of the CXCL12-CXCR4 axis and possibly also other chemokine systems. Although not specifically demonstrated by the authors, DPP-IV most likely inactivated CXCL12 proteolytically, resulting in the downregulation of its downstream effectors, but in addition it downregulated the mRNAs of CXCL12 and CXCR4 and several other chemokines including non-DPP-IV substrates [103].

FAP was originally described to be typically expressed in the stromal compartment of tumors (see section 2.2), but several reports, including ours, also show its expression in the transformed elements. A prototypical example is the LOX melanoma cell line, where FAP co-localizes with the urokinase plasminogen activator receptor (uPAR) on the invadopodia and likely contributes to the pericellular proteolysis and invasiveness of these cells [119, 120, 47, 121, 122]. Somewhat surprisingly, Ramirez-Montagut et al. [123] were able to show that in mouse melanoma cells FAP may actually act as a tumor suppressor with the main effects on cell growth and survival independently of its enzymatic activity. These results are in agreement with Rettig et al., who observed loss of FAP during Ras mediated transformation of melanocytes [124] and with the fact that FAP is upregulated upon reintroduction of DPP-IV into melanoma cells with the resulting tumor suppressing effects [99]. Similarly, FAP negative subclones in osteosarcoma were tumorigenic and grew to high densities in contrast to non-tumorigenic FAP positive subclones [124].

Breast cancer cells also express FAP in vivo [15, 125]. FAP is associated with their decreased dependence on growth factors in vitro and formation of more rapidly growing and more vascularized tumors in a xenotransplantation model [125-127]. Interestingly and somewhat in contrast to the previously published data in other cancer types, the tumor promoting activities in breast cancer cells may be independent of the intrinsic enzymatic activity of FAP [128]. FAP is also expressed in the tumor cells of mesenchymal origin in malignant and benign tumors, but is probably rather linked to their myofibroblastic differentiation than to their malignant potential [129]. Epithelial cancer cells e.g. in gastric [130], esophageal [131], colorectal [132] and cervical cancer [133] were also demonstrated to be FAP positive. The function of FAP in these cells is unclear but in analogy to other cancers it is presumed to be linked to their invasiveness.

There is limited data on the expression and in particular the function of DPP8, DPP9 and DPP-II in cancer cells. Yu et al. described increased DPP9 mRNA in testicular cancers on a small patient sample [52], both DPP8 and DPP9 are expressed in human breast, ovarian and hepatic cancer cells as well as in lymphoma cells lines [52, 134] and chronic B cell leukemia cells [135]. Interestingly, transgenic DPP9 was shown to induce apoptosis in hepatoma cells and decrease the EGF mediated activation of Akt [56]. These effects were dependent on the enzymatic activity of DPP9, but in addition to that, both DPP9 and DPP8 were demonstrated to interact with Ras [56]. In Ewing sarcoma cells, DPP8 and DPP9 seem to exert similar effects as DPP-IV (see above) due to their similar enzymatic activity [98] and efficient cleavage of NP Y [77](Figure 1.). Whether DPP8 and DPP9 regulate the adhesion and migration [55] of malignant cells remains to be established. Lower DPP-II catalytic histochemistry staining was suggested as a favorable prognostic marker in chronic lymphocytic leukemia (CLL) [136]. In addition, DPP-II inhibition leads to induction of apoptosis in CLL cells in approximately 60% of patients, which is associated with the presence of other established positive prognostic markers and a clinically more benign disease course [137]. Whether DPP-II is functionally involved in the pathogenesis in CLL and/or other cancers is currently not known.

2.2. Expression and role of dipeptidyl peptidase-IV and related proteases in the stromal compartment of tumors

Tumor stroma is composed of an extracellular matrix and a diverse set of cell types that significantly contribute to tumor progression [138]. Among others, the stroma is an important source of tumor associated proteases including the DASH molecules.

Vascular and lymphatic endothelial cells express DPP-IV in cell culture as well as in situ [139, 140], but the expression is variable and several reports show no DPP-IV staining of cell vessels [141]. Similarly ambiguous are the data regarding the function of DPP-IV in endothelial cells: it is speculated to contribute to their interaction with the extracellular matrix proteins, convert NP Y to its pro-angiogenic form and promote their migration and invasion [50, 142-144]. Contrarily, a recent report showed that DPP-IV ablation using either genetic or pharmacologic approaches may increase endothelial cell proliferation and migration induced by the inflammatory cytokines TNF-α or IL-1β [139]. These somewhat conflicting results may be due to regional differences in the proteolytic makeup of endothelial cells as well as differing functions of DPP-IV depending on the presence of its "molecular partners" and microenvironmental stimuli. FAP mRNA was also detected in endothelial cells cultured in vitro [145]. Interestingly, Ghilardi et al. [146] observed higher FAP expression in endothelial cells derived from ovarian and renal carcinoma compared to cells derived from normal tissues. The functions of FAP in endothelial cells are mostly speculative but it may (probably together with DPP-IV) contribute to the degradation of extracellular matrix [50]. FAP may be also expressed by pericytes [138], although in some cancer models its expression was restricted to isolated infiltrating stromal cells rather than pericytes [147].

Expression of DPP-IV in the normal and cancer associated fibroblasts is rather variable [148-151], but cultured fibroblasts and myofibroblasts in the majority of epithelial cancers strongly express FAP [15, 152, 153]. Stimuli leading to the upregulation of FAP may involve inflammatory mediators such as TGF beta, Il1 and oncostatin M [43, 154], factors secreted by tumor cells (i.e. PDGF-BB, TGF-beta1 and Wnt5a in melanoma cells [155]) and the transcription factor EGR1 [156]. Pathophysiologically, FAP likely participates in the turnover and modification of the extracellular matrix [157]. Lee et al. [158] found that fibroblasts engineered to express FAP seeded on gelatin produced matrices with changed composition and structure, which promoted the migratory behavior of pancreatic carcinoma cells. These changes were mediated by the enzymatic activity of FAP as demonstrated by using a FAP inhibitor naphthalenecarboxy-Gly-boroPro [158]. FAP inhibition was also shown to block the growth of lung and colon cancer in a mouse model by increased accumulation of collagen, decreased myofibroblast content and vessel density [159] suggesting its crucial role for the effective establishment of tumor stroma. Other mechanisms may also contribute to the important role of FAP in tumor microenvironment. By selectively depleting the FAP positive stromal cells, Kraman et al. demonstrated that they are crucial for the suppression of antitumor immune response [160]. Whether FAP is just an "innocent by-stander" marker of these cells, or plays a direct role in this process remains to be established. In multiple myeloma, the stromal FAP expression is important in promoting the survival of myeloma cells [18, 161], but the mechanisms are unknown. The expression of FAP in tumors is in general associated with a more aggressive disease course and shorter patient survival [153, 162, 163]. Surprisingly, one study in breast cancer [164] described longer overall survival and the disease free interval in patients with higher stromal FAP expression.

Immune cells are another important constituent of the tumor microenvironment that may express DPP-IV, DPP8 and DPP9, but do not express FAP [135, 165, 166]. In cancer patients, changes in the DPP-IV levels are frequently seen in serum and in lymphocytes [80] and cytokines such as TGF-β may contribute to these changes in peripheral blood lymphocytes as documented in patients with oral cancer [167]. Despite the well established role of DPP-IV in human lymphocyte proliferation and activation [33], its function, as well as the possible significance of DPP8 and DPP9 in mediating or suppressing effective antitumor responses is unknown. Talabostat (PT-100), an inhibitor of DPP-IV and FAP, was demonstrated to stimulate the immune response to several experimental tumors, but the mechanisms were not dependent on the inhibition of DPP-IV [168].

In conclusion, the expression of DPP-IV and related proteases is frequently deregulated in the parenchymal and/or stromal compartment in human malignancies. The molecules may promote or suppress tumor progression depending on the tumor type and the presence of their substrates and/or interactors in the microenvironment, which are characteristic for individual tumors. This highly context dependent role is the likely explanation for the conflicting data reported on their role in cancer [27, 74, 169]. The mechanisms seem to involve proteolytic processing as well as non-proteolytic protein-protein interactions and modification of intracellular signaling pathways. Similar mechanisms likely operate for the intracellular proteases DPP8 and DPP9, but the evidence for their role in human cancers is currently limited.

3. Dipeptidyl peptidase-IV and related proteases in the pathogenesis of brain tumors

3.1. Expression of DPP-IV and related proteases in glioma cell lines

In astrocytoma cells, DPP-IV was first detected using immunohistochemistry by Medeiros [170]. Subsequent work in our laboratory revealed the presence of DPP-IV-like enzymatic activity together with the expression of mRNA for DPP-IV, FAP and DPP-8 and 9 in permanent glioma cell lines C6, U373, T98G, U251, U87, U138, U118 and in human glioma primary cell cultures as well as in glioma stem-like cells ([118, 171-175] and unpublished data). The DPP-IV-like enzymatic activity in the permanent glioma cell lines is only partially inhibited by a highly specific DPP-IV inhibitor sitagliptin. In U87, U138 and U118 lines 30, 60 and 85% respectively of the total enzymatic activity is inhibited and can therefore be attributed to the canonical DPP-IV. In contrast, only 12-15% of the DPP-IV-like enzymatic activity in U373, T98G, U251 cells is inhibited by sitagliptin (Busek et al. unpublished data). These results correspond well with the relatively high DPP-IV mRNA expression in the U87, U138 and U118 cell lines [175, 176].

FAP is also expressed in glioma cells. The early work by Rettig et al. [177] detected FAP in 19 out of 22 of astrocytoma cell lines by immunohistochemistry using the F19 monoclonal antibody. Similarly Mentlein et al. [176] showed high FAP mRNA expression in 6 out of 7 glioma cell lines. According to our data, the expression of FAP may be more variable [118] with substantial variation in individual primary cell cultures as well as permanent cell lines. In the panel of glioma cell lines examined in our studies, FAP expression mirrored the expression of DPP-IV and was substantially higher in U87, U138 and U118 cell lines than in U373, T98G, U251 lines [175]. Therefore, although FAP is significantly less efficient in cleaving the H-Gly-Pro-AMC substrate compared to DPP-IV [48], it may partly contribute to the sitagliptin resistant DPP-IV-like enzymatic activity in some of the glioma cells lines. Interestingly, we have consistently observed a positive correlation between the mRNA expression of the two transmembrane proteases DPP-IV and FAP in glioma cell lines as well as in glioma primary cell cultures [178]. Moreover, the expression of both DPP-IV and FAP increased concomitantly in glioma cells cultured in serum free media and decreased after the addition of serum to the starved cells [178] suggesting that similar pathways regulate their expression in this model, most likely on the transcription and/or mRNA stability levels [178]. The mRNAs for the ubiquitous intracellular enzymes DPP8 and DPP9 are expressed in similar quantities in the glioma cell lines tested in our laboratory and probably make the largest contribution to the residual DPP-IV-like enzymatic activity after inhibition with sitagliptin (Busek et al. unpublished data).

It is currently unclear to what extent the in vitro cell culture conditions and the standard process of glioma cell line establishment may influence the observed expression of DPP-IV and especially FAP, a known phenotypic marker of mesenchymal cells such as activated fibroblasts [15]. The typical media supplemented with 10% fetal calf serum are known to promote the mesenchymal phenotype in cultured cells ("mesenchymal drift"; [179]) which could lead to the upregulation of FAP. Xenotransplants generated by orthotopic implantation of the glioma cells into immunodeficient mice exhibited higher DPP-IV-like enzymatic activity compared to the contralateral hemisphere (Figure 2) and the enzymatic activity was in part sensitive to a specific DPP-IV inhibitor. DPP-IV as well as FAP could be detected on the mRNA level as well as by immunohistochemistry in the xenotransplants from the U87 and U138 cells (data not shown), which suggests that their expression in glioma cells is retained under the conditions closely mimicking the microenvironment of human gliomas.

http://dx.doi.org/10.5772/53888

Similarly, Li et al. [180] were able to demonstrate the enzymatic activity of FAP in a U87 tumor model, although the subcutaneous implantation used in their study exposed the glioma cells to somewhat unnatural microenvironment. Orthotopic xenotransplantation of freshly isolated glioma cells or expanded glioma stem-like cells are necessary to determine whether the expression of FAP in particular is maintained in glioma cells in situ. Such experimental approach would be suitable for the preclinical tests of therapies targeting this protease.

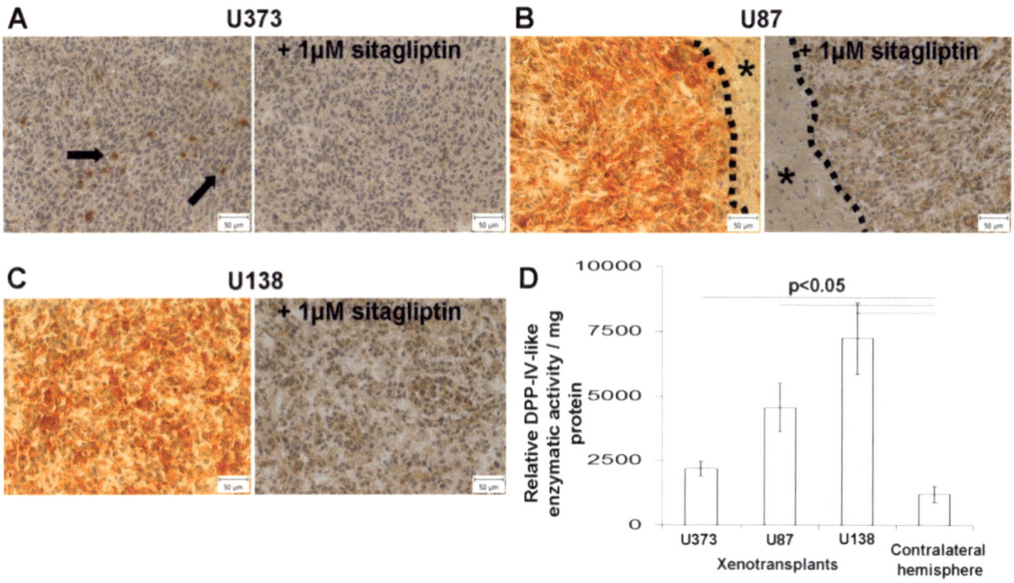

Figure 2. DPP-IV-like enzymatic activity detected by catalytic histochemistry in orthotopic glioma xenotransplants (A-C). 10^6 cells of the indicated cell lines were used for intracerebral implantation into immunodeficient mice [118]. DPP-IV-like enzymatic activity (red precipitate) was detected by incubating 10μm frozen sections with 7-(glycyl-l-prolylamido)-4-methoxy-β-naphthylamide hydrochloride as a substrate and Fast Blue B in PBS (pH 7.4) at 4°C overnight [181]. 1μM sitagliptin was used to inhibit the enzymatic activity of canonical DPP-IV (CD26), nuclei were counterstained with haematoxylin. Only small areas of DPP-IV-like enzymatic activity (arrows) can be detected in U373 tumors (A). In (B), the dashed line marks the interface between the diffusely stained tumor tissue and surrounding normal brain (asterisk). (D) DPP-IV-like enzymatic activity in homogenates from the xenotransplants compared to the contralateral hemisphere. H-Gly-Pro-7-amino-4-methylcoumarin was used as a substrate at pH 7.5 and 37°C [118].

3.2. Expression of DPP-IV and related proteases in normal brain and human astrocytic tumors

The data on the expression of DPP-IV, DPP-II, FAP and DPP8 and 9 in the human brain is limited. Using immunohistochemistry, Bernstein et al. detected abundant expression of DPP-IV in the immature central nervous system with much lower expression in adults [246]. In rats, mice and ginea-pigs, the expression of DPP-IV was studied in more detail and DPP-IV was detected in the capillaries, meninges as well as certain neuronal structures (see [175] and references therein). By means of its enzymatic activity, DPP-IV is speculated to participate on nociception and behavior regulation most likely by inactivating biologically active peptides such as SP, endomorphin-2 and NP Y [182-184]. DPP-IV may also be involved in the pathogenesis of ischemia-reperfusion injury. Roehnert et al. [185] described the appearance of DPP-IV immunoreactivity in rat microglia, astrocytes and neurons following unilateral transient occlusion of the medial carotid artery. Interestingly, intracranial administration of a specific DPP-IV inhibitor sitagliptin led to a 21.1±5.8% decrease in infarct size suggesting neuroprotection in this model [185].

Enzymatic activity attributed to DP-II was detected in brain homogenates [186, 187] and histochemically in specific neuronal populations in rat brain by Gorenstein et al. [188]. Later studies demonstrated its presence in glial cells [189] and speculated its association with astrocyte differentiation [190].

DPP8 and 9 are also expressed in the brain tissue [13, 52] and are probably responsible for a significant part of the DPP-IV-like enzymatic activity detected in human brain tissue homogenates [87]. In rats, DPP8 was detected in neurons, but not astroglial cells and microglia by immunohistochemistry [185].

On the contrary, FAP protein is most likely absent in non-tumorous human brain: Rettig et al. [177] failed to detect its expression in human autopsy material using the F19 antibody; similarly, samples obtained from patients with pharmacoresistant epilepsy show no staining using several anti FAP antibodies ([87] and unpublished data). Although FAP mRNA can be detected by sensitive RT-qPCR assays [87, 176], it is probably not being translated or the protein levels are bellow the detection limit of the methods used.

In gliomas the DPP-IV-like enzymatic activity is substantially higher compared to the non-tumorous brain [87, 191] and DPP8 and 9 represent the major part in both cases [87]. In contrast to DPP8 and 9, the expression of DPP-IV and FAP is significantly increased in gliomas compared to the non-tumorous brain. According to The Cancer Genome Atlas ([192], http://cancergenome.nih.gov/) DPP-IV and FAP mRNA are upregulated more than two times compared to controls in 200 of 424 (47%) and in 162 of 424 (38%) glioblastoma patients respectively. In our patient cohort ([87] and unpublished data) DPP-IV and FAP mRNA were upregulated 9.9 and 4.6 fold respectively in newly diagnosed glioblastoma (N=28) compared to controls (pharmacoresistant epilepsy, N=15). Using RT-qPCR, Mentlein et al. also observed upregulation of DPP-IV and FAP in a small cohort of glioblastoma patients compared to the autopsy material [176]. Similarly, increased FAP expression in grade IV tumors and especially in gliosarcomas was observed by Mikheeva et al. [193].

Using catalytic histochemistry, Mares et al. could show that the DPP-IV-like enzymatic activity in grade II astrocytomas was mainly localized perivascularly and in mononuclear-like cells in the parenchyma [191]. In grade IV tumors (glioblastomas), the proportion of these stained cells was markedly increased and in addition, the DPP-IV-like enzymatic activity was present in spindle shaped, smooth muscle- or pericyte-like cells around hyperplastic vessels, and in tumor parenchyma [191]. Interestingly, the overall DPP-IV-like enzymatic activity determined by catalytic histochemistry correlated negatively ($r= -0.30$, $p= 0.04$) with the proliferation marker Ki67 [191]. Immunohistochemistry staining with DPP-IV and FAP specific antibodies revealed minimal positivity in non-tumorous brain with frequent fiber-like positivity in glioblastomas, occasionally close to the capillaries [191]. Mentlein et al. showed that at least part of the FAP expressing cells also coexpressed GFAP and Ki67 [176]. Collectively, these data demonstrate that the expression of DPP-IV and FAP as well as the DPP-IV-like enzymatic activity is increased in a substantial part of glioblastomas. Both the transformed as well as stromal cells such as reactive astrocytes, cells in the vessel wall and infiltrating immune cells may contribute to this increased expression.

3.3. Possible functions of DPP-IV and FAP in the glioma microenvironment

Glioblastomas are highly heterogenous both histologically and on the molecular level [194, 195]. The transformed cells themselves represent a mixture of cell types that may originate from the stochastic clonal expansion or from a more hierarchical organization of gliomas as postulated by the cancer stem cell hypothesis [196, 197]. In addition to the transformed cells, a variety of host cells contributes to the glioma microenvironment. This stromal compartment is an important contributor to the malignant phenotype of glioma cells and comprises of microglia/macrophages, lymphocytes, neural precursor cells, neurons, pericytes/vascular smooth muscle cells, reactive astrocytes and endothelial cells [198].

Given the marked increase of the expression of DPP-IV and FAP mRNA in glioblastoma tissue homogenates and the increase of the DPP-IV-like enzymatic activity in the microvasculature and parenchyma, the proteases seem to be functionally important for the transformed as well as nontransformed cells.

3.3.1. DPP-IV as a possible regulator of glioma cell growth

The DPP-IV-like enzymatic activity may influence signaling of various soluble mediators involved in the pathogenesis of gliomas (Table 1).

DPP-IV substrate	Role in gliomagenesis
CCL3L1 (LD78beta)	Enhances glioma cell proliferation[199].
CCL5	Possible role in the recruitment of microglia/macrophages [200], promotion of glioma invasion and angiogenesis [201].
CCL22	Recruitment of immunosuppressive Treg cells [202, 203].
CXCL9	Increased expression in glioblastoma [204], promotes glioma cell growth [205].
CXCL10	Pro-proliferative signaling through ERK1/2 in glioma cells [205, 206].
CXCL11	A ligand for CXCR7, which mediates prosurvival signaling in glioma cells [207, 208].
CXCL12	Promotion of glioma invasion, growth and angiogenesis (for review see [209])
SP	Promotion of glioma growth and secretion of cytokines (reviewed in [210, 211]).
PACAP, VIP	Stimulation of glioma cell growth [212, 213].

Table 1. DPP-IV substrates implicated in the pathogenesis of gliomas

Although DPP-IV and FAP exhibit similar dipeptidyl peptidase activity on small fluorogenic substrates, a recent study found substantial differences in their ability to cleave peptide substrates [79]. All peptides (with the exception of VIP) listed in Table 1 are cleaved rapidly by recombinant DPP-IV; in contrast FAP can only cleave SP effectively and does not cleave chemokines, PACAP or VIP [79](Figure 1). Given that, DPP-IV is the main candidate for influencing the functions of these mediators in gliomas.

By removing the N-terminal dipeptide from the biologically active peptides, DPP-IV in general diminishes their activity and/or increases their susceptibility to cleavage by other proteases [73]. Given that the majority of the substrates listed in Table 1 are thought to promote the malignant phenotype of glioma cells, DPP-IV would be somewhat paradoxically expected to suppress it. Indeed, we have previously shown the ability of DPP-IV to abrogate the calcium mediated signaling of SP in glioma cells [214]. We also observed that higher DPP-IV-like enzymatic activity in primary glioma cell cultures correlated with their slower growth [118]. In addition, overexpression of the transgenic DPP-IV in several glioma cell lines decreased their proliferation, led to a cell cycle block and a 50% decrease of the size of xenotransplanted tumors in immunodeficient mice [118]. Interestingly, our microarray data suggested that expression of several molecules linked to glioma pathogenesis was perturbed in glioma cells with forced expression of DPP-IV [118]. This included e.g. downregulated expression of transcripts encoding membrane growth factor receptors (PDGFRA, CALCRL, GRPR) and adhesion molecules (CD97, COL8A1, COL13A1, NLGN1, NLGN4X, PCDH20, SCARF2, NrCAM) as well as molecules typically overexpressed in gliomas (e.g. CALCRL, COL8A1, HAS2, NES, RRM2 [192], http://cancergenome.nih.gov). On the contrary, several tumor suppressors e.g. BEX2, RAP1GAP, DUSP26, SYT13, TSPYL2 were upregulated ([118] and references therein). In order to determine whether the observed in vitro and in vivo growth inhibitory effects were mediated by the enzymatic activity, the experiments were done in parallel with cells transfected with an enzymatically inactive mutant DPP-IV due to a single amino acid ($Ser^{630} \rightarrow Ala^{630}$) substitution in the active site [118]. These studies revealed similarly decreased growth of glioma cells overexpressing the enzymatically inactive DPP-IV providing evidence that these effects were independent of the enzymatic activity [118]. In summary, our studies demonstrate that DPP-IV may modify the function of its substrates through proteolysis, but likely has also an enzymatic activity independent growth inhibitory effect in glioma cells. The detailed molecular mechanism(s) for these effects however remain to be identified.

These data strongly argue that DPP-IV in glioma cells in vivo is unlikely to directly promote the malignant potential of the expressing cells. However, DPP-IV did not suppress the malignant phenotype of glioma cells completely in our studies – albeit the tumors were smaller with lower percentage of Ki67 positive nuclei, they exhibited an infiltrative growth pattern similar to controls [118]. We also observed a highly infiltrative growth of the xenotransplanted glioma stem-like cells expressing DPP-IV (Busek et al. unpublished). Several possibilities exist to explain these seeming contradictions: i) DPP-IV expression / enzymatic activity may reflect a mechanism striving to prevent the inappropriate proliferation of malignant cells. In support of this possibility, Mares et al. [191] observed an inverse correlation between the DPP-IV-like enzymatic activity and Ki67 in glioblastoma tissues. On the other hand, these less proliferative cells may be more resistant to conventional adjuvant therapies and therefore contribute to tumor recurrence. ii) Glioblastomas are highly heterogeneous and likely composed of several interacting subpopulations establishing a complex "ecosystem" [197]. DPP-IV may contribute to the interaction with other tumor clones and/or stromal compartment by local proteolytic processing of biologically active peptides with an overall increased tumor growth despite its growth inhibitory effects in the expressing subpopulation. Such a role of DPP-IV could not have been identified using conventional cell-line based xenotransplantation models in immunodeficient animals utilized in our studies. iii) DPP-IV expression may also be linked to the microenvironment typical of glioblastomas. The grade IV tumors characteristically contain necrotic areas and exhibit enormous stimulation of angiogenesis caused by hypoxia. Hypoxia also promotes the aggressiveness of glioma cells through the transcription factor HIF-1α (hypoxia inducible factor-1α) [215]. DPP-IV was demonstrated to be regulated by hypoxia in several systems although with variable outcomes. In extravillous trophoblast cells, the hypoxia induced increase of DPP-IV was associated with their decreased invasiveness [216]. In colon and gastric cancer cell lines, DPP-IV was increased in a HIF-1α dependent manner in response to hypoxia in vitro and in xenotransplants depleted of VEGF [217]. The purpose of this induction of DPP-IV in the response to hypoxia is not clear. The data from other experimental systems nevertheless suggest that by promoting the expression of DPP-IV together with the angiogenic receptor Y2, ischemia may enhance the angiogenic response to NPY [218, 219].

In addition to the transformed glioma cells, DPP-IV is also increased in the microvasculature [191]. Here, DPP-IV may contribute to neoangiogenesis by promoting the proliferation and invasiveness of endothelial cells.

In summary, higher expression of DPP-IV is typical for glioblastomas. Although the function of the protease cannot be currently ascribed with certainty, it may negatively affect glioma cell proliferation even independent of its enzymatic activity [118] and participate on the pericellular proteolysis with possible paracrine effects on other tumor subpopulations including stromal cells. The functional significance of DPP-IV upregulation in the glioma stromal compartment remains to be established.

3.3.2. Implications of FAP for glioma migration, ECM remodeling and angiogenesis

Several reports suggest a possible role of FAP in glioma cell migration not only because of its role in the extracranial malignancies (section 2.1). Lal et al. [220] studied the phenotypic and molecular changes caused by the introduction of the activating mutant form of EGFR (EGFRvIII) into glioma cells with low EGFR expression. They observed increased invasiveness of the EGFRvIII transduced cells, which was accompanied by upregulation of several transcripts encoding proteins of the extracellular matrix and proteases, including FAP [220]. A similarly designed study tested the effects of the introduction of IGFBP2, a molecule with pleiotrophic roles in glioblastoma [221], into the SNB19 glioma cell line. Here, increased invasion was also observed and FAP was among the 28 significantly induced genes with a 4.5 to 16 fold increase in different clones according to the microarray data [222]. Likewise, introduction of TWIST1, a basic helix-loop-helix domain-containing transcription factor implicated in EMT (epithelial mesenchymal transition) and cancer metastasis [223], into glioma cells promoted their invasion and among other genes activated the expression of FAP [193]. Tatenhorst et al. [247] took a different approach and compared the expression profile in two subpopulations isolated from the U373 glioma cell line based on their differing migratory rates on Matrigel. FAP was the top upregulated gene (11.7 fold) in the clone with high migration in vitro. Although these studies do not provide direct evidence that FAP contributes to the high migration and invasiveness characteristic for glioma cells, they strongly suggest an association of FAP expression with the glioma migratory phenotype and its activation in response to molecular abnormalities frequently occurring in glioblastomas. Mentlein et al. [176] addressed the role of FAP in glioma migration directly by siRNA mediated downregulation in the A746 glioma cell line. No effect on cell migration was noted in the transwell assay when uncoated or Matrigel coated inserts were used [176]. However, the cells invaded slightly less efficiently through the gelatin coated inserts and their invasion through brevican, a chondroitin sulfate proteoglycan abundantly present in the adult human brain, was reduced by almost 50% [176]. The underlying mechanisms remain to be established. The extracellular matrix of gliomas is substantially different from the extracranial malignancies: the fibrillary proteins (e.g. collagens, fibronectin, laminin) are much less abundant and mostly present in the perivascular space. Instead, hyaluronic acid and associated proteins such as versican and brevican prevail [224, 225]. Although Mentlein et al. [176] demonstrated that FAP cleaved brevican, the cleavage by the recombinant protease was inefficient and required prolonged incubations. Thus, the siRNA mediated downregulation of FAP in glioma cells could instead have effects on other ECM degrading systems. FAP is known to be part of multiprotein complexes in invadopodia [153, 226] and it was demonstrated to physically interact with uPAR in a β1-integrin dependent manner [121]. Interestingly, simultaneous downregulation of uPAR and cathepsin B was shown to downregulate FAP in glioma cells [227]. FAP therefore seems to act in cooperation with other proteolytic systems and its presence may influence the remodeling of glioma ECM not only by its intrinsic gelatinolytic activity but also by its possible role in the formation and/or stabilization of invadopodia.

Another interesting but unexplored aspect is the possible role of FAP in the promotion of angiogenesis of glioblastomas. The expression of FAP in endothelial cells [145, 146], higher microvessel densities in breast cancer xenotransplants engineered to express FAP [127] and the decreased microvessel density in response to FAP ablation in a lung cancer model consistently imply its role in angiogenesis. This may be –similarly to DPP-IV– via the processing of NP Y 1-36 to an angiogenic NP Y 3-36 [228]. In addition, FAP expressing fibroblasts are able to modify collagen type I matrices in a way that promotes the invasion of tumor cells (see section 2.2, [158]). Possibly, FAP may participate on the transformation of the glioma extracellular matrix into an environment that would be more supportive for the migration of endothelial cells [15].

Glioblastomas typically contain necrotic areas surrounded by pseudopalisades. A model for the pathogenesis of this typical morphological feature of glioblastoma has been proposed [229, 230] and postulates that thrombotic occlusion of the central vessel results in hypoxia, which than drives the migration of the surrounding glioma cells and robustly stimulates angiogenesis. Several mechanisms likely contribute to the vaso-occlusive process including the leakage of plasma clotting factors through the damaged vessels and their contact with a procoagulant tumor environment (see [231] for review). FAP was previously demonstrated to be identical with α2-antiplasmin cleaving enzyme [42]. Upon conversion by FAP, α2-antiplasmin is more effectively incorporated into fibrin and protects the fibrin clot from plasmin degradation [232]. By this mechanism, FAP may contribute to the prothrombogenic state in glioblastoma with resulting development of necrosis and stimulation of angiogenesis. The speculated mechanisms listed above are mediated by the DPP-IV-like or prolyl- endopeptidase enzymatic activities of FAP. In addition, FAP has probably other, enzymatic activity independent pro-angiogenic effects as recently demonstrated in breast cancer using catalytically inactive mutant FAP [15, 128].

4. DPP-IV and FAP as possible markers and treatment targets in gliomas?

Glioblastomas have dismal prognosis and despite the multimodality treatment the majority of patients die within 10-14 months [248, 249]. Regardless of ongoing efforts, the pathogenesis of glioblastoma remains unknown and therefore specific targeted therapies are currently not available. Despite their rather peculiar role in cancer pathogenesis, both DPP-IV and FAP were suggested as diagnostic and prognostic markers and therapeutic targets for tumors outside of the central nervous system (reviewed in [15, 88]). DPP-IV staining was suggested as a useful adjunct marker for the differentiation of malignant melanomas from deep penetrating nevi [101] and benign and malignant diseases of the thyroid gland [93, 233]. To the best of our knowledge, there is only one study suggesting a possible prognostic relevance of DASH molecules in the brain tumors. Shaw et al. [234] studied the expression signature that was related to the chemosensitivity of oligodendroglial tumors and observed that FAP was downregulated several fold in tumors that were chemosensitive and/or exhibited the prognostically favorable 1p/19q loss [234].

Preclinical studies with DPP-IV targeting antibodies suggest that DPP-IV may be a new therapeutic target in malignant mesothelioma [96, 97], renal carcinoma [235] and some hematologic malignancies [236]. The highly selective expression of FAP in the tumor microenvironment and its expected direct pathogenetic participation on tumor progression has also raised interest in its possible therapeutic exploitation with a simultaneous impact not only on the transformed cells, but also on the stromal elements („stroma targeted therapies") [138]. Experimentally, FAP specific antibodies were utilized for the targeting of TNF alpha carrying nanoparticles [237] or in the form of a chimeric protein with the extracellular domain of the ligand of the TNF receptor 4-1BB to enhance the local T cell-mediated antitumor responses [238]. Further, induction of immune response against FAP leads to a decreased tumor growth and an enhanced effect of cytostatic therapy in several experimental models [239-242]. FAP activated cytotoxic prodrugs have also been designed [243] and the inhibition of FAP enzymatic activity by specific low molecular weight inhibitors was tested in experimental myeloma treatment [18].

Several important issues arise when designing treatment modalities targeting the DASH molecules by enzyme inhibitors or antibodies. In the case of DPP-IV, its almost ubiquitous presence, combined with multiple tissue specific biological roles, increases the risk of on-target side effects. In this respect, the restricted expression of FAP seems to be a substantial advantage. Further, the similar enzymatic properties of DASH proteases represent a possible source of off-target side effects [19]. Such a problem may be avoided by using highly specific inhibitors as documented by the successful introduction of DPP-IV inhibitors into clinical practice for the treatment of diabetes mellitus [244]. On the other hand, the moonlighting nature of the DASH molecules (combination of enzymatic and non-enzymatic functions), might hypothetically represent an advantage for their targeting as the non-enzymatic functions would remain untouched when using low molecular weight inhibitors to block the enzymatic functions.

In conclusion, given the emerging role of DPP-IV and FAP in the processes of gliomagenesis and the precedent evidence for their possible therapeutic exploitation in extracranial malignancies, they seem to be promising candidates for the targeting of gliomas.

Acknowledgements

This work was supported by grants IGA 12237-5/2011, PRVOUK-P27/LF1/1 and UNCE 204013.

Author details

Petr Busek and Aleksi Sedo

Laboratory of Cancer Cell Biology, Institute of Biochemistry and Experimental Oncology, 1st Faculty of Medicine, Charles University in Prague, Czech Republic

References

[1] Albesiano, E., J.E. Han, and M. Lim, Mechanisms of local immunoresistance in glioma. Neurosurg Clin N Am, 2010. 21(1): 17-29.

[2] Waziri, A., Glioblastoma-derived mechanisms of systemic immunosuppression. Neurosurg Clin N Am, 2010. 21(1): 31-42.

[3] Mentlein, R., Cell-surface peptidases. Int Rev Cytol, 2004. 235: 165-213.

[4] Rao, J.S., Molecular mechanisms of glioma invasiveness: the role of proteases. Nat Rev Cancer, 2003. 3(7): 489-501.

[5] Lakka, S.S., C.S. Gondi, and J.S. Rao, Proteases and glioma angiogenesis. Brain Pathol, 2005. 15(4): 327-41.

[6] Fukuda, M.E., et al., Cathepsin D is a potential serum marker for poor prognosis in glioma patients. Cancer Res, 2005. 65(12): 5190-4.

[7] Takano, S., et al., Detection of failure of bevacizumab treatment for malignant glioma based on urinary matrix metalloproteinase activity. Brain Tumor Pathol, 2010. 27(2): 89-94.

[8] Hsu, D.W., J.T. Efird, and E.T. Hedley-Whyte, Prognostic role of urokinase-type plasminogen activator in human gliomas. Am J Pathol, 1995. 147(1): 114-23.

[9] Hopsu-Havu, V.K. and G.G. Glenner, A new dipeptide naphthylamidase hydrolyzing glycyl-prolyl-beta-naphthylamide. Histochemie, 1966. 7(3): 197-201.

[10] Nagatsu, I., T. Nagatsu, and T. Yamamoto, Hydrolysis of amino acid beta-naphthylamides by aminopeptidases in human parotid salva and human serum. Experientia, 1968. 24(4): 347-8.

[11] Lambeir, A.M., et al., Dipeptidyl-peptidase IV from bench to bedside: an update on structural properties, functions, and clinical aspects of the enzyme DPP IV. Critical Reviews in Clinical Laboratory Sciences, 2003. 40(3): 209-94.

[12] Sedo, A., et al., Dipeptidyl peptidase IV in the human lung and spinocellular lung cancer. Physiological Research, 1991. 40(3): 359-62.

[13] Abbott, C.A., et al., Cloning, expression and chromosomal localization of a novel human dipeptidyl peptidase (DPP) IV homolog, DPP8. Eur J Biochem, 2000. 267(20): 6140-50.

[14] Tang, H.K., et al., Biochemical properties and expression profile of human prolyl dipeptidase DPP9. Arch Biochem Biophys, 2009. 485(2): 120-7.

[15] Kelly, T., et al., Fibroblast activation protein-alpha: a key modulator of the microenvironment in multiple pathologies. Int Rev Cell Mol Biol, 2012. 297: 83-116.

[16] Maes, M.B., S. Scharpe, and I. De Meester, Dipeptidyl peptidase II (DPPII), a review. Clinica Chimica Acta, 2007. 380(1-2): 31-49.

[17] McNicholas, K., T. Chen, and C.A. Abbott, Dipeptidyl peptidase (DP) 6 and DP10: novel brain proteins implicated in human health and disease. Clin Chem Lab Med, 2009. 47(3): 262-7.

[18] Pennisi, A., et al., Inhibitor of DASH proteases affects expression of adhesion molecules in osteoclasts and reduces myeloma growth and bone disease. Br J Haematol, 2009. 145(6): 775-87.

[19] Lankas, G.R., et al., Dipeptidyl peptidase IV inhibition for the treatment of type 2 diabetes: potential importance of selectivity over dipeptidyl peptidases 8 and 9. Diabetes, 2005. 54(10): 2988-94.

[20] Bezerra, G.A., et al., Structures of Human DPP7 Reveal the Molecular Basis of Specific Inhibition and the Architectural Diversity of Proline-Specific Peptidases. PLoS One, 2012. 7(8): e43019

[21] Dubois, V., et al., Dipeptidyl peptidase 9 (DPP9) from bovine testes: identification and characterization as the short form by mass spectrometry. Biochim Biophys Acta, 2010. 1804(4): 781-8.

[22] Ansorge, S., et al., Recent insights into the role of dipeptidyl aminopeptidase IV (DPIV) and aminopeptidase N (APN) families in immune functions. Clin Chem Lab Med, 2009. 47(3): 253-61.

[23] Rummey, C. and G. Metz, Homology models of dipeptidyl peptidases 8 and 9 with a focus on loop predictions near the active site. Proteins, 2007. 66(1): 160-71.

[24] Sedo, A. and R. Malik, Dipeptidyl peptidase IV-like molecules: homologous proteins or homologous activities? Biochimica et Biophysica Acta, 2001. 1550(2): 107-16.

[25] Barinka, C., et al., Substrate specificity, inhibition and enzymological analysis of recombinant human glutamate carboxypeptidase II. Journal of Neurochemistry, 2002. 80(3): 477-87.

[26] Friedrich, D., et al., Does human attractin have DP4 activity? Biological Chemistry, 2007. 388(2): 155-62.

[27] Yu, D.M., et al., The dipeptidyl peptidase IV family in cancer and cell biology. FEBS Journal, 2010. 277(5): 1126-44.

[28] Durinx, C., et al., Molecular characterization of dipeptidyl peptidase activity in serum - Soluble CD26/dipeptidyl peptidase IV is responsible for the release of X-Pro dipeptides. European Journal of Biochemistry, 2000. 267(17): 5608-5613.

[29] Morimoto, C. and S.F. Schlossman, The structure and function of CD26 in the T-cell immune response. Immunological Reviews, 1998. 161: 55-70.

[30] Sato, K. and N.H. Dang, CD26: A novel treatment target for T-cell lymphoid malignancies? International Journal of Oncology, 2003. 22(3): 481-497.

[31] Agarwal, S., K.L. Holton, and R. Lanza, Efficient differentiation of functional hepatocytes from human embryonic stem cells. Stem Cells, 2008. 26(5): 1117-27.

[32] Darmoul, D., et al., Dipeptidyl peptidase IV (CD 26) gene expression in enterocyte-like colon cancer cell lines HT-29 and Caco-2. Cloning of the complete human coding sequence and changes of dipeptidyl peptidase IV mRNA levels during cell differentiation. Journal of Biological Chemistry, 1992. 267(7): 4824-33.

[33] Dang, N.H. and C. Morimoto, CD26: an expanding role in immune regulation and cancer. Histology & Histopathology, 2002. 17(4): 1213-26.

[34] Fan, H., et al., Dipeptidyl peptidase IV/CD26 in T cell activation, cytokine secretion and immunoglobulin production. Advances in Experimental Medicine & Biology, 2003. 524: 165-74.

[35] Fleischer, B., CD26: a surface protease involved in T-cell activation. Immunol Today, 1994. 15(4): 180-4.

[36] Franco, R., et al., Enzymatic and extraenzymatic role of ecto-adenosine deaminase in lymphocytes. Immunol Rev, 1998. 161: 27-42.

[37] Gorrell, M.D., V. Gysbers, and G.W. McCaughan, CD26: a multifunctional integral membrane and secreted protein of activated lymphocytes. Scandinavian Journal of Immunology, 2001. 54(3): 249-64.

[38] Gonzalez-Gronow, M., et al., Dipeptidyl peptidase IV (DPP IV/CD26) is a cell-surface plasminogen receptor. Frontiers in Bioscience, 2008. 13: 1610-8.

[39] Loster, K., et al., The cysteine-rich region of dipeptidyl peptidase IV (CD 26) is the collagen-binding site. Biochemical & Biophysical Research Communications, 1995. 217(1): 341-8.

[40] Cheng, H.C., M. Abdel-Ghany, and B.U. Pauli, A novel consensus motif in fibronectin mediates dipeptidyl peptidase IV adhesion and metastasis. Journal of Biological Chemistry, 2003. 278(27): 24600-7.

[41] Lee, K.N., et al., A novel plasma proteinase potentiates alpha2-antiplasmin inhibition of fibrin digestion. Blood, 2004. 103(10): 3783-8.

[42] Lee, K.N., et al., Antiplasmin-cleaving enzyme is a soluble form of fibroblast activation protein. Blood, 2006. 107(4): 1397-404.

[43] Milner, J.M., et al., Fibroblast activation protein alpha is expressed by chondrocytes following a pro-inflammatory stimulus and is elevated in osteoarthritis. Arthritis Res Ther, 2006. 8(1): R23.

[44] Bauer, S., et al., Fibroblast activation protein is expressed by rheumatoid myofibroblast-like synoviocytes. Arthritis Res Ther, 2006. 8(6): R171.

[45] Levy, M.T., et al., Fibroblast activation protein: a cell surface dipeptidyl peptidase and gelatinase expressed by stellate cells at the tissue remodelling interface in human cirrhosis. Hepatology, 1999. 29(6): 1768-78.

[46] Garinchesa, P., L.J. Old, and W.J. Rettig, Cell-Surface Glycoprotein of Reactive Stromal Fibroblasts as a Potential Antibody Target in Human Epithelial Cancers. Proceedings of the National Academy of Sciences of the United States of America, 1990. 87(18): 7235-7239.

[47] Aoyama, A. and W.T. Chen, A 170-kDa membrane-bound protease is associated with the expression of invasiveness by human malignant melanoma cells. Proceedings of the National Academy of Sciences of the United States of America, 1990. 87(21): 8296-300.

[48] Aertgeerts, K., et al., Structural and kinetic analysis of the substrate specificity of human fibroblast activation protein alpha. J Biol Chem, 2005. 280(20): 19441-4.

[49] Ghersi, G., et al., Regulation of fibroblast migration on collagenous matrix by a cell surface peptidase complex. J Biol Chem, 2002. 277(32): 29231-41.

[50] Ghersi, G., et al., The protease complex consisting of dipeptidyl peptidase IV and seprase plays a role in the migration and invasion of human endothelial cells in collagenous matrices. Cancer Research, 2006. 66(9): 4652-4661.

[51] Ajami, K., et al., Dipeptidyl peptidase 9 has two forms, a broad tissue distribution, cytoplasmic localization and DPIV-like peptidase activity. Biochim Biophys Acta, 2004. 1679(1): 18-28.

[52] Yu, D.M., et al., The in vivo expression of dipeptidyl peptidases 8 and 9. J Histochem Cytochem, 2009. 57(11): 1025-40.

[53] Pitman, M.R., et al., Dipeptidyl peptidase 8 and 9--guilty by association? Front Biosci, 2009. 14: 3619-33.

[54] Geiss-Friedlander, R., et al., The cytoplasmic peptidase DPP9 is rate-limiting for degradation of proline-containing peptides. J Biol Chem, 2009. 284(40): 27211-9.

[55] Yu, D.M., et al., Extraenzymatic functions of the dipeptidyl peptidase IV-related proteins DP8 and DP9 in cell adhesion, migration and apoptosis. FEBS Journal, 2006. 273(11): 2447-60.

[56] Yao, T.W., et al., A novel role of dipeptidyl peptidase 9 in epidermal growth factor signaling. Mol Cancer Res, 2011. 9(7): 948-59.

[57] Maes, M.B., et al., Dipeptidyl peptidase 8/9-like activity in human leukocytes. Journal of Leukocyte Biology, 2007. 81(5): 1252-1257.

[58] Andersen, K.J. and J.K. McDonald, Lysosomal heterogeneity of dipeptidyl peptidase II active on collagen-related peptides. Ren Physiol Biochem, 1989. 12(1): 32-40.

[59] McDonald, J.K. and C. Schwabe, Dipeptidyl peptidase II of bovine dental pulp. Initial demonstration and characterization as a fibroblastic, lysosomal peptidase of the serine class active on collagen-related peptides. Biochim Biophys Acta, 1980. 616(1): 68-81.

[60] Mele, D.A., et al., Dipeptidyl peptidase 2 is an essential survival factor in the regulation of cell quiescence. Cell Cycle, 2009. 8(15): 2425-34.

[61] Bista, P., et al., Lymphocyte quiescence factor Dpp2 is transcriptionally activated by KLF2 and TOB1. Mol Immunol, 2008. 45(13): 3618-23.

[62] Danilova, O.V., et al., Neurogenin 3-specific dipeptidyl peptidase-2 deficiency causes impaired glucose tolerance, insulin resistance, and visceral obesity. Endocrinology, 2009. 150(12): 5240-8.

[63] Mele, D.A., J.F. Sampson, and B.T. Huber, Th17 differentiation is the default program for DPP2-deficient T-cell differentiation. Eur J Immunol, 2011. 41(6): 1583-93.

[64] Chiravuri, M., et al., A novel apoptotic pathway in quiescent lymphocytes identified by inhibition of a post-proline cleaving aminodipeptidase: a candidate target protease, quiescent cell proline dipeptidase. J Immunol, 1999. 163(6): 3092-9.

[65] Underwood, R., et al., Sequence, purification, and cloning of an intracellular serine protease, quiescent cell proline dipeptidase. J Biol Chem, 1999. 274(48): 34053-8.

[66] Wada, K., et al., Differential expression of two distinct forms of mRNA encoding members of a dipeptidyl aminopeptidase family. Proc Natl Acad Sci U S A, 1992. 89(1): 197-201.

[67] Qi, S.Y., et al., Cloning and characterization of dipeptidyl peptidase 10, a new member of an emerging subgroup of serine proteases. Biochem J, 2003. 373(Pt 1): 179-89.

[68] Jerng, H.H., A.D. Lauver, and P.J. Pfaffinger, DPP10 splice variants are localized in distinct neuronal populations and act to differentially regulate the inactivation properties of Kv4-based ion channels. Mol Cell Neurosci, 2007. 35(4): 604-24.

[69] Du, J., et al., Expression of Dpp6 in mouse embryonic craniofacial development. Acta Histochem, 2011. 113(6): 636-9.

[70] van Es, M.A., et al., Genetic variation in DPP6 is associated with susceptibility to amyotrophic lateral sclerosis. Nat Genet, 2008. 40(1): 29-31.

[71] Jones, S., et al., Core signaling pathways in human pancreatic cancers revealed by global genomic analyses. Science, 2008. 321(5897): 1801-6.

[72] Low, S.K., et al., Genome-wide association study of pancreatic cancer in Japanese population. PLoS One, 2010. 5(7): e11824.

[73] Mentlein, R., Dipeptidyl-peptidase IV (CD26)-role in the inactivation of regulatory peptides. Regulatory Peptides, 1999. 85(1): 9-24.

[74] Busek, P., R. Malik, and A. Sedo, Dipeptidyl peptidase IV activity and/or structure homologues (DASH) and their substrates in cancer. International Journal of Biochemistry & Cell Biology, 2004. 36(3): 408-21.

[75] Sedo, A., et al., Dipeptidyl peptidase IV activity and/or structure homologs: contributing factors in the pathogenesis of rheumatoid arthritis? Arthritis Research & Therapy, 2005. 7(6): 253-69.

[76] Jeffery, C.J., Moonlighting proteins: old proteins learning new tricks. Trends Genet, 2003. 19(8): 415-7.

[77] Bjelke, J.R., et al., Dipeptidyl peptidases 8 and 9: specificity and molecular characterization compared with dipeptidyl peptidase IV. Biochemical Journal, 2006. 396(2): 391-9.

[78] Ajami, K., et al., Stromal cell-derived factors 1alpha and 1beta, inflammatory protein-10 and interferon-inducible T cell chemo-attractant are novel substrates of dipeptidyl peptidase 8. FEBS Lett, 2008. 582(5): 819-25.

[79] Keane, F.M., et al., Neuropeptide Y, B-type natriuretic peptide, substance P and peptide YY are novel substrates of fibroblast activation protein-alpha. FEBS J, 2011. 278(8): 1316-32.

[80] Cordero, O.J., F.J. Salgado, and M. Nogueira, On the origin of serum CD26 and its altered concentration in cancer patients. Cancer Immunol Immunother, 2009. 58(11): 1723-47.

[81] Gomez, N., et al., Dipeptidyl peptidase IV inhibition improves cardiorenal function in overpacing-induced heart failure. Eur J Heart Fail, 2012. 14(1): 14-21.

[82] Brandt, I., et al., Dipeptidyl-peptidase IV converts intact B-type natriuretic peptide into its des-SerPro form. Clin Chem, 2006. 52(1): 82-7.

[83] Marchetti, C., et al., High mobility group box 1 is a novel substrate of dipeptidyl peptidase-IV. Diabetologia, 2012. 55(1): 236-44.

[84] de Meester, I., et al., Dipeptidyl peptidase IV substrates. An update on in vitro peptide hydrolysis by human DPPIV. Advances in Experimental Medicine & Biology, 2003. 524: 3-17.

[85] Tagore, D.M., et al., Peptidase substrates via global peptide profiling. Nat Chem Biol, 2009. 5(1): 23-5.

[86] Huang, C.H., et al., Cleavage-site specificity of prolyl endopeptidase FAP investigated with a full-length protein substrate. J Biochem, 2011. 149(6): 685-92.

[87] Stremenova, J., et al., Expression and enzymatic activity of dipeptidyl peptidase-IV in human astrocytic tumours are associated with tumour grade. International Journal of Oncology, 2007. 31(4): 785-92.

[88] Sedo, A., et al., Dipeptidyl peptidase-IV and related molecules: markers of malignancy? Expert Opinion on Medical Diagnostics, 2008. 2: 677-689.

[89] Havre, P.A., et al., The role of CD26/dipeptidyl peptidase IV in cancer. Frontiers in Bioscience, 2008. 13: 1634-45.

[90] Sato, T., et al., CD26 regulates p38 mitogen-activated protein kinase-dependent phosphorylation of integrin beta1, adhesion to extracellular matrix, and tumorigenicity of T-anaplastic large cell lymphoma Karpas 299. Cancer Research, 2005. 65(15): 6950-6.

[91] Aytac, U. and N.H. Dang, CD26/dipeptidyl peptidase IV: a regulator of immune function and a potential molecular target for therapy. Current Drug Targets - Immune Endocrine & Metabolic Disorders, 2004. 4(1): 11-8.

[92] Cro, L., et al., CD26 expression in mature B-cell neoplasia: its possible role as a new prognostic marker in B-CLL. Hematol Oncol, 2009. 27(3): 140-7.

[93] Hirai, K., et al., Dipeptidyl peptidase IV (DPP IV/CD26) staining predicts distant metastasis of 'benign' thyroid tumor. Pathology International, 1999. 49(3): 264-265.

[94] Yamaguchi, U., et al., Distinct gene expression-defined classes of gastrointestinal stromal tumor. J Clin Oncol, 2008. 26(25): 4100-8.

[95] Pang, R., et al., A subpopulation of CD26+ cancer stem cells with metastatic capacity in human colorectal cancer. Cell Stem Cell, 2010. 6(6): 603-15.

[96] Amatya, V.J., et al., Overexpression of CD26/DPPIV in mesothelioma tissue and mesothelioma cell lines. Oncol Rep, 2011. 26(6): 1369-75.

[97] Inamoto, T., et al., Humanized Anti-CD26 Monoclonal Antibody as a Treatment for Malignant Mesothelioma Tumors. Clin Cancer Res, 2007. 13(14): 4191-4200.

[98] Lu, C., et al., Dipeptidyl peptidases as survival factors in Ewing sarcoma family of tumors: implications for tumor biology and therapy. J Biol Chem, 2011. 286(31): 27494-505.

[99] Wesley, U.V., et al., A role for dipeptidyl peptidase IV in suppressing the malignant phenotype of melanocytic cells. Journal of Experimental Medicine, 1999. 190(3): 311-322.

[100] Houghton, A.N., et al., Cell surface antigens of human melanocytes and melanoma. Expression of adenosine deaminase binding protein is extinguished with melanocyte transformation. Journal of Experimental Medicine, 1988. 167(1): 197-212.

[101] Roesch, A., et al., Loss of dipeptidyl peptidase IV immunostaining discriminates malignant melanomas from deep penetrating nevi. Modern Pathology, 2006. 19(10): 1378-85.

[102] Pethiyagoda, C.L., D.R. Welch, and T.P. Fleming, Dipeptidyl peptidase IV (DPPIV) inhibits cellular invasion of melanoma cells. Clinical & Experimental Metastasis, 2000. 18(5): 391-400.

[103] Arscott, W.T., et al., Suppression of neuroblastoma growth by dipeptidyl peptidase IV: relevance of chemokine regulation and caspase activation. Oncogene, 2009. 28(4): 479-91.

[104] Wesley, U.V., M. McGroarty, and A. Homoyouni, Dipeptidyl peptidase inhibits malignant phenotype of prostate cancer cells by blocking basic fibroblast growth factor signaling pathway. Cancer Research, 2005. 65(4): 1325-34.

[105] Wesley, U.V., S. Tiwari, and A.N. Houghton, Role for dipeptidyl peptidase IV in tumor suppression of human non small cell lung carcinoma cells. International Journal of Cancer, 2004. 109(6): 855-66.

[106] Wilson, M.J., et al., Dipeptidylpeptidase IV activities are elevated in prostate cancers and adjacent benign hyperplastic glands. Journal of Andrology, 2000. 21(2): 220-226.

[107] Wilson, M.J., et al., Elevation of dipeptidylpeptidase iv activities in the prostate peripheral zone and prostatic secretions of men with prostate cancer: possible prostate cancer disease marker. Journal of Urology, 2005. 174(3): 1124-8.

[108] Sedo, A., E. Krepela, and E. Kasafirek, Dipeptidyl peptidase IV, prolyl endopeptidase and cathepsin B activities in primary human lung tumors and lung parenchyma. Journal of Cancer Research & Clinical Oncology, 1991. 117(3): 249-53.

[109] Asada, Y., et al., Expression of dipeptidyl aminopeptidase IV activity in human lung carcinoma. Histopathology, 1993. 23(3): 265-70.

[110] McIntosh, C.H., Dipeptidyl peptidase IV inhibitors and diabetes therapy. Frontiers in Bioscience, 2008. 13: 1753-73.

[111] Herman, G.A., et al., Effect of single oral doses of sitagliptin, a dipeptidyl peptidase-4 inhibitor, on incretin and plasma glucose levels after an oral glucose tolerance test in patients with type 2 diabetes. J Clin Endocrinol Metab, 2006. 91(11): 4612-9.

[112] Masur, K., et al., DPPIV inhibitors extend GLP-2 mediated tumour promoting effects on intestinal cancer cells. Regulatory Peptides, 2006. 137(3): 147-55.

[113] Sun, Y.X., et al., CD26/dipeptidyl peptidase IV regulates prostate cancer metastasis by degrading SDF-1/CXCL12. Clin Exp Metastasis, 2008. 25(7): 765-76.

[114] Kajiyama, H., et al., Dipeptidyl peptidase IV overexpression induces up-regulation of E-cadherin and tissue inhibitors of matrix metalloproteinases, resulting in decreased invasive potential in ovarian carcinoma cells. Cancer Research, 2003. 63(9): 2278-83.

[115] Kajiyama, H., et al., Prolonged survival and decreased invasive activity attributable to dipeptidyl peptidase IV overexpression in ovarian carcinoma. Cancer Research, 2002. 62(10): 2753-7.

[116] Kajiyama, H., et al., The expression of dipeptidyl peptidase IV (DPPIV/CD26) is associated with enhanced chemosensitivity to paclitaxel in epithelial ovarian carcinoma cells. Cancer Sci, 2010. 101(2): 347-54.

[117] Gonzalez-Gronow, M., et al., Angiostatin directly inhibits human prostate tumor cell invasion by blocking plasminogen binding to its cellular receptor, CD26. Experimental Cell Research, 2005. 303(1): 22-31.

[118] Busek, P., et al., Dipeptidyl peptidase-IV inhibits glioma cell growth independent of its enzymatic activity. Int J Biochem Cell Biol, 2012. 44(5): 738-47.

[119] Goldstein, L.A., et al., Molecular cloning of seprase: a serine integral membrane protease from human melanoma. Biochimica et Biophysica Acta, 1997. 1361(1): 11-9.

[120] Gilmore, B.F., et al., Dipeptide proline diphenyl phosphonates are potent, irreversible inhibitors of seprase (FAPalpha). Biochemical & Biophysical Research Communications, 2006. 346(2): 436-46.

[121] Artym, V.V., et al., Molecular proximity of seprase and the urokinase-type plasminogen activator receptor on malignant melanoma cell membranes: dependence on beta1 integrins and the cytoskeleton. Carcinogenesis, 2002. 23(10): 1593-601.

[122] Monsky, W.L., et al., A potential marker protease of invasiveness, seprase, is localized on invadopodia of human malignant melanoma cells. Cancer Research, 1994. 54(21): 5702-10.

[123] Ramirez-Montagut, T., et al., FAPalpha, a surface peptidase expressed during wound healing, is a tumor suppressor. Oncogene, 2004. 23(32): 5435-46.

[124] Rettig, W.J., et al., Regulation and heteromeric structure of the fibroblast activation protein in normal and transformed cells of mesenchymal and neuroectodermal origin. Cancer Research, 1993. 53(14): 3327-35.

[125] Kelly, T., et al., Seprase, a membrane-bound protease, is overexpressed by invasive ductal carcinoma cells of human breast cancers. Modern Pathology, 1998. 11(9): 855-63.

[126] Goodman, J.D., T.L. Rozypal, and T. Kelly, Seprase, a membrane-bound protease, alleviates the serum growth requirement of human breast cancer cells. Clinical & Experimental Metastasis, 2003. 20(5): 459-70.

[127] Huang, Y., S. Wang, and T. Kelly, Seprase promotes rapid tumor growth and increased microvessel density in a mouse model of human breast cancer. Cancer Res, 2004. 64(8): 2712-6.

[128] Huang, Y., et al., Fibroblast activation protein-alpha promotes tumor growth and invasion of breast cancer cells through non-enzymatic functions. Clin Exp Metastasis, 2011. 28(6): 567-79.

[129] Dohi, O., et al., Histogenesis-specific expression of fibroblast activation protein and dipeptidylpeptidase-IV in human bone and soft tissue tumours. Histopathology, 2009. 55(4): 432-40.

[130] Mori, Y., et al., The expression of a type II transmembrane serine protease (Seprase) in human gastric carcinoma. Oncology, 2004. 67(5-6): 411-9.

[131] Goscinski, M.A., et al., Seprase, dipeptidyl peptidase IV and urokinase-type plasminogen activator expression in dysplasia and invasive squamous cell carcinoma of the esophagus. A study of 229 cases from Anyang Tumor Hospital, Henan Province, China. Oncology, 2008. 75(1-2): 49-59.

[132] Iwasa, S., et al., Increased expression of seprase, a membrane-type serine protease, is associated with lymph node metastasis in human colorectal cancer.[erratum appears in Cancer Lett. 2005 Sep 28;227(2):227][republished in Cancer Lett. 2005 Sep 28;227(2): 229-36; PMID: 16196122]. Cancer Letters, 2003. 199(1): 91-8.

[133] Jin, X., et al., Expression patterns of seprase, a membrane serine protease, in cervical carcinoma and cervical intraepithelial neoplasm.[erratum appears in Anticancer Res. 2003;23:5371-2]. Anticancer Research, 2003. 23(4): 3195-8.

[134] Wilson, C.H. and C.A. Abbott, Expression profiling of dipeptidyl peptidase 8 and 9 in breast and ovarian carcinoma cell lines. Int J Oncol, 2012. 41(3): 919-32.

[135] Sulda, M.L., et al., Expression and prognostic assessment of dipeptidyl peptidase IV and related enzymes in B-cell chronic lymphocytic leukemia. Cancer Biol Ther, 2010. 10(2): 180-9.

[136] Klener, P., et al., Possible Prognostic-Significance of the Assessment of Dipeptidyl-peptidase-Ii in Peripheral-Blood Lymphocytes of Patients with Chronic Lymphocytic-Leukemia. Neoplasma, 1987. 34(5): 581-586.

[137] Danilov, A.V., et al., Dipeptidyl peptidase 2 apoptosis assay determines the B-cell activation stage and predicts prognosis in chronic lymphocytic leukemia. Exp Hematol, 2010. 38(12): 1167-77.

[138] Pure, E., The road to integrative cancer therapies: emergence of a tumor-associated fibroblast protease as a potential therapeutic target in cancer. Expert Opin Ther Targets, 2009. 13(8): 967-73.

[139] Takasawa, W., et al., Inhibition of dipeptidyl peptidase 4 regulates microvascular endothelial growth induced by inflammatory cytokines. Biochem Biophys Res Commun, 2010. 401(1): 7-12.

[140] Matheeussen, V., et al., Expression and spatial heterogeneity of dipeptidyl peptidases in endothelial cells of conduct vessels and capillaries. Biol Chem, 2011. 392(3): 189-98.

[141] Arwert, E.N., et al., Upregulation of CD26 expression in epithelial cells and stromal cells during wound-induced skin tumour formation. Oncogene, 2011. 31(8): 992-1000.

[142] Shin, J.W., G. Jurisic, and M. Detmar, Lymphatic-specific expression of dipeptidyl peptidase IV and its dual role in lymphatic endothelial function. Exp Cell Res, 2008. 314(16): 3048-56.

[143] Cheng, H.C., et al., Lung endothelial dipeptidyl peptidase IV promotes adhesion and metastasis of rat breast cancer cells via tumor cell surface-associated fibronectin. Journal of Biological Chemistry, 1998. 273(37): 24207-15.

[144] Ghersi, G., et al., Critical role of dipeptidyl peptidase IV in neuropeptide Y-mediated endothelial cell migration in response to wounding. Peptides, 2001. 22(3): 453-8.

[145] Aimes, R.T., et al., Endothelial cell serine proteases expressed during vascular morphogenesis and angiogenesis. Thromb Haemost, 2003. 89(3): 561-72.

[146] Ghilardi, C., et al., Identification of novel vascular markers through gene expression profiling of tumor-derived endothelium. BMC Genomics, 2008. 9: 201.

[147] Kidd, S., et al., Origins of the tumor microenvironment: quantitative assessment of adipose-derived and bone marrow-derived stroma. PLoS One, 2012. 7(2): e30563.

[148] Atherton, A.J., et al., Dipeptidyl peptidase IV expression identifies a functional subpopulation of breast fibroblasts. Int J Cancer, 1992. 50(1): 15-9.

[149] Atherton, A.J., et al., Ectoenzyme regulation by phenotypically distinct fibroblast sub-populations isolated from the human mammary gland. J Cell Sci, 1994. 107 (Pt 10): 2931-9.

[150] Moehrle, M.C., et al., Aminopeptidase-M and Dipeptidyl Peptidase-Iv Activity in Epithelial Skin Tumors - a Histochemical-Study. Journal of Cutaneous Pathology, 1995. 22(3): 241-247.

[151] Kacar, A., et al., Stromal expression of CD34, alpha-smooth muscle actin and CD26/DPPIV in squamous cell carcinoma of the skin: a comparative immunohistochemical study. Pathol Oncol Res, 2012. 18(1): 25-31.

[152] Park, J.E., et al., Fibroblast activation protein, a dual specificity serine protease expressed in reactive human tumor stromal fibroblasts. Journal of Biological Chemistry, 1999. 274(51): 36505-12.

[153] O'Brien, P. and B.F. O'Connor, Seprase: An overview of an important matrix serine protease. Biochimica Biophysica Acta, 2008. 1784(9):1130-45.

[154] Rettig, W.J., et al., Fibroblast activation protein: purification, epitope mapping and induction by growth factors. International Journal of Cancer, 1994. 58(3): 385-92.

[155] Waster, P., et al., Ultraviolet exposure of melanoma cells induces fibroblast activation protein-alpha in fibroblasts: Implications for melanoma invasion. Int J Oncol, 2011.

[156] Zhang, J., M. Valianou, and J.D. Cheng, Identification and characterization of the promoter of fibroblast activation protein. Front Biosci (Elite Ed), 2010. 2: 1154-63.

[157] Christiansen, V.J., et al., Effect of fibroblast activation protein and alpha2-antiplasmin cleaving enzyme on collagen types I, III, and IV. Arch Biochem Biophys, 2007. 457(2): 177-86.

[158] Lee, H.O., et al., FAP-overexpressing fibroblasts produce an extracellular matrix that enhances invasive velocity and directionality of pancreatic cancer cells. BMC Cancer, 2011. 11: 245.

[159] Santos, A.M., et al., Targeting fibroblast activation protein inhibits tumor stromagenesis and growth in mice. J Clin Invest, 2009. 119(12): 3613-25.

[160] Kraman, M., et al., Suppression of antitumor immunity by stromal cells expressing fibroblast activation protein-alpha. Science, 2010. 330(6005): 827-30.

[161] Ge, Y., et al., Fibroblast activation protein (FAP) is upregulated in myelomatous bone and supports myeloma cell survival. British Journal of Haematology, 2006. 133(1): 83-92.

[162] Cohen, S.J., et al., Fibroblast activation protein and its relationship to clinical outcome in pancreatic adenocarcinoma. Pancreas, 2008. 37(2): 154-8.

[163] Saadi, A., et al., Stromal genes discriminate preinvasive from invasive disease, predict outcome, and highlight inflammatory pathways in digestive cancers. Proc Natl Acad Sci U S A. 107(5): 2177-82.

[164] Ariga, N., et al., Stromal expression of fibroblast activation protein/seprase, a cell membrane serine proteinase and gelatinase, is associated with longer survival in patients with invasive ductal carcinoma of breast. Int J Cancer, 2001. 95(1): 67-72.

[165] Balaziova, E., et al., Dipeptidyl peptidase-IV activity and/or structure homologs (DASH): contributing factors in the pathogenesis of rheumatic diseases? Advances in Experimental Medicine & Biology, 2006. 575: 169-74.

[166] Bank, U., et al., Outside or inside: role of the subcellular localization of DP4-like enzymes for substrate conversion and inhibitor effects. Biol Chem, 2011. 392(3): 169-87.

[167] Uematsu, T., et al., Effects of oral squamous cell carcinoma-derived TGF-beta1 on CD26/DPPIV expression in T cells. Anticancer Research, 2004. 24(2B): 619-24.

[168] Adams, S., et al., PT-100, a small molecule dipeptidyl peptidase inhibitor, has potent antitumor effects and augments antibody-mediated cytotoxicity via a novel immune mechanism. Cancer Research, 2004. 64(15): 5471-80.

[169] Sulda, M.L., C.A. Abbott, and M. Hildebrandt, DPIV/CD26 and FAP in cancer: a tale of contradictions. Advances in Experimental Medicine & Biology, 2006. 575: 197-206.

[170] Medeiros Mdos, S., et al., Hydrolysis of atrial and brain natriuretic peptides by the human astrocytoma clone D384 and the neuroblastoma line SH-SY5Y. Neuroendocrinology, 1991. 54(3): 295-302.

[171] Sedo, A., et al., Dipeptidyl peptidase IV in two human glioma cell lines. European Journal of Histochemistry, 2001. 45(1): 57-63.

[172] Sedo, A., R. Malik, and E. Krepela, Dipeptidyl peptidase IV in C6 rat glioma cell line differentiation. Biological Chemistry, 1998. 379(1): 39-44.

[173] Sedo, A. and R.P. Revoltella, Detection of dipeptidyl peptidase IV in glioma C6 and neuroblastoma SK-N-SH cell lines. Biochemistry & Cell Biology, 1995. 73(1-2): 113-5.

[174] Malik, R., et al., Dipeptidyl peptidase-IV activity and/or structure homologues (DASH) in transformed neuroectodermal cells. Advances in Experimental Medicine & Biology, 2003. 524: 95-102.

[175] Busek, P., J. Stremenova, and A. Sedo, Dipeptidyl peptidase-IV enzymatic activity bearing molecules in human brain tumors-good or evil? Frontiers in Bioscience, 2008. 13: 2319-26.

[176] Mentlein, R., et al., Expression and role of the cell surface protease seprase/fibroblast activation protein-alpha (FAP-alpha) in astroglial tumors. Biol Chem, 2011.

[177] Rettig, W.J., et al., Differential expression of cell surface antigens and glial fibrillary acidic protein in human astrocytoma subsets. Cancer Research, 1986. 46(12 Pt 1): 6406-12.

[178] Balaziova, E., et al., Coupled expression of dipeptidyl peptidase-IV and fibroblast activation protein-alpha in transformed astrocytic cells. Mol Cell Biochem, 2011. 354(1-2): 283-9.

[179] Paulus, W., C. Huettner, and J.C. Tonn, Collagens, integrins and the mesenchymal drift in glioblastomas: a comparison of biopsy specimens, spheroid and early monolayer cultures. Int J Cancer, 1994. 58(6): 841-6.

[180] Li, J., et al., An Activatable Near Infrared Fluorescent Probe for In Vivo Imaging of Fibroblast Activation Protein-alpha. Bioconjug Chem, 2012. 23: 1704-1711.

[181] Lojda, Z., Proteinases in pathology. Usefulness of histochemical methods. J Histochem Cytochem, 1981. 29(3A Suppl): 481-93.

[182] Guieu, R., et al., CD26 modulates nociception in mice via its dipeptidyl-peptidase IV activity. Behavioural Brain Research, 2006. 166(2): 230-5.

[183] Sakurada, C., et al., Degradation of endomorphin-2 at the supraspinal level in mice is initiated by dipeptidyl peptidase IV: an in vitro and in vivo study. Biochemical Pharmacology, 2003. 66(4): 653-61.

[184] Karl, T., et al., Extreme reduction of dipeptidyl peptidase IV activity in F344 rat substrains is associated with various behavioral differences. Physiology & Behavior, 2003. 80(1): 123-34.

[185] Rohnert, P., et al., Dipeptidyl peptidase IV, aminopeptidase N and DPIV/APN-like proteases in cerebral ischemia. J Neuroinflammation, 2012. 9: 44.

[186] Mentlein, R. and G. Struckhoff, Purification of two dipeptidyl aminopeptidases II from rat brain and their action on proline-containing neuropeptides. Journal of Neurochemistry, 1989. 52(4): 1284-93.

[187] Frerker, N., et al., Neuropeptide Y (NPY) cleaving enzymes: structural and functional homologues of dipeptidyl peptidase 4. Peptides, 2007. 28(2): 257-68.

[188] Gorenstein, C., V.T. Tran, and S.H. Snyder, Brain peptidase with a unique neuronal localization: the histochemical distribution of dipeptidyl-aminopeptidase II. Journal of Neuroscience, 1981. 1(10): 1096-102.

[189] Stevens, B.R., et al., Dipeptidyl peptidase-II activity in cultured astroglial cells from neonatal rat brain. Brain Research, 1987. 406(1-2): 113-7.

[190] Struckhoff, G., Dipeptidyl peptidase II in astrocytes of the rat brain. Meningeal cells increase enzymic activity in cultivated astrocytes. Brain Research, 1993. 620(1): 49-57.

[191] Mares, V., et al., Compartment- and malignance-dependent up-regulation of gamma-glutamyltranspeptidase and dipetidylpeptidase-IV activity in human brain gliomas. Histol Histopathol, 2012. 27(7): 931-40.

[192] Network, C.G.A.R., Comprehensive genomic characterization defines human glioblastoma genes and core pathways. Nature, 2008. 455(7216): 1061-8.

[193] Mikheeva, S.A., et al., TWIST1 promotes invasion through mesenchymal change in human glioblastoma. Mol Cancer, 2010. 9: 194.

[194] Huse, J.T., H.S. Phillips, and C.W. Brennan, Molecular subclassification of diffuse gliomas: seeing order in the chaos. Glia, 2011. 59(8): 1190-9.

[195] Verhaak, R.G., et al., Integrated genomic analysis identifies clinically relevant subtypes of glioblastoma characterized by abnormalities in PDGFRA, IDH1, EGFR, and NF1. Cancer Cell, 2010. 17(1): 98-110.

[196] Venere, M., et al., Cancer stem cells in gliomas: identifying and understanding the apex cell in cancer's hierarchy. Glia, 2011. 59(8): 1148-54.

[197] Bonavia, R., et al., Heterogeneity maintenance in glioblastoma: a social network. Cancer Res, 2011. 71(12): 4055-60.

[198] Charles, N.A., et al., The brain tumor microenvironment. Glia, 2012. 59(8): 1169-80.

[199] Kouno, J., et al., Up-regulation of CC chemokine, CCL3L1, and receptors, CCR3, CCR5 in human glioblastoma that promotes cell growth. Journal of Neuro-Oncology, 2004. 70(3): 301-7.

[200] Pham, K., et al., CCL5, CCR1 and CCR5 in murine glioblastoma: immune cell infiltration and survival rates are not dependent on individual expression of either CCR1 or CCR5. J Neuroimmunol, 2012. 246(1-2): 10-7.

[201] Soroceanu, L., et al., Human cytomegalovirus US28 found in glioblastoma promotes an invasive and angiogenic phenotype. Cancer Res, 2011. 71(21): 6643-53.

[202] Jacobs, J.F., et al., Prognostic significance and mechanism of Treg infiltration in human brain tumors. J Neuroimmunol, 2010. 225(1-2): 195-9.

[203] Jordan, J.T., et al., Preferential migration of regulatory T cells mediated by glioma-secreted chemokines can be blocked with chemotherapy. Cancer Immunol Immunother, 2008. 57(1): 123-31.

[204] Sreekanthreddy, P., et al., Identification of potential serum biomarkers of glioblastoma: serum osteopontin levels correlate with poor prognosis. Cancer Epidemiol Biomarkers Prev, 2010. 19(6): 1409-22.

[205] Liu, C., et al., Chemokine receptor CXCR3 promotes growth of glioma. Carcinogenesis, 2011. 32(2): 129-37.

[206] Maru, S.V., et al., Chemokine production and chemokine receptor expression by human glioma cells: role of CXCL10 in tumour cell proliferation. J Neuroimmunol, 2008. 199(1-2): 35-45.

[207] Hattermann, K., et al., The chemokine receptor CXCR7 is highly expressed in human glioma cells and mediates antiapoptotic effects. Cancer Res, 2010. 70(8): 3299-308.

[208] Calatozzolo, C., et al., Expression of the new CXCL12 receptor, CXCR7, in gliomas. Cancer Biol Ther, 2011. 11(2): 242-53.

[209] Jiang, Z., et al., Contribution of SDF-1alpha/CXCR4 Signaling to Brain Development and Glioma Progression. Neurosignals, 2012.

[210] Lazarczyk, M., E. Matyja, and A. Lipkowski, Substance P and its receptors -- a potential target for novel medicines in malignant brain tumour therapies (mini-review). Folia Neuropathol, 2007. 45(3): 99-107.

[211] Palma, C. and C.A. Maggi, The role of tachykinins via NK1 receptors in progression of human gliomas. Life Sciences, 2000. 67(9): 985-1001.

[212] Dufes, C., et al., Effects of the vasoactive intestinal peptide (VIP) and related peptides on glioblastoma cell growth in vitro. J Mol Neurosci, 2003. 21(2): 91-102.

[213] Sharma, A., et al., A vasoactive intestinal peptide antagonist inhibits the growth of glioblastoma cells. J Mol Neurosci, 2001. 17(3): 331-9.

[214] Busek, P., et al., Modulation of substance P signaling by dipeptidyl peptidase-IV enzymatic activity in human glioma cell lines. Physiological Research, 2008. 57(3): 443-9.

[215] Kaur, B., et al., Hypoxia and the hypoxia-inducible-factor pathway in glioma growth and angiogenesis. Neuro Oncol, 2005. 7(2): 134-53.

[216] Sato, Y., et al., Involvement of dipeptidyl peptidase IV in extravillous trophoblast invasion and differentiation. J Clin Endocrinol Metab, 2002. 87(9): 4287-96.

[217] Dang, D.T., et al., Hypoxia-inducible factor-1 target genes as indicators of tumor vessel response to vascular endothelial growth factor inhibition. Cancer Res, 2008. 68(6): 1872-80.

[218] Lee, E.W., et al., Neuropeptide Y induces ischemic angiogenesis and restores function of ischemic skeletal muscles. Journal of Clinical Investigation, 2003. 111(12): 1853-62.

[219] Tilan, J., et al., Differential functions of neuropeptide Y in Ewing's sarcoma - hypoxia as a switch Cancer Research Proceedings of the 103rd Annual Meeting of the American Association for Cancer Research; 2012 Mar 31-Apr 4; Chicago, IL. Philadelphia (PA): AACR, 2012. 72(8 Suppl:Abstract nr 3950).

[220] Lal, A., et al., Mutant epidermal growth factor receptor up-regulates molecular effectors of tumor invasion. Cancer Res, 2002. 62(12): 3335-9.

[221] Fukushima, T. and H. Kataoka, Roles of insulin-like growth factor binding protein-2 (IGFBP-2) in glioblastoma. Anticancer Res, 2007. 27(6A): 3685-92.

[222] Wang, H., et al., Insulin-like growth factor binding protein 2 enhances glioblastoma invasion by activating invasion-enhancing genes. Cancer Res, 2003. 63(15): 4315-21.

[223] Qin, Q., et al., Normal and disease-related biological functions of Twist1 and underlying molecular mechanisms. Cell Res, 2012. 22(1): 90-106.

[224] Bellail, A.C., et al., Microregional extracellular matrix heterogeneity in brain modulates glioma cell invasion. Int J Biochem Cell Biol, 2004. 36(6): 1046-69.

[225] Viapiano, M.S., S.E. Lawler, and E.G. Meir, Glioma Invasion: Mechanisms and Therapeutic Challenges. CNS Cancer, B.A. Teicher, Editor. 2009, Humana Press. 1219-1252.

[226] Mueller, S.C., et al., A novel protease-docking function of integrin at invadopodia. Journal of Biological Chemistry, 1999. 274(35): 24947-52.

[227] Gondi, C.S., et al., Expression of seprase on the cellular surface is dependent on uP-AR and cathepsin B expression levels in gliomas. AACR Meeting Abstracts, 2006. 2006(1): 389-d-390.

[228] Zukowska-Grojec, Z., et al., Neuropeptide Y: a novel angiogenic factor from the sympathetic nerves and endothelium. Circulation Research, 1998. 83(2): 187-95.

[229] Brat, D.J. and E.G. Van Meir, Vaso-occlusive and prothrombotic mechanisms associated with tumor hypoxia, necrosis, and accelerated growth in glioblastoma. Lab Invest, 2004. 84(4): 397-405.

[230] Rong, Y., et al., 'Pseudopalisading' necrosis in glioblastoma: a familiar morphologic feature that links vascular pathology, hypoxia, and angiogenesis. J Neuropathol Exp Neurol, 2006. 65(6): 529-39.

[231] Rong, Y., D.J. Brat, and E.G. Meir, Vaso-occlusive Mechanisms that Intiate Hypoxia and Necrosis in Glioblastoma: The Role of Thrombosis and Tissue Factor. CNS Cancer, B.A. Teicher, Editor. 2009, Humana Press. 507-528.

[232] Lee, K.N., et al., Enhancement of fibrinolysis by inhibiting enzymatic cleavage of precursor alpha2-antiplasmin. J Thromb Haemost, 2011. 9(5): 987-96.

[233] Aratake, Y., et al., Diagnostic utility of galectin-3 and CD26/DPPIV as preoperative diagnostic markers for thyroid nodules. Diagnostic Cytopathology, 2002. 26(6): 366-372.

[234] Shaw, E.J., et al., Gene expression in oligodendroglial tumors. Anal Cell Pathol (Amst), 2010. 33(2): 81-94.

[235] Inamoto, T., et al., Anti-CD26 Monoclonal Antibody-Mediated G1-S Arrest of Human Renal Clear Cell Carcinoma Caki-2 Is Associated with Retinoblastoma Substrate Dephosphorylation, Cyclin-Dependent Kinase 2 Reduction, p27kip1 Enhancement, and Disruption of Binding to the Extracellular Matrix. Clin Cancer Res, 2006. 12(11): 3470-3477.

[236] Ho, L., et al., In vitro and in vivo antitumor effect of the anti-CD26 monoclonal antibody 1F7 on human CD30+ anaplastic large cell T-cell lymphoma Karpas 299. Clin Cancer Res, 2001. 7(7): 2031-40.

[237] Messerschmidt, S.K., et al., Targeted lipid-coated nanoparticles: delivery of tumor necrosis factor-functionalized particles to tumor cells. J Control Release, 2009. 137(1): 69-77.

[238] Muller, D., K. Frey, and R.E. Kontermann, A novel antibody-4-1BBL fusion protein for targeted costimulation in cancer immunotherapy. J Immunother, 2008. 31(8): 714-22.

[239] Liao, D., et al., Cancer associated fibroblasts promote tumor growth and metastasis by modulating the tumor immune microenvironment in a 4T1 murine breast cancer model. PLoS One, 2009. 4(11): e7965.

[240] Loeffler, M., et al., Targeting tumor-associated fibroblasts improves cancer chemotherapy by increasing intratumoral drug uptake. Journal of Clinical Investigation, 2006. 116(7): 1955-62.

[241] Lee, J., et al., Tumor immunotherapy targeting fibroblast activation protein, a product expressed in tumor-associated fibroblasts. Cancer Research, 2005. 65(23): 11156-63.

[242] Fassnacht, M., et al., Induction of CD4(+) and CD8(+) T-cell responses to the human stromal antigen, fibroblast activation protein: implication for cancer immunotherapy. Clinical Cancer Research, 2005. 11(15): 5566-71.

[243] Lebeau, A.M., et al., Targeting the cancer stroma with a fibroblast activation protein-activated promelittin protoxin. Mol Cancer Ther, 2009. 8(5):1378-86.

[244] Neumiller, J.J., L. Wood, and R.K. Campbell, Dipeptidyl peptidase-4 inhibitors for the treatment of type 2 diabetes mellitus. Pharmacotherapy, 2010. 30(5): 463-84.

[245] Vanhoof, G., et al., Proline motifs in peptides and their biological processing. FASEB Journal, 1995. 9(9): 736-44.

[246] Bernstein, H.G., et al., Immunolocalization of dipeptidyl aminopeptidase (DAP IV) in the developing human brain. International Journal of Developmental Neuroscience, 1987. 5(3): 237-42.

[247] Tatenhorst, L., et al., Regulators of G-protein signaling 3 and 4 (RGS3, RGS4) are associated with glioma cell motility. J Neuropathol Exp Neurol, 2004. 63(3): 210-22.

[248] Van Meir, E.G., et al., Exciting new advances in neuro-oncology: the avenue to a cure for malignant glioma. CA Cancer J Clin, 2010. 60(3): 166-93.

[249] Jones, T.S. and E.C. Holland, Standard of care therapy for malignant glioma and its effect on tumor and stromal cells. Oncogene, 2012. 31(16): 1995-2006.

Chapter 9

Apoptotic Events in Glioma Activate Metalloproteinases and Enhance Invasiveness

Albert Magro

Additional information is available at the end of the chapter

http://dx.doi.org/10.5772/52359

1. Introduction

A cancer of the brain that arises from supporting tissue (glial cells) is referred to as a glioma. Glioblastomas are fast growing gliomas and can be referred to as a Grade IV astrocytomas or glioblastoma multiformes (GBMs). GBMs that affect the brain do not readily spread to parts of the body outside of the brain, but they are highly invasive and invade surrounding tissue in the brain. The persistent invasiveness, which is extremely difficult to reverse, is what makes GBMs so deadly. Therapeutic regimens for GBM and other high grade gliomas have fallen short of providing effective treatment. Clinical studies comparing chemotherapeutic agents have indicated increased tumor shrinkage and a very slight increase in median survival times, but no evidence for an increase in survival rates [1, 2]. More recent clinical studies employing surgery with the use of chemotherapeutic regimens in combination with radiation therapy or by receptor mediated growth hormone deprivation are slightly more effective in increasing median survival times, but again have had limited success in increasing the overall survival rate in patients being treated for primary or recurrent GBM [3-7]. Clinicians and neurosurgeons are diligently pursuing new treatments and provide hope for patients and their families [8, 9]. However, the difficulties of complete resection, the resistance to radiation and other therapies and particularly the intractable malignant invasiveness still remains at the root of the very poor survival prognosis for patients with GBM and other high grade gliomas. Despite extensive studies regarding the clinical aspects of GBM very little is known about the behavior of GBM during apoptosis. The ideas pursued in this paper are relevant to apoptotic cells within a glioma enhancing the invasiveness of the apoptotic resistant cells and thus contributing to the tumor's malignant properties.

Apoptosis is a type of cell death in which there is a multipath sequence of programmed events within the cell. These events require energy and lead to a suicidal self-destruction of the cell without releasing intracellular components to the surrounding area. The apoptotic process is accompanied by numerous biochemical changes within the cell that are manifested by morphological changes which include blebbing, cell shrinkage, chromatin condensation and DNA fragmentation. The etymological origins of the word apoptosis is a Greek term meaning "falling off" and first appeared in a publication in 1972 by Kerr and his colleagues [10]. Over the past four decades apoptosis has been extensively studied [11]. Apoptosis is considered an essential physiological process in eukaryotes which impacts embryonic development, tissue homeostasis, wound healing, elimination of cells by the immune response and is an important process in the elimination of malignant or potentially malignant cells. For a tumor mass to arise, the cells within the cancerous tumor in some way had to escape apoptosis. The cancerous cell type that emerges requires clinical treatment by surgical, radiological and chemotherapeutic techniques. It is well known that all radiological and pharmacological treatments of cancerous cells are treatments that induce cell death by apoptosis. In fact, other than surgery, malignant cell types require a clinical treatment that induces cell death by apoptosis because the cellular debris and inflammation produced by massive necrosis of an extensive tumor would be systemically injurious to the patient. Thus, capable investigations of some of the mechanisms associated with apoptotic cell death in Glioblastomas can of themselves be significant. Beyond that however, the fact that Glioblastomas are usually highly invasive, but in general do not metastasize is what renders studies about invasiveness particularly relevant to clinical treatments of Glioblastomas [12]. In light of this, any contribution to furthering the understanding about the invasiveness of Glioblastomas would be significant and is likely to be well received.

Metalloproteinases are a group of enzymes that can break down proteins such as collagen and other extracellular matrix proteins. Because these enzymes need zinc or calcium to work properly, they are called metalloproteinases. It has been known for some time that metalloproteinases play an important role in the degradation of the extracellular matrix (ECM) [13, 14]. However, the basic action of metalloproteinases, which is the cleavage of proteins, has proven sufficiently sophisticated to orchestrate various functions in addition to degradation of the ECM [15, 16]. The metalloproteinase family includes: matrix metalloproteinases (MMPs) [17, 18], membrane type matrix metalloproteinases (MT-MMPs) [19, 20], a disintegrin and metalloproteinases (ADAMs) [21] and a disintegrin and metalloproteinases with thrombospondin type 1 motif (ADAMTs) [22]. The MMPs and the ADAMTs are secreted while the activated ADAMs and MT-MMPs remain anchored to the cell. All four of the metalloproteinase families have the ability to act on ECM proteins and growth factor receptors as substrates. The metalloproteinases have the capacity to regulate tumorigenesis [23], angiogenesis [24, 25], tumor growth [26], and invasiveness [16]. Metalloproteinases are naturally inhibited by specific tissue inhibitors of metalloproteinases (TIMPs) [27]. Thus, over the last two decades, it has become clear that metalloproteinases do more than degrade structural ECM proteins. Metalloproteinases are produced in an inactive zymogen form. One of the aims of this present report is to focus on the role of apoptosis with regard to the secretion and activation of metalloproteinases. Although metalloproteinases have been extensively studied, the total relevance of secreted MMPs or MT-MMPs with regard to invasiveness and malignancy of Glioblastomas is not completely resolved at present. It might be anticipated that metalloproteinases have important and yet to be discovered roles with regard to the invasiveness of Glioblastomas.

Anoikis is a form of cell death induced by inadequate or inappropriate cell–matrix interactions whereupon there is a loss of cell adhesion signals [28]. In the case of noncancerous cells, as they lose contact with the extracellular matrix an anoikic cell death response is initiated. Anoikic cell death proceeds via apoptotic programs and can be considered a natural protection against cells being detached and subsequently migrating from their primary site and becoming established outside of their normal environment. With regard to cancerous cells many of them are anoikic resistant. Anoikis is regulated by a variety of signaling pathways depending on the cell type [29]. The circumventing of anoikic cell death by cancer cells enables the cancer cells to migrate from their primary site and enter new environments and survive [30, 31]. Despite the fact that in general Glioblastomas do not metastasize, there is motivation to know more about the secretion and activity of metalloproteinases in anoikic resistant glioma cells. A focus of this present report is to address the question of whether apoptotic and anoikic resistant LN18 cells are an important factor with regard to metalloproteinase secretion and activation of the zymogen form. The question is significant given the nonhomogeneous state of a tumor which most likely consists of a mixture of apoptotic and non-apoptotic cells. As cells within a tumor become apoptotic micro cavities will be formed and not all of the cells will receive a full complement of cell adhesion signals. Thus, whether treated by radiation, chemotherapeutics or natural defenses, a tumor is most likely to exist as a milieu of dying apoptotic cells, anoikic resistant cells, and non-apoptotic cells that are resistant to treatment. The question of whether MMPs are activated or secreted from apoptotic or anoikic resistant cells is relevant to the possibility that loosely attached cells or therapeutically induced apoptotic cells can interact with apoptotic resistant cells and thus contribute to angiogenesis, tumor growth and the invasiveness of Glioblastomas. Experiments within this report have been done with the view that anoikis and the escape from anoikis are worthy of investigation in the context of MMP secretion; particularly in the context of the effects of activated MMPs upon GBM invasiveness.

2. Overall purpose

This report will first provide evidence that the apoptotic state of LN18 glioblastoma cells can be readily delineated and as such provides a convenient *in vitro* model to study effects of apoptotic cells upon the malignant properties of gliomas. In the context of metalloproteinase activation, an objective is to point out that in late apoptosis LN18 cells manifest a degradation of surface determinants including: growth factor receptors EGFR and IGF1-R, histocompatibility markers such as HLA-ABC, and a variety of cluster determinants including alpha and beta integrins. The degradation of surface determinants like integrins and growth factor receptors could be viewed as a full commitment to apoptosis through a decrease in survival signals. However, the perspective presented here is that Glioblastomas that lose growth factor signals and cell adhesion signals, even if dying, still have the capacity to affect the malignancy of those GBM cells within the tumor that are in a non-apoptotic state. In addition, it has been presumed that GBM cells going into apoptosis is a condition that is totally beneficial to the patient. However, an aim of this report is to point out that there may be a down side to apoptosis that is worthy of consideration. In addition, anoikic resistance is thought of mostly in terms of cells traveling through the circulatory system and surviving to be the root cause of metastases [32]. Yet, anoikic resistant cells that lose their adhesion signals *in situ* may be supportive of the deadly invasive characteristics of the malignant non-apoptotic cells within the GBM tumor. More specifically the explorations of this report are intended to:

- present evidence for the presence and increased activation of metalloproteinases in LN18 glioblastoma cells as they proceed through apoptosis,
- address the possibility that MMP secretion increases in LN18 cells that are devoid of cell adhesion signals and,
- call attention to the idea that within the milieu of a glioblastoma, apoptosis may have a role in enhancing the invasiveness of the non-apoptotic cells.

3. Methods

3.1. Cell culture conditions

The LN18 cell line (ATTC CRL-2610) was established in 1976 from a patient with a high grade right temporal lobe glioma. The cells are poorly differentiated, are adherent, and grow well in culture [33]. For cell maintenance, the cells were incubated at 37°C in an atmosphere of 5% CO_2, 95% air, and 100% humidity. Cells were maintained in 75 cm^2 flasks in Dulbecco's Modified Eagle Medium free of phenol red and supplemented with the dipeptide L-alanyl-L-glutamine (2mM), non-essential amino acids, pyruvate (100μg/ml), penicillin (100 units/ml), streptomycin (100μg/ml), amphotericin B (0.25μg/ml), HEPES (25mM), and fetal bovine serum (10%). Media and all tissue culture reagents were purchased from Invitrogen. Cells were plated from a trypsin digest (0.25% trypsin, EDTA). All plastic ware used for tissue culture and other experimentation including flasks, 96, 24 and 6 well plates were purchased from Fisher (Costar). Numerical data represent 3 to 4 replicates per sample. When establishing significant differences between samples (α=0.05) the data were analyzed by One Way Anova/Tukey Tests.

3.2. Apoptotic inducing agents

The apoptotic inducing agents used in the report are MK886 and staurosporine. MK886 is a molecule reported to inhibit both five lipoxygenase activating protein (FLAP) [39] and peroxisome proliferator activated receptor-α (PPAR-α) [34]. Staurosporine has been reported to inhibit protein kinase c [35]. Both MK886 and staurosporine are proven apoptotic inducing agents [36-40]. MK886 and staurosporine were purchased from Sigma. Apoptosis was induced by micro molar levels of inducing agent solubilized in DMSO and diluted to the appropriate concentration in the Dulbecco's reaction medium

3.3. Antibodies and reagents

Mouse monoclonal primary antibodies used for flow cytometry included: mouse anti-KLH (Biolegend), mouse anti-β actin, mouse anti-integrins and mouse anti-HLA-ABC (Upstate, Chemicon, Linco) and goat anti-mouse-IgG conjugated to phycoerythrin (Jackson Laboratories).

4. Assays for apoptosis for LN18 cells in a monolayer

Classical apoptotic morphology was used as a manifestation of apoptosis. Early apoptosis was determined by phosphatidylserine (PS) translocation to the outer membrane as measured by flow cytometry manifested by annexin binding in the absence of propidium iodide uptake (Roche, Annexin-V-FLOUS kit) or annexin binding in the absence of uptake of 7-aminoactiomycin D (Molecular Probes).

Apoptosis was also detected by measuring the degradation and loss of activity of Poly(ADP-ribose) polymerase (PARP). The functional activity of PARP was determined using a PARP Activity Assay kit (R&D Systems). PARP activity extracted from cells and activated was measured by determining the level of incorporation of biotin labeled NAD into histones that are coated onto a microtiter plate. The color development was measured with a computer-assisted MR4000 Dynatech Microplate Reader at 450nm.

Late apoptosis was measured by the release of nucleosome histone complexes from the nucleus into the cytosol. The Cell Death ELISA kit (Roche) was used. The method includes a microtiter plate which has its wells streptavidin coated. The primary immunoreagent is a biotin labeled anti-histone antibody which binds to the streptavidin coated plate and histones within the experimental sample. The secondary antibody is a peroxidase conjugated anti-DNA that was added after sample addition. The assay detects soluble cytoplasmic DNA-histone complexes resulting from apoptotic nucleosomes that are tightly bound with core histones that appear in the cytosol before the plasma membrane disintegrates. The ELISA color development was measured with a computer-assisted MR4000 Dynatech Microplate Reader at 405nm.

Late apoptosis was also measured by the electrophoretic manifestation of DNA degradation. DNA extraction for electrophoresis was done according to the procedure described by Gong et al. [41]. Essentially, the cells were prefixed in 70% ethanol and the DNA was extracted with 0.2 M phosphate-citrate buffer at pH 7.8. The extract was sequentially treated with RNase A and proteinase K and then subjected to electrophoresis. After 12 hours of treatment with MK886 the DNA was extracted from $3x10^6$ LN18 cells and loaded in a 20μL volume into a 4% agarose gel. The gel was run at 85volts for 1h. The gels where subsequently stained with 0.4μg/ml of ethidium bromide and photographed under UV exposure in an Alpha Innotech Fluorchem 8800 photo imager.

Measuring the degree of nuclear condensation and fragmentation by staining with the DNA binding fluorescent dye 4',6-diamidino-2-phenylindole (DAPI) was another indicator of apoptosis that was used.

4.1. Flow cytometry to detect surface proteins and apoptosis

The surface proteins of apoptotic cells were compared to the surface proteins of non-apoptotic cells. Following treatment the apoptotic and non-apoptotic cells were suspended, centrifuged and washed. The cells were then suspended in the appropriate buffer and reacted with the primary antibodies (mouse @ ITGA2, mouse @ ITGB2 or mouse @ HLA-ABC). Following incubation with the primary antibody the cells were rewashed and incubated with goat @ mouse IgG conjugated to phycoerythrin. The cells were then washed and assayed by flow cytometry. To measure apoptosis the dyes annexinV conjugated to fluorescein isothiocyanate (annexin –FITC) and 7-Amino-actinomycinD (7-AAD) were used. Dyes were added in the appropriate buffer. Following labeling, cells were analyzed with Becton-Dickinson FACSCalibur (San Jose, CA) using CellQuest Pro software.

4.2. Real time RT-PCR

The RNA was isolated from cells using TRIZOL Reagent (Life Technologies). Reverse transcriptase generated c-DNAs were obtained using random hexamers with the high capacity archive kit from Applied Biosystems. C-DNAs were allowed to form for 2h at 37°C. Negative controls were generated by omitting the reverse transcriptase in the cDNA generating step. For the PCR step, the primers and Taq-Man fluorescent probes were purchased from Applied Biosystems. The primers were designed to span an intron to avoid amplification of any contaminating DNA. Real time PCR was performed using the Applied Biosystems Gene Amp 5700 system with the Taq-Man Universal PCR Master Mix. Relative mRNA levels were measured using the threshold cycle (Ct). The threshold cycle was defined as the cycle number that first gives detection of the PCR amplicon above a fixed threshold baseline set within the log phase of the plot of fluorescence versus cycle number. The amplicons were generated over 40 cycles where each cycle consisted of a 15 sec dissociation step at 92°C and a polymerization step at 60°C for 1 min. The ΔCt was calculated by subtracting the Ct value for the housekeeping gene β-actin (ACTB) from the Ct value for the gene of interest for the same c-DNA sample. The ΔCt of the vehicle (DMSO) control cells was then compared to the ΔCt of the MK886 treated cells.

4.3. ELISA assay of matrix metalloproteinase proteins released from LN18 cells

The level of each MMP protein released into the supernatant from non-adherent anoikic LN18 cells incubated in polyhema coated flasks was measured by a sandwich ELISA (R&D Systems). Monoclonal antibodies specific for the human MMP were immobilized onto the surface of the wells of a plastic 96 well microtiter plate. 100μl of undiluted samples were added and following incubation (2h @ RT), the unbound material was washed away (4X) and a biotinylated goat anti-human MMP conjugated to horseradish peroxidase (HRP) was added and incubated for 2h @ RT. The cells were then washed 4X. The substrate tetra-methyl-benzidine (TMB) was added and allowed to develop for 30min. Sulfuric acid was added as a stopping solution. A BMG Labtech FLUOstar OPTIMA plate reader at 450nm was used to quantify the absorbance that resulted from the developed color of the substrate.

4.4. Fluorometric assay of metalloproteinase activity

The enzymatic activity of released MMPs from suspended LN18 cells was tested using the Fluorescence Resonance Energy Transfer (FRET) peptide QXL520 -Arg-Pro-Leu-Ala-Leu-Trp-Arg-Lys(5-FAM)-NH2 (ANASPEC). The hydrolysis of the FRET peptide by the pure recombinant MMP3 was used as a control. The fluorescence was monitored in microtiter plates using a FLUOStar OPTIMA Fluorometer at an Ex/Em=490nm/520nm. The complete activation of the released MMPs was insured by the use of 1mM of 4-aminophenylmercuric acetate (APMA).

4.5. Matrigel measure of LN18 cell invasiveness

The invasiveness was measured *in vitro* using a BD Falcon matrigel matrix system. This system consists of a 24-multiwell plate where each well has an insert consisting of an 8.0μ pore size polyethylene terephthalate (PET) membrane that has been uniformly coated with a layer of matrigel which serves as a reconstituted matrix *in vitro*. The coating process occludes the pores of the PET membrane and thereby blocks the non-invasive cells from migrating through the membrane. In contrast, invasive cells are able to degrade the matrigel coating of the membrane and migrate through the 8.0μ pores of the PET membrane. The invasive non-apoptotic LN18 cells were stained with the lipophilic fluorescent dye DiI (Molecular Probes). Since the PET membrane effectively blocks the passage of light from 490-700nm at >99% efficiency only those stained cells that pass through the PET membrane are detected. Fluorescently-labeled cells that have not passed through the matrigel and the PET membrane are not detected by the bottom reading fluorescent plate reader. The chemoattractant in the lower chambers of the 24 well plate (below the matrigel insert) was DMEM medium that is 0.5% fetal bovine serum (FBS). Invasiveness was monitored using a FLUOStar OPTIMA plate reading fluorometer at an Ex/Em=549nm/565nm for 2h at 37°C.

5. Results

5.1. Characterization of apoptosis induced by MK886 in a monolayer of LN18 cells

DNA fragmentation is a classic indicator of apoptosis. Figure1 is a photographed UV exposure of DNA agarose gels. The DNA was extracted from control LN18 cells and MK886 treated LN18 cells while in a monolayer. Following electrophoresis of the extracted DNA the gels were stained with ethidium bromide. Column A is the electrophoretic pattern of a 100bp standard. The following columns are the electrophoretic patterns for the medium control (column B), 10μM of MK886 for 12h (column C), 25μM of MK886 for 12h (column D) and 50μM of MK886 for 12h (column E). DNA fragmentation is a very late event in the apoptotic process. Not all cell types respond the same in the fragmentation of DNA. Some cell types give a very clear laddering and others produce more of a smearing of DNA similar to that found in states of necrosis. For apoptotic processes the nuclear DNA would have been previously condensed during the earlier stages of apoptosis distinguishing it from necrosis. The asynchrony and slowness of apoptotic entry can also contribute to the formation of wider smeared bands of degraded DNA. We have found that the more compact a monolayer of LN18 cells is the slower is the apoptotic entry as indicated by the slower development of morphological changes of rounding up and blebbing of the cells. The electrophoretic patterns of Figure 1 show that there is more degradation of DNA when LN18 cells are treated with increasing concentrations of MK886.

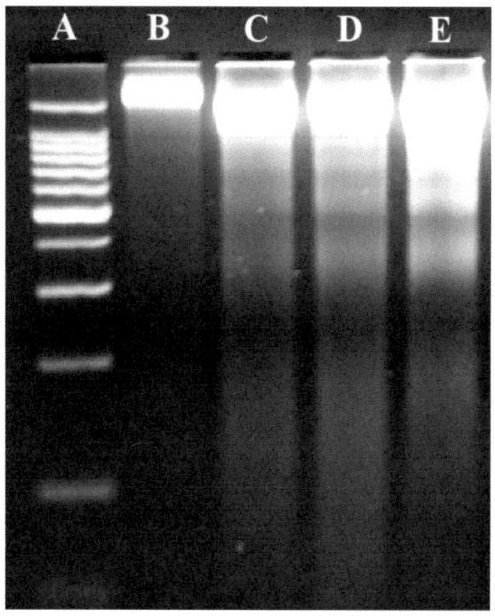

Figure 1. Electrophoretic patterns of DNA fragmentation of apoptotic LN18 cells. Column A: 100 bp standard. Column B: non-apoptotic control. Columns C-E: increasing concentrations of apoptotic MK886 inducing agent of 10, 25 & 50 μM respectively for 12h.

Another classical indicator of apoptosis is the degradation and loss of enzymatic activity of Poly(ADP-ribose) polymerase (PARP). PARP is a family of multifunctional enzymes the most dominant of which are PARP-1 and PARP-2. One of the major roles of PARP-1 is the post-translational modification of nuclear proteins induced by DNA strand-breaks that contributes to the survival of injured proliferating cells [42]. The catalytic activity of PARP is immediately stimulated by DNA strand-breaks [43]. As delineated in the Methods, activated PARP-1 cleaves NAD into nicotinamide and ADP-ribose and catalyzes the transfer of ADP-ribose units from NAD+ to target nuclear proteins. Apoptosis initiates a caspases degradation of PARP which is manifested by a decrease in PARP's enzymatic activity [44]. The data of Table 1 show the activity of PARP for control cells held in medium and MK886 treated cells at 10, 25 and 50μM of MK886. The decrease in activity of PARP is indicated by the decrease in color development as demonstrated by the decrease in absorbance at 450nm. In addition to the measures of apoptosis shown here, MK886 induced apoptosis in monolayer LN18 cells has been shown to be caspases dependent and is exhibited by the release of nucleosomes, annexinV binding to phosphatidylserine in the presence and absence of nuclear staining, changes in morphology and changes in the fluorescent intensity of mitotracker deep red indicating changes in mitochondrial oxidative function [45]. The alteration of the mitochondrial function implies that apoptosis is induced in the LN18 cells via a mitochondrial pathway.

http://dx.doi.org/10.5772/52359

Treatment	$A_{450\,nm}$
Medium	0.756 +/- 0.136
Medium W/O bio-NAD	0.155 +/- 0.058
10 μM MK886	0.481 +/- 0.173
25 μM MK886	0.308 +/- 0.079
50 μM MK886	0.296 +/- 0.094

[1]LN18 cells were treated for 10h at indicated MK886 concentrations while in a monolayer

Table 1. MK886 Treatment of LN18 Cells Inhibits PARP Activity[1]

5.2. Degradation of surface determinants of monolayered LN18 cells in late apoptosis

The data presented here and the previous assessments of the time course and characteristics of apoptosis in monolayered LN18 cells render the system useful for further studies about the role of apoptosis and anoikis in enhancing GBN malignancy. LN18 cells losing contact with the extracellular matrix as they proceed through apoptosis is of interest. Integrins are a class of molecules relevant to cell adhesion to extracellular matrix proteins. Integrins exist as heterodimers consisting of linked alpha and beta chains forming a family of 24 distinct integrins. Integrins were first recognized as a family of receptors in a seminal paper put forth by Hynes in 1987 [46]. Since that time, it has become established that integrins have roles in addition to being receptors for cell adhesion proteins [47, 48]. Integrins act as membrane transduction receptors with the ability to promote a variety of signals to the cytoskeleton which activate many intracellular signaling pathways. An important property in the resistance to apoptosis is the ability of the beta1 integrin subunit (designated ITGB1 or Integrin β1) to bind extracellular domains and promote the formation of the Focal adhesion kinase-1 (FAK) complex. The FAK complex in turn results in activating the PI 3-kinase/Akt signaling pathway which promotes survival and delivers anti-apoptotic signals [49]. This raises the possibility that in the normal process of apoptosis there is a commitment by the apoptotic LN18 cells to degrade those surface determinants that promote survival signals and resistance to apoptosis.

Figure 2 and Figure 3 are both composites of flow cytometry histograms (Curves A, B and C) showing phycoerythrin fluorescence intensity vs. cell counts. The curves were obtained by using mouse primary IgG antibodies specific for the integrin in question followed by goat anti-mouse-IgG conjugated to phycoerythrin. The intent of Figure 2 is to illustrate the density of the integrin subunit IGA2 ($\alpha 2$) on the surface of the LN18 cell as the cell progresses through apoptosis. The subunit $\alpha 2$ in combination with the subunit ITGB1 (β1) forms the dimer receptor that binds collagen which is a ubiquitous extracellular matrix protein [50, 51].

Similarly to Figure 2, Figure 3 illustrates the density of the integrin subunit ITGB5 (β) on the surface of the LN18 cell vs. cell count as the cell progresses through apoptosis. The integrin subunit β5 in combination with αV recognizes the short motif Arg-Gly-Asp (RGD motif) which can be found in many proteins of the extracellular matrix [52]. Curves labeled A (green) of Figures 2 and 3 show the non-specific labeling that was obtained by using mouse anti-KLH as a primary antibody. Curves labeled B (purple) of Figures 2 and 3 indicate the fluorescence obtained by the mouse antibodies specific for each growth factor receptor for LN18 cells in mid apoptosis. For curves B, the cells were treated for 10h while in a monolayer with 50µM of MK886. The bimodal curve indicates that the population consists of cells that have high and low density of integrin determinants on the surface of the cells. Curves labeled C (red) indicate the fluorescence obtained by the mouse antibodies specific for each growth factor receptor for LN18 cells treated with MK886 for 15h. A clear down shift in the intensity of the growth factor histograms can be seen for the 15h MK886 treated cells (red) as compared to the cells treated for 10 h (purple). The down shift in integrin fluorescence intensities of the 15h MK886 treated cells fall almost completely into the region of non-specific binding indicating a high degree of degradation of the integrin determinants.

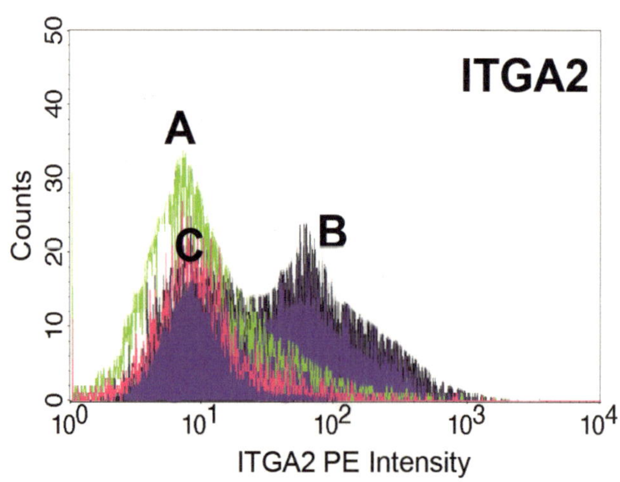

Figure 2. Flow cytometry histograms showing the density of integrin-α 5 on the surface of LN18 cells in mid and late apoptosis. Curve A: @KLH non-binding control. Curve B: bimodal histogram of LN18 cells in mid apoptosis. Curve C: LN18 cells in late apoptosis.

http://dx.doi.org/10.5772/52359

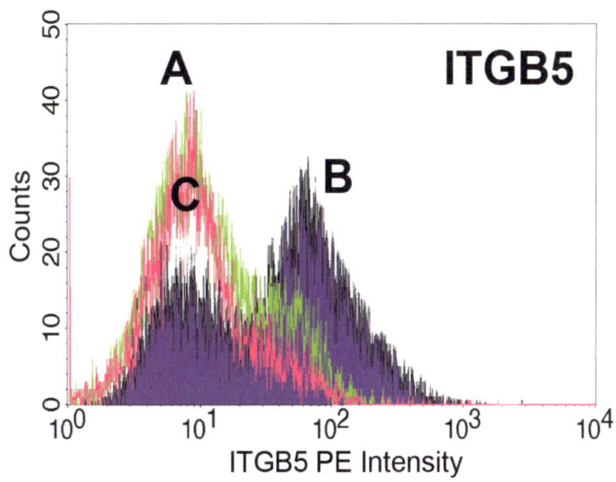

Figure 3. Flow cytometry histograms showing the density of integrin-β 5 on the surface of LN18 cells in mid and late apoptosis. Curve A: @KLH non-binding control. Curve B: bimodal histogram of LN18 cells in mid apoptosis. Curve C: LN18 cells in late apoptosis.

5.3. RT–PCR of integrins

It is possible that the observed decrease in the density of the integrins on the surface of the LN18 cells is due to a decrease in expression rather than a degradation of the integrin determinants. To answer this we measured the expression of a number of integrins in control LN18 cells as compared to apoptotic LN18 cells. Table 2 shows the results obtained by real time reverse transcriptase polymerase chain reaction (real time RT-PCR) as a measure of message for specific integrins. The data were obtained from an amplification plot of the fluorescence signal versus cycle number. The numbers in the columns of Table 2 show the cycles to threshold (Ct values) for β-actin and the specific integrin subunits listed in column 1. The β-actin was used as a housekeeping control. The data of Table 2 show the Ct value for non-treated LN18 cells (2nd column) and cells exposed to 50μM MK886 for 10h (3rd column). The changes in Ct values (ΔCt) for each mRNA were obtained by subtracting the Ct value of the DMSO control cells from the Ct value for the MK886 treated cells at 10h and 15h. The Ct values for β-actin and the integrin subunits increased by about a cycle indicating a slight decrease of message as the LN18 cells proceeded through apoptosis. This slight increase in cycle number to threshold could not account for the large decreases in surface integrins shown in Figures 2 and 3. A normed (ΔΔCt) was calculated for each sample by subtracting the ΔCt value of β-actin from the ΔCt value for the gene of interest. The Ct values for the calculation of the 10h ΔΔCt values (4th column) are shown above, but the Ct values at 15h for the calculation of the 15h ΔΔCt values (5th column) are not shown.

Gene Designation	Ct Control 10h	Ct MK886 10h	ΔΔCt MK886 10h	ΔΔCt MK886 15h
β- ACTIN (ACTB)	17	18	NA	NA
INTEGRIN-α 5 (ITGA5)	19	20	0	1
INTEGRIN-α V (ITGAV)	19	20	0	-1
INTEGRIN-β 1 (ITGB1)	19	20	0	0
INTEGRIN- β 3 (ITGB3)	23	24	0	0
INTEGRIN- β 5 (ITGB5)	20	21	0	1

Table 2. Effect of MK886 on the level of specific mRNAs in LN18 cells

5.4. Degradation of LN18 cell surface determinants is mediated by metalloproteinases

There is the question of whether the degradation of surface determinants due to apoptosis is specific or whether there is a gross loss of surface determinants as the cells progress through apoptosis. An additional question is, are there specific proteases that are activated that degrade the surface determinants of LN18 cells as they go into apoptosis? Human leukocyte antigens ABC (HLA-ABC) are within the major histocompatibility complex class1 and are virtually ubiquitous in tissues. Thus, the HLA-ABC complex was chosen to determine if they also are degraded in apoptotic cells and if the degradation can be reversed by various protease inhibitors.

The flow cytometry output of Table 3 was obtained by using mouse primary IgG antibodies specific for HLA-ABC determinants followed by goat @mouse IgG conjugated to phycoerythrin. The first column of Table 3 is a list of protease inhibitors. The numerical values within the columns of Table 3 represent the integrated fluorescence intensity of the phycoerythrin dye where a decrease in integrated intensity indicates a decrease in the density of HLA-ABC determinants on the surface of the LN18 cell. The data of Table 3 show that as LN18 cells progress through apoptosis, induced by 50μM of MK886, there is a decrease in the surface determinants of HLA-ABC as compared to vehicle control cells (2nd column vs. 3rd column). For the non-apoptotic controls (2nd column) the proteolytic inhibitors were added at 7h after the initiation of the incubation. For the apoptotic MK886 treated cells (3rd column) no proteolytic inhibitors were added. For the cells that had both MK886 and proteolytic inhibitor added, the proteolytic inhibitor was added 7h after the MK886 was added (4th column). The cells were allowed to incubate for an additional 6h after the addition of the protease inhibitors. It can be seen from the third column of Table 3 as compared to the second column that treatment with the matrix metalloproteinase inhibitors GM6001 and MM-2 MM-9 demonstrated a significant inhibition of the apoptotic loss of HLA-ABC determinants. Some of the proteasome inhibitors severely exacerbated the LN18 cell's loss of determinants while the calpain inhibitors had little to no effect. Similar effects were obtained for the cell surface receptors EGFR, INGF1-R and INGF2-R (not shown). Serine protease inhibitors such as aprotinin and soybean trypsin inhibitor partially reversed surface determinant degradation induced by apoptosis indicating that degradation of surface determinants is the result of a combination or interplay of serine proteases and metalloproteinases (not shown). The reversal of the degradation of cluster determinants by metalloproteinase inhibitors is relevant to the studies showing matrix metalloproteinase secretion from LN18 glioblastoma cells in suspension.

Type of Proteolytic Inhibitor	Control No MK886	MK886 50μM	50μM MK886 Plus Inhibitor
ZVAD-FMK (50μM)	3299	2001	2335
CALPAIN III (50μM)	3449	2465	2350
CALPEPTIN (50μM)	2690	1647	1425
MG-132 (50μM)	2858	1791	TOO LOW
PSI (50μM)	2880	2089	1003
GM6001 (10μM)	2907	1914	2854
MM-2 MM-9 (50μM)	3069	1722	2759
PD 150606 (50μM)	3822	2153	742
ALLN,MG101 (50μM)	3534	1795	211
ZVAD-FMK (50μM) Broad caspases inhibitor			
CALPAIN III (50μM) Inhibits calpain 1&2			
CALPEPTIN (50μM) Inhibits calpain 1&2 and papain			
MG-132 (50μM) Proteasome inhibitor that also inhibits NF-κB			
PSI (50μM) Proteasome inhibitor that also inhibits NF-κB and chymotrypsin			
GM6001 (10μM) Broad matrix metalloproteinase inhibitor			
MM-2 MM-9 (50μM) Broad matrix metalloproteinase inhibitor			
PD 150606 (50μM) Calpain 1 inhibitor: directed against the calcium binding site			
ALLN,MG101 (50μM) Inhibits Calpain 1&2 , cysteine proteases, proteasomes, IκB-α, IκB-β, ubiquitin-proteasome complexes, arrests cell cycle at G_1/S			

Table 3. Effect of Proteolytic Inhibitors upon Apoptotic Decrease of the HLA-ABC Determinants on the Surface of LN18 Cells

5.5. Apoptosis induced by MK886 and staurosporine in LN18 cells held in suspension and devoid of integrin signaling

The panels of Figure 4 are flow cytometry outputs and are plots of annexin conjugated to fluorescein isothiocyanate (annexinV-FITC) versus 7-amino-actinomycinD (7AAD) staining of the LN18 cells. The flow cytometry data of annexinV-FITC versus 7AAD is a classical test for apoptosis. The data of Figure 4 are a measure of the degree of apoptosis in LN18 glioblastoma cells while suspended in polyhema coated flasks. Panel A of Figure 4 illustrates vehicle control cells which were iced while in suspension and then immediately stained. Pharmacologically induced apoptosis of the suspended cells was brought about by treating the cells with 50μM of MK886 for 8h (panel B) and for 10h (panel C). Numbers denoted in quadrants of each panel represent the percentage of cells in each quadrant. Viable cells that are not positive for annexinV-FITC or 7AAD are neither apoptotic nor necrotic and are represented in the lower left quadrant. Necrotic cells devoid of apoptosis that stained positive for 7AAD, but not for annexinV-FITC, are represented in the upper left quadrant. Apoptotic cells devoid of necrosis that stained for annexinV-FITC, but not 7AAD, are in the lower right quadrant and late apoptotic/necrotic cells that stained for both annexinV-FITC and 7AAD are represented in the upper right quadrant. Panel A of Figure 4 shows that 90% of control cells are devoid of annexinV-FITC or 7AAD staining indicating no initial necrosis or apoptosis. LN18 cells in suspension devoid of extracellular signaling rapidly go into apoptosis. It can be seen that 67% of the cells are stained positive for annexinV-FITC by 6h (sum of the 2 right quadrants of panel B) due to treatment with MK886. When the LN18 cells are in suspension devoid of integrin signaling, they proceed into apoptosis much more rapidly than when in a monolayer. After 8h of stimulation with MK886, 77% of the cells stain positive with annexinV-FITC (sum of the 2 right quadrants of panel C). The data of Figure 4 are relevant to those experiments which show that LN18 cells rendered apoptotic while in suspension enhance the invasiveness of non-apoptotic LN18 cells.

Nucleosomes are essentially DNA-histone complexes which in non-apoptotic cells are confined to the nucleus. An additional well established test for apoptosis is the release of nucleosomes from the nucleus into the cytosol. To further demonstrate apoptosis for cells that lack integrin stimulation, LN18 cells were treated with a variety of concentrations of staurosporine while in suspension in polyhema coated flasks. The data of Table 4 show the results of assaying for the release of DNA-histone complexes from the nucleus into the cytosol for LN18 cells in polyhema coated flasks. The LN18 cells were treated with staurosporine at the concentrations indicated for 8h. The cells were then centrifuged and washed and then treated with lysis buffer. The supernatants of the lysed cells were then transferred to a streptavidin coated 96 well microtiter plates and tested for DNA-histone complexes by ELISA using anti-histone-biotin-antibody followed by peroxidase conjugated to anti-DNA. The development of peroxidase substrate was measured by reading a Dynatech Microplate Reader at 405nm. It can be seen that 1μM of staurosporine can induce the release of a significant amount of histone-associated DNA-fragments into the cytosol by 8h. Furthermore, the release of DNA fragments was inhibited by the broad caspases inhibitor ZVAD-FMK, indicating that staurosporine-induced degradation of DNA in LN18 cells is caspases dependent.

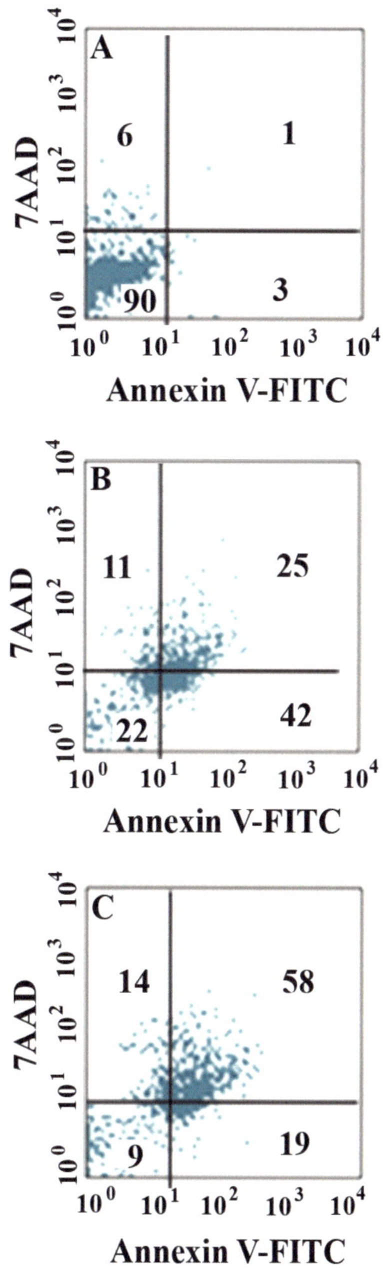

Figure 4. Flow cytometry data showing nuclear staining vs. translocated phosphatidylserine (PS) staining as LN18 cells proceed through MK886 induced apoptosis while in suspension and devoid of integrin stimulation.

Staurosporine Concentration	$A_{405\,nm}$	SD
Medium Control	0.145	+/-0.051
0.5 μM	0.297	+/-0.081
1.0 μM	0.643	+/-0.073
2.0 μM	0.862	+/-0.136
2.0 μM + 50μM ZVAD-FMK	0.197	+/-0.026

[1]LN18 cells were treated for 8h at indicated staurosporine concentrations.

Table 4. Apoptotic Release of Nucleosome from LN18 Cells Treated with Staurosporine while Suspended in Polyhema Coated Flasks[1]

The LN18 cells shown in the micrograph labeled Figure 5 were incubated in suspension with 1uM staurosporine for 6h. After the incubation the cells were harvested by centrifugation and then fixed in 70% ethanol. The cells were then centrifuged and washed and suspended in 2ml of phosphate buffered saline. For the assay 10ul of stock (0.1mg/ml) 4,6-diamidino-2-phenyl-indole (DAPI) was added to the 2ml PBS. After completion of the staining with DAPI, the cells were observed on a slide with an inverted microscope set for DAPI. The arrows of the micrograph labeled Figure 5 show nuclear condensation within LN18 cells. Nuclear condensation is another established indicator of apoptosis. The condensation correlates with the nucleosome release and is clear indication that both staurosporine and MK886 induce late apoptotic effects in LN18 cells that are not integrin stimulated as early as 8-10h.

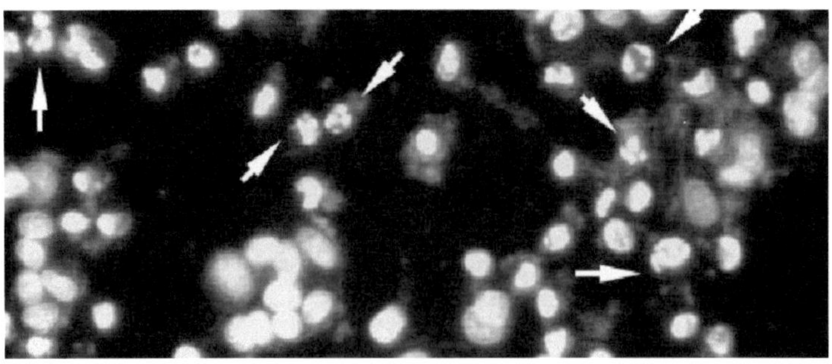

Figure 5. The arrows within the micrograph show nuclear condensation within LN18 cells in suspension upon the induction of apoptosis by treating the cells with 1μM Staurosporine for 6h.

5.6. LN18 cells that are devoid of integrin stimulation release matrix metalloproteinases

Cells held in suspension in polyhema coated flasks are devoid of those extracellular matrix transduction signals that are derived from cells bring stimulated by extracellular matrix proteins. The data of Figures 6 and 7 were accumulated by an ELISA technique as presented in the Methods. The data show the release of MMP13 (Figure 6) and the lack of release of MMP8 (Figure 7). The MMPs were released in the absence of pharmacological stimulation (MK886 or staurosporine) by LN18 glioblastoma cells when there is merely a loss of cell adhesion signals brought about by incubating the cells in suspension in polyhema coated flasks. The samples for the Figures 6 and 7 are as follows: Bar A is the medium control; Bar B is the supernatant of the ice control where the cells were suspended, but not allowed to progress at 37⁰C; Bars C through G illustrate dose responses for pure MMP13 (Figure 6) and pure MMP8 (Figure 7) which are 0.5ng/ml (Bar C), 1.0ng/ml (Bar D), 2.0ng/ml (Bar E), 4.0ng/ml (Bar F), and 6.0ng/ml (Bar G). Bars H through J are the supernatants of LN18 cells suspended in polyhema coated flasks at 1.5 x 10^6 cells/ml in Dulbecco's medium with 2% FBS for 2hrs (Bar H), 4hrs (Bar I), 6hrs (Bar J) at 37⁰C. Bar K is the response from LN18 cells held for 6hrs in suspension, but in the presence of 1.78 x 10^{-4} M cycloheximide. Other metalloproteinases released from LN18 cells while being held in suspension include MMP1, MMP2 and MMP3 (not shown).

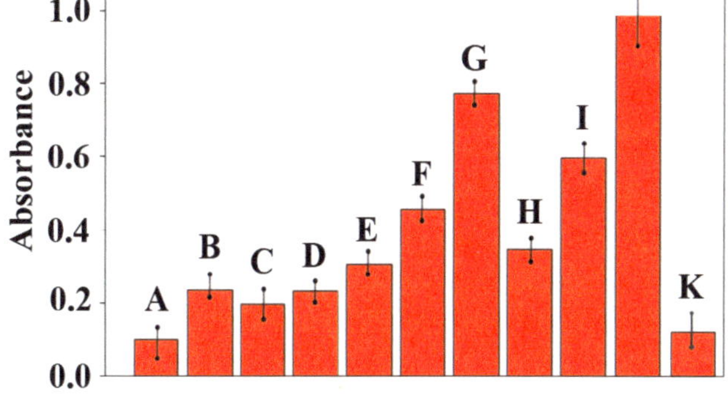

Figure 6. ELISA measurement of released MMP13 from LN18 cells in suspension. Bars A&B are controls. Bars C &D are the dose responses for pure MMP13. Bars H-J are measures of the MMP13 released from cells held in suspension for 2, 4 & 6h respectively. Bar K is the cycloheximide control at 6h.

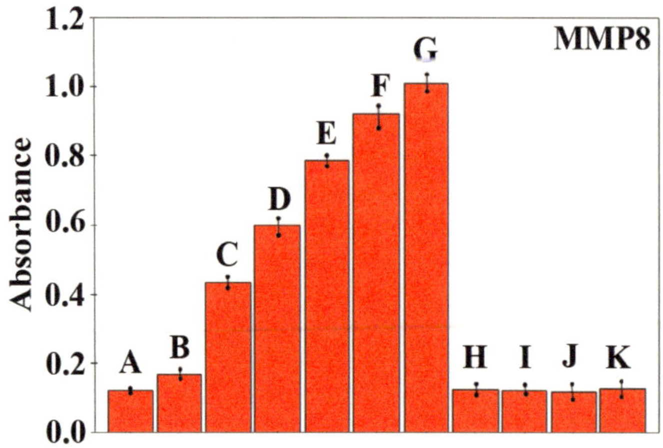

Figure 7. ELISA measurement of released MMP8 from LN18 cells in suspension. Bars A&B are controls. Bars C&D are the dose responses for pure MMP8. Bars H-J are measures of the MMP8 released from cells held in suspension for 2, 4 & 6h respectively. Bar K is the cycloheximide control at 6h.

As determined by RT-PCR there was a slight increase in message (one to two cycles) for the metalloproteinases shown in Figures 6 and 7 when the cells were held in suspension for 6h at 37ºC (not shown). Examining Bars H-J of Figure 6 as compared to cells not allowed to progress at 37ºC in suspension (ice control Bar B) it can be seen that there is a significant amount of MMP13 release from the LN18 cells held in suspension. Whether the zymogen form of the MMPs is stored in the cytosol was not determined but it appears from Bar K that, even if much of the metalloproteinase are stored in the cytosol prior to secretion, translation is essential indicating that the production of some type of protein is required for secretion to proceed. Figure 7 shows a lack of secretion of MMP8. In addition to MMP8, MMP7 and MMP9 were not secreted in amounts that were detectable (not shown).

5.7. Metalloproteinase inhibitors block the MMP activity released from LN18 cells held in suspension

The data of Figure 8 illustrate the inhibition of the total metalloproteinase activity released into the supernatant from LN18 cells held in suspension. The cells were incubated in polyhema coated flasks in the presence of DMEM supplemented with 1% FBS and growth hormones for 6hrs. As described in the Methods, the MMP activity in the supernatant of the suspended cells was measured fluorometrically using the broad MMP substrate QXL520 -Arg-Pro-Leu-Ala-Leu-Trp-Arg-Lys(5-FAM)-NH2. The total secreted metalloproteinase activity included a variety of MMPs secreted from the LN18 cells including that of MMP-1, -2, -3 (not shown) in addition to MMP13 (shown in Figure 6). Bar A is the metalloproteinase activity of the supernatant of cells left on ice (control blank). Bar B is supernatant of the 6hr incubation positive control showing the secreted enzymatic activity tested in the absence of inhibitors. For the remaining samples, the supernatant of the 6hr suspended cells containing the secreted

http://dx.doi.org/10.5772/52359

metalloproteinases was tested for enzymatic activity in the presence of the following inhibitors: 10mM EDTA (Bar C); 5mM EDTA (Bar D); 5mM of the zinc chelator 1,10 phenanthroline (Bar E); 2.5mM of 1,10 phenanthroline (Bar F); 50μM of the broad metalloproteinase inhibitor GM6001 (Bar G); and, 25μM of GM6001 (Bar H). Bar I shows the effect of the solvent isopropyl alcohol (12.5%), which was used to dissolve the 1,10 phenanthroline. Bar J shows the effect of the solvent DMSO (12.5%), which was used to dissolve the GM6001. The data indicate that metalloproteinases secreted from the suspended LN18 cells have enzymatic activity that was inhibited by a variety of known MMP inhibitors.

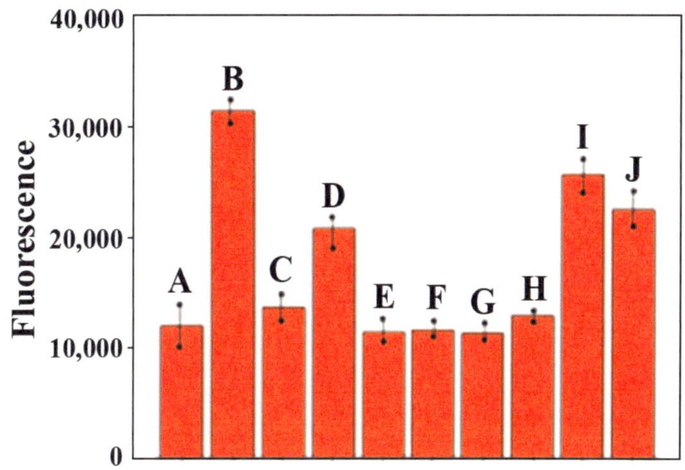

Figure 8. Inhibition of metalloproteinase activity secreted from LN18 cells. Bar A is the non-releasing ice control. Bar B is the non-inhibited sample. Bars C-H show reduced activity by a variety of known metalloproteinase inhibitors. Bars I & J are solvent controls.

5.8. Effect of apoptotic LN18 cells upon the invasiveness of non–apoptotic LN18 cells

The invasiveness was measured *in vitro* using a BD Falcon matrigel matrix system. This system consists of a 24-multiwell plate where each well has an insert consisting of an 8.0μ pore size polyethylene terephthalate (PET) membrane that has been uniformly coated with a layer of matrigel which serves as a reconstituted matrix *in vitro.* The coating procedure occludes the pores of the PET membrane. Those cells capable of degrading the matrigel coating of the PET membrane will migrate through the 8.0μ pores of the PET membrane. For clarification, a diagram of one well of the 24 well plate matrigel system is shown in Figure 9.

The system requires a chemoattractant in the lower chamber. Constituents within fetal bovine serum (FBS) are known to act as chemoattractants, which enables the cells to migrate from the serum free upper chamber toward the lower chamber. Various concentrations of FBS were tested and it was determined that 0.5% FBS in Dulbecco's medium was an effective concentration (not shown). The invasive cells are stained with the lipophilic fluorescent dye DiI (Molecular Probes). Since the PET membrane effectively blocks the passage of light from

490-700nm at >99% efficiency, only those stained cells that pass through the PET membrane were detected. Fluorescently-labeled cells that have not passed through the matrigel and the PET membrane were not detected by the bottom reading fluorescent plate reader. Invasiveness was monitored using a FLUOStar OPTIMA plate reading fluorometer at an Ex/Em=549nm/565nm for 2h at 37°C. It was determined that $2x10^5$ stained LN18 cells in the upper chamber that were capable of migrating into the lower chamber gave a strong fluorometric signal.

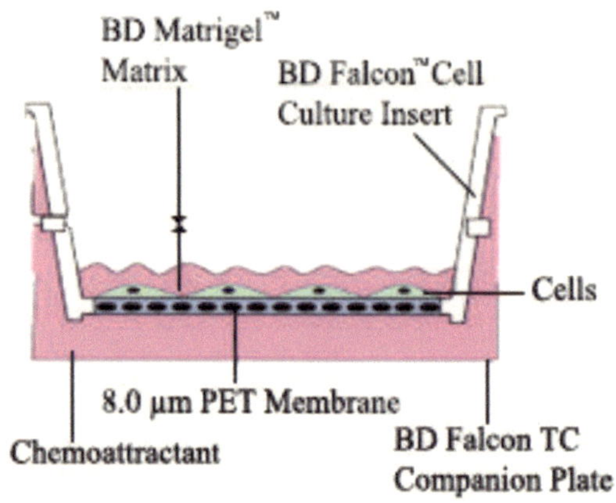

Figure 9. Diagram of one well of the 24 well plate matrigel system.

The intent of using the matrigel invasive system was to measure the effect various numbers of apoptotic LN18 cells have upon the invasiveness of a fixed number of stained non-apoptotic LN18 cells. Figure 10 shows the effect of combining in the upper chamber a variety of apoptotic LN18 cells upon $2x10^5$ of the invasive, non-apoptotic, Dil stained LN18 cells. Before mixing the two cell populations apoptosis was induced separately from the non-apoptotic cell population. The apoptotic population was obtained by stimulating the LN18 cells with 1µM of staurosporine for 8h. The apoptotic LN18 cells were then washed but not stained. The non-apoptotic cells were stained with DiI and the mixtures of the non-apoptotic and apoptotic cells were aliquoted into the upper chambers in Dulbecco's medium supplemented with growth factors and 0.5% bovine serum albumin (BSA) but devoid of FBS. Dulbecco's medium supplemented with 0.5% FBS was the chemoattractant within the lower chamber. Samples A through D represent the following cell mixtures where in each case only the $2x10^5$ non-apoptotic cell populations were stained with DiI. Sample A is $1.7x10^5$ unstained apoptotic LN18 cells + $2x10^5$ non-apoptotic dil stained LN18 cells with no FBS in the lower chamber (no chemoattractant control). Sample B is $1.7x10^5$ unstained non-apoptotic LN18 cells + $2x10^5$ non-apoptotic Dil stained LN18 cells (non-apoptotic equal cell count control). Sample C is $2.7x10^5$ unstained apoptotic LN18 cells + $2x10^5$ non-apoptotic Dil stained LN18 cells. Sample D is $4.7x10^5$ unstained apoptotic LN18 cells + $2x10^5$ non-apoptotic Dil stained LN18 cells. Only sample A was devoid of FBS in the lower chamber. It can be seen from samples C and D of Figure 10 that increasing populations of apoptotic LN18 cells enhance the invasiveness of the of the non-apoptotic LN18 cells.

http://dx.doi.org/10.5772/52359

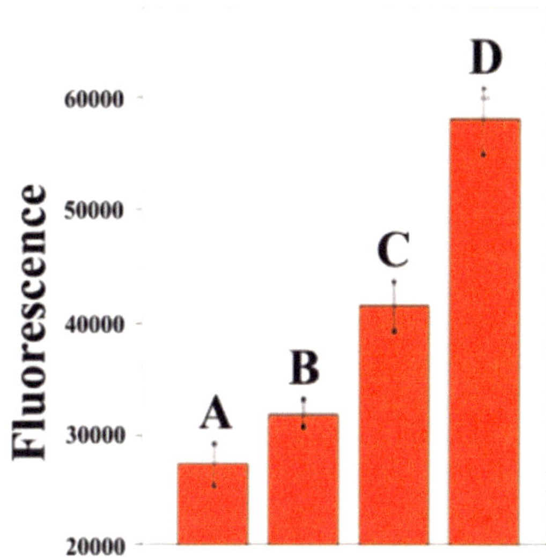

Figure 10. Enhanced invasiveness of non-apoptotic LN18 cells by the presences of apoptotic LN18 cells. Bar A no chemoattractant control. Bar B invasiveness of non-apoptotic cells in the absence of apoptotic cells. Bars C&D increased invasiveness of the non-apoptotic cells by increasing populations of apoptotic cells.

6. Conclusions

The main focus of this report was examining the effects of apoptotic glioblastoma cells upon the non-apoptotic glioblastoma cell population. Overall, the data show that the effects are in large part mediated by metalloproteinases.

A summary of the findings of this study are as follows:

- Apoptosis induced in LN18 cells, that are in a monolayer and integrin stimulated, is accompanied by an enhanced activation of metalloproteinases on the surface of the LN18 cells.
- Matrix metalloproteinases are secreted from LN18 cells that are in suspension and devoid of integrin signals, even in the absence of the pharmacological stimulation of apoptosis.
- The matrix metalloproteinase released from LN18 cells can be made to exhibit enzymatic activity which is reversed by metalloproteinase inhibitors.
- As LN18 glioblastoma cells progress through apoptosis, there is a degradation of surface determinants including, growth factor receptors, histocompatibility markers such as HLA-ABC, and a variety of cluster determinant including alpha and beta integrins. The degradation takes place in mid to late apoptosis. Metalloproteinase inhibitors blocked the degradation of surface determinants even when added after the cells where fully committed to apoptosis.

- By the use of Real-Time RT-PCR, it was determined that, overall, the down-regulation of surface proteins that takes place in late apoptosis is not mediated by an interruption of transcription mechanisms.
- Apoptotic LN18 glioblastoma cells when mixed with non-apoptotic LN18 cells enhance the invasiveness of the non-apoptotic LN18 cells

As aforementioned, when a malignancy is diagnosed and is subjected to primary treatment some of the cells will be more resistant to apoptosis than others which will inherently result in a mixture of apoptotic and viable non-apoptotic tumor cells. The existence of a mixture of apoptotic and non-apoptotic tumor cells is particularly true during recurrence and the required therapy that inevitably induces apoptosis which leads to a population of apoptotic cells within the tumor. As treatment progresses beyond the primary stage, mutated cells and resistant cells that escape apoptosis will proliferate. Thus, the sustained cell population of a tumor will consist of non-apoptotic cells capable of invading surrounding tissue while coexisting with a dying population of apoptotic cells. This view that recurrent GBM tumors consist of cells that are refractory to treatment while being highly invasive, and exist as a mixed population of apoptotic and non-apoptotic cells, was the stimulus for this study.

There have been elegant studies comparing non-cancerous glial cells to gliomas and demonstrating elevated membrane-type metalloproteinases in gliomas [53]. There are also studies demonstrating membrane-type metalloproteinases expression and function during glioma invasion [54, 55]. These studies have provided a footing and direction for this present study. The important idea here is that there are metalloproteinase activating processes that are taking place in apoptotic and anoikic cells. What is different about the approach proposed here is that we are not comparing glioma cells to normal glial cells, but rather investigating the presence of, and activity of, metalloproteinases in glioma cells as they progress through apoptosis.

It can be concluded from the data of this report that the membrane bound metalloproteinases in LN18 glioblastoma cells are surprisingly active during the late phases of pharmacologically induced apoptosis. In addition, matrix metalloproteinases are secreted from LN18 glioblastoma cells in early anoikis. One of the hallmarks for the induction of anoikis is the absence of cell adhesion signals. It can be assumed that the secreted matrix metalloproteinases, when activated, have effects on the pericellular matrix and adjacent cells. Even if the anoikic cells are apoptotic resistant, because metalloproteinases are secreted in early anoikis, apoptotic resistant cells devoid of adhesion signals could have the capacity to affect the surrounding matrix and nearby cells.

Most metalloproteinases are synthesized and secreted in a latent zymogen form. Furin-like proteases are known to act as sheddases acting on membrane type metalloproteinases [56]. Also there are type II transmembrane serine proteases (TTSPs), and possibly other proteases, present on the surface of glioma cells [57-59]. From the data presented here, it is reasonable to suspect that during the process of apoptosis there are secreted furins and possibly membrane-bound TTSPs that are capable of converting latent membrane bound or secreted metalloproteinases to their active form.

To reiterate, the conventional assumption is that ongoing apoptosis within a malignant tumor is desirable with no effects that may be harmful to the patient. What has been presented here

http://dx.doi.org/10.5772/52359

raises the possibility that within the mixed cell population of LN18 glioma cells and non-apoptotic LN18 cells, the apoptotic dying cells are capable of enhancing the invasiveness of the LN18 cells that are not apoptotic. As far as we know, investigating the invasive synergy between a mixture of apoptotic and non-apoptotic cells is somewhat neglected as an approach. The data of this study can be distinctive and be complementary to other studies directed toward the long standing problem of the malignant invasiveness of high grade gliomas.

7. Future studies

We look to identify which membrane type metalloproteinases (MT-MMPs and ADAMs) are on the surface of the LN18 glioblastoma cells and whether there is an increase in synthesis and their presence during apoptosis. One would surmise that inhibition of metalloproteinase activity would be an effective clinical treatment. There have been a good number of clinical trials for a variety of cancers determining the effectiveness of metalloproteinase inhibition upon patient improvement and survival rates [60-65] Unfortunately such studies have been disappointing particularly those clinical trials that have focused on glioblastomas [66,67]. The role of metalloproteinases with regard to invasiveness of GBM appears to be more complex than the ability of metalloproteinases to degrade the extracellular matrix (ECM). The experiments presented here raise questions about the role of furins, serine proteases, anoikis and apoptosis and their interrelationship to metalloproteinases and invasiveness. To expand upon the ideas presented here there is a need to determine whether the synthesis, secretion and presence of furins and TTSPs increase with apoptosis and whether these proteases are responsible for the activation of the latent zymogen form of metalloproteinases. Investigating the interplay between furins, TTSPs and the increased presence and activation of metalloproteinases during apoptosis in the context of the ability of apoptotic glioblastoma cells to enhance the invasiveness and motility of glioblastoma cells is a natural extension of what was presented here. Of particular interest is whether the apoptotic cells are acting on the extracellular matrix or there are direct effects upon the invading non-apoptotic cells. Findings utilizing the LN18 glioblastoma cell line will need to be tested in a variety of available glioma cell lines.

Acknowledgements

Supported by NIH Grant 5P20RR016477 to the West Virginia IDeA Network for Biomedical Research Excellence

Author details

Albert Magro*

Department of Biology Fairmont State University, Fairmont, West Virginia, USA

References

[1] Surawicz TS, Davis F, Freels S, Laws Jr, ER, Menck H R. Brain tumor survival: results from the national cancer data base. Journal of Neuro-Oncology 1998;40:151–160.

[2] Yung WK, Albright RE, Olson J, et al. A phase II study of temozolomide vs. carbazine in patients with glioblastoma multiforme at first relapse. British Journal of Cancer 2000;83:588-593.

[3] Kanu OO, Mehta A, Di C, Lin N, Bortoff K, Bigner DD, Yan H, Adamson DC. Glioblastoma multiforme: a review of therapeutic targets. Expert Opinion on Therapeutic Targets. 2009;13:701-18.

[4] Salvati, M, D'Elia, A, Formichella, AI, and Frati, A. Insights into pharmacotherapy of malignant glioma in adults. Expert Opinion Pharmacotherapy 2009;10(14) 2279-2290.

[5] Minniti,G, Muni, R, Lanzetta, G. Marchetti, P, and Enrici, RM. Chemotherapy for glioblastoma: current treatment and future perspectives for cytotoxic and targeted agents Anticancer Research 2009;12 5171-5184.

[6] Stupp R, Mason WP, van den Bent MJ, Weller M, Fisher B, & Taphoorn MJ, et. al. Radiotherapy plus concomitant and adjuvant temozolomide for glioblastoma. *New England Journal of Med.* 2005;352(10): 987-996.

[7] Lo, HW. EGFR-targeted therapy in malignant glioma: novel aspects and mechanisms of drug resistance. Current Molecular Pharmacology 2010;3(1) 37-52.

[8] Salacz ME, Watson KR, Schomas DA. Glioblastoma. Part II: Future directions. Mo Med. 2011;108:289-291.

[9] Jain A, Lai JCK, Chowdhury GMI, Behar K and Bhushan A. Glioblastoma: Current Chemotherapeutic Status and Need for New Targets and Approaches in Brain Tumors. In: Abujarma, AL. (ed.) Current and Emerging Therapeutic Strategies 2011. p146-176.

[10] Kerr JF, Wyllie AH, Currie AR. Apoptosis: a basic biological phenomenon with wide-ranging implications in tissue kinetics. British Journal of Cancer 1972;26(4): 239–257.

[11] Elmore, S. Apoptosis: A Review of Programmed Cell Death. Toxicologic Pathology 2007;35(4): 495–516.

[12] Giese A, Bjerkvig R, Berens ME, Westphal M. Cost of migration: invasion of malignant gliomas and implications for treatment. Journal of Clinical Oncology 2003;21: 1624-1636.

[13] Werb Z. ECM and cell surface proteolysis: regulating cellular ecology. Cell 1997;91: 439-442.

[14] Mott JD, Werb Z. Regulation of matrix biology by matrix metalloproteinases. Current Opinion in Cell Biology 2004;16: 558-564.

[15] Handsley MM, Edwards DR. Metalloproteinases and their inhibitors in tumor angiogenesis. International Journal of Cancer 2005;115: 849-860.

[16] Egeblad M, Werb Z. New functions for the matrix metalloproteinases in cancer progression. Nature Reviews Cancer 2002;2: 161-174.

[17] Massova I, Kotra LP, Fridman R, Mobashery S. Matrix metalloproteinases: Structures, evolution, and diversification. The FASEB Journal 1998;12: 1075–95.

[18] Nagase H, Woessner Jr JF. Matrix Metalloproteinases. Journal of Biological Chemistry 1999;274(31): 21491–21494.

[19] Seiki, M. Membrane-type 1 matrix metalloproteinase: A key enzyme for tumor invasion. Cancer Letters 2003;194(1): 1–11.

[20] Sohail A, Sun Q, Zhao H, Bernardo MM, Cho JA, Fridman R. MT4-(MMP17) and MT6-MMP (MMP25), A unique set of membrane-anchored matrix metalloproteinases: properties and expression in cancer. Cancer Metastasis Review 2008;27: 289-302.

[21] Edwards DR, Handsley MM, Pennington CJ. The ADAM metalloproteinases. Molecular Aspects of Medicine 2008;5: 258-89.

[22] Tang BL. ADAMTS: a novel family of extracellular matrix proteases. International Journal of Biochemistry and Cell Biology 2001; 33: 33-44.

[23] Hua H, Li M, Luo T, Yin Y, Jiang Y. Matrix metalloproteinases in tumorigenesis: an evolving paradigm. Cellular and Molecular Life Sciences 2001;68(23): 3853-68.

[24] Deryugina EI, Quigley JP. Pleiotropic roles of matrix metalloproteinases in tumor angiogenesis: Contrasting, overlapping and compensatory functions. Biochimica et Biophysica Acta 2010;1803(1): 103–120.

[25] Handsley MM, Edwards DR. Metalloproteinases and their inhibitors in tumor angiogenesis. International Journal of Cancer 2005;115: 849-860.

[26] Gialeli C, Theocharis AD, Karamanos NK. Roles of matrix metalloproteinases in cancer progression and their pharmacological targeting. FEBS Journal 2011;278(1): 16-27.

[27] Brew K, Nagase H. The tissue inhibitors of metalloproteinases (TIMPs): an ancient family with structural and functional diversity. Biochimica et Biophysica Acta 2010;1803: 55-71.

[28] Frisch SM, Francis H. Disruption of epithelial cell-matrix interactions induces apoptosis. Journal of Cell Biology 1994;124(4): 619–626.

[29] Frisch SM, Screaton RA. Anoikis mechanisms. Current Opinion Cell Biology 2001;(5): 555-62.

[30] Taddei ML, Giannoni E, Fiaschi T, Chiarugi P. Anoikis: an emerging hallmark in health and diseases. Journal of Pathology 2012;226(2): 380–393.

[31] Simpson CD, Anyiwe K, Schimmer AD. Anoikis resistance and tumor metastasis. Cancer Letters 2008;272(2): 177–185.

[32] Kim Y-N, Koo KH, Sung JY, Yun U-J, Kim H. Anoikis Resistance: An Essential Prerequisite for Tumor Metastasis. International Journal of Cell Biology 2012; Article ID 306879, 11 page doi:10.1155/2012/306879.

[33] Diserens AC, de Tribolet N, Martin-Achard A, et al. Characterization of an established human malignant glioma cell line: LN-18. Acta Neuorpathologic 1981;53: 21-28.

[34] Kehrer JP, Biswal SS, Thuillier P, Datta K, Fischer SM, Vanden Heuvel JP. Inhibition of peroxisome-proliferator-activated receptor (PPAR) alpha by MK886. Biochemical Journal 2001;356: 899-906.

[35] Vegesna RV, Wu HL, Mong S, Crooke ST. Staurosporine inhibits protein kinase C and prevents phorbol ester-mediated eukotriene D4 receptor desensitization in RBL-1 cells. Molecular Pharmacology 1988;33(5): 537-542.

[36] Datta K, Biswal SS, Kehrer JP. The 5-lipoxygenase-activating protein (FLAP) inhibitor, MK886, induces apoptosis ndependently of FLAP. Biochemistry Journal 1999;340(2): 371–375.

[37] Anderson KM, Seed T, Jajeh A, Dudeja P, Byun T, Meng J, Ou D, Bonomi P, Harris JE. An in vivo inhibitor of 5-lipoxygenase, MK886, at micromolar concentration induces apoptosis in U937 and CML cells. Anticancer Research 1996;16(5A): 2589-2599.

[38] Lim JY, Oh JH, Jung JR, Kim SM, Ryu CH, Kim HT, Jeun SS. MK886-induced apoptosis depends on the 5-LO expression level n human malignant glioma cells. Journal of Neuro-Oncology 2010;97(3): 339-46.

[39] Belmokhtar CA, Hillion J, Ségal-Bendirdjian E. Staurosporine induces apoptosis through both caspase-dependent and caspase-independent mechanisms. *Oncogene* 2001;20: 3354-3362.

[40] Kabir J, Lobo M, Zachary I. Staurosporine induces endothelial cell apoptosis via focal adhesion kinase dephosphorylation and focal adhesion disassembly independent of focal adhesion kinase proteolysis. Journal of Biochemistry 2002;367: 145-155.

[41] Gong JP, Traganos F, Darzynkiewicz Z. A Selective Procedure for DNA Extraction from Apoptotic Cells Applicable for Gel Electrophoresis and Flow Cytometry. Analytical Biochemistry 1994;218(2): 314–319.

[42] D'Amours D, Desnoyers S, D'Silva I, Poirier GG. Poly(ADP-ribosyl)ation reactions in the regulation of nuclear functions. Biochemical Journal 1999;342(2): 249-268.

[43] Amé JC, Spenlehauer C, de Murcia G. The PARP superfamily. Bioessays. 2004;26(8): 882-93.

[44] Simbulan-Rosenthal CM, Rosenthal DS, Iyer S, Boulares AH, Smulson ME. Transient poly(ADP-ribosyl)ation of nuclear proteins and role of poly(ADP-ribose) polymerase in the

[45] Magro AM, Magro AD, Cunningham C, Miller MR. Down-regulation of vinculin upon MK886-induced apoptosis in LN18 glioblastoma cells. Neoplasma 2007;54(6): 517-526.

[46] Hynes, R.O. Integrins: a family of cell surface receptors. Cell 1987;48: 549–554.

[47] Hynes, R.O. Integrins: versatility, modulation, and signaling in cell adhesion. Cell 1992;69, 11–25.

[48] Hynes, R.O. Integrins: Bidirectional, Allosteric Signaling Machines. Cell 2002; 673–687.

[49] Kennedy SG, Wagner AJ, Conzev S, et. al. The PI 3- kinase/Akt signaling pathway delivers an anti-apoptotic signal. Genes and Development 1997;11: 701-713.

[50] Hemler ME. Integrin associated proteins. Current Opinion Cell Biology 1998;10: 578–585.

[51] Plow EF, Haas TA, Zhang L, Loftus J, Smith JW. Ligand binding to integrins. Journal of Biological Chemistry 2000;275: 21785–21788.

[52] van der Flier A, Sonnenberg A. Function and interactions of integrins. Cell Tissue Research 2001;305: 285–298.

[53] Nuttall RK, Pennington CJ, Taplin J, Wheal A, Yong VW, Forsyth PA, Edwards DR. (2003) Elevated membrane-type matrix metalloproteinases in gliomas revealed by profiling proteases and inhibitors in human cancer cells. Molecular Cancer Research 2003;1: 333-45.

[54] Belien AT, Paganetti PA, Schwab ME. Membranetype1 matrix metalloprotease (MT1-MMP) enables invasive migration of glioma cells in central nervous system white matter. Journal of Cell Biology 1999;144: 373–384.

[55] Fillmore HL, VanMeter TE, Broaddus WC. Membrane-type matrix metalloproteinases (MTMMPs):expression and function during glioma invasion. Journal of Neuro-Oncology 2001;53: 187-202.

[56] Wang X, Pei D. Shedding of membrane type matrix metalloproteinase by a furin-type convertase: a potential mechanism for down-regulation. Journal of Biological Chemistry 2001;276(38): 35953-35960.

[57] Hooper JD, Clements JA, Quigley JP, Antalis TM. Type II transmembrane serine proteases. Insights into an emerging class of cell surface proteolytic enzymes. Journal of Biological Chemistry 2001;276: 857-860.

[58] Netzel-Arnett S, Hooper JD, Szabo R, Madison EL, Quigley JP, Bugge TH, Antalis TM. Membrane anchored serine proteases: a rapidly expanding group of cell surface

proteolytic enzymes with potential roles in cancer. Cancer Metastasis Review 2003;22: 237-258.

[59] Bugge, TH, Antalis,TM, Wu Q. Type II Transmembrane Serine Proteases. The Journal of Biological Chemistry 2009;284: 23177-23181.

[60] Wojtowicz-Praga S, Torri J, Johnson M, Steen V, Marshall J, Ness E, Dickson R, Sale M, Rasmussen HS, Chiodo TA, Hawkins MJ. Phase I trial of Marimastat, a novel matrix metalloproteinase inhibitor, administered orally to patients with advanced lung cancer. Journal of Clinical Oncology 1998;16: 2150-2156.

[61] Bramhall SR, Rosemurgy A, Brown PD, Bowry C, Buckels JA. Marimastat as first-line therapy for patients with unresectable pancreatic cancer: A randomized trial. Journal of Clinical Oncology 2001;19: 3447-3455.

[62] Bramhall SR, Schulz J, Nemunaitis J, Brown PD, Baillet M, Buckels JA. A double-blind placebo-controlled, randomized study comparing gemcitabine and marimastat with gemcitabine and placebo as first line therapy in patients with advanced pancreatic cancer. British Journal of Cancer 2002;87: 161-167.

[63] Bramhall SR, Hallissey MT, Whiting J, Scholefield J, Tierney G, Stuart RC, Hawkins RE, McCulloch P, Maughan T, Brown PD, Baillet M and Fielding JWL. Marimastat as maintenance therapy for patients with advanced gastric cancer: A randomized trial. British Journal of Cancer 2002;86: 1864-1870.

[64] Miller KD, Gradishar W, Schuchter L, Sparano JA, Cobleigh M, Robert N, Rasmussen H and Sledge GW. A randomized phase II pilot trial of adjuvant marimastat in patients with early-stage breast cancer. Annals of Oncology 2002;13: 1220-1224.

[65] Sparano JA, Bernardo P, Stephenson P, Gradisha WJ, Ingle JN, Zucker S and Davidson NE. Randomized Phase III Trial of Marimastat Versus Placebo in Patients With Metastatic Breast Cancer Who Have Responding or Stable Disease After First-Line Chemotherapy: Eastern Cooperative Oncology GroupTrial E2196. Journal of Clinical Oncology 2004;22(5): 4683-4690.

[66] Groves MD, Puduvalli VK, Hess KR, Jaeckle KA, Peterson P, Yung WKA and Levin VA. Phase II Trial of Temozolomide Plus the Matrix Metalloproteinase Inhibitor, Marimastat, in Recurrent and Progressive Glioblastoma Multiforme. Journal of Clinical Oncology 2002;20(5): 1383-1388.

[67] Levin VA, Phuphanich S, Yung WKA, Forsyth PA, Del Maestro R, Perry JR, Fuller GN and Baillet M. Randomized, double-blind, placebo-controlled trial of marimastat in glioblastoma multiforme patients following surgery and irradiation. Journal of Neuro-Oncology 2006;78(3): 295-302.

Chapter 10

The Distribution and Significance of IDH Mutations in Gliomas

Marta Mellai, Valentina Caldera,
Laura Annovazzi and Davide Schiffer

Additional information is available at the end of the chapter

http://dx.doi.org/10.5772/52357

1. Introduction

The discovery of somatic isocitrate dehydrogenase (IDH) mutations in gliomas is an example of the powerful impact of the next-generation sequencing on the comprehension of both tumor biology and human diseases.

IDHs catalyze the oxidative decarboxylation of isocitrate to α-ketoglutarate with production of NADH/NADPH. Thus, they are key enzymes in the Krebs cycle. For this family of metabolic genes, no previous role in human cancer has been described. However, in a recent genome-wide study, recurrent somatic mutations in the IDH1 gene have been identified in patients affected by Glioblastoma Multiforme (GBM) [1]. In successive studies, IDH mutations have also been found in low-grade gliomas, as well as in acute myeloid leukemia.

The aim of this chapter is to review the findings on the epidemiology and significance of IDH mutations in human gliomas, from the discovery to the current knowledge about their molecular pathogenesis.

Special attention will be paid to the powerful diagnostic and prognostic relevance of the IDH mutations in the clinical practice of neuro-oncology.

2. Function of isocitrate dehydrogenases

2.1. Isocitrate dehydrogenase enzymatic activity and structure

IDHs are enzymes catalyzing the oxidative decarboxylation of isocitrate to α-ketoglutarate (α-KG) in the Krebs cycle. During this process, NAD^+ or $NADP^+$ are respectively reduced to

NADH or NADPH, depending on the isoform that catalyzes the reaction. A scheme of this reaction is shown in Figure 1. In mammalian tissues, three different isoforms have been described: cytosolic NADP(+)-specific IDH (IDH1), mitochondrial NADP(+)-specific IDH (IDH2), and mitochondrial NAD(+)-specific IDH (IDH3).

The IDH1 and IDH2 isoforms are structurally related with 70% of sequence identity [2]. Both function as homodimers, are NADP+ dependent [3] and show a moderate expression in a variety of tissues, including brain [4]. IDH1 is active in cytosol and peroxisomes [5] while IDH2 has a mitochondrial localization [6].

The IDH3 isoform is NAD^+ dependent, functions as heterodimer and is structurally unrelated to IDH1 and IDH2 [7,8]. It is composed of three subunits (α, β and γ) organized in a multi-tetrameric structure (2α, 1β and 1γ). α-subunit has a catalytic function whereas β- and γ-subunits have a regulatory function [9,10]. IDH3 is localized in the mitocondria [11].

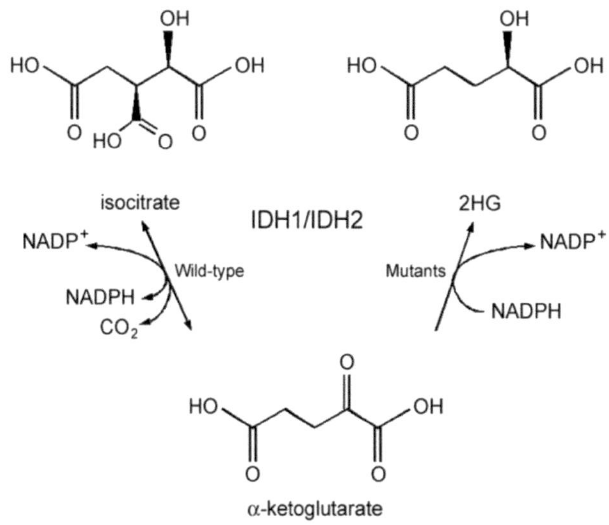

Figure 1. Enzymatic activity of wild-type and mutant IDH isoforms.

The activity of IDH1 and IDH2 in normal cells is regulated by the availability of substrate and cofactors. A key feature of this kinetic regulatory mechanism is the directionality of the enzymatic activity. Reactions catalyzed by IDH1 and IDH2 are reversible but not the similar reaction catalyzed by IDH3.

The crystal structure of mammalian IDH1 and IDH2 enzymes is well-known [2,12]. The structure of the wild-type IDH1 homodimer is reported in Figure 2.

In the IDH1 homodimer, each homolog comprises a large domain, a clasp domain and a small domain. Each homodimer contains two asymmetric and identical active sites, each composed of a cleft formed by the large and small domain of the other IDH1 homolog. The active sites are exposed to solvent and are accessible to the substrate and cofactors. The clasp holds the two subunits together to form the active site. IDH1 shifts between an inactive open, a transitional semi-open and a catalytically active closed conformation. It dimerizes with two active sites in the inactive open conformation, which is maintained by intramolecular interactions between Ser94 and Asp279 residues, blocking access to the active site. Asp279 resides in the position where the isocitrate normally forms hydrogen bonds with Ser94. During the two-step catalysis of the oxidative decarboxylation of isocitrate to α-KG, IDH1 adopts the active closed conformation where the steric hindrance by Asp279 to magnesium (Mg^{2+})-isocitrate complex binding is relieved and the latter binds between the large and small domains of the enzyme [2]. The reaction proceeds with production of α-KG and NADPH, followed by either the reoccupation of the active site by another Mg^{2+}-isocitrate complex or by restoring Ser94-Asp279 interactions in the inactive open conformation.

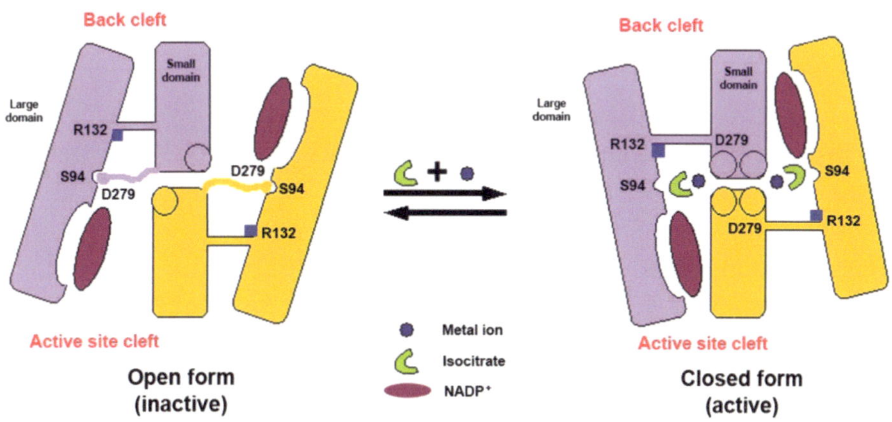

Figure 2. Structure of the wild-type IDH1 homodimer.

2.2. Function of isocitrate dehydrogenases in cellular metabolism

IDHs play prominent but distinctive roles in a variety of cellular metabolic functions [13]. The main functions of IDH1 are the lipid synthesis and the cellular glucose sensing [14] while IDH2 participates in the control of both the mitochondrial redox balance and cellular oxidative damage [15]. IDH3 plays an integral role in cellular energy metabolism.

In addition, IDHs contribute to the cellular protection generating the reducing equivalent NAPDH and, on the other hand, they regulate the function of a variety of α-KG-dependent processes [16-18]. Several cellular enzymes use α-KG, partially produced by IDH reactions with isocitrate, as co-substrate. α-KG is required for the optimal function of 5-methylcytosine (5mC) hydroxylases and histone methyltransferases that are crucial in the regulation of epigenetic processes [18-22].

Likewise, α-KG plays an important role in the degradation of hypoxia-inducible factor-1 alpha (HIF-1α), through a prolyl hydroxylase domain-containing protein (PHD)-mediated pathway [23], and in the glia-specific glutamine and glutamate metabolism [24].

2.3. Function of isocitrate dehydrogenases in response to oxidative stress

In mammalian cells, the activity of IDHs increases in response to a variety of oxidative insults, with concomitant decrease of IDH3, α-KG dehydrogenase and succinate dehydrogenase functions [13]. NADPH plays a major role in the cellular protection against oxidative damage due to free oxygen radicals, and from both gamma and ultraviolet radiations [16,17,25,26]. It is also essential for the regeneration of glutathione (GSH) that neutralizes free radicals and reactive oxygen species (ROS), and for the activity of the thioredoxin system. Although the pentose phosphate pathway is the main source of NADPH, IDH1 and IDH2 enzymes are as much important.

Further evidences do exist for their role in cell protection from different insults. IDH1 and IDH2 deficiency leads to increased lipid peroxidation, oxidative DNA damage, intracellular peroxide generation and decreased survival of a fibroblast cell line after exposure to oxidative agents [16].

3. Epidemiology of IDH mutations in human malignancies and genetic disorders

3.1. IDH mutations in GBMs

Mutations in the IDH1 gene were identified in a recent genome-wide analysis where 20661 protein coding genes were systematically sequenced on 22 patients affected by WHO (World Health Organization) grade IV GBM. Among the several candidate genes not previously associated with GBM, the IDH1 gene on chromosome 2q33.3 was the most interesting one [1]. Somatic and recurrent IDH1 mutations affecting the highly conserved arginine (R) residue at codon 132 in the enzyme's active site were found with a frequency of 12%. They occurred in a large fraction of younger patients and, especially, in secondary GBMs. They were also associated with a significant increase in patient overall survival (OS).

In agreement with the current WHO classification of the central nervous system (CNS) tumors [27], GBMs are considered to be secondary (sGBMs) or primary (pGBM) tumors according to the histologically verified presence or not of a previous low-grade glioma.

In a small group of GBM patients without IDH1 mutations, somatic recurrent mutations were identified in the IDH2 gene, even though at lower frequency. They affected codon R172, homologous to R132 of the IDH1 gene [28].

In contrast to sGBMs, IDH1 or IDH2 mutations were only found in a minority of pGBMs (<5-10%) [1,28,29]. The recurrence of IDH1 and IDH2 mutations among GBM patients was confirmed by following studies on larger series in Caucasian patients [30-44] as well as in Japanese, Indian, Korean, Brazilian and Chinese patients [45-49].

In pediatric GBMs, somatic IDH mutations were only rarely identified (approximately 16%) [28,29,50-52]. Pediatric malignant gliomas in patients ≥14 years showed a higher frequency

http://dx.doi.org/10.5772/52357

(about 35%) of IDH mutations in comparison with children malignant gliomas [52]. This finding suggests that the biology of histologically similar high-grade gliomas in younger pediatric patients differs from adults.

Stabilized GBM cell lines (both neurospheres and adherent cells) did not show IDH1 or IDH2 mutations [53]. This finding is not surprising considering that the majority of GBM cell lines that develop in *in vitro* culture originate from pGBMs.

The frequency of IDH mutations in high-grade gliomas is summarized in Table 1.

Tumor type, (WHO grade)	Total cases	IDH1 and IDH2 mutations detected	%, range	Reference
Pilocytic astrocytoma (I)	221	5	2.3 (0-5.9)	28[*],30,32-34,39,42,43,59
Diffuse astrocytoma (II)	608	455	75 (30.7-100)	28[*], 30,32-34,36,38-43,45,46,56
Anaplastic astrocytoma (III)	566	330	58 (44.4-87.5)	28[*],30,32-36,38-42,45,46
Oligodendroglioma (II)	597	366	61 (42.9-100)	28[*],30,32-34,36,38-42,46
Anaplastic oligodendroglioma (III)	561	346	62 (46-100)	28[*],30,32-36,38-42,45,46,57
Oligoastrocytoma (II)	207	149	72 (49-100)	28[*],30,32,33,36,38,41,42,46
Anaplastic oligoastrocytoma (III)	297	202	66 (63-100)	28[*],30,32,33,36,38,42,45,46
Primary glioblastoma (IV)	2362	170	7.2 (1.8-19.4)	28[*],31-37,38-43,45-49
Secondary glioblastoma (IV)	335	250	75 (15.4-84.6)	28[*],31-36,38-42,45,46,48
Giant cell glioblastoma (IV)	18	4	22 (20-25)	28[*]
Pediatric glioblastoma (IV)	69	2	3 (0-7.6)	30,50-52
Gliomatosis cerebri	15	5	33	58

[*] Combined results from Balss and Hartmann studies due to duplication of some cases. Abbreviations: WHO, World Health Organization; IDH, isocitrate dehydrogenase.

Table 1. Table 1. Frequency of IDH1 and IDH2 mutations in high- and low-grade gliomas.

3.2. IDH mutations in low-grade gliomas

After the discovery of IDH mutations in sGBMs, a great interest arose in verifying whether these mutations were also present among low-grade gliomas. As expected, IDH1 or IDH2 mutations recur in >65-80% of WHO grade II and III astrocytomas [28,30,32-36,38-43,45,46,54-56], and even more (approximately 70-85%) in WHO grade II and III oligoastrocytomas and oligodendrogliomas [28-30,32-36,38-43,45,46,5-59].

Mutations in the IDH1 gene have also been found in some cases of gliomatosis cerebri [58].

In contrast to diffuse gliomas, IDH mutations are very rare or absent in a variety of WHO grade I and II CNS tumors, such as pilocytic astrocytomas, subependymal giant cell tumors, gangliogliomas, ependymomas and pleiomorphic xanthoastrocytomas

[28-30,32-34,39,42,43,59-62]. The frequency of IDH1 and IDH2 mutations in low-grade gliomas is reported in Table 1.

Relatively rare neuronal and glioneuronal tumors as central neurocytomas, dysembryoplastic neuroepithelial tumors and rosette-forming glioneuronal tumors, as well as embryonal tumors as medulloblastomas, do not show IDH mutations [28,32,33,42,59-64].

Mutations in the IDH genes were not detected among non-glial brain tumors, with the exception of adult (but not children) primitive neuroectodermal tumors (sPNETs) [29,42,65,66], and maybe two cases of atypical meningiomas [67,68].

3.3. IDH mutations in other malignancies

IDH1 and IDH2 mutations are relatively glioma specific. However, they have been reported at lower frequency in some other mesenchymal tumors, especially haematopoietic malignancies and chondroid neoplasms [69-74]. IDH mutations were identified in approximately 8% of patients with acute myeloid leukemia (AML), in some myelodysplastic syndromes and myeloproliferative neoplasms [70-72]. Among AML patients, they were mainly found in tumors without cytogenetic abnormalities, and typically affect the IDH2 gene, at codons R140 or R172 [70-74]. Unlike gliomas, rare instances of AML patients with mutations in both IDH1 and IDH2 genes have been reported [75].

IDH1 mutations have also been described as a frequent event (56%) in endochondromas, as well as in central or differentiated chondrosarcomas [69], but not in peripheral chondrosarcomas or osteochondromas [76]. The majority of IDH mutations in chondroid neoplasms are represented by the p.R132C substitution [69].

Mutations in the IDH1 and IDH2 genes are extremely rare in most of other human malignances [35,47]. Rare IDH1 mutations, mostly characterized by the p.R132C substitution, have been described in prostatic adenocarcinomas, thyroid carcinomas, melanomas and B-acute lymphoblastic leukemia [45,77-79]. No IDH mutations were detected in brain metastases of colorectal cancers [80].

3.4. IDH mutations in hereditary diseases

L-2- and D-2-hydroxyglutaric aciduria (L-2-HGA and D-2-HGA, respectively) are rare neurometabolic disorders with mendelian inheritance caused by mutations in the L-2-hydroxyglutarate dehydrogenase (L2HGDH) or D-2-hydroxyglutarate dehydrogenase (type I D2HGDH) genes. Both are characterized by elevated levels of 2-hydroxyglutarate (2-HG) in body fluids including urine, plasma and cerebrospinal fluid [81,82]. L-2-HGA is the most common and severe of the two, and mainly affects the CNS. In contrast, symptoms associated to D-2-HG may be mild to nearly absent. Interestingly, heterozygous mutations at codon R140 of the IDH2 gene were found in a subset of D2HGDH (type II D2HGDH) patients with normal D2HGDH enzymatic activity, no D2HGDH gene mutations but with increased D2HGDH levels in body fluids [83,84].

Although IDH mutations result in D-2-HG accumulation, L-2-HGA but not D-2-HGA patients have unexpectedly been reported to have a higher risk of malignant brain tumors [85-87].

Somatic mosaic IDH1 and IDH2 mutations have also been found associated in humans to multiple endochondromatosis, Ollier disease and Maffucci symdrome [88,89]. Patients with Ollier disease/Maffucci syndrome develop multiple central cartilaginous tumors with an uncertain inheritance (possibly dominant inheritance with reduced penetrance); interestingly, some of them develop gliomas and AML. A model in which IDH1 and IDH2 mutations are early post-zygotic events in individuals affected by these syndromes has been proposed, suggesting their implication in tumorigenesis [88].

4. Molecular genetics of IDH mutations in gliomas

4.1. Spectrum of IDH mutations

Five genes encoding human isocitrate dehydrogenases have been identified. IDH1 on 2q33.3 encodes for the IDH1 isoform [90], IDH2 on 15q26.1 for the IDH2 isoform [91], IDH3A on 15q25.1 for the α-subunit of the IDH3 isoform [92], IDH3B on 20p13 for the β-subunit [93] and IDH3G on Xq28 for the γ-subunit [94].

All the identified mutations in gliomas affect either the IDH1 or the IDH2 gene. IDH3A, IDH3B and IDH3G genes have not been implicated to date in gliomas [95].

All IDH1 and IDH2 mutations are somatic, heterozygous and missense changes. They typically affect codon R132 in the IDH1 gene and its homologous R172 in the IDH2 gene, both within the enzyme's substrate binding site. In contrast to ALM, in gliomas mutations in the IDH1 and IDH2 genes are always mutually exclusive.

Over 90% of the reported mutations affect the IDH1 gene and, among them, different types of mutations have been described. The p.R132H substitution accounts for about 92.4%, followed by p.R132C for 3.2%, p.R132G for 2.1%, p.R132G for 1.6% and p.R132L for <1% [28,30-39,41-48,56,57,59]. The rare p.R132V nucleotide substitution, originally proposed as somatic mutation, was later labeled as single nucleotide polymorphism (SNP) [29,78].

Interestingly, >90% of IDH1 mutations at codon R132 leads to a histidine change, suggesting a significant selective advantage in favor of this particular point mutation.

A single report has recently identified a predicted new mutation at codon R100 (p.R100Q), located in the enzyme's active site, in two WHO grade III oligodendrogliomas and in one WHO grade II astrocytoma [54]. Two other very rare IDH1 mutations (p.R49C and p.G97D) have only been described in a single pediatric GBM patient [50].

Mutations in the IDH2 gene are less common in gliomas, accounting for 3-5% or less of all the identified mutations [30,31,34,39,42-45,56,57,59]. The p.R172K mutation accounts for about 60%, followed by p.R172M for 26.7%, p.R172W for 11.1%, p.R172S for 2.2% [30,31,34,39,42-45, 56,57,59]. Rare nonsense IDH2 mutations have been described in a single study, with uncertain significance [39].

The type and frequency of the identified mutations at codons IDH1 R132 and IDH2 R172 are summarized in Table 2. All are reported at the Catalogue of Somatic Mutations in Cancer (COSMIC database) (http://www.sanger.ac.uk/cosmic/).

Gene	Nucleotide change	Amino acid change	Total mutated cases	%	Reference
IDH1			1791		
	c.G395A	p.R132H	1655	92.4	28,30-39,41-48,56,59
	c.C394T	p.R132C	58	3.2	28,30-39,41-48,56,59
	c.C394G	p.R132G	38	2.1	28,30-39,41-48,56,59
	c.C394A	p.R132S	29	1.6	28,30-39,41-48,56,59
	c.G395T	p.R132L	11	0.6	28,30-39,41-48,56,59
IDH2			45		
	c.G515A	p.R172K	27	60	30,31,34,39,42-45,56,57,59
	c.G515T	p.R172M	12	26.7	30,31,34,39,42-45, 56,57,59
	c.A514T	p.R172W	5	11.1	30,31,34,39,42-45,56,57,59
	c.G516T	p.R172S	1	2.2	30,31,34,39,42-45,56,57,59

The reported nucleotide and amino acid numbering for the IDH1 and IDH2 genes is relative to the transcription start site (+1) corresponding to the A of the ATG on the respective GenBank reference sequences NM_005896 and NM_002168. Abbreviations: IDH, isocitrate dehydrogenase.

Table 2. Type and frequency of IDH1 R132 and IDH2 R172 mutations in gliomas.

4.2. Association with clinical and histological features

The occurrence of IDH mutations correlates with some clinical and histopathological features of gliomas. The strongest significant association is between IDH mutations and patient's age at diagnosis in most glioma tumor subtypes [28,30,31,36,42,46,49]. Generally, the mean age of patients with IDH mutations is significantly lower in comparison with patients without IDH mutations. In contrast, in pediatric high-grade gliomas, patients with IDH1 mutations are older than children with wild-type tumors [28].

In GBMs, the average time from the first clinical symptom to the histological diagnosis is significantly longer in patients with IDH mutations than in wild-type patients, consistently with a slower growth and less aggressive tumor [31].

In adult patients, IDH mutations are significantly and inversely associated with the histological malignancy grade [28,36]. Interestingly, they show a non-random distribution within the glioma subtypes [30]. The p.R132C mutation in the IDH1 gene is strongly associated with the astrocytic phenotype while IDH2 mutations mainly affect oligodendroglial tumors [30,41]. When astrocytomas develop in patients affected by Li-Fraumeni syndrome, they always show the p.R132C mutation [55], suggesting that precursor cells, which for definition already carry a germline tumor protein *p53* (TP53) mutation, specifically acquire this relatively uncommon IDH1 mutation.

In GBMs, the occurrence of an oligodendroglial component is significantly more frequent in tumors with IDH mutations, as well as large ischemic and pseudopalisading necroses are typical hallmarks of wild-type tumors [31].

Finally, a preferential distribution of IDH mutations within different regions of the brain has been reported in two recent large-scale studies. WHO grade II-III gliomas and pGBMs with IDH1 mutations are mainly located in the frontal lobe (73.5%) rather than in the temporal lobe (41.7%) [49,96]. This distribution, similar to that of 1p/19q co-deletion, provides further evidence for the distinctiveness of gliomas from different brain lobes. The absence of IDH mutations also identify, among WHO grade II gliomas, a novel tumor subtype characterized by a predominant insular location, greater tumor size, infiltrative aspects on magnetic resonance imaging (MRI) and dismal prognosis [56].

4.3. Association with genetic and epigenetic alterations

IDH mutations show significant associations with some of the typical genetic and epigenetic changes of gliomas. IDH mutations are tightly associated with the 1p/19q co-deletion and the methylguanine-DNA methyltransferase (MGMT) promoter hypermethylation status [33,36,37,42,57,97,98].

Interestingly, they are inversely correlated with the specific genetic alterations of pGBMs, such as the epidermal growth factor receptor (EGFR) amplification, the cyclin-dependent kinase inhibitor 2A or 2B (CDKN2A/CDKN2B) deletion and the phosphatase and tensin homolog (PTEN) mutations [28,32]. The mutual exclusion with EGFR amplification coincides with the rarity of IDH mutations in pGBMs [33,36,37,42,57,98].

Furthermore, astrocytic tumors and GBMs with IDH mutations typically show a higher rate of TP53 mutations in comparison with wild-type tumors [28,32,33,46,98].

The strong association between IDH mutations and the 1p/19q co-deletion in oligodendrogliomas corresponds to approximately 100% concordance in the occurrence of both genetic alterations, as confirmed by three independent large-scale studies [28,98,99]. In oligodendrocytic tumors, IDH mutations also correlate with somatic mutations in the homolog of the *Drosophila capicua* (CIC) gene on chromosome 19q13.2, suggesting a putative role of the latter in the pathogenesis of this tumor subtype [100,101]. Interestingly, a significant association was also found with the epithelial membrane protein 3 (EMP3) promoter hypermethylation status [personnal data].

IDH mutations and the KIAA1549- v-raf murine sarcoma viral oncogene homolog B1 (BRAF) fusion gene are considered two mutually exclusive genetic events in diffuse and pilocytic astrocytomas, respectively. However, in a series of 185 adult diffuse gliomas, IDH mutations coexist with the KIAA1549-BRAF fusion gene, mainly in oligodendroglial tumors [102].

4.4. Timing and relationships with gliomagenesis

The majority of tumors with IDH mutations also harbor either TP53 mutations or 1p/19q co-deletion [28,29,32]. The concurrence of IDH and TP53 mutations is typically observed in WHO grade II and III astrocytic tumors, as well as in sGBMs. The concomitance of IDH mutations with 1p/19q co-deletion is mainly found in WHO grade II and III oligodendrogliomas. WHO grade II and III oligoastrocytic tumors mostly show IDH mutations in association with TP53 mutations and 1p/19q co-deletion.

The temporal sequence of the genetic and epigenetic events during gliomagenesis has recently been determined [33]. A series of paired initial and recurrent tumors from 51 patients was screened for the occurrence of both IDH1 and TP53 mutations, and 1p/19q co-deletion. In this study, diffuse astrocytomas and oligodendrogliomas with IDH1 mutations at first surgery developed, respectively, either TP53 mutations or 1p/19q co-deletion, at recurrence. In this series, no tumor developed IDH1 mutations after the acquisition of either TP53 mutations or 1p/19q co-deletion [33]. This finding validates the chronological order proposed for the genetic events during gliomagenesis with IDH1 mutations as the earliest genetic event, interesting the common glial precursor cell population, even before EGFR amplification [36,57]. The successive acquisition of TP53 mutations or 1p/19q co-deletion may lead, respectively, to the astrocytic or oligodendroglial differentiation. This hypothesis is further supported by the significant association of IDH mutations with 1p/19q co-deletion in oligodendrogliomas and with TP53 mutations in astrocytomas [57,99].

In contrast, pilocytic astrocytomas showing the KIAA1549-BRAF fusion gene should derive from different progenitors.

Interestingly, IDH mutations do occur in sGBMs, but not in pGBMs. This difference must be referred to the different origin of the two tumor subtypes. sGBM develops from a previous astrocytoma, whereas pGBM is a *de novo* tumor. They differ for the genetic configuration, age, and growth speed [103], but not for location and phenotype; at the most, they can differ for the spreading modalities [104]. It is not known how *de novo* tumors arise, whereas it is believed that secondary ones originate through anaplasia, *i.e.* through dedifferentiation of tumor cells which follows mutation accumulation [27]. Generally, it is known that GBMs originate either from Neural Stem Cells (NSCs) or from astrocytes [105] and this could correspond to the distinction between pGBMs and sGBMs. Obviously, it is likely that the two GBM subtypes must originate *ab initio* from the same Cancer Stem Cells (CSCs). The development of GBM in the emisphere, far away from the sub-ventricular zone (SVZ), could be in contrast with its origin from NSCs of the same region, but this can be got over if we refer to the concept of both asymmetric division and migration of progenitors [106]. A path has been traced from mitotically active precursors to the developed tumors [107], which recognizes in transiently dividing progenitors and in somatic stem cells, the elements where mutations accumulate; they also express EGFR, present in normal progenitors of the SVZ [108]. These cells are the possible source of pGBMs, whereas for sGBMs it is mandatory to refer to a previous astrocytoma [109,110].

A genetic model for the origin and progression of the different glioma subtypes is shown in Figure 3.

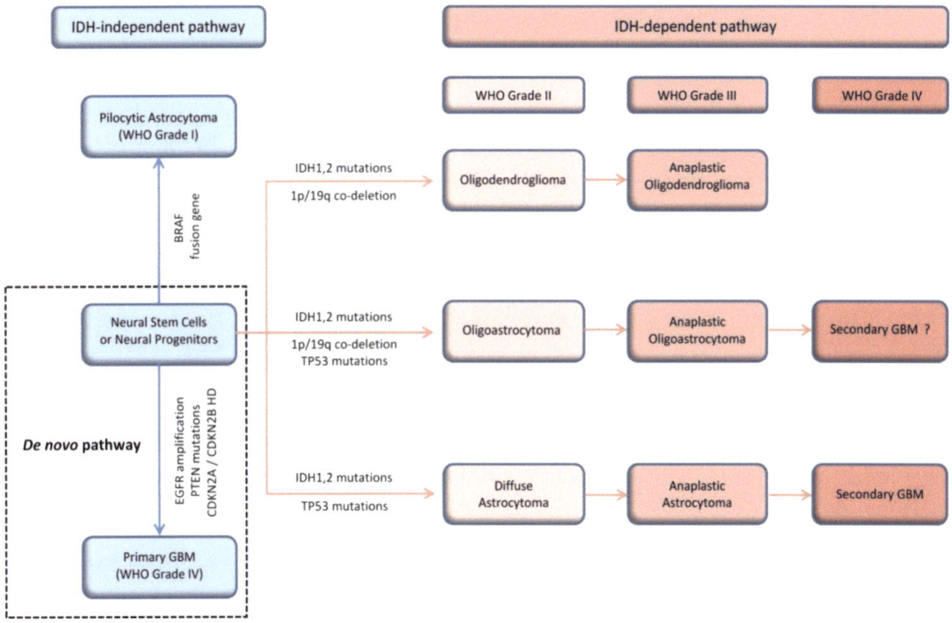

Abbreviations: IDH, isocitrate dehydrogenase; BRAF, v-raf murine sarcoma viral oncogene homolog B1; CDKN2A/B, cyclin-dependent kinase inhibitors 2A and 2B; EGFR, epidermal growth factor receptor; PTEN, phosphatase and tensin homolog; TP53, tumor protein *p53*; HD, homozygous deletion; GBM, glioblastoma multiforme; WHO, World Health Organization.

Figure 3. Model for the development of astrocytic and oligodendrocytic tumors. Two different pathways have been proposed, according to the IDH mutation status [111]. In the IDH-dependent pathway, WHO grade II astrocytomas and oligodendrogliomas arise by first acquisition of IDH mutations and successive development of either TP53 mutations or 1p/19q co-deletion. They further progress to WHO grade III astrocytomas or oligodendrogliomas and, ultimately, become secondary GBMs. WHO grade II and III oligoastrocytomas show genetic changes common to both astrocytomas or oligodendrogliomas. In the IDH-independent pathway, primary GBMs de novo develop irrespective of IDH mutations, by acquisition of the following genetic alterations: EGFR amplification, PTEN mutations and CDKN2A/CDKN2B homozygous deletion. Pilocytic astrocytomas arise by acquisition of the KIAA1549-BRAF fusion gene (modified from Ref.111).

4.5. Association with the Proneuronal glioma subtype

Gene expression profiling studies of high-grade gliomas have permitted a subclassification of tumors according to a molecular signature [112]. In a recent study on 115 WHO grade II and III astrocytomas, three distinct subgroups termed Proneuronal, Proliferative and Mesenchymal have been identified, in agreement with similarities in expression profiling of survival-related genes [112]. The Proneuronal group is characterized by a better prognosis and by expression of genes associated with normal brain and neurogenesis. The Proliferative group has a markedly better prognosis and shows expression of genes associated with both proliferation and angiogenesis, whereas the Mesenchymal group has a poorer prognosis and expresses genes associated to mesenchymal origin. Most WHO grade III gliomas, as well as

75% of low-grade gliomas, were classified as Proneuronal. Interestingly, IDH mutations were significantly associated to the latter subgroup.

Recently, the Cancer Genome Atlas (TCGA) Research Network has been hired to generate the comprehensive catalogue of genomic abnormalities occurring during tumorigenesis in the majority of human cancers [113]. Among them, GBM was chosen as the pilot disease for this project. Based on gene expression profiling of 206 GBMs, the following four clinically relevant subtypes were identified: Classical, Proneuronal, Neuronal and Mesenchymal. Aberrations and gene expression of EGFR, neurofibromatosis type I (NF1) and platelet-derived growth factor receptor A (PDGFRA)/IDH1 each defines the Classical, Mesenchymal and Proneuronal subtype [113]. Notably, most sGBMs were classified as Proneuronal. The successive up-dated TGCA report confirmed the association with this favorable GBM subtype [114].

An independent study by array-based comparative genomic hybridization (CGH) analysis identified distinct genomic and expression profiles between pGBMs and sGBMs [44]. Few pGBMs with IDH1 mutations have similar expression profiles as sGBMs with IDH1 mutations [44].

Similar findings were described in low-grade gliomas [115]. In a series of 101 diffuse astrocytic gliomas, IDH mutation status discriminated molecularly and clinically distinct low-grade glioma subsets, where tumors with IDH mutations show TP53 mutations, PDGFRA overexpression, and better survival. In contrast, tumors without IDH mutations show EGFR amplification, PTEN loss, and unfavorable disease outcome. Furthermore, global expression profiling revealed three robust molecular subclasses within lower grade diffuse astrocytic gliomas, two of which mainly characterized by IDH mutations and TP53 mutations and one prevailingly wild-type. The former can be distinguished from each other on the basis of TP53 mutations, DNA copy number abnormalities, and links to distinct stages of neurogenesis in the SVZ [115].

4.6. Association with the G-CIMP hypermethylated phenotype

In a genome-wide DNA methylation analysis in human gliomas distinct methylation profiles have been associated with gene expression subtypes [114]. Interestingly, a specific glioma CpG island methylator phenotype (G-CIMP) was found, able to define a distinct molecular subclass of tumors. G-CIMP is analogous to the CpG island methylator phenotype (CIMP) previously described in a number of human malignances, including AML and colorectal carcinoma [116]. Similarly to these, G-CIMP is characterized by a high number of hypermethylated *loci*. The G-CIMP prevails among low-grade gliomas, shows distinct copy number alterations and correlates with better survival and younger age [114].

Notably, it is strongly associated with IDH mutations and the Proneuronal subtype [114,117,118]. The significant association between IDH mutations and MGMT promoter hypermethylation found by us [42,97] and by others [33,36,37,57] in low-grade gliomas is in line with this finding.

Remarkably, IDH mutations alone are sufficient to establish the G-CIMP, by remodelling the methylome and the transcriptome. Introduction of mutant IDH1 into primary human astrocytes alters specific histone marks, induces extensive DNA hypermethylation and reshapes the methylome [119].

As for gliomas, IDH mutations have also been found associated with peculiar DNA hypermethylation pattern in AML [116]. In the latter, hypermethylation may be alternatively caused by inhibition of the oncogene family member 2 (TET2). TET2 encodes an α-KG-dependent dioxygenase that catalyzes the formation of 5-hydroxymethylcytosine (5hmC), with subsequent DNA demethylation [120,121].

5. Molecular pathogenesis of IDH mutations

5.1. Biochemistry of mutant isocitrate dehydrogenases

All the identified IDH mutations in gliomas are amino acid substitutions at codon R132 in the IDH1 and codon R172 in the IDH2 gene. Both residues are highly conserved and involved in the formation of the active site of the two enzymes.

During the two-step catalysis of the oxidative decarboxylation of isocitrate to α-KG, IDH adopts an active closed conformation where the Mg^{2+}-isocitrate substrate complex binds between large and small domains of the enzyme [2]. The active site is composed of two groups of key residues. The first consists of two essential catalytic residues in IDH1, tyrosine (Y) 140 and lysine (K) 212, that participate in the acid-base catalysis during decarboxylation of isocitrate and are evolutionarily highly conserved [122]. The second consists of a triad of arginines (R100, R109 and R132 in IDH1 and R140, R149 and R172 in IDH2) in the Mg^{2+}-isocitrate complex recognition site that forms a salt-bridge with the substrate [77].

Modelling studies on human cytosolic IDH1 structure suggest that substitutions at R132 would impair interactions of the enzyme with the substrate [23]. Among all the amino acid residues involved in the binding with isocitrate, R132 only forms three hydrogen bonds with the α- and β-carboxyl of isocitrate, while all the others no more than one or two. Therefore, substitutions at R132 may weaken the hydrogen bond of IDH1 to substrate. Since R132 contacts Asp297 in the transitional semi-open conformation of IDH1, it may be important in the transition from open to closed conformation [19]. In this regard, R172, as well as R140 in IDH2, is equivalent to R132. These chemical factors may explain why mutations in the IDH1 and IDH2 genes exclusively affect these amino acids.The position, rather than the nature of the amino acid substitution, seems to affect the IDH activity, by conferring a selective advantage to tumor cells with IDH mutations [77].

To date, all the identified mutations have been tested, and all of them impair the normal IDH enzymatic activity [23,32]. The enzymatic activity of IDH mutant proteins is significantly reduced, irrespective of the nature of the amino acid substitution [35,111]. Any amino acid substitutions in one of the two homologue arginines R100 or R132 in IDH1 and R140 and R172 in IDH2 lead to the same gain of function in both proteins. Interestingly, the third conserved arginine (R109 in IDH1 and R149 in IDH2) of the triad has never been reported to be mutated [54].

Recently, IDH1 mutations at codons R100 (in adult glioma) and G97 (in pediatric GBM and colon cancer cell lines), as well as at the predicted Y139, have been found to be associated with D-2-HG production [124]. In contrast, IDH1 SNPs V71I and V178I, as well as several single report non-synonymous substitutions, have no effect on cellular D-2-HG levels and retain the wild-type ability for isocitrate-dependent NADPH production [123].

5.2. Dominant negative enzymatic activity

The mechanism by which IDH1 and IDH2 mutations mediate oncogenesis in gliomas is not completely clarified [20,24,124]. However, two hypotheses have been proposed (Figure 4) [125-128]. Both IDH1 and IDH2 mutant enzymes show a loss of function in the forward reaction leading to a reduced production of α-KG and NAPDH [23] and a gain of function in the reverse reaction leading to an increased production of D-2-HG [19]. Both loss- and gain-of function reactions may have significant implications for cellular metabolism in glioma tumor cells.

In agreement with the loss of function hypothesis, IDH mutations may dominantly inhibit the wild-type copy of the homodimer. By *in vitro* studies, it was found that the IDH1 wild-type/ mutant heterodimer exhibits only 4% of the enzymatic activity of the IDH1 wild-type homodimer, with a reduced production of α-KG and NADPH [23]. Neverthless, this dominant negative inhibition by the mutant proteins may not be observed for all the known IDH mutant types [129]. Definite evidence that dominant negative activity occurs *in vivo* is lacking [73, 128].

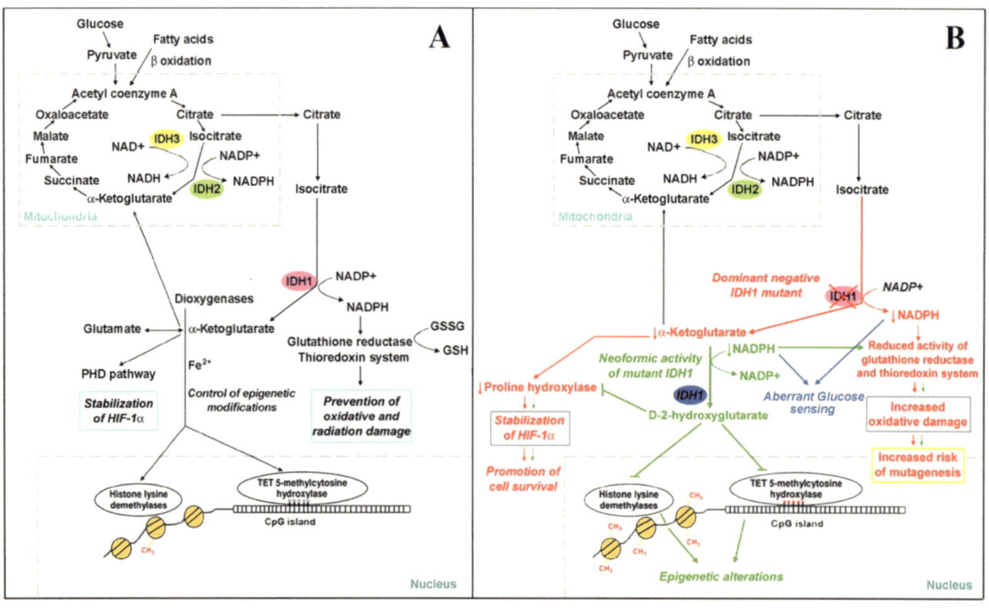

Figure 4. Functions of normal (A) and mutant (B) isocitrate dehydrogenase (IDH) enzymes (modified from Ref.126).

5.3. Neomorphic enzymatic activity

The only consequence universally recognized for all types of IDH mutations is the acquisition of a neomorphic enzymatic activity to reduce α-KG to the new metabolite D-2-HG [19]. This finding is in favor of the oncogenetic function of the IDH mutant proteins. Furthermore, the mutation pattern with hot-spot missense nucleotide substitutions in a heterozygous status is typical of activated oncogenes, for example v-ki-ras2 kirsten rat sarcoma viral oncogene homolog (KRAS) and BRAF [128]. Thus, IDH1 and IDH2 genes may function as oncogenes rather than tumor suppressor genes, and IDH1 and IDH2 mutations as oncogenic driver rather than passenger mutations [77]. Moreover, the 2q34 region, in which IDH1 maps, is one of the most stable chromosomal regions in gliomas, with rare deletions described.

The specific orientation by which the hydride transfer takes place in the IDH1 active site results in the production of the R(-) enantiomer of 2-HG, that is equivalent to the D-isomer [77]. Interestingly, the IDH mutant proteins only produce D-2-HG but not its enantiomer L-2-HG [19]. This unique feature may be useful to understand the mechanism by which IDH mutations contribute to gliomagenesis [127].

The occurrence of IDH mutations results in an increased (approximately 100-fold) amount of D-2-HG [19,73]. D-2-HG is structurally similar to α-KG and then it functions as a competitive inhibitor of multiple α-KG-dependent enzymes with important roles in cancer. They are mainly dioxygenases, which use α-KG as co-substrate to catalyze a variety of reactions, including the repair of alkylated DNA, the response to hypoxia and the biosynthesis of collagene or L-carnitine [130]. Three relevant classes of dioxygenases are PHDs, histone demethylases and the TET family of 5mC hydroxylases [131].

5.4. Hypoxia signaling pathway

PHD promotes the degradation of the HIF-1α. The latter is a transcription factor of crucial importance in the cellular response to hypoxia. It activates the transcription of genes involved in apoptosis, cell survival, and angiogenesis, most notably vascular endothelial growth factor (VEGF) [23]. A variety of human cancers show up-regulation of HIF-1α, probably associated with the VEGF-mediated angiogenesis. D-2-HG produced by the IDH mutant enzymes may compete with α-KG and inhibit the PHD-mediated degradation of HIF-1α. Increased HIF-1α levels may induce VEGF expression and consequently promote angiogenesis and enhancement of tumor growth [23]. In favor of this hypothesis, induction of R132H mutant IDH1 up-regulates HIF-1α inducible genes including VEGF in U87MG glioma cells [23]. However, the up-regulation of HIF-1α in glioma tissues with IDH1 mutations has not been replicated by others [132]. Moreover, WHO grade II and III gliomas are not so vascularized and do not show angiogenesis, as it would expect for tumors that activate this hypoxia signaling pathway.

5.5. Genome-wide epigenetic deregulation

IDH mutations may promote tumorigenesis by genome-wide epigenetic deregulation through the inhibition of demethylation of 5mC and histones. A member of the α-KG-dependent dioxygenases is the TET family of 5mC hydroxylases [18,131]. TET2 is a putative tumor suppressor gene at chromosome 4q24 that plays an important role in the regulation of DNA methylation by conversion of 5mC into 5hmC. The great majority of DNA methylation sites are 5mC at CpG dinucleotides and 5hmC is regarded as an intermediate product of DNA demethylation. D-2-HG produced by the IDH mutant proteins may inhibit TET2-mediated demethylation, leading to a global hypermethylation [131].

Interestingly, a subset of AML patients with TET mutations, which are mutually exclusive with IDH mutations, show the same hypermethylation phenotype of patients with IDH mutations, suggesting that IDH-mutant tumors may be mediated by TET2 inhibition [120]. This finding also suggests that IDH and TET2 mutations may be functionally redundant.

The tight association between the occurrence of IDH mutations and the before mentioned G-CIMP in gliomas, as well as with the CIMP in AML, is a strong evidence in favour of this hypothesis. Not least is the direct evidence that IDH mutations alone establish G-CIMP, as recently reported [119]. Moreover, overexpression of R132H mutant IDH1 or R172K mutant IDH2 in 293T cells leads to increased D-2-HG and to a significant up-regulation of global 5mC levels [120].

An alternative epigenetic mechanism involved in the regulation of gene expression is represented by histone lysine methyltransferases that mediate the methylation of histone proteins [131]. Increased D-2-HG levels may result in alterations of the methylation status of lysine residues in histones, such as H3K9, H3K27 and H3K79 [132]. D-2-HG-producing IDH mutants can prevent the histone demethylation required for lineage-specific progenitor cells to differentiate into completely differentiated cells [133]. The introduction of either mutant IDH or cell-permeable 2-HG is associated with repression of the inducible expression of lineage-specific differentiation genes and with a block in cell differentation. Notably, the aberrant histone methylation may precede and occur independently of DNA methylation [133].

Overall, by these two mechanisms IDH mutations may induce DNA hypermethylation at a number of target genes and globally deregulate gene expression.

5.6. Response to oxidative insults

An alternative hypothesis is related to the IDH function in the cellular protection by generation of the reducing equivalent NADPH. The latter plays an important role in the protection of cell from oxidative damage and radiation-induced stress by contributing to GSH reductase and thioredoxin systems.

Human brain is highly susceptible to oxidative stress because of high oxygen consumption, relative lack of antioxidant enzymes and large amount of iron, a well-known pro-oxidant [134]. The main source of DNA damage in brain is represented by ROS produced during normal cellular metabolism [135]. GSH is the most important antioxidant against the oxidative stress caused by ROS. NAPDH is required for the reduction of glutathione disulfide (GSSG) to GSH by glutathione reductase and for the maintenance of the antioxidant status of GSH in the cell. The cytosolic IDH1 contributes to the NADPH pool in the cell, even though two other cytosolic enzymes, glucose 6-phosphate dehydrogenase (G6PD) and the malic enzyme, also generate NADPH [16].

http://dx.doi.org/10.5772/52357

Under oxidative stress conditions, the activity of NAD+-dependent IDHs increases. IDH mutations reduce the ability of IDH to produce NADPH from NADP+ [19,23,32,111], but also deplete NADPH by consuming it as cofactor to convert α-KG in D-2-HG with NADP+ production [19]. Cells with reduced NADP-dependent IDH activity have increased oxidative DNA damage, higher GSSG to total GSH ratio and reduced survival on exposure to oxidative stress [16].

Oxidative DNA damage may promote the occurrence of other genetic changes, for example TP53 mutations or t(1;19) translocation favoring, respectively, the differentiation of the astrocytic or oligodendrocytic lineage. Furthermore, DNA damage may lead to DNA double-strand breaks [136] and ROS accumulation has been shown to induce unbalanced translocation in leukemia cells [137]. This finding may explain the high prevalence of t(1;19) translocation (corresponding to the total 1p/19q co-deletion) in oligodendrogliomas with IDH mutations.

This hypothetical model may also explain why D-2-HGA patients do not develop gliomas, because mutations in the D2HGDH gene in these patients would not affect the redox system *via* GSH [127].

5.7. Aberrant glucose sensing

A possible selective advantage for tumor cells could derive from the role of IDH1 in the glucose sensing. IDH1 participates in a glucose-sensing pathway in pancreatic islets [138] by signaling the presence of high glucose to downstream members of this pathway by raising the NADPH levels. IDH1 and IDH2 mutant proteins consume NADPH to convert α-KG to D-2-HG decreasing the cytosolic NADPH level. This may be wrongly considered as signal of a low nutrient status in the glucose-sensing pathway. Cells may compensate this status by increasing cellular nutrient consumption or by blocking cellular differentiation. The former is known as a typical tumor hallmark and it may give tumor cells a selective growth advantage. Indeed, both glioma and AML tumor cells are relative undifferentiated [73]. The block of differentiation, finally, may benefit tumor cells by self-renewal.

6. Assessment of IDH mutation status

Currently, different methods are available to determine the IDH mutation status. They analyze either the nucleotide sequence of the gene or the altered structure of the protein.

6.1. Gene sequencing

Practical guidelines are available for a reliable detection of IDH mutations with molecular genetics techniques. In this regard, crucial aspects are the availability of tumor tissue, the tumor cell content and the quality of the respective genomic DNA (gDNA). The amount of tumor tissue available for the genetic analysis is often limited, especially for stereotactic biopsies. It also depends on the modality of tissue dissection, by manual macrodissection or laser capture microdissection (LCM).

The content in tumor cells is a critical point because contaminating cells from adjacent normal brain tissue, lymphocyte infiltrates, microglial and endothelial cells may dilute the mutant allele below the detection threshold level leading to false negative results. Consequently, each tumor sample should be as pure as possible and should reflect the highest percentage of tumor cells. This can be particularly problematic in tumor biopsy specimens. Prior to gDNA extraction, the identification and selection of tumor areas as proliferating, by haematoxylin and eosin (H&E) staining and microscopic examination, is therefore mandatory.

Among DNA-based methods, conventional Sanger sequencing is the most frequently used. It is a relatively inexpensive method for laboratories with access to an automated sequencer and it represents to date the "gold standard" for the detection of IDH mutations. It allows to identify all the possible sequence variations in the amplified region with a sensitivity of approximately 20% of the mutant allele in a wild-type background. Typically, Sanger sequencing is carried out on formalin or RCL2 fixed paraffin embedded tumor tissue, rather than on fresh frozen tissue, because the latter is frequently unavailable. The effects on gDNA quality of the different variables affecting tissue fixation are not to be neglected.

Bi-directional Sanger sequencing on at least two replicates is strongly recommended [139].

Representative electropherograms of IDH1 and IDH2 mutations detected in our previous study [42] are shown in Figures 5,6.

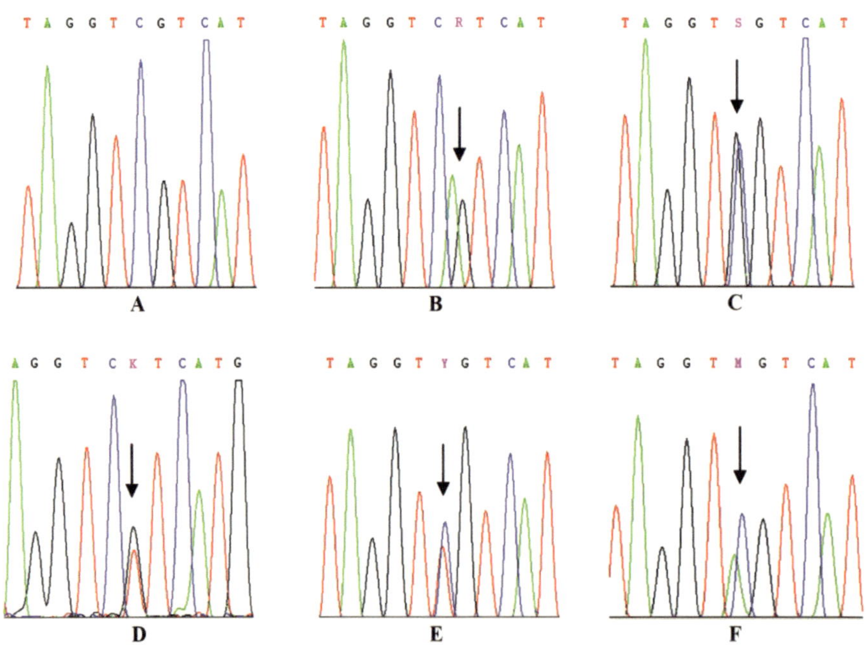

Figure 5. Electropherograms of representative mutations in the IDH1 gene. A – IDH1 wild-type; B – c.G395A (p.R132H); C – c.C394G (p.R132G); D – c.G395T (p.R132L); E – c.C394T (p.R132C); F – c.C394A (p.R132S).

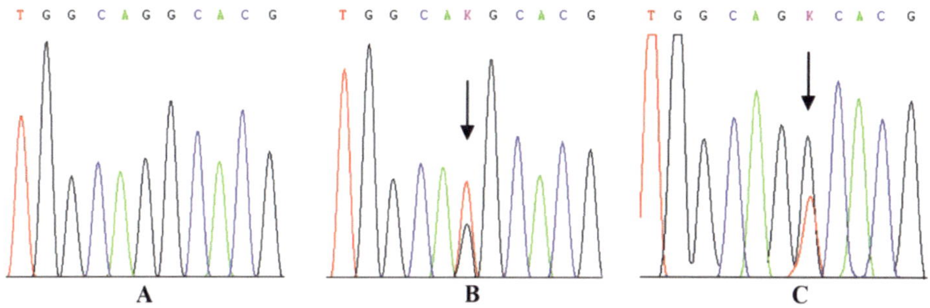

Figure 6. Electropherograms of representative mutations in the IDH2 gene. A – IDH2 wild-type; B – c.G515T (p.R172M); C – c.G516T (p.R172S).

Alternatively to Sanger sequencing, several studies have successively applied pyrosequencing technique [40,140]. The tightly clustered nature of the IDH mutations makes them ideal candidates for pyrosequencing. This technique allows a quantitative analysis and high throughput, with a sensitivity of 5-7% of the mutant allele in a wild-type background.

6.2. Alternative molecular techniques

Alternative methods to assess the IDH mutation status exist. They include derived cleaved amplified polymorphic sequence (dCAPS) [141], PCR-based restriction length polymorphism assays [142], cold PCR high resolution melting (HRM) [143], post-PCR fluorescence melting curve analysis (FMCA) [39] and SNaPshot assays [144]. The two latter methods are characterized by a sensitivity of approximately 2 and 5%, respectively.

Among the above mentioned techniques, melting curve analysis is currently approved for clinical use in the detection of BRAF and KRAS point mutations [62].

Anyway, the choice of the detection method both depends on the researcher's expertise and the laboratory facilities.

6.3. Immunohistochemistry

Two monoclonal antibodies (Mab), H09 (referred in some papers as anti-mIDH1^{R132H}) and IMab-1, have been developed to recognize the mutant-specific epitope of the IDH1 R132H mutant protein [145,146]. These antibodies can be used for both immunohistochemical analyses of tumor tissue and Western blotting analyses of tumor cell lysates. However, the latter procedure is not used in the clinical practice. Currently, the clone H09 antibody is the only commercially available (Dianova, Hamburg, Germany), with satisfactory results in the routine immunohistochemistry of formalin or RCL2 fixed paraffin embedded tissues [29,34,38,42,43].

The sensitivity and specificity of the clone H09 to detect positive tumor cells has been widely demonstrated in several studies and approaches 100% [38,42,145]. In comparison with IMab-1, clone H09 shows superior staining results [139].

Recently, a new Mab (SMab-1) directed to the p.R132S mutation of the IDH1 gene has been developed [148]. SMab-1 seems to show a specificity similar to that of clone H09 in both immunohistochemistry and immunocytochemistry; further studies are required to validate its use. The monoclonal antibody SMab-1 should be soon commercially available.

While the current clone H09 is highly specific for the IDH1 p.R132H mutation, it does not detect the other rare substitutions in the IDH1 or IDH2 genes [38]. For this reason, Sanger sequencing of the relevant exons of the IDH1 and IDH2 genes is always recommended to exclude the occurrence of other types of mutations in immunonegative cases [42,59,62,56,148].

The immunohistochemical analysis of the IDH1 p.R132H mutation can be manually performed or by automated immunostaining instruments. The Euro-CNS research committee has recently proposed practical guidelines to standardize the diagnostic IDH test with clone H09 by both procedures [139]. The "Vienna protocol", established at the Institute of Neurology, Medical University of Vienna (Austria), is recommended for manual immunostaining. In contrast, the "Heidelberg protocol", established at the Department of Neuropathology, Institute of Pathology, Ruprecht-Karls-Universität Heidelberg (Germany), is recommended for automatic immunostaining on Ventana BenchMark immunostainers (Ventana Medical Systems, Tucson, AZ, USA) [139].

6.4. Immunoreactivity of the IDH1 R132H mutant protein

In our experience, as well as in the experience of others, the anti-mIDH1^{R132H} immunoreactivity is cytoplasmic and perinuclear. In a variable percentage of cases, the staining is diffuse in the glia-fibrillary network. In some instances, an additional slightly weaker nuclear staining can be observed, although IDH1 is physiologically located in cytoplasm and peroxisomes. Normal cells, endothelial cells and lymphocytes are immunonegative.

In positive diffuse astrocytomas, all the cells show immunoreactivity (Figure 7A). The gemistocytic cells of astrocytomas are weakly positive with a reduced reaction in the center of the cells (Figure 7B). In this case, the doubt that it is not a specific reaction cannot be excluded.

In oligodendrogliomas, the staining is intense and perinuclear (Figure 7C). The minigemistocytes show a more compact staining of the cytoplasm. In oligodendroglial tumors with a sharp boundary with the normal tissue, the protein expression abruptly ceases at the tumor border; only isolated and rare positive cells are scattered in the normal tissue. In infiltrating tumors, a gradient of positive cells at the border with normal tissue is clearly visible (Figure 7D). In these tumors, tumor cells positive for the clone H09 are mixed with and distinguishable from normal oligodendrocytes (Figure 8E). The latter can be identified for their Cyclin D1 positive expression, being the two stainings complementary. In gliomas, only cycling cells such as tumor oligodendrocytes and reactive and tumor astrocytes express Cyclin D1 while all the other cells are immunonegative. In contrast, normal oligodendrocytes of the cortex and white matter, and microglial cells exhibit a Cyclin D1 positive nuclear staining [149,150]. Applied to oligoastrocytomas, the analysis of Cyclin D1 could prevent the identification of tumor cells as normal oligodendrocytes. In tumors with high cell density, oligodendrocytes appear compacted with a round cytoplasm, whereas in infiltrated areas they acquire an elongated form with polar processes, similar to that observed by silver impregnation (Figure 8B).

http://dx.doi.org/10.5772/52357

The majority of perivascular oligodendrocytes (Figure 8A) and perineuronal satellites are positive with elegant images (Figure 8C), with some exceptions (Figure 8D). Some of them are immunonegative for clone H09 but immunopositive for Cyclin D1.

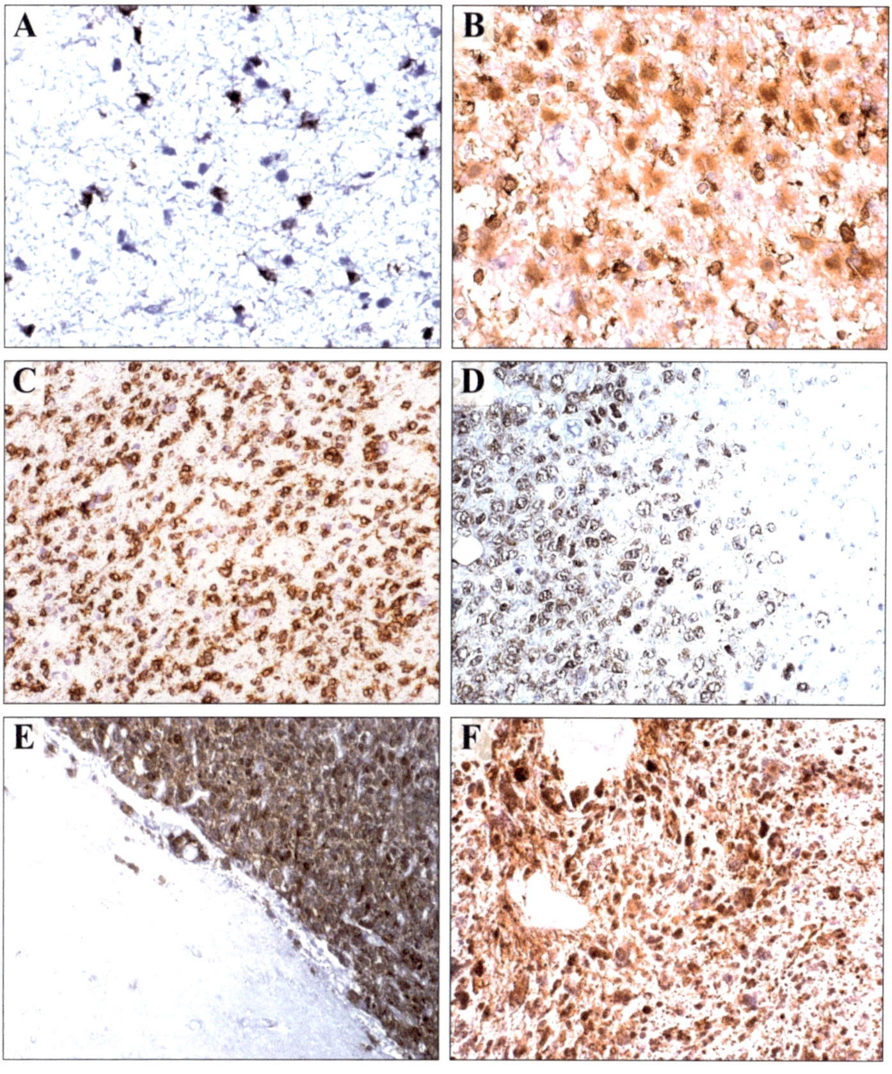

Figure 7. Anti-mIDH1^{R132H} immunohistochemistry. A – Diffuse astrocytoma, immunoreactive cells; B – Gemistocytic astrocytoma, immunoreactive cells; C – Oligodendroglioma, diffuse immunoreactivity of the cells; D – Oligodendroglioma, gradient of immunoreactivity toward the cortex; E – sGBM, sharp border; F – sGBM, immunoreactive cells. All DAB, x200.

In GBMs, positive cells may be polymorphous and the tumor borders could be either sharp or with a gradient of positive cells (Figures 7E,F). Cells crowded around vessels are strongly positive. Giant cells could be either positive or negative.

Pilocytic astrocytomas rarely show immunoreactivity. Reactive astrocytes could be easily recognized for their H09-negative and GFAP-positive immunostaining (Figure 8F).

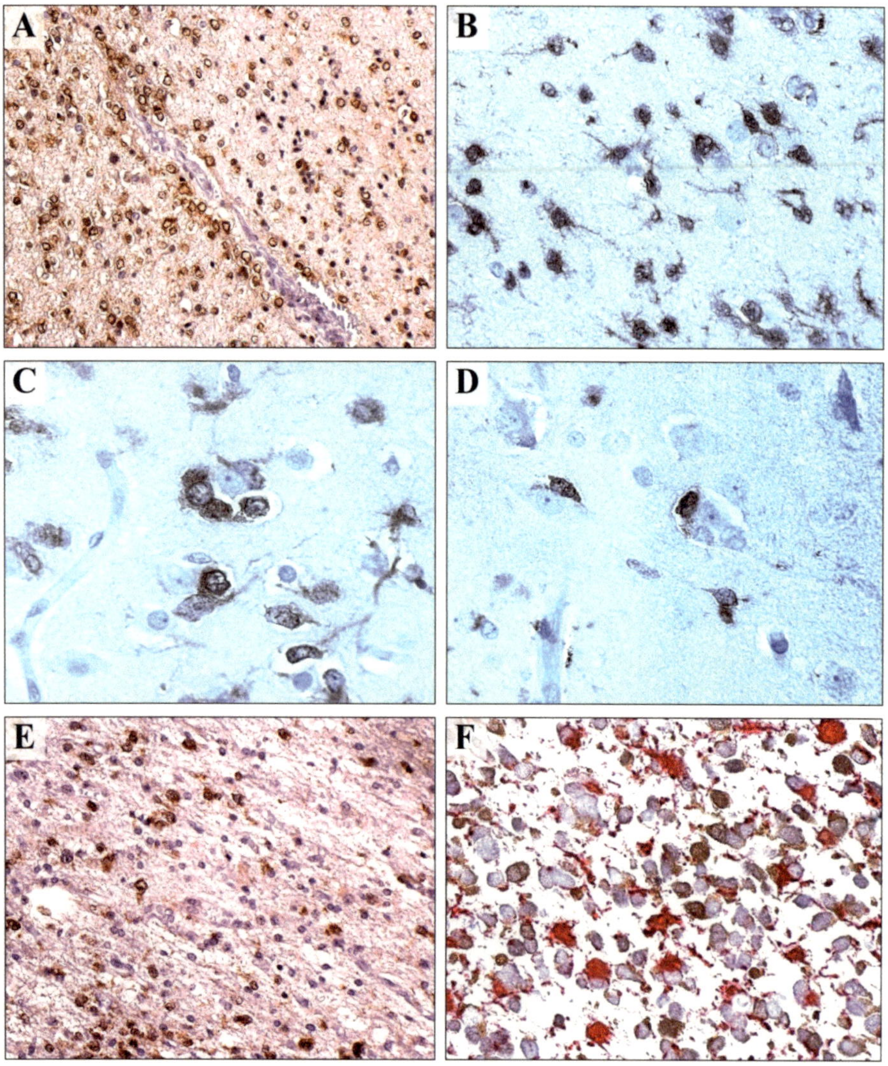

Figure 8. Anti-mIDH1^{R132H} immunohistochemistry. A – Oligodendroglioma, pericapillary cell crowding. DAB, x200; B – Oligodendroglioma, various cell forms in the tumor periphery. DAB, x400; C – Oligodendroglioma, positive perineuronal satellites. DAB, x400; D – Oligodendroglioma, positive and negative perineuronal satellites. DAB, x400; E – Oligodendroglioma, positive and negative cells in an infiltrated area. DAB, x200; F – Double immunohistochemistry showing mIDH1^{R132H}-positive tumor oligodendrocytes and GFAP-positive reactive astrocytes. DAB and Alkaline Phosphatase Red, respectively, x400.

7. Diagnostic, prognostic, predictive and therapeutic considerations

7.1. Diagnostic relevance of IDH mutation assessment

The anti-mIDH1^{R132H} immunohistochemical evaluation is of great utility in the diagnosis of human brain tumors. As already reported, it allows differential diagnosis between gliomas and non-neoplastic CNS lesions (astrocytosis or therapy-induced changes) [151,152], between gliomas and non-glial CNS tumors, and within glioma subtypes [88,90,153].

In our experience, it is useful in the further following diagnostic situations.

1. In small stereotactic biopsies with hypercellular white matter, to recognize tumor infiltration, because single tumor cells can be detected among normal cells in the infiltrating nervous tissue. This is especially relevant in oligodendrogliomas, where it allows to identify the pattern of the tumor infiltration. A clear-cut distinction can be made between tumors with a sharp border with the normal tissue and the infiltrating tumors, where a gradient of tumor cells can be observed toward the normal tissue. Perineuronal and pericapillary satellitoses are immunopositive for the clone H09, with the exception of some cells that may remain unstained. The latter should represent normal perineuronal satellites joined by tumor cells. However, this finding leaves unresolved the question whether the increased number of satellites corresponds to infiltrating cells or whether they derive by transformation of normal satellites. In infiltrating oligodendrogliomas, Cyclin D1 positive normal oligodendrocytes are recognizable by H09-positive tumor oligodendrocytes. This finding may be useful when an oligoastrocytoma must be distinguished from an astrocytoma infiltrating the white matter, contributing to the resolution of the diagnostic ambiguity of these tumors.
2. To discriminate between tumor astrocytes and reactive astrocytes. The latter point is sometimes of paramount importance, especially when the diagnosis must be carried out on small samples, for example in stereotactic biopsies where infiltrative cells must be recognized among normal cells. Immunoreactivity for the clone H09 is a strong evidence for the tumor nature of positive cells among normal or reactive cells. However, the absence of immunoreactivity does not exclude the occurrence of a glioma.
3. In the differential diagnosis between diffuse astrocytomas, frequently immunopositive, and pilocytic or pleomorphic astrocytomas, both typically immunonegative.
4. Among GBMs, to differentiate primary from secondary tumors (see 4.4). Interesting is the diagnostic utility of the IDH status, together with the assessment of TP53 mutation status, in the recognizing of secondary gliosarcoma [154].
5. To discriminate gemystocytes that show variable immunopositivity with usually a less stained center, from minigemistocytes of oligodendrogliomas, in contrast, uniformly and intensely stained [38,145].
6. In the diagnostic ambiguity of oligoastrocytomas or of a tumor with astrocytes, where it is important to identify the normal or tumor nature of oligodendrocytes and the tumor or normal reactive nature of astrocytes [155].

7.2. Prognostic significance of IDH mutations

The occurrence of IDH mutations predicts significantly longer survival for patients affected by GBMs and by WHO grade III astrocytomas and oligodendrogliomas. This was reported in the original discovery of IDH mutations in GBMs [1] and successively confirmed in a large study on WHO grade II and III astrocytomas, oligodendrogliomas and GBMs [28]. Later, the association of IDH mutations with a better patient overall survival (OS) and progression-free survival (PFS) has been confirmed by several reports [36,37,42,57,156-160].

In a recent and partially retrospective study, including the NOA-04 trial cohort of anaplastic astrocytomas and GBMs, IDH mutations are the most powerful single prognostic factor for improved OS, followed by age, tumor type and MGMT promoter hypermethylation [161]. The most favorable outcome is observed in anaplastic astrocytomas with IDH1 mutations, followed by GBMs with IDH1 mutations, anaplastic astrocytomas without IDH1 mutations and GBMs without IDH1 mutations [162].

Likewise, IDH mutations also confer an independent favorable prognosis in WHO grade III oligodendrogliomas, as reported by the European Organization for Research and Treatment (EORTC) trial 2951 [57].

In GBMs, a significant association of IDH1 mutations with OS and PFS was found in primary tumors [37,49] with limited independent prognostic effect [45,159].

In low-grade gliomas, however, the prognostic role of IDH mutations is still controversial, although patients with IDH mutations tend to show a longer survival [36,98,163]. In independent studies on WHO grade II and III gliomas, IDH mutations are prognostic on OS [30,36,56] and PFS [56]. However, in the largest series of low-grade gliomas so far analyzed, no prognostic role of IDH mutations was found in diffuse astrocytomas and oligodendrogliomas [164], in agreement with two recent reports on low-grade astrocytomas [165,166]. Furthermore, patients with low-grade gliomas without IDH1 mutations have a dismal prognosis [56].

In Japanese glioma patients, IDH mutations were significantly associated with increased OS and PFS in WHO grade III tumors but not in WHO grade II [68,98] or in GBMs [98].

In two recent reports on gliomatosis cerebri IDH mutations are strongly correlated to better OS [167,168].

Anyway, the prognostic significance of IDH mutations may be secondary to their prevalence among younger patients, and age is a well-known prognostic factor in gliomas [27]. An explanation for the better prognosis may potentially be related to the biological effect of the IDH mutations. Indeed, IDH1 R132H mutant enzyme seems to impede both migration and growth of stabilized transfected glioma cell lines [169].

In conclusion, the consistent finding of a more favorable outcome in malignant glioma patients with IDH mutations suggests the evaluation of IDH mutation status for prognostic considerations in the clinical setting [139].

7.3. Predictive significance of IDH mutations

Generally, IDH mutations do not show correlations with response to antineoplastic therapy in GBMs [37], anaplastic gliomas [159,161], anaplastic oligodendrogliomas [57] or progressive low-grade gliomas [156]. However, IDH mutations correlate with a higher rate of responses to up-front Temozolomide (TMZ) in a series of 84 low-grade glioma patients, independently from the 1p/19q co-deletion [157]. They also show evidence for differential responsiveness to genotoxic therapy of low-grade glioma patients [163]. The occurrence of IDH mutations is associated with favorable PFS and OS in a cohort of WHO grade II gliomas who received radiotherapy or chemotherapy at diagnosis but not in a cohort of low-grade diffuse gliomas initially treated with surgery alone. In a single report, IDH mutations predict response to TMZ in sGBMs [170].

Interestingly, patients with IDH mutations treated for recurrent gliomas have a longer OS from the time of recurrence when treated with the VEGF (receptor) (VEGF(R))-targeted agents sunitinib malate and bevacizumab, rather than with the EGFR-targeted blocking monoclonal antibody cetuximab. This finding supports the hypothesis that IDH1 mutation may benefit from VEGF(R)- versus EGFR-targeted therapy at the time of recurrence [158].

7.4. Therapeutic significance of IDH mutations

As before mentioned, the impact of IDH mutations on both radio- and chemotherapy responses in gliomas has not yet been clarified. Anyway, a higher therapeutic sensitivity is expected for IDH mutant rather than wild-type tumor cells.

No therapy that specifically targets IDH mutations is currently available. However, mutant IDH enzymes are attractive candidate for a target therapy in gliomas and there is increasing interest in the development of IDH-related therapies. The standard goal should be the block of the D-2-HG oncometabolite by inhibition of IDH mutant enzymes. Restoring normal IDH function, replacing depleted α-KG and/or depleting D-2-HG should be beneficial for glioma patients.

Importantly, in the design of inhibitor molecules for IDH mutant proteins in gliomas, compound selection criteria should include consideration for blood-brain barrier penetration. To date, only few reports of inhibitors against dehydrogenases are available. Among them, inositol monophosphate dehydrogenase (IMPDH) inhibitors only have been introduced into clinical development [171].

A recent intriguing possibility is the opportunity to *in vivo* measure D-2-HG levels on glioma patients. Different methods are available, including direct liquid-chromatography-mass spectrometry (LC-MS), gas chromatography-mass spectrometry (GC-MS) and non invasive imaging techniques as proton magnetic resonance spectroscopy (MRS). Preliminary data in the use of D-2-HG as pharmacodynamic biomarker seem to be promising. Interestingly, D-2-HG levels detected by MRS in glioma patients correlates with the occurrence of IDH mutations [172-175]. However, in a small series of gliomas, D-2-HG levels in serum do not correlate with IDH mutations [176], in contrast to previous findings in AML [177].

In conclusion, IDH mutations identify in gliomas a biologically distinct tumor identity [109]. Suggestions are in favor of the hypothesis that rare pGBMs with IDH mutations might be sGBMs progressed by clinically undetected preceding gliomas of lower malignancy grade. Likewise, sGBMs without IDH mutations might be pGBMs, unrecognized because of inappropriate histological sampling [111]. Anyway, GBMs with IDH mutations seems to be a distinct entity [111] and stratification of GBMs patients according the IDH mutation status should be mandatory.

8. Conclusions

The discovery of recurrent somatic IDH mutations in gliomas is the most significant advance in the field of neuro-oncology in the recent years. This finding emphasizes the putative role of the IDH1 and IDH2 metabolic genes in the molecular pathogenesis of gliomas and, more importantly, the translational relevance of the IDH mutations.

Currently, they are considered a strong prognostic marker for glioma patients, independently from the other well-known prognostic factors. For this reason, the knowledge of the IDH mutation status has a great importance for the diagnosis and prognosis of patients, especially when affected by WHO grade III gliomas and GBMs.

This finding suggests revisions of the current WHO classification of human brain tumors with the addition of the IDH mutation status, as well as the KIAA1549/BRAF fusion gene for pilocytic astrocytomas and the total 1p/19q co-deletion for oligodendrogliomas. Common opinion is in favor of a molecular stratification over the conventional WHO grading for prognostic and therapeutic considerations in both low- and high-grade glioma patients. This may also contribute to solve the ambiguity in the histophatological diagnosis of oligoastrocytoma [155,164].

One of the major question remains the molecular pathogenesis of WHO grade II and III gliomas without IDH mutations, which often do not show alterations in genes typically involved in gliomas, as TP53 mutations or CDKN2A homozygous deletion. Whole-genome or exome sequencing by the next generation sequencing technology may be useful in future to identify the molecular basis of these tumors and to a better comprehension of the molecular pathogenesis of gliomas.

Author details

Marta Mellai*, Valentina Caldera, Laura Annovazzi and Davide Schiffer

*Address all correspondence to: marta.mellai@cnbo.it

Neuro-Bio-Oncology Research Center/ Policlinico di Monza Foundation, Consorzio di Neuroscienze, University of Pavia, Vercelli, Italy

References

[1] Parsons, D. W, Jones, S, Zhang, X, Lin, J. C, Leary, R. J, Angenendt, P, Mankoo, P, Carter, H, Siu, I. M, Gallia, G. L, Olivi, A, Mclendon, R, Rasheed, B. A, Keir, S, Nikolskaya, T, Nikolsky, Y, Busam, D. A, Tekleab, H, Diaz, L, A Jr, Hartigan, J, Smith, D. R, Strausberg, R. L, Marie, S. K, Shinjo, S. M, Yan, H, Riggins, G. J, Bigner, D. D, Karchin, R, Papadopoulos, N, Parmigiani, G, Vogelstein, B, Velculescu, V. E, & Kinzler, K. W. (2008). An integrated genomic analysis of human glioblastoma multiforme. Science., , 321, 1807-1812.

[2] Xu, X, Zhao, J, Xu, Z, Peng, B, Huang, Q, Arnold, E, & Ding, J. (2004). Structures of human cytosolic NADP-dependent isocitrate dehydrogenase reveal a novel self-regulatory mechanism of activity. J Biol Chem., , 279, 33946-33957.

[3] Kelly, J. H, & Plaut, G. W. (1981). Physical evidence for the dimerization of the triphosphopyridine-specific isocitrate dehydrogenase from pig heart. J Biol Chem., , 256, 330-334.

[4] Jennings, G. T, Sechi, S, Stevenson, P. M, Tuckey, R. C, Parmelee, D, & Mcalisterhenn, L. (1994). Cytosolic NADP(+)-dependent isocitrate dehydrogenase. Isolation of rat cDNA and study of tissue-specific and developmental expression of mRNA. J Biol Chem., , 269, 23128-23134.

[5] Geisbrecht, B. V, & Gould, S. J. (1999). The human PICD gene encodes a cytoplasmic and peroxisomal NADP(+)-dependent isocitrate dehydrogenase. J Biol Chem., , 274, 30527-30533.

[6] Park, S. Y, Lee, S. M, Shin, S. W, & Park, J. W. (2008). Inactivation of mitochondrial NADP+-dependent isocitrate dehydrogenase by hypochlorous acid. Free Radic Res., , 42, 467-473.

[7] Nichols, B. J, Hall, L, Perry, A. C, & Denton, R. M. (1993). Molecular cloning and deduced amino acid sequences of the gamma-subunits of rat and monkey NAD(+)-isocitrate dehydrogenases. Biochem J., , 295, 347-350.

[8] Nichols, B. J, Perry, A. C, Hall, L, & Denton, R. M. (1995). Molecular cloning and deduced amino acid sequences of the alpha- and beta- subunits of mammalian NAD(+)-isocitrate dehydrogenase. Biochem J., , 310, 917-922.

[9] Ramachandran, N, & Colman, R. F. (1980). Chemical characterization of distinct subunits of pig heart DPN-specific isocitrate dehydrogenase. J Biol Chem., , 255, 8859-8864.

[10] Weiss, C, Zeng, Y, Huang, J, Sobocka, M. B, & Rushbrook, J. I. (2000). Bovine NAD+-dependent isocitrate dehydrogenase: alternative splicing and tissue-dependent expression of subunit 1. Biochemistry., , 39, 1807-1816.

[11] Haselbeck, R. J, & McAlister-Henn, L. (1993). Function and expression of yeast mitochondrial NAD- and NADP-specific isocitrate dehydrogenases. J Biol Chem., , 268, 12116-12122.

[12] Ceccarelli, C, Grodsky, N. B, Ariyaratne, N, Colman, R. F, & Bahnson, B. J. (2002). Crystal structure of porcine mitochondrial NADP+-dependent isocitrate dehydrogenase complexed with Mn2+ and isocitrate. Insights into the enzyme mechanism. J Biol Chem., , 277, 43454-43462.

[13] Mailloux, R. J, Bériault, R, Lemire, J, Singh, R, Chénier, D. R, Hamel, R. D, & Appanna, V. D. (2007). The tricarboxylic acid cycle, an ancient metabolic network with a novel twist. PLoS One., , 2, e690.

[14] Shechter, I, Dai, P, Huo, L, & Guan, G. (2003). IDH1 gene transcription is sterol regulated and activated by SREBP-1a and SREBP-2 in human hepatoma HepG2 cells: evidence that IDH1 may regulate lipogenesis in hepatic cells. J Lipid Res., , 44, 2169-2180.

[15] Hartong, D. T, Dange, M, Mcgee, T. L, Berson, E. L, Dryja, T. P, & Colman, R. F. (2008). Insights from retinitis pigmentosa into the roles of isocitrate dehydrogenases in the Krebs cycle. Nat Genet., , 40, 1230-1234.

[16] Lee, S. M, Koh, H. J, Park, D. C, Song, B. J, Huh, T. L, & Park, J. W. (2002). Cytosolic NADP(+)-dependent isocitrate dehydrogenase status modulates oxidative damage to cells. Free Radic Biol Med., , 32, 1185-1196.

[17] Nakamura, H. (2005). Thioredoxin and its related molecules: update 2005. Antioxid Redox Signal., , 7, 823-828.

[18] Chowdhury, R, Yeoh, K. K, Tian, Y. M, Hillringhaus, L, Bagg, E. A, Rose, N. R, Leung, I. K, Li, X. S, Woon, E. C, Yang, M, Mcdonough, M. A, King, O. N, Clifton, I. J, Klose, R. J, Claridge, T. D, Ratcliffe, P. J, Schofield, C. J, & Kawamura, A. (2011). The oncometabolite 2-hydroxyglutarate inhibits histone lysine demethylases. EMBO Rep., , 12, 463-469.

[19] Dang, L, White, D. W, Gross, S, Bennett, B. D, Bittinger, M. A, Driggers, E. M, Fantin, V. R, Jang, H. G, Jin, S, Keenan, M. C, Marks, K. M, Prins, R. M, Ward, P. S, Yen, K. E, Liau, L. M, Rabinowitz, J. D, Cantley, L. C, Thompson, C. B, Vander Heiden, M. G, & Su, S. M. (2009). Cancer-associated IDH1 mutations produce 2-hydroxyglutarate. Nature., , 462, 739-744.

[20] Reitman, Z. J, Parsons, D. W, & Yan, H. (2010). IDH1 and IDH2: not your typical oncogenes. Cancer Cell., , 17, 215-216.

[21] Frezza, C, Tennant, D. A, & Gottlieb, E. (2010). IDH1 mutations in gliomas: when an enzyme loses its grip. Cancer Cell., , 17, 7-9.

[22] Cyr, A. R, & Domann, F. E. (2011). The redox basis of epigenetic modifications: from mechanisms to functional consequences. Antioxid Redox Signal., , 15, 551-589.

[23] Zhao, S, Lin, Y, Xu, W, Jiang, W, Zha, Z, Wang, P, Yu, W, Li, Z, Gong, L, Peng, L, Ding, Y, Lei, J, Guan, Q, & Xiong, Y. (2009). Glioma-derived mutations in IDH1 dominantly inhibit IDH1 catalytic activity and induce HIF-1alpha. Science., , 324, 261-265.

[24] Reitman, Z. J, Jin, G, Karoly, E. D, Spasojevic, I, Yang, J, Kinzler, K. W, He, Y, Bigner, D. D, Vogelstein, B, & Yan, H. (2011). Profiling the effects of isocitrate dehydrogenase 1 and 2 mutations on the cellular metabolome. Proc Natl Acad Sci U S A., , 108, 3270-3275.

[25] Jo, S. H, Lee, S. H, Chun, H. S, Lee, S. M, Koh, H. J, Lee, S. E, Chun, J. S, Park, J. W, & Huh, T. L. (2002). Cellular defense against UVB-induced phototoxicity by cytosolic NADP(+)-dependent isocitrate dehydrogenase. Biochem Biophys Res Commun., , 292, 542-549.

[26] Yang, E. S, Richter, C, Chun, J. S, Huh, T. L, Kang, S. S, & Park, J. W. (2002). Inactivation of NADP(+)-dependent isocitrate dehydrogenase by nitric oxide. Free Radic Biol Med., , 33, 927-937.

[27] Louis, D. N, Ohgaki, H, Wiestler, O. D, & Cavenee, W. K. (2007). WHO Classification of Tumors of the Central Nervous Systems (4th edition). Lyon: International Agency for Research on Cancer (IARC).

[28] Yan, H, Parsons, D. W, Jin, G, Mclendon, R, Rasheed, B. A, Yuan, W, Kos, I, Batinic-haberle, I, Jones, S, Riggins, G. J, Friedman, H, Friedman, A, Reardon, D, Herndon, J, Kinzler, K. W, Velculescu, V. E, Vogelstein, B, & Bigner, D. D. (2009). IDH1 and IDH2 mutations in gliomas. N Engl J Med., , 360, 765-773.

[29] Balss, J, Meyer, J, Mueller, W, Korshunov, A, Hartmann, C, & von Deimling, A. (2008). Analysis of the IDH1 codon 132 mutation in brain tumors. Acta Neuropathol., , 116, 597-602.

[30] Hartmann, C, Meyer, J, Balss, J, Capper, D, Mueller, W, Christians, A, Felsberg, J, Wolter, M, Mawrin, C, Wick, W, Weller, M, Herold-Mende, C, Unterberg, A, Jeuken, J. W, Wesseling, P, Reifenberger, G, & von Deimling, A. (2009). Type and frequency of IDH1 and IDH2 mutations are related to astrocytic and oligodendroglial differentiation and age: a study of 1,010 diffuse gliomas. Acta Neuropathol., , 118, 469-474.

[31] Nobusawa, S, Watanabe, T, Kleihues, P, & Ohgaki, H. (2009). IDH1 mutations as molecular signature and predictive factor of secondary glioblastomas. Clin Cancer Res., , 15, 6002-6007.

[32] Ichimura, K, Pearson, D. M, Kocialkowski, S, Bäcklund, L. M, Chan, R, Jones, D. T, & Collins, V. P. (2009). IDH1 mutations are present in the majority of common adult gliomas but rare in primary glioblastomas. Neuro Oncol., , 11, 341-347.

[33] Watanabe, T, Nobusawa, S, Kleihues, P, & Ohgaki, H. (2009). IDH1 mutations are early events in the development of astrocytomas and oligodendrogliomas. Am J Pathol., , 174, 1149-1153.

[34] Horbinski, C, Kofler, J, Kelly, L. M, Murdoch, G. H, & Nikiforova, M. N. (2009). Diagnostic use of IDH1/2 mutation analysis in routine clinical testing of formalin-fixed, paraffin-embedded glioma tissues. J Neuropathol Exp Neurol., , 68, 1319-1325.

[35] Bleeker, F. E, Lamba, S, Leenstra, S, Troost, D, Hulsebos, T, Vandertop, W. P, Frattini, M, Molinari, F, Knowles, M, Cerrato, A, Rodolfo, M, Scarpa, A, Felicioni, L, Buttitta, F, Malatesta, S, Marchetti, A, & Bardelli, A. (2009). IDH1 mutations at residue p.R132 (IDH1(R132)) occur frequently in high-grade gliomas but not in other solid tumors. Hum Mutat., , 30, 7-11.

[36] Sanson, M, Marie, Y, Paris, S, Idbaih, A, Laffaire, J, Ducray, F, El Hallani, S, Boisselier, B, Mokhtari, K, Hoang-Xuan, K, & Delattre, J. Y. (2009). Isocitrate dehydrogenase 1 codon 132 mutation is an important prognostic biomarker in gliomas. J Clin Oncol., , 27, 4150-4154.

[37] Weller, M, Felsberg, J, Hartmann, C, Berger, H, Steinbach, J. P, Schramm, J, Westphal, M, Schackert, G, Simon, M, Tonn, J. C, Heese, O, Krex, D, Nikkhah, G, Pietsch, T, Wiestler, O, Reifenberger, G, von Deimling, A, & Loeffler, M. (2009). Molecular predictors of progression-free and overall survival in patients with newly diagnosed glioblastoma: a prospective translational study of the German Glioma Network. J Clin Oncol., , 27, 5743-5750.

[38] Capper, D, Weissert, S, Balss, J, Habel, A, Meyer, J, Jäger, D, Ackermann, U, Tessmer, C, Korshunov, A, Zentgraf, H, Hartmann, C, & von Deimling, A. (2010). Characterization of R132H mutation-specific IDH1 antibody binding in brain tumors. Brain Pathol., , 20, 245-254.

[39] Horbinski, C, Kelly, L, Nikiforov, Y. E, Durso, M. B, & Nikiforova, M. N. (2010). Detection of IDH1 and IDH2 mutations by fluorescence melting curve analysis as a diagnostic tool for brain biopsies. J Mol Diagn., , 12, 487-492.

[40] Felsberg, J, Wolter, M, Seul, H, Friedensdorf, B, Göppert, M, Sabel, M. C, & Reifenberger, G. (2010). Rapid and sensitive assessment of the IDH1 and IDH2 mutation status in cerebral gliomas based on DNA pyrosequencing. Acta Neuropathol., , 119, 501-507.

[41] Gravendeel, L. A, Kloosterhof, N. K, Bralten, L. B, Van Marion, R, Dubbink, H. J, Dinjens, W, Bleeker, F. E, Hoogenraad, C. C, Michiels, E, Kros, J. M, van den Bent, M, Smitt, P. A., & French, P. J. (2010). Segregation of non-p.R132H mutations in IDH1 in distinct molecular subtypes of glioma. Hum Mutat., , 31, E1186-E1199.

[42] Mellai, M, Piazzi, A, Caldera, V, Monzeglio, O, Cassoni, P, Valente, G, & Schiffer, D. (2011). IDH1 and IDH2 mutations, immunohistochemistry and associations in a series of brain tumors. J Neurooncol., , 105, 345-357.

[43] Takano, S, Tian, W, Matsuda, M, Yamamoto, T, Ishikawa, E, Kaneko, M. K, Yamazaki, K, Kato, Y, & Matsumura, A. (2011). Detection of IDH1 mutation in human glio-

mas: comparison of immunohistochemistry and sequencing. Brain Tumor Pathol., , 28, 115-123.

[44] Toedt, G, Barbus, S, Wolter, M, Felsberg, J, Tews, B, Blond, F, Sabel, M. C, Hofmann, S, Becker, N, Hartmann, C, Ohgaki, H, von Deimling, A, Wiestler, O. D, Hahn, M, Lichter, P, Reifenberger, G, & Radlwimmer, B. (2011). Molecular signatures classify astrocytic gliomas by IDH1 mutation status. Int J Cancer., , 128, 1095-1103.

[45] Sonoda, Y, Kumabe, T, Nakamura, T, Saito, R, Kanamori, M, Yamashita, Y, Suzuk, H, & Tominaga, T. (2009). Analysis of IDH1 and IDH2 mutations in Japanese glioma patients. Cancer Sci., , 100, 1996-1998.

[46] Jha, P, Suri, V, Sharma, V, Singh, G, Sharma, M. C, Pathak, P, Chosdol, K, Jha, P, Suri, A, Mahapatra, A. K, Kale, S. S, & Sarkar, C. (2011). IDH1 mutations in gliomas: first series from a tertiary care centre in India with comprehensive review of literature. Exp Mol Pathol., , 91, 385-393.

[47] Kang, M. R, Kim, M. S, Oh, J. E, Kim, Y. R, Song, S. Y, Seo, S. I, Lee, J. Y, Yoo, N. J, & Lee, S. H. (2009). Mutational analysis of IDH1 codon 132 in glioblastomas and other common cancers. Int J Cancer., , 125, 353-355.

[48] Uno, M, Oba-Shinjo, S. M, Silva, R, Miura, F, Clara, C. A, Almeida, J. R, Malheiros, S. M, Bianco, A. M, Brandt, R, Ribas, G. C, Feres, H, Dzik, C, Rosemberg, S, Stavale, J. N, Teixeira, M. J, & Marie, S. K. (2011). IDH1 mutations in a Brazilian series of glioblastoma. Clinics (Sao Paulo)., , 66, 163-165.

[49] Yan, W, Zhang, W, You, G, Bao, Z, Wang, Y, Liu, Y, Kang, C, You, Y, Wang, L, & Jiang, T. (2012). Correlation of IDH1 mutation with clinicopathologic factors and prognosis in primary glioblastoma: a report of 118 patients from China. PLoS One., , 7, e30339.

[50] Paugh, B. S, Qu, C, Jones, C, Liu, Z, Adamowicz-Brice, M, Zhang, J, Bax, D. A, Coyle, B, Barrow, J, Hargrave, D, Lowe, J, Gajjar, A, Zhao, W, Broniscer, A, Ellison, D. W, Grundy, R. G, & Baker, S. J. (2010). Integrated molecular genetics profiling of pediatric high-grade gliomas reveals key differences with the adult disease. J Clin Oncol., , 28, 3061-3068.

[51] Antonelli, M, Buttarelli, F. R, Arcella, A, Nobusawa, S, Donofrio, V, Oghaki, H, & Giangaspero, F. (2010). Prognostic significance of histological grading, p53 status, YKL-40 expression, and IDH1 mutations in pediatric high-grade gliomas. J Neurooncol., , 99, 209-215.

[52] Pollack, I. F, Hamilton, R. L, Sobol, R. W, Nikiforova, M. N, & Lyons-Weiler, M. A. LaFramboise, W. A, Burger, P. C, Brat, D. J, Rosenblum, M. K, Holmes, E. J, Zhou, T, Jakacki, R. I, & Children's Oncology Group. (2011). IDH1 mutations are common in malignant gliomas arising in adolescents: a report from the Children's Oncology Group. Childs Nerv Syst., , 27, 87-94.

[53] Caldera, V, Mellai, M, Annovazzi, L, Piazzi, A, Lanotte, M, Cassoni, P, & Schiffer, D. (2011). Antigenic and genotypic similarity between primary glioblastomas and their derived neurospheres. J Oncol., , 314962.

[54] Pusch, S, Sahm, F, Meyer, J, Mittelbronn, M, Hartmann, C, & von Deimling, A. (2011). Glioma IDH1 mutation patterns off the beaten track. Neuropathol Appl Neurobiol., , 37, 428-430.

[55] Watanabe, T, Vital, A, Nobusawa, S, Kleihues, P, & Ohgaki, H. (2009). Selective acquisition of IDH1 R132C mutations in astrocytomas associated with Li-Fraumeni syndrome. Acta Neuropathol., , 117, 653-656.

[56] Metellus, P, Coulibaly, B, Colin, C, De Paula, A. M, Vasiljevic, A, Taieb, D, Barlier, A, Boisselier, B, Mokhtari, K, Wang, X. W, Loundou, A, Chapon, F, Pineau, S, Ouafik, L, Chinot, O, & Figarella-Branger, D. (2010). Absence of IDH mutation identifies a novel radiologic and molecular subtype of WHO grade II gliomas with dismal prognosis. Acta Neuropathol., , 120, 719-729.

[57] van den Bent, M. J, Dubbink, H. J, Marie, Y, Brandes, A. A, Taphoorn, M. J, Wesseling, P, Frenay, M, Tijssen, C. C, Lacombe, D, Idbaih, A, van Marion, R, Kros, J. M, Dinjens, W. N, Gorlia, T, & Sanson, M. (2010). IDH1 and IDH2 mutations are prognostic but not predictive for outcome in anaplastic oligodendroglial tumors: a report of the European Organization for Research and Treatment of Cancer Brain Tumor Group. Clin Cancer Res., , 16, 1597-1604.

[58] Narasimhaiah, D, Miquel, C, Verhamme, E, Desclée, P, Cosnard, G, & Godfraind, C. (2012). IDH1 mutation, a genetic alteration associated with adult gliomatosis cerebri. Neuropathology., , 32, 30-37.

[59] Korshunov, A, Meyer, J, Capper, D, Christians, A, Remke, M, Witt, H, Pfister, S, von Deimling, A, & Hartmann, C. (2009). Combined molecular analysis of BRAF and IDH1 distinguishes pilocytic astrocytoma from diffuse astrocytoma. Acta Neuropathol., , 118, 401-405.

[60] Horbinski, C, Kofler, J, Yeaney, G, Camelo-Piragua, S, Venneti, S, Louis, D. N, Perry, A, Murdoch, G, & Nikiforova, M. N. (2011). Isocitrate dehydrogenase 1 analysis differentiates gangliogliomas from infiltrative gliomas. Brain Pathol., , 21, 564-574.

[61] Huse, J. T, Nafa, K, Shukla, N, Kastenhuber, E. R, Lavi, E, Hedvat, C. V, Ladanyi, M, & Rosenblum, M. K. (2011). High frequency of IDH-1 mutation links glioneuronal tumors with neuropil-like islands to diffuse astrocytomas. Acta Neuropathol., , 122, 367-369.

[62] von Deimling, A, Korshunov, A, & Hartmann, C. (2011). The next generation of glioma biomarkers: MGMT methylation, BRAF fusions and IDH1 mutations. Brain Pathol., , 21, 74-87.

[63] Solis, O. E, Mehta, R. I, Lai, A, Mehta, R. I, Farchoukh, L. O, Green, R. M, Cheng, J. C, Natarajan, S, Vinters, H. V, Cloughesy, T, & Yong, W. H. (2011). Rosette-forming

glioneuronal tumor: a pineal region case with IDH1 and IDH2 mutation analyses and literature review of 43 cases. J Neurooncol., , 102, 477-484.

[64] Ishizawa, K, Hirose, T, Sugiyama, K, Kageji, T, Nobusawa, S, Homma, T, Komori, T, & Sasaki, A. (2012). Pathologic diversity of glioneuronal tumor with neuropil-like islands: a histological and immunohistochemical study with a special reference to isocitrate dehydrogenase 1 (IDH1) in 5 cases. Clin Neuropathol., , 31, 67-76.

[65] Hayden, J. T, Frühwald, M. C, Hasselblatt, M, Ellison, D. W, Bailey, S, & Clifford, S. C. (2009). Frequent IDH1 mutations in supratentorial primitive neuroectodermal tumors (sPNET) of adults but not children. Cell Cycle., , 8, 1806-1807.

[66] Gessi, M, Setty, P, Bisceglia, M, zur Muehlen, A, Lauriola, L, Waha, A, Giangaspero, F, & Pietsch, T. (2011). Supratentorial primitive neuroectodermal tumors of the central nervous system in adults: molecular and histopathologic analysis of 12 cases. Am J Surg Pathol., , 35, 573-582.

[67] Ishida, A, Shibuya, M, Komori, T, Nobusawa, S, Niimura, K, Matsuo, S, & Hori, T. (2013). Papillary tumor of the pineal region: a case involving isocitrate dehydrogenase (IDH) genotyping. Brain Tumor Pathol., , 30, 45-49.

[68] Ikota, H, Nobusawa, S, Tanaka, Y, Yokoo, H, & Nakazato, Y. (2011). High-throughput immunohistochemical profiling of primary brain tumors and non-neoplastic systemic organs with a specific antibody against the mutant isocitrate dehydrogenase 1 R132H protein. Brain Tumor Pathol., , 28, 107-114.

[69] Amary, M. F, Bacsi, K, Maggiani, F, Damato, S, Halai, D, Berisha, F, Pollock, R, O'Donnell, P, Grigoriadis, A, Diss, T, Eskandarpour, M, Presneau, N, Hogendoorn, P. C, Futreal, A, Tirabosco, R, & Flanagan, A. M. (2011). IDH1 and IDH2 mutations are frequent events in central chondrosarcoma and central and periosteal chondromas but not in other mesenchymal tumours. J Pathol., , 224, 334-343.

[70] Mardis, E. R, Ding, L, Dooling, D. J, Larson, D. E, Mclellan, M. D, Chen, K, Koboldt, D. C, Fulton, R. S, Delehaunty, K. D, McGrath, S. D, Fulton, L. A, Locke, D. P, Magrini, V. J, Abbott, R. M, Vickery, T. L, Reed, J. S, Robinson, J. S, Wylie, T, Smith, S. M, Carmichael, L, Eldred, J. M, Harris, C. C, Walker, J, Peck, J. B, Du, F, Dukes, A. F, Sanderson, G. E, Brummett, A. M, Clark, E, McMichael, J. F, Meyer, R. J, Schindler, J. K, Pohl, C. S, Wallis, J. W, Shi, X, Lin, L, Schmidt, H, Tang, Y, Haipek, C, Wiechert, M. E, Ivy, J. V, Kalicki, J, Elliott, G, Ries, R. E, Payton, J. E, Westervelt, P, Tomasson, M. H, Watson, M. A, Baty, J, Heath, S, Shannon, W. D, Nagarajan, R, Link, D. C, Walter, M. J, Graubert, T. A, DiPersio, J. F, Wilson, R. K, & Ley, T. J. (2009). Recurring mutations found by sequencing an acute myeloid leukemia genome. N Engl J Med., , 361, 1058-1066.

[71] Andrulis, M, Capper, D, Luft, T, Hartmann, C, Zentgraf, H, & von Deimling, A. (2010). Detection of isocitrate dehydrogenase 1 mutation R132H in myelodysplastic

syndrome by mutation-specific antibody and direct sequencing. Leuk Res., , 34, 1091-1093.

[72] Patel, K. P, Ravandi, F, Ma, D, Paladugu, A, Barkoh, B. A, Medeiros, L. J, & Luthra, R. (2011). Acute myeloid leukemia with IDH1 or IDH2 mutation: frequency and clinico-pathologic features. Am J Clin Pathol., , 135, 35-45.

[73] Ward, P. S, Patel, J, Wise, D. R, Abdel-Wahab, O, Bennett, B. D, Coller, H. A, Cross, J. R, Fantin, V. R, Hedvat, C. V, Perl, A. E, Rabinowitz, J. D, Carroll, M, Su, S. M, Sharp, K. A, Levine, R. L, & Thompson, C. B. (2010). The common feature of leukemia-associated IDH1 and IDH2 mutations is a neomorphic enzyme activity converting alpha-ketoglutarate to 2-hydroxyglutarate. Cancer Cell., , 17, 225-234.

[74] Green, A, & Beer, P. (2010). Somatic mutations of IDH1 and IDH2 in the leukemic transformation of myeloproliferative neoplasms. N Engl J Med., , 362, 369-370.

[75] Paschka, P, Schlenk, R. F, Gaidzik, V. I, Habdank, M, Krönke, J, Bullinger, L, Späth, D, Kayser, S, Zucknick, M, Götze, K, Horst, H. A, Germing, U, Döhner, H, & Döhner, K. (2010). IDH1 and IDH2 mutations are frequent genetic alterations in acute myeloid leukemia and confer adverse prognosis in cytogenetically normal acute myeloid leukemia with NPM1 mutation without FLT3 internal tandem duplication. J Clin Oncol., , 28, 3636-3643.

[76] Arai, M, Nobusawa, S, Ikota, H, Takemura, S, & Nakazato, Y. (2012). Frequent IDH1/2 mutations in intracranial chondrosarcoma: a possible diagnostic clue for its differentiation from chordoma. Brain Tumor Pathol., , 29, 201-206.

[77] Dang, L, Jin, S, & Su, S. M. (2010). IDH mutations in glioma and acute myeloid leukemia. Trends Mol Med., , 16, 387-397.

[78] Rakheja, D, Mitui, M, Boriack, R. L, & DeBerardinis, R. J. (2011). Isocitrate dehydrogenase 1/2 mutational analyses and 2-hydroxyglutarate measurements in Wilms tumors. Pediatr Blood Cancer., , 56, 379-383.

[79] Tang, J. Y, Chang, C. C, Lin, P. C, & Chang, J. G. (2012). Isocitrate dehydrogenase mutation hot spots in acute lymphoblastic leukemia and oral cancer. Kaohsiung J Med Sci., , 28, 138-144.

[80] Holdhoff, M, Parsons, D. W, & Diaz, L. A. Jr. (2009). Mutations of IDH1 and IDH2 are not detected in brain metastases of colorectal cancer. J Neurooncol., , 94, 297.

[81] Struys, E. A. (2006). Unravelling the biochemical pathway and the genetic defect. J Inherit Metab Dis., , 29, 21-29.

[82] van Schaftingen, E, Rzem, R, & Veiga-da-Cunha, M. (2009). L:-2-Hydroxyglutaric aciduria, a disorder of metabolite repair. J Inherit Metab Dis., , 32, 135-142.

[83] Kranendijk, M, Struys, E. A, van Schaftingen, E, Gibson, K. M, Kanhai, W. A, van Der Knaap, M. S, Amiel, J, Buist, N. R, Das, A. M, de Klerk, J. B, Feigenbaum, A. S, Grange, D. K, Hofstede, F. C, Holme, E, Kirk, E. P, Korman, S. H, Morava, E, Morris,

A, Smeitink, J, Sukhai, R. N, Vallance, H, Jakobs, C, & Salomons, G. S. (2010). IDH2 mutations in patients with D-2-hydroxyglutaric aciduria. Science., , 330, 336.

[84] Kranendijk, M, Struys, E. A, Gibson, K. M, Wickenhagen, W. V, Abdenur, J. E, Buechner, J, Christensen, E, de Kremer, R. D, Errami, A, Gissen, P, Gradowska, W, Hobson, E, Islam, L, Korman, S. H, Kurczynski, T, Maranda, B, Meli, C, Rizzo, C, Sansaricq, C, Trefz, F. K, Webster, R, Jakobs, C, & Salomons, G. S. (2010). Evidence for genetic heterogeneity in D-2-hydroxyglutaric aciduria. Mutat., , 31, 279-283.

[85] Kölker, S, Mayatepek, E, & Hoffmann, G. F. (2002). White matter disease in cerebral organic acid disorders: clinical implications and suggested pathomechanisms. Neuropediatrics., , 33, 225-231.

[86] Wajner, M, Latini, A, Wyse, A. T, & Dutra-Filho, C. S. (2004). The role of oxidative damage in the neuropathology of organic acidurias: insights from animal studies. J Inherit Metab Dis., , 27, 427-448.

[87] Aghili, M, Zahedi, F, & Rafiee, E. (2009). Hydroxyglutaric aciduria and malignant brain tumor: a case report and literature review. J Neurooncol., , 91, 233-236.

[88] Amary, M. F, Damato, S, Halai, D, Eskandarpour, M, Berisha, F, Bonar, F, McCarthy, S, Fantin, V. R, Straley, K. S, Lobo, S, Aston, W, Green, C. L, Gale, R. E, Tirabosco, R, Futreal, A, Campbell, P, Presneau, N, & Flanagan, A. M. (2011). Ollier disease and Maffucci syndrome are caused by somatic mosaic mutations of IDH1 and IDH2. Nature Genet., , 43, 1262-1265.

[89] Pansuriya, T. C, van Eijk, R, d'Adamo, P, van Ruler, M. A, Kuijjer, M. L, Oosting, J, Cleton-Jansen, A. M, van Oosterwijk, J. G, Verbeke, S. L, Meijer, D, van Wezel, T, Nord, K. H, Sangiorgi, L, Toker, B, Liegl-Atzwanger, B, San-Julian, M, Sciot, R, Limaye, N, Kindblom, L. G, Daugaard, S, Godfraind, C, Boon, L. M, Vikkula, M, Kurek, K. C, Szuhai, K, French, P. J, & Bovée, J. V. (2011). Somatic mosaic IDH1 and IDH2 mutations are associated with enchondroma and spindle cell hemangioma in Ollier disease and Maffucci syndrome. Nature Genet., , 43, 1256-1261.

[90] Narahara, K, Kimura, S, Kikkawa, K, Takahashi, Y, Wakita, Y, Kasai, R, Nagai, S, Nishibayashi, Y, & Kimoto, H. (1985). Probable assignment of soluble isocitrate dehydrogenase (IDH1) to 2q33.3. Hum Genet., , 71, 37-40.

[91] Grzeschik, K. H. (1976). Assignment of a gene for human mitochondrial isocitrate dehydrogenase (ICD-M, EC 1.1.1.41) to chromosome 15. Hum Genet., , 34, 23-28.

[92] Huh, T. L, Kim, Y. O, Oh, I. U, Song, B. J, & Inazawa, J. (1996). Assignment of the human mitochondrial NAD+-specific isocitrate dehydrogenase alpha subunit (IDH3A) gene to 15q25.1-->q25.2 by in situ hybridization. Genomics., , 32, 295-296.

[93] Kim, Y. O, Park, S. H, Kang, Y. J, Koh, H. J, Kim, S. H, Park, S. Y, Sohn, U, & Huh, T. L. (1999). Assignment of mitochondrial NAD(+)-specific isocitrate dehydrogenase be-

ta subunit gene (IDH3B) to human chromosome band 20p13 by in situ hybridization and radiation hybrid mapping. Cytogenet Cell Genet., , 86, 240-241.

[94] Brenner, V, Nyakatura, G, Rosenthal, A, & Platzer, M. (1997). Genomic organization of two novel genes on human Xq28: compact head to head arrangement of IDH gamma and TRAP delta is conserved in rat and mouse. Genomics., , 44, 8-14.

[95] Krell, D, Assoku, M, Galloway, M, Mulholland, P, Tomlinson, I, & Bardella, C. (2011). Screen for IDH1, IDH2, IDH3, D2HGDH and L2HGDH mutations in glioblastoma. PLoS One., , 6, e19868.

[96] Ren, X, Cui, X, Lin, S, Wang, J, Jiang, Z, Sui, D, Li, J, & Wang, Z. (2012). Co-deletion of chromosome 1p/19q and IDH1/2 mutation in glioma subsets of brain tumors in Chinese patients. PLoS One., , 7, e32764.

[97] Mellai, M, Monzeglio, O, Piazzi, A, Caldera, V, Annovazzi, L, Cassoni, P, Valente, G, Cordera, S, Mocellini, C, & Schiffer, D. (2012). MGMT promoter hypermethylation and its associations with genetic alterations in a series of 350 brain tumors. J Neurooncol., , 107, 617-631.

[98] Mukasa, A, Takayanagi, S, Saito, K, Shibahara, J, Tabei, Y, Furuya, K, Ide, T, Narita, Y, Nishikawa, R, Ueki, K, & Saito, N. (2012). Significance of IDH mutations varies with tumor histology, grade, and genetics in Japanese glioma patients. Cancer Sci., , 103, 587-592.

[99] Labussière, M, Idbaih, A, Wang, X. W, Marie, Y, Boisselier, B, Falet, C, Paris, S, Laffaire, J, Carpentier, C, Crinière, E, Ducray, F, El Hallani, S, Mokhtari, K, Hoang-Xuan, K, Delattre, J. Y, & Sanson, M. (2010). All the 1p/19q codeleted gliomas are mutated on IDH1 or IDH2. Neurology., , 74, 1886-1890.

[100] Bettegowda, C, Agrawal, N, Jiao, Y, Sausen, M, Wood, L. D, Hruban, R. H, Rodriguez, F. J, Cahill, D. P, McLendon, R, Riggins, G, Velculescu, V. E, Oba-Shinjo, S. M, Marie, S. K, Vogelstein, B, Bigner, D, Yan, H, Papadopoulos, N, & Kinzler, K. W. (2011). Mutations in CIC and FUBP1 contribute to human oligodendroglioma. Science., , 333, 1453-1455.

[101] Yip, S, Butterfield, Y. S, Morozova, O, Chittaranjan, S, Blough, M. D, An, J, Birol, I, Chesnelong, C, Chiu, R, Chuah, E, Corbett, R, Docking, R, Firme, M, Hirst, M, Jackman, S, Karsan, A, Li, H, Louis, D. N, Maslova, A, Moore, R, Moradian, A, Mungall, K. L, Perizzolo, M, Qian, J, Roldan, G, Smith, E. E, Tamura-Wells, J, Thiessen, N, Varhol, R, Weiss, S, Wu, W, Young, S, Zhao, Y, Mungall, A. J, Jones, S. J, Morin, G. B, Chan, J. A, Cairncross, J. G, & Marra, M. A. (2012). Concurrent CIC mutations, IDH mutations, and 1p/19q loss distinguish oligodendrogliomas from other cancers. J Pathol., , 226, 7-16.

[102] Badiali, M, Gleize, V, Paris, S, Moi, L, Elhouadani, S, Arcella, A, Morace, R, Antonelli, M, Buttarelli, F, Figarella-Branger, D, Kim, Y. H, Ohgaki, H, Mokhtari, K, Sanson, M,

& Giangaspero, F. (2012). KIAA1549-BRAF fusions and IDH mutations can coexist in diffuse gliomas of adults. Brain Pathol., , 22, 841-847.

[103] Kleihues, P, & Ohgaki, H. (1999). Primary and secondary glioblastomas: from concept to clinical diagnosis. Neuro Oncol., , 1, 44-51.

[104] Uchida, K, Mukai, M, Okano, H, & Kawase, T. (2004). Possible oncogenicity of subventricular zone neural stem cells: case report. Neurosurgery., , 55, 977-978.

[105] Dai, C, Celestino, J. C, Okada, Y, Louis, D. N, Fuller, G. N, & Holland, E. C. (2011). PDGF autocrine stimulation dedifferentiates cultured astrocytes and induces oligodendrogliomas and oligoastrocytomas from neural progenitors and astrocytes in vivo. Genes Dev., , 15, 1913-1925.

[106] Berger, F, Gay, E, Pelletier, L, Tropel, P, & Wion, D. (2004). Development of gliomas: potential role of asymmetrical cell division of neural stem cells. Lancet Oncol., , 5, 511-514.

[107] Bachoo, R. M, Maher, E. A, Ligon, K. L, Sharpless, N. E, Chan, S. S, You, M. J, Tang, Y, Defrances, J, Stover, E, Weissleder, R, Rowitch, D. H, Louis, D. N, & Depinho, R. A. (2002). Epidermal growth factor receptor and Ink4a/Arf: convergent mechanisms governing terminal differentiation and transformation along the neural stem cell to astrocyte axis. Cancer Cell., , 1, 269-277.

[108] Doetsch, F, Petreanu, L, Caille, I, Garcia-Verdugo, J. M, & Alvarez-Buylla, A. (2002). EGF converts transit-amplifying neurogenic precursors in the adult brain into multipotent stem cells. Neuron., , 36, 1021-1034.

[109] Schiffer, D, Mellai, M, Annovazzi, L, Piazzi, A, Monzeglio, O, & Caldera, V. (2012). Glioblastoma cancer stem cells: basis for a functional hypothesis. Stem Cell Discovery., , 2, 122-131.

[110] Lai, A, Kharbanda, S, Pope, W. B, Tran, A, Solis, O. E, Peale, F, Forrest, W. F, Pujara, K, Carrillo, J. A, Pandita, A, Ellingson, B. M, Bowers, C. W, Soriano, R. H, Schmidt, N. O, Mohan, S, Yong, W. H, Seshagiri, S, Modrusan, Z, Jiang, Z, Aldape, K. D, Mischel, P. S, Liau, L. M, Escovedo, C. J, Chen, W, Nghiemphu, P. L, James, C. D, Prados, M. D, Westphal, M, Lamszus, K, Cloughesy, T, & Phillips, H. S. (2011). Evidence for sequenced molecular evolution of IDH1 mutant glioblastoma from a distinct cell of origin. J Clin Oncol., , 29, 4482-4490.

[111] Yan, H, Bigner, D. D, Velculescu, V, & Parsons, D. W. (2009). Mutant metabolic enzymes are at the origin of gliomas. Cancer Res., , 69, 9157-9159.

[112] Phillips, H. S, Kharbanda, S, Chen, R, Forrest, W. F, Soriano, R. H, Wu, T. D, Misra, A, Nigro, J. M, Colman, H, Soroceanu, L, Williams, P. M, Modrusan, Z, Feuerstein, B. G, & Aldape, K. (2006). Molecular subclasses of high-grade glioma predict prognosis, delineate a pattern of disease progression, and resemble stages in neurogenesis. Cancer Cell., , 9, 157-173.

[113] Verhaak, R. G, Hoadley, K. A, Purdom, E, Wang, V, Qi, Y, Wilkerson, M. D, Miller, C. R, Ding, L, Golub, T, Mesirov, J. P, Alexe, G, Lawrence, M, O'Kelly, M, Tamayo, P, Weir, B. A, Gabriel, S, Winckler, W, Gupta, S, Jakkula, L, Feiler, H. S, Hodgson, J. G, James, C. D, Sarkaria, J. N, Brennan, C, Kahn, A, Spellman, P. T, Wilson, R. K, Speed, T. P, Gray, J. W, Meyerson, M, Getz, G, Perou, C. M, & Hayes, D. N; Cancer Genome Atlas Research Network. (2010). Integrated genomic analysis identifies clinically relevant subtypes of glioblastoma characterized by abnormalities in PDGFRA, IDH1, EGFR, and NF1. Cancer Cell., , 17, 98-110.

[114] Noushmeher, H, Weisenberger, D. J, Diefes, K, Phillips, H. S, Pujara, K, Berman, B. P, Pan, F, Pelloski, C. E, Sulman, E. P, Bhat, K. P, Verhaak, R. G, Hoadley, K. A, Hayes, D. N, Perou, C. M, Schmidt, H. K, Ding, L, Wilson, R. K, Van Den Berg, D, Shen, H, Bengtsson, H, Neuvial, P, Cope, L. M, Buckley, J, Herman, J. G, Baylin, S. B, Laird, P. W, & Aldape, K; Cancer Genome Atlas Research Network. (2010). Identification of a CpG island methylator phenotype that defines a distinct subgroup of gliomas. Cancer Cell., , 17, 510-522.

[115] Gorovets, D, Kannan, K, Shen, R, Kastenhuber, E. R, Islamdoust, N, Campos, C, Pentsova, E, Heguy, A, Jhanwar, S. C, Mellinghoff, I. K, Chan, T. A, & Huse, J. T. (2012). IDH mutation and neuroglial developmental features define clinically distinct subclasses of lower grade diffuse astrocytic glioma. Clin Cancer Res., , 18, 2490-2501.

[116] Figueroa, M. E, Lugthart, S, Li, Y, Erpelinck-Verschueren, C, Deng, X, Christos, P. J, Schifano, E, Booth, J, van Putten, W, Skrabanek, L, Campagne, F, Mazumdar, M, Greally, J. M, Valk, P. J, Löwenberg, B, Delwel, R, & Melnick, A. (2010). DNA methylation signatures identify biologically distinct subtypes in acute myeloid leukemia. Cancer Cell., , 17, 13-27.

[117] Christensen, B. C, Smith, A. A, Zheng, S, Koestler, D. C, Houseman, E. A, Marsit, C. J, Wiemels, J. L, Nelson, H. H, Karagas, M. R, Wrensch, M. R, Kelsey, K. T, & Wiencke, J. K. (2011). DNA methylation, isocitrate dehydrogenase mutation, and survival in glioma. J Natl Cancer Inst., , 103, 143-153.

[118] Laffaire, J, Everhard, S, Idbaih, A, Crinière, E, Marie, Y, De Reyniès, A, Schiappa, R, Mokhtari, K, Hoang-Xuan, K, Sanson, M, Delattre, J. Y, Thillet, J, & Ducray, F. (2011). Methylation profiling identifies 2 groups of gliomas according to their tumorigenesis. Neuro Oncol., , 13, 84-98.

[119] Turcan, S, Rohle, D, Goenka, A, Walsh, L. A, Fang, F, Yilmaz, E, Campos, C, Fabius, A. W, Lu, C, Ward, P. S, Thompson, C. B, Kaufman, A, Guryanova, O, Levine, R, Heguy, A, Viale, A, Morris, L. G, Huse, J. T, Mellinghoff, I. K, & Chan, T. A. (2012). IDH1 mutation is sufficient to establish the glioma hypermethylator phenotype. Nature., , 483, 479-483.

[120] Figueroa, M. E, Abdel-Wahab, O, Lu, C, Ward, P. S, Patel, J, Shih, A, Li, Y, Bhagwat, N, Vasanthakumar, A, Fernandez, H. F, Tallman, M. S, Sun, Z, Wolniak, K, Peeters, J. K, Liu, W, Choe, S. E, Fantin, V. R, Paietta, E, Löwenberg, B, Licht, J. D, Godley, L. A,

Delwel, R, Valk, P. J, Thompson, C. B, Levine, R. L, & Melnick, A. (2010). Leukemic IDH1 and IDH2 mutations result in a hypermethylation phenotype, disrupt TET2 function, and impair hematopoietic differentiation. Cancer Cell., , 18, 553-567.

[121] Ito, S, D'Alessio, A. C, Taranova, O. V, Hong, K, Sowers, L. C, & Zhang, Y. (2010). Role of TET proteins in 5mC to 5hmC conversion, ES-cell self-renewal and inner cell mass specification. Nature., , 466, 1129-1133.

[122] Kim, T, Lee, P, & Colman, R. F. (2003). Critical role of Lys212 and Tyr140 in porcine NADP-dependent isocitrate dehydrogenase. J Biol Chem., , 278, 49323-49331.

[123] Ward, P. S, Cross, J. R, Lu, C, Weigert, O, Abel-Wahab, O, Levine, R. L, Weinstock, D. M, Sharp, K. A, & Thompson, C. B. (2012). Identification of additional IDH mutations associated with oncometabolite R(-)-2-hydroxyglutarate production. Oncogene., , 31, 2491-2498.

[124] Thompson, C. B. (2009). Metabolic enzymes as oncogens or tumor suppressors. N Engl J Med., , 360, 813-815.

[125] Guo, C, Pirozzi, C. J, Lopez, G. Y, & Yan, H. (2011). Isocitrate dehydrogenase mutations in gliomas: mechanisms, biomarkers and therapeutic target. Curr Opin Neurol., , 24, 648-652.

[126] Gupta, R, Webb-Myers, R, Flanagan, S, & Buckland, M. E. (2011). Isocitrate dehydrogenase mutations in diffuse gliomas: clinical and aetiological implications. J Clin Pathol., , 64, 835-844.

[127] Ichimura, K. (2012). Molecular pathogenesis of IDH mutations in gliomas. Brain Tumor Pathol., , 29, 131-139.

[128] Reitman, Z. J, & Yan, H. (2010). Isocitrate dehydrogenase 1 and 2 mutations in cancer: alterations at a crossroads of cellular metabolism. J Natl Cancer Inst., , 102, 932-941.

[129] Jin, G, Reitman, Z. J, Spasojevic, I, Batinic-Haberle, I, Yang, J, Schmidt-Kittler, O, Bigner, D. D, & Yan, H. (2011). 2-hydroxyglutarate production, but not dominant negative function, is conferred by glioma-derived NADP-dependent isocitrate dehydrogenase mutations. PLoS One., , 6, e16812.

[130] Hausinger, R. P. (2004). FeII/alpha-ketoglutarate-dependent hydroxylases and related enzymes. Crit Rev Biochem Mol Biol., , 39, 21-68.

[131] Xu, W, Yang, H, Liu, Y, Yang, Y, Wang, P, Kim, S. H, Ito, S, Yang, C, Wang, P, Xiao, M. T, Liu, L. X, Jiang, W. Q, Liu, J, Zhang, J. Y, Wang, B, Frye, S, Zhang, Y, Xu, Y. H, Lei, Q. Y, Guan, K. L, Zhao, S. M, & Xiong, Y. (2011). Oncometabolite 2-hydroxyglutarate is a competitive inhibitor of α-ketoglutarate-dependent dioxygenases. Cancer Cell., , 19, 17-30.

[132] Williams, S. C, Karajannis, M. A, Chiriboga, L, Golfinos, J. G, von Deimling, A, & Zagzag, D. (2011). R132H-mutation of isocitrate dehydrogenase-1 is not sufficient for HIF-1α upregulation in adult glioma. Acta Neuropathol., , 121, 279-281.

[133] Lu, C, Ward, P. S, Kapoor, G. S, Rohle, D, Turcan, S, Abdel-Wahab, O, Edwards, C. R, Khanin, R, Figueroa, M. E, Melnick, A, Wellen, K. E, O'Rourke, D. M, Berger, S. L, Chan, T. A, Levine, R. L, Mellinghoff, I. K, & Thompson, C. B. (2012). IDH mutation impairs histone demethylation and results in a block to cell differentiation. Nature., , 483, 474-478.

[134] Dringen, R, Bishop, G. M, Koeppe, M, Dang, T. N, & Robinson, S. R. (2007). The pivotal role of astrocytes in the metabolism of iron in the brain. Neurochem Res., , 32, 1884-1890.

[135] Townsend, D. M, Tew, K. D, & Tapiero, H. (2003). The importance of glutathione in human disease. Biomed Pharmacother., , 57, 145-155.

[136] Lieber, M. R. (2008). The mechanism of human nonhomologous DNA end joining. J Biol Chem., , 283, 1-5.

[137] Koptyra, M, Cramer, K, Slupianek, A, Richardson, C, & Skorski, T. (2008). BCR/ABL promotes accumulation of chromosomal aberrations induced by oxidative and genotoxic stress. Leukemia., , 22, 1969-1972.

[138] Ronnebaum, S. M, Ilkayeva, O, Burgess, S. C, Joseph, J. W, Lu, D, Stevens, R. D, Becker, T. C, Sherry, A. D, Newgard, C. B, & Jensen, M. V. (2006). A pyruvate cycling pathway involving cytosolic NADP-dependent isocitrate dehydrogenase regulates glucose-stimulated insulin secretion. J Biol Chem., , 281, 30593-30602.

[139] Preusser, M, Capper, D, & Hartmann, C. ; Euro-CNS Research Committee. (2011). IDH testing in diagnostic neuropathology: review and practical guideline article invited by the Euro-CNS research committee. Clin Neuropathol., , 30, 217-230.

[140] Setty, P, Hammes, J, Rothämel, T, Vladimirova, V, Kramm, C. M, Pietsch, T, & Waha, A. (2010). A pyrosequencing-based assay for the rapid detection of IDH1 mutations in clinical samples. J Mol Diagn., , 12, 750-756.

[141] Meyer, J, Pusch, S, Balss, J, Capper, D, Mueller, W, Christians, A, Hartmann, C, & von Deimling, A. (2010). PCR- and restriction endonuclease-based detection of IDH1 mutations. Brain Pathol., , 20, 298-300.

[142] Bujko, M, Kober, P, Matyja, E, Nauman, P, Dyttus-Cebulok, K, Czeremszynska, B, Bonicki, W, & Siedlecki, J. A. (2010). Prognostic value of IDH1 mutations identified with PCR-RFLP assay in glioblastoma patients. Mol Diagn Ther., , 14, 163-169.

[143] Boisselier, B, Marie, Y, Labussière, M, Ciccarino, P, Desestret, V, Wang, X, Capelle, L, Delattre, J. Y, & Sanson, M. (2010). COLD PCR HRM: a highly sensitive detection method for IDH1 mutations. Hum Mutat., , 31, 1360-1365.

[144] Perizzolo, M, Winkfein, B, Hui, S, Krulicki, W, Chan, J. A, & Demetrick, D. J. (2012). IDH mutation detection in formalin-fixed paraffin-embedded gliomas using multiplex PCR and single-base extension. Brain Pathol., , 22, 619-624.

[145] Capper, D, Zentgraf, H, Balss, J, Hartmann, C, & von Deimling, A. (2009). Monoclonal antibody specific for IDH1 R132H mutation. Acta Neuropathol., , 118, 599-601.

[146] Kato, Y, Jin, G, Kuan, C. T, McLendon, R. E, Yan, H, & Bigner, D. D. (2009). A monoclonal antibody IMab-1 specifically recognizes IDH1R132H, the most common glioma-derived mutation. Biochem Biophys Res Commun., , 390, 547-551.

[147] Kaneko, M. K, Tian, W, Takano, S, Suzuki, H, Sawa, Y, Hozumi, Y, Goto, K, Yamazaki, K, Kitanaka, C, & Kato, Y. (2011). Establishment of a novel monoclonal antibody SMab-1 specific for IDH1-R132S mutation. Biochem Biophys Res Commun., , 406, 608-613.

[148] Tabatabai, G, Stupp, R, van den Bent, M. J, Hegi, M. E, Tonn, J. C, Wick, W, & Weller, M. (2010). Molecular diagnostics of gliomas: the clinical perspective. Acta Neuropathol., , 120, 585-592.

[149] Cavalla, P, Dutto, A, Piva, R, Richiardi, P, Grosso, R, & Schiffer, D. (1998). Cyclin D1 expression in gliomas. Acta Neuropathol., , 95, 131-135.

[150] Bosone, I, Cavalla, P, Chiadò-Piat, L, Vito, N. D, & Schiffer, D. (2001). Cyclin D1 expression in normal oligodendroglia and microglia cells: its use in the differential diagnosis of oligodendrogliomas. Neuropathology., , 21, 155-161.

[151] Capper, D, Sahm, F, Hartmann, C, Meyermann, R, von Deimling, A, & Schittenhelm, J. (2010). Application of mutant IDH1 antibody to differentiate diffuse glioma from nonneoplastic central nervous system lesions and therapy-induced changes. Am J Surg Pathol., , 34, 1199-1204.

[152] Camelo-Piragua, S, Jansen, M, Ganguly, A, Kim, J. C, Louis, D. N, & Nutt, C. L. (2010). Mutant IDH1-specific immunohistochemistry distinguishes diffuse astrocytoma from astrocytosis. Acta Neuropathol., , 119, 509-511.

[153] Capper, D, Reuss, D, Schittenhelm, J, Hartmann, C, Bremer, J, Sahm, F, Harter, P. N, Jeibmann, A, & von Deimling, A. (2011). Mutation-specific IDH1 antibody differentiates oligodendrogliomas and oligoastrocytomas from other brain tumors with oligodendroglioma-like morphology. Acta Neuropathol., , 121, 241-252.

[154] Romeike, B. F, Chen, Y, Walter, J, & Petersen, I. (2011). Diagnostic utility of IDH1- and p53-analysis in secondary gliosarcoma. Clin Neuropathol., , 30, 231-234.

[155] Schiffer, D. (2006). Brain tumor pathology: current diagnostic hotspots and pitfalls. The Netherlands: Springer.

[156] Dubbink, H. J, Taal, W, van Marion, R, Kros, J. M, van Heuvel, I, Bromberg, J. E, Zonnenberg, B. A, Zonnenberg, C. B, Postma, T. J, Gijtenbeek, J. M, Boogerd, W, Groenendijk, F. H, Smitt, P. A, Dinjens, W. N, & van den Bent, M. J. (2009). IDH1

mutations in low-grade astrocytomas predict survival but not response to temozolomide. Neurology., , 73, 1792-1795.

[157] Houillier, C, Wang, X, Kaloshi, G, Mokhtari, K, Guillevin, R, Laffaire, J, Paris, S, Boisselier, B, Idbaih, A, Laigle-Donadey, F, Hoang-Xuan, K, Sanson, M, & Delattre, J. Y. (2010). IDH1 or IDH2 mutations predict longer survival and response to temozolomide in low-grade gliomas. Neurology., , 75, 1560-1566.

[158] Lv, S, Teugels, E, Sadones, J, Quartier, E, Huylebrouck, M, Four, D. U, Mercier, S, L. E, Witte, M, D. E, Salmon, O, Michotte, I, Grève, A, D. E, & Neyns, J. B. (2011). Correlation between IDH1 gene mutation status and survival of patients treated for recurrent glioma. Anticancer Res., , 31, 4457-4463.

[159] Qi, S. T, Yu, L, Lu, Y. T, Ou, Y. H, Li, Z. Y, Wu, L. X, & Yao, F. (2011). IDH mutations occur frequently in Chinese glioma patients and predict longer survival but not response to concomitant chemoradiotherapy in anaplastic gliomas. Oncol Rep., , 26, 1479-1485.

[160] Schittenhelm, J, Mittelbronn, M, Meyermann, R, Melms, A, Tatagiba, M, & Capper, D. (2011). Confirmation of R132H mutation of isocitrate dehydrogenase 1 as an independent prognostic factor in anaplastic astrocytoma. Acta Neuropathol., , 122, 651-652.

[161] Wick, W, Hartmann, C, Engel, C, Stoffels, M, Felsberg, J, Stockhammer, F, Sabel, M. C, Koeppen, S, Ketter, R, Meyermann, R, Rapp, M, Meisner, C, Kortmann, R. D, Pietsch, T, Wiestler, O. D, Ernemann, U, Bamberg, M, Reifenberger, G, von Deimling, A, & Weller, M. (2009). NOA-04 randomized phase III trial of sequential radiochemotherapy of anaplastic glioma with procarbazine, lomustine, and vincristine or temozolomide. J Clin Oncol., , 27, 5874-5880.

[162] Hartmann, C, Hentschel, B, Wick, W, Capper, D, Felsberg, J, Simon, M, Westphal, M, Schackert, G, Meyermann, R, Pietsch, T, Reifenberger, G, Weller, M, Loeffler, M, & von Deimling, A. (2010). Patients with IDH1 wild type anaplastic astrocytomas exhibit worse prognosis than IDH1-mutated glioblastomas, and IDH1 mutation status accounts for the unfavorable prognostic effect of higher age: implications for classification of gliomas. Acta Neuropathol., , 120, 707-718.

[163] Hartmann, C, Hentschel, B, Tatagiba, M, Schramm, J, Schnell, O, Seidel, C, Stein, R, Reifenberger, G, Pietsch, T, von Deimling, A, Loeffler, M, & Weller, M. ; German Glioma Network. (2011). Molecular markers in low-grade gliomas: predictive or prognostic? Clin Cancer Res., , 17, 4588-4599.

[164] Kim, Y. H, Nobusawa, S, Mittelbronn, M, Paulus, W, Brokinkel, B, Keyvani, K, Sure, U, Wrede, K, Nakazato, Y, Tanaka, Y, Vital, A, Mariani, L, Stawski, R, Watanabe, T, De Girolami, U, Kleihues, P, & Ohgaki, H. (2010). Molecular classification of low-grade diffuse gliomas. Am J Pathol., , 177, 2708-2714.

[165] Juratli, T. A, Kirsch, M, Robel, K, Soucek, S, Geiger, K, von Kummer, R, Schackert, G, & Krex, D. (2012). IDH mutations as an early and consistent marker in low-grade as-

trocytomas WHO grade II and their consecutive secondary high-grade gliomas. J Neurooncol., , 108, 403-410.

[166] Ahmadi, R, Stockhammer, F, Becker, N, Hohlen, K, Misch, M, Christians, A, Dictus, C, Herold-Mende, C, Capper, D, Unterberg, A, von Deimling, A, Wick, W, & Hartmann, C. (2012). No prognostic value of IDH1 mutations in a series of 100 WHO grade II astrocytomas. J Neurooncol., , 109, 15-22.

[167] Desestret, V, Ciccarino, P, Ducray, F, Crinière, E, Boisselier, B, Labussière, M, Polivka, M, Idbaih, A, Kaloshi, G, von Deimling, A, Hoang-Xuan, K, Delattre, J. Y, Mokhtari, K, & Sanson, M. (2011). Prognostic stratification of gliomatosis cerebri by IDH1 R132H and INA expression. J Neurooncol., , 105, 219-224.

[168] Glas, M, Bähr, O, Felsberg, J, Rasch, K, Wiewrodt, D, Schabet, M, Simon, M, Urbach, H, Steinbach, J. P, Rieger, J, Fimmers, R, Bamberg, M, Nägele, T, Reifenberger, G, Weller, M, & Herrlinger, U. ; Neuro-Oncology Group of the German Cancer Society. (2011). NOA-05 phase 2 trial of procarbazine and lomustine therapy in gliomatosis cerebri. Ann Neurol., , 70, 445-453.

[169] Bralten, L. B, Kloosterhof, N. K, Balvers, R, Sacchetti, A, Lapre, L, Lamfers, M, Leenstra, S, De Jonge, H, Kros, J. M, Jansen, E. E, Struys, E. A, Jakobs, C, Salomons, G. S, Diks, S. H, Peppelenbosch, M, Kremer, A, Hoogenraad, C. C, Smitt, P. A, & French, P. J. (2011). IDH1 R132H decreases proliferation of glioma cell lines in vitro and in vivo. Ann Neurol., , 69, 455-463.

[170] SongTao, Q, Lei, Y, Si, G, YanQing, D, HuiXia, H, XueLin, Z, LanXiao, W, & Fei, Y. (2012). IDH mutations predict longer survival and response to temozolomide in secondary glioblastoma. Cancer Sci., , 103, 269-273.

[171] Jain, J, Almquist, S. J, Shlyakhter, D, & Harding, M. W. (2001). VX-497: a novel, selective IMPDH inhibitor and immunosuppressive agent. J Pharm Sci., , 90, 625-637.

[172] Pope, W. B, Prins, R. M, Albert Thomas, M, Nagarajan, R, Yen, K. E, Bittinger, M. A, Salamon, N, Chou, A. P, Yong, W. H, Soto, H, Wilson, N, Driggers, E, Jang, H. G, Su, S. M, Schenkein, D. P, Lai, A, Cloughesy, T. F, Kornblum, H. I, Wu, H, Fantin, V. R, & Liau, L. M. (2012). Non-invasive detection of 2-hydroxyglutarate and other metabolites in IDH1 mutant glioma patients using magnetic resonance spectroscopy. J Neurooncol., , 107, 197-205.

[173] Choi, C, Ganji, S. K, DeBerardinis, R. J, Hatanpaa, K. J, Rakheja, D, Kovacs, Z, Yang, X. L, Mashimo, T, Raisanen, J. M, Marin-Valencia, I, Pascual, J. M, Madden, C. J, Mickey, B. E, Malloy, C. R, Bachoo, R. M, & Maher, E. A. (2012). 2-hydroxyglutarate detection by magnetic resonance spectroscopy in IDH-mutated patients with gliomas. Nat Med., , 18, 624-629.

[174] Kalinina, J, Carroll, A, Wang, L, Yu, Q, Mancheno, D. E, Wu, S, Liu, F, Ahn, J, He, M, Mao, H, & van Meir, E. G. (2012). Detection of "oncometabolite" 2-hydroxyglutarate

by magnetic resonance analysis as a biomarker of IDH1/2 mutations in glioma. J Mol Med (Berl)., , 90, 1161-1171.

[175] Andronesi, O. C, Kim, G. S, Gerstner, E, Batchelor, T, Tzika, A. A, Fantin, V. R, Vander Heiden, M. G, & Sorensen, A. G. (2012). Detection of 2-hydroxyglutarate in IDH-mutated glioma patients by in vivo spectral-editing and 2D correlation magnetic resonance spectroscopy. Sci Transl Med., , 4, 116ra4.

[176] Capper, D, Simon, M, Langhans, C. D, Okun, J. G, Tonn, J. C, Weller, M, Deimling, A. V, & Hartmann, C. ; German Glioma Network. (2012). 2-Hydroxyglutarate concentration in serum from patients with gliomas does not correlate with IDH1/2 mutation status or tumor size. Int J Cancer., , 131, 766-768.

[177] Gross, S, Cairns, R. A, Minden, M. D, Driggers, E. M, Bittinger, M. A, Jang, H. G, Sasaki, M, Jin, S, Schenkein, D. P, Su, S. M, Dang, L, Fantin, V. R, & Mak, T. W. (2010). Cancer-associated metabolite 2-hydroxyglutarate accumulates in acute myelogenous leukemia with isocitrate dehydrogenase 1 and 2 mutations. J Exp Med., , 207, 339-344.

Chapter 11

Deregulation of Cell Polarity Proteins in Gliomagenesis

Khamushavalli Geevimaan and
Phanithi Prakash Babu

Additional information is available at the end of the chapter

http://dx.doi.org/10.5772/52365

1. Introduction

Gliomas are the most common central nervous system neoplasms that arise from the transformation of astrocytes or their precursor cells. Glial tumors develop as a result of stepwise accumulation of genetic alterations, which disrupt the cell cycle arrest pathways or activate various signal transduction pathways. Despite recent advances in treatment modalities such as surgical techniques, radiation therapy, chemotherapy and targeted gene therapy, their prognosis remains poor. Gliomas are graded from I to IV according to the 2007 World Health Organization (WHO) malignancy scale. Grade I lesions are benign and quite constrained with a slow propagation rate and they constitute the most common glioma of children, pilocytic astrocytoma. Grade II tumors, called diffuse astrocytoma have a slow growth rate and a high degree of cellular differentiation, with their ability to diffuse into normal brain parenchyma and progress toward more malignant form. Grade III tumors include anaplastic astrocytoma, which are characterized by a higher cellular density and the plentiful persistence of atypia and mitotic cells. Grade IV tumors are the most frequent malignant gliomas and they are characterized as glioblastoma with high recurrence rate. GBMs include two subtypes, primary GBMs arise `*de novo*' and secondary GBMs develop due to accumulation of mutations in lower grade gliomas. EGFR amplification, LoH 10q, $p16^{Ink4A}$ deletion and PTEN mutations are the common genetic alterations associated with primary GBMs whereas p53 mutations and PDGFR amplifications are frequent in secondary GBMs (Ohgaki and Kleihues., 2007; Holland., 2001). These genetic alterations disrupt the cell cycle arrest pathways or activate various signal transduction pathways. Mutation of the p53, retinoblastoma (RB) and PTEN, deletion of $p16^{Ink4A}$, activation of the Ras and Akt pathways, and amplification of CDK4 and EGFR contribute to the development of gliomas (Cavenee., 1992; Hayashi et al., 1997).

Cell polarity is an essential phenomenon in several biological processes that contribute to normal tissue integrity and maturity. Several studies in different genetic models has identified and revealed different roles of polarity complexes in maintenances of stem cell population and their asymmetric division (Knoblich., 2010), T-cell function like migration in response to chemokines and antigens (Krummel and Macara., 2006), neuronal cell axon and dendritic specification (Arimura and Kaibuchi., 2007) and cell polarity is crucial for epithelial cell and tissue polarization for maintenance of multicellular structures and perform normal physiological functions like secretion, absorption and distribution of cytoplasmic and membrane proteins in appropriate positions within the cell in order to conduct proper signals.

2. Cell polarity regulators and their deregulation in cancer

Proficient research work in organisms like *Caenorhabditis elegans* and *Drosophila melanogaster* has led to discovery of three different polarity complexes which are asymmetrically distributed within the cell. They are Partitioning defective (Par) complex consists of Par3, Par6 and an atypical protein kinase C, Crumbs complex consists of Crumbs, Pals1 (Protein associated with Lin seven 1) and Pals1-associated tight junction protein (PATJ) and Scribble complex consists of Scribble, Discs large (Dlg) and Lethal giant larvae (Lgl). Crumbs polarity complex and the Partitioning defective (Par) polarity complex are localized to the apical cortex, whereas members of the Scribble polarity complex are localized at the basolateral regions of the cell (Bilder and Perrimon., 2000; Humbert et al., 2006).

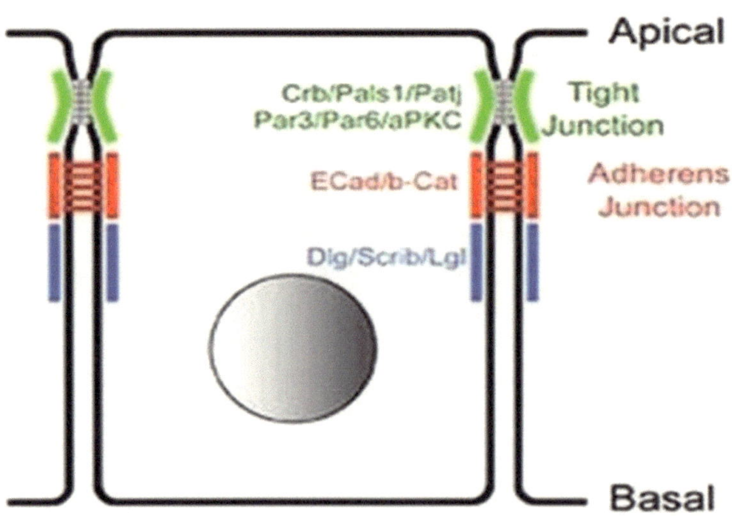

Figure 1. Localization of cell polarity complexes in epithelial cell. Par complex consisting of Par3, Par6, aPKC and Crumbs complex consisting of Crb, Palsl, PAT J are localized apically in the region of tight junctions (T Js). Scribble complex consisting of Scrib, Dlg and Lgl is localized basolaterally in the region of adherens Junction. (this illustrationis reproduced fiom I)Djiane laboratory)

2.1. PAR polarity complex

Par complex was initially identified in *C.elegans* and it consists of two scaffold proteins, PAR6 and PAR3 and an atypical protein kinase C, aPKC. In mammals Par6 protein is encoded by three different genes PAR6A/C, PAR6B and PAR6D/G, Par3 is encoded by *PAR3A* and *PAR3B* genes and two *aPKC* genes, *aPKCλ/ι* and *aPKCζ* encode two different proteins. Par3 and Par6 interact with each other via their PDZ domains and the interaction between Par 3 protein to aPKC/Par6 is dynamic and aPKC-dependent phosphorylation can expel Par3 from the aPKC/Par6 unit (Horikoshi et al., 2009). PAR complex is essential for defining the appropriate apico-lateral axis and assembly of tight junction proteins at their respective position.

2.2. Crumb polarity complex

Crumbs polarity complex was identified in *Drosophila* and in mammals it consists of trans-membrane protein CRB encoded by *CRB1, 2,* and *3* genes along with two cytoplasmic scaffolding proteins PALS1 and PATJ. CRB1 connect to PDZ domains of Pals1 and PATJ through C-terminal ERLI motif. Pals1 is a member of the membrane-associated guanylate kinase (MAGUK) family, which has a PDZ domain, two L27 domains, a SH3 domain and a guanylate kinase domain. PATJ has 10 PDZ domains and one L27N domain (Tepass and Knust., 1993). CRB complex is involved in formation of tight junctions and differentiation of the apical membrane.

2.3. SCRIB polarity complex:

Scribble, Dlg and Lgl were identified in Drosophila as tumor suppressors, in mammals SCRIB is also called VARTUL. Scribble is a member of LAP family with leucine-rich repeats and PDZ domains, while Dlg in mammals exists in five isoforms and it is a member of the MAGUK family containing PDZ domains. Lgl which exists as Lgl1 and Lgl2 in mammals does not contain PDZ domains but has WD40 domains, which is thought to mediate interactions with phosphorylated serine and tyrosine (Dow et al. 2007).

Interaction among these three complexes dictates them to localize in their respective positions, for example Lgl1 and 2 can compete with Par3 for binding to a module of Par6 and aPKC and aPKC phosphorylate Lgl releasing it from the Par6/aPKC dimer, ensuing its localization to the basolateral region of cells (Betschinger et al. 2003). These complexes induce their function by regulating cytoskeleton architecture and there is a substantial data showing direct link with small GTPases of the Rho family and Cdc42, Rac1 and RhoA, control the cytoskeletal changes in cells by switching between an active GTP-bound state and an inactive GDP-bound state. For example Par3 can bind the Rac-activator Tiam1 during tight junction formation and Par6/Par3 regulates Cdc42-mediated Rac1 activation through Tiam1 in neuronal cells (Nishimura et al. 2005). These multifaceted interactions between polarity proteins and with small GTPases is essential for maintenance of polarity and carrying out normal physiological functions of the cell and any aberrant regulation in any of these proteins is related to tumor genesis.

Cell polarity proteins regulate cancer cell properties like proliferation, apoptosis, and epithelial-mesenchymal transition. Studies have shown that Par6 induces growth factor independent proliferation of human mammary epithelial cells by activating MAPK signaling through aPKC and Cdc42/Rac (Muthuswamy et al. 2008). aPKC can regulate cell proliferation through ERK and SRC-3 dependent manner (Castoria et al. 2004 and Yi et al. 2008) and knock down of aPKC in MCF-7 breast cancer cell line inhibited cell proliferation. Down regulation of Scribble induces JNK-dependent cell death (Brumby and Richardson. 2003) and in similar manner inhibition of aPKC increases apoptosis of MDCK cell by activating GSK3β (Kim et al., 2007). Acquisition of mesenchymal property by cancer cells during metastasis is due to change in the cell architecture which is regulated by cell polarity proteins. Research in genetic model *Drosophila* led to discovery that Scribble, DLg, Lgl, Par and Cdc42 cooperate with Rasv12 during invasion (Pagliarini and Xu. 2003). TGFβ signaling has been shown to phosphorylate Par6 protein which leads to RhoA degradation through Smurf1 (Wang et al., 2003). ZEB1 which is a transcriptional regulator of EMT represses the expression of polarity proteins like Crumbs, Lgl2 and PATJ ultimately leading to mesenchymal transition (Aigner et al., 2007).

Cancer is a multistep process whereby cells first acquire benign over proliferation due to genetic assaults, followed by inhibition of apoptosis and increased cell proliferation. The conversion of benign to malignant form is accompanied by loss in cell-cell to contact and apical-basal polarity which ultimately leads to EMT associated with invasion into different parts from the site of cancer. During cancer progression steps these different polarity complexes are either aberrantly expressed or mislocalised from their respective locations. Genetic studies in model organisms and *in vitro* cell culture has shown that these polarity complexes append to take apart in diverse hierarchy of human cancer. aPKC is over expressed in various human cancers like non-small cell lung cancer, ovarian cancer and its expression level correlates with over expression of Cyclin E and with their poor prognosis (Regala et al., 2005 and Eder et al., 2005). In human esophageal squamous cell carcinoma Par3 gene is homozygously lost with reduced protein expression (Zen et al., 2009). Par6 is regarded as a tumor promoter as it is over expressed in human breast cancer and its interaction with TGFβ receptor implicates its role in EMT (Ozdamar et al., 2005).

However contribution of Crumb complex for tumor progression is not completely elucidated. Few studies have shown that Crb-3 expression negatively correlates with metastatic behavior of cells as its decreased expression is associated with increased expression of vimentin and reduced expression of E-cadherin (Bhat et al., 1999). Assembly of Crumb complex leads to phosphorylation of transcription effector molecule of Hippo signaling pathway TAZ/YAP which in turn leads to inhibition of TGF-β-SMAD signaling essential for vimentin expression (Varels et al., 2010). ZEB1 and SNAIL represses the Crumb complex activity. PATJ and Pals1 are required for tight junction (TJ) assembly. PATJ is targeted for degradation by human papiloma virus (HPV) oncoprotein during development of cervical cancer (Javier. 2008). Till date there is no evidence for role of Pals1 in cancer, however few studies in mice model have shown that Pals1 is essential for survival since its loss results in embryonic lethality.

Scribble complex, regarded as fly tumor suppressor genes and basolateral polarity complex are regulated at different levels in human cancers. Dlg and Lgl proteins are down regulated and mislocalised in tumors of breast, prostate, lung, ovary, cervical and liver.scribble and Dlg are targeted for degradation by viral oncoproteins from HPV(Thomas et al., 2005), Human T-cell leukemia (HTLV) (Okajima et al., 2008) and their expression levels are correlated with loss of tissue architecture. Scribble is miss localized in cervical, colon, endometrial and prostate cancer (Nakagawa et al., 2004, Gardiol et al., 2006, Ouyang et al., 2010 and Pearson et al., 2011). In *Drosophila* genetic study, it has been exposed that loss of Scribble function alone is not sufficient to induce tumor, instead Scrib mutant cells expressing oncogenic Raf, Ras or Notch results in loss of apical-basal polarity, neoplastic overgrowth and metastasis.

3. Cell polarity in glial cell

Glial cells include myelinating oligodendrocytes, Schwann cells and astrocytes and they execute diverse functions that are vital for the development, functioning and regeneration of neurons. Unlike epithelial cells which require cell polarity for polarization of cellular components and neurons for axon and dendrite specification, glial cells require cell polarity for migration and myelination.

Oligodendrocytes and Schwann cells are responsible for myelination of neurons, it requires proper sorting of proteins and lipids and polarized membrane trafficking to organize myelin domains and maintain this highly polarized phenotype (DeBruin and Harauz. 2007). Astrocytes are the cells which carry out major functions in brain including interactions with neurons and blood vessels (Schipke and Kettenmann., 2004), migration towards inflammation called astrogliosis (Ridet et al. 1997) which requires polarization of astrocytes into front-rear axis. Astrocytes polarize and migrate by interacting with extra cellular matrix components. Upon interaction of ECM with integrin receptors on astorcytes, activates intracellular signaling through small G proteins like Rac and Cdc42 for controlled polarization and orientation (Heasman and Ridley. 2008). Guanine exchange factors are in charge for the GDP–GTP exchange and therefore are the major regulators of small G proteins activity. It has been shown that cell polarity protein Scrib plays a crucial role in astrocyte migration by binding with Rac and Cdc42-specific exchange factor βPIX and controlling the localization of Cdc42 at leading edge of migratory processes (Osmani et al. 2006). Besides Scrib other evolutionary conserved polarity proteins like Par protein complex is implicated in astrocyte migration. Par6-aPKC complex controls and regulates the microtubule organization during astrocyte migration. The GTP-bound form of Cdc4 binds to Par6 and activates aPKC kinase at leading edge of astrocyte (Etienne-Manneville et al., 2005).

4. Loss of cell polarity during gliomagenesis

Previously loss of cell polarity was regarded as post effect of cancer, but recent research work led to discovery that cell polarity is lost and responsible for tumorigenesis and its progression. Loss of cell polarity in brain tumors is not well documented and very few works like Klezovitch et al. have show that loss of cell polarity causes severe brain dysplasia using Lgl1 knockout mice. We analyzed total of 50 astrocytic tumor samples from Krishna Institute of Medical Sciences (Hyderabad, India), they were classified histopathologically according to the WHO classification: 16 pilocytic astrocytoma (PILO; grade I), 8 diffuse astrocytomas (DA; grade II), 7 anaplastic astrocytomas (AA; grade III), and 19 glioblastoma multiforme (GBM; grade IV) and one normal brain sample was obtained during autopsy for the expression of Scribble polarity complex in astocytic tumors. All samples were obtained from patients after taking the informed consent form patients or their guardians. Using western blotting and immuno histochemical examination we found that protein levels of Scrib was negatively associated with increase in the tumor grade and in few GBM samples Scrib was completely absent. Immuno fluorescence staining as shown in Fig. 2, 3, 4 revealed that in control brain astrocytes, Scrib was localized at the end of astrocyte processes and it was mislocalised in low grade tumors with complete absence in GBM (Khamushavalli et al., unpublished data).

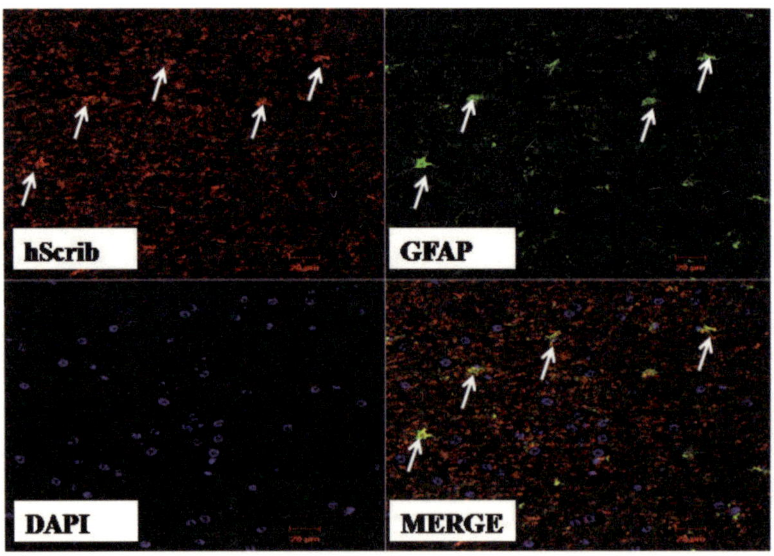

Figure 2. Localization of hSrib in control astrocytes: Paraffin-embedded control brain section was prepared from autopsy brain specimen. Secations were incubated with anti-rabbit-hScrib and anti-mouse-GFAP specific primary antibodies (1:100 dilution) overnight at 4°C and anti-rabbit-TRITC and anti-mouse-FITC secondary antibodies were used for 1 h at room temperature. DAPI was used for the detection of nuclei and fluorescence was captured under Leica confocal microscope. Representative figure showed the localization of hScrib in GFAP positive astrocyte processes.

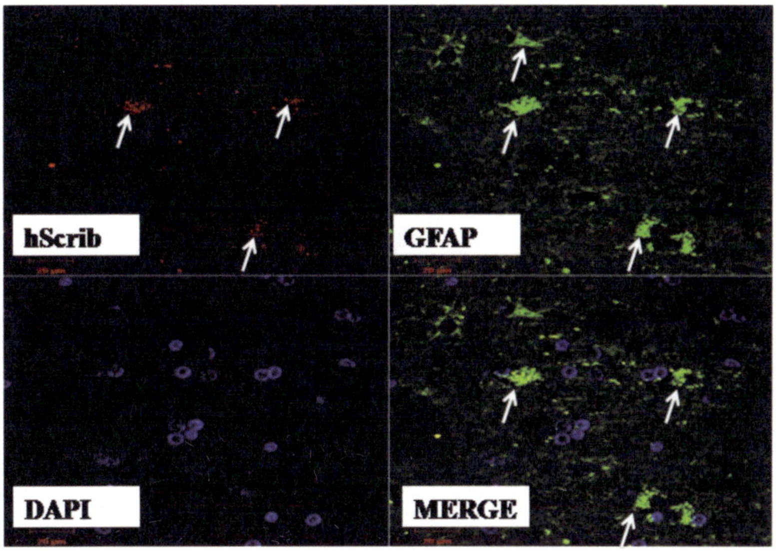

Figure 3. Localization of hScrib in grade II astrocytoma: Paraffin-embedded grade II astrocytoma section was prepared and incubated with anti-rabbit-hScrib and anti-mouseGFAP specific primary antibodies (1:100 delution) overnight at 4°C and anti-rabbit-TRITC and anti-mouse-FITC secondary antibodies were used for 1 h at room temperature. DAPI was used for the detection of nuclei and fluorescence was captured under Leica confocal microscope. Representative figure showed the diffuse localization and low level expression of hScrib in GFAP positive astrocytes.

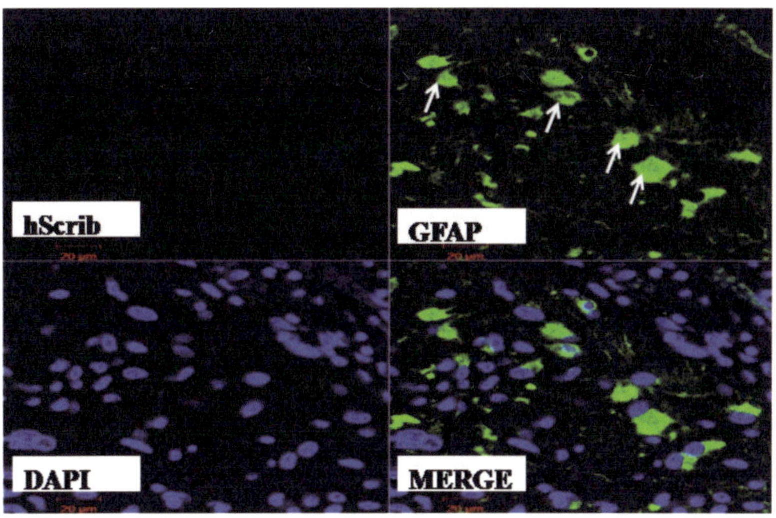

Figure 4. Localization of hScrib in grade IV astrocytoma: Paraffin-embedded grade II astrocytoma section was prepared and incubated with anti-rabbit-hScrib and anti-mouseGFAP specific primary antibodies (1:100 delution) overnight at 4°C and anti-rabbit-TRITC and anti-mouse-FITC secondary antibodies were used for 1 h at room temperature. DAPI was used for the detection of nuclei and fluorescence was captured under Leica confocal microscope. Representative figure showed the loss of hScrib in GFAP positive astrocytes

5. Conclusion

Loss of cell architecture and cell-cell contacts is the hall mark of metastasis, and these process are regulated by cell polarity proteins. Recent work in different cancers has revealed the expressional loss and mislocalisation of cell polarity proteins and their potential role as tumor suppressors. Till date there is no report explaining the role of these polarity proteins in glioma and the above results indicate that cell polarity proteins do have role in glioamgenesis and further research is necessary to elucidate how these proteins are deregulated during glioma prosression.

Acknowledgements

The authors would like to acknowledge funding from DBT, CSIR, ICMR, DST and DST nano UoH project. We thank CSIR for fellowship to Khamushavalli Geevimaan.

Author details

Khamushavalli Geevimaan and Phanithi Prakash Babu*

Department of Biotechnology, School of Lifesciences, University of Hyderabad, Hyderabad, India

References

[1] Ohgaki, H, & Kleihues, P. (2007). Genetic pathways to primary and secondary glioblastoma. Am. J. Pathol. , 170, 1445-1453.

[2] Holland, E. C. (2001). Gliomagenesis: genetic alterations and mouse models. Nat. Rev. Genet. , 2, 120-129.

[3] Cavenee, W. K. (1992). Accumulation of genetic defects during astrocytoma progression. Cancer. , 70, 1788-1793.

[4] Hayashi, Y, Ueki, K, Waha, A, Wiestler, O. D, Louis, D. N, & Von Deimling, A. (1997). Association of EGFR gene amplification and CDKN2 (MTS1) gene deletion in glioblastoma multiforme. Brain Pathol. 7:871-875., 16.

[5] Knoblich, J. A. (2010). Asymmetric cell division: recent developments and their implications for tumour biology. Nat Rev Mol Cell Biol. , 11, 849-860.

[6] Krummel, M. F, & Macara, I. (2006). Maintenance and modulation of T cell polarity. Nat Immunol. , 7, 1143-1149.

[7] Arimura, N, & Kaibuchi, K. (2007). Neuronal polarity: from extracellular signals to intracellular mechanisms. Nat Rev Neurosci. , 8, 194-205.

[8] Bilder, D, Li, M, & Perrimon, N. (2000). Cooperative regulation of cell polarity and growth by Drosophila tumor suppressors. Science. , 289, 113-116.

[9] Humbert, P. O, Dow, L. E, & Russell, S. M. The Scribble and Par complexes in polarity and migration: friends or foes? Trends Cell Biol. , 16, 622-630.

[10] Horikoshi, Y, Suzuki, A, Yamanaka, T, Sasaki, K, Mizuno, K, Sawada, H, et al. (2009). Interaction between PAR-3 and the aPKC-PAR-6 complex is indispensable for apical domain development of epithelial cell. J Cell Sci. , 122, 1595-1606.

[11] Tepass, U, & Knust, E. (1993). Crumbs and stardust act in a genetic pathway that controls the organization of epithelia in Drosophila melanogaste. Dev Biol. , 159, 311-326.

[12] Dow, L. E, Kauffman, J. S, Caddy, J, Zarbalis, K, Peterson, A. S, Jane, S. M, Russell, S. M, & Humbert, P. O. (2007). The tumour-suppressor Scribble dictates cell polarity during directed epithelial migration: regulation of Rho GTPase recruitment to the leading edge. Oncogene. , 26, 2272-2282.

[13] Betschinger, J, Mechtler, K, & Knoblich, J. A. (2003). The Par complex directs asymmetric cell division by phosphorylating the cytoskeletal protein Lgl. Nature. , 422, 326-330.

[14] Nishimura, T, Yamaguchi, T, Kato, K, Yoshizawa, M, Nabeshima, Y, Ohno, S, et al. (2005). PAR-6-PAR-3 mediates Cdc42-induced Rac activation through the Rac GEFs STEF/Tiam1. Nat Cell Biol. , 7, 270-277.

[15] Nolan, M. E, Aranda, V, Lee, S, Lakshmi, B, Basu, S, Allred, D. C, & Muthuswamy, S. K. (2008). The polarity protein Par6 induces cell proliferation and is over expressed in breast cancer. Cancer Res., 68, 8201-8209.

[16] Castoria, G, & Migliaccio, A. Di Domenico, M., Lombardi, M., De Falco, A., Varricchio, L., Bilancio, A., Barone, M.V., Auricchio, F. (2004). Role of atypical protein kinase C in estradiol-triggered G1/S progression of Mcf-7 cells. Mol Cell Biol. , 24, 7643-7653.

[17] Yi, P, Feng, Q, Amazit, L, Lonard, D. M, Tsai, S. Y, Tsai, M. J, & Malley, O. B.W. (2008). Atypical protein kinase C regulates dual pathways for degradation of the oncogenic coactivator Src-3/Aib1. Mol Cell. , 29, 465-476.

[18] Brumby, A. M, & Richardson, H. E. (2003). Scribble mutants cooperate with oncogenic Ras or notch to cause neoplastic overgrowth in Drosophila. EMBO J. , 22, 5769-5779.

[19] Kim, M, Datta, A, Brakeman, P, Yu, W, & Mostov, K. E. (2007). Polarity proteins Par6 and APKC regulate cell death through GSK-3beta in 3d epithelial morphogenesis. J Cell Sci, , 120, 2309 2317.

[20] Pagliarini, R. A, & Xu, T. (2003). A genetic screen in Drosophila for metastatic behavior. Science. , 302, 1227-1231.

[21] Wang, H. R, Zhang, Y, Ozdamar, B, Ogunjimi, A. A, Alexandrova, E, Thomsen, G. H, & Wrana, J. L. (2003). Regulation of cell polarity and protrusion formation by targeting Rhoa for degradation. Science. , 302, 1775-1779.

[22] Aigner, K, Dampier, B, Descovich, L, Mikula, M, Sultan, A, Schreiber, M, Mikulits, W, Brabletz, T, Strand, D, Obrist, P, et al. (2007). The transcription factor Zeb1 ([Delta]Ef1) promotes tumour cell dedifferentiation by repressing master regulators of epithelial polarity. Oncogene. , 26, 6979-6988.

[23] Regala, R. P, Weems, C, Jamieson, L, Khoor, A, Edell, E. S, Lohse, C. M, et al. (2005). Atypical protein kinase C iota is an oncogene in human non-small cell lung cancer. Cancer Res. , 65, 8905-8911.

[24] Eder, A. M, Sui, X, Rosen, D. G, Nolden, L. K, Cheng, K. W, Lahad, J. P, et al. (2005). Atypical PKCiota contributes to poor prognosis through loss of apical-basal polarity and cyclin E overexpression in ovarian cancer. Proc Natl Acad Sci U S A. , 102, 12519-12524.

[25] Zen, K, Yasui, K, Gen, Y, Dohi, O, Wakabayashi, N, Mitsufuji, S, et al. (2009). Defective expression of polarity protein PAR-3 gene (PARD3) in esophageal squamous cell carcinoma. Oncogene. , 28, 2910-2918.

[26] Ozdamar, B, Bose, R, Barrios-rodiles, M, Wang, H. R, Zhang, Y, & Wrana, J. L. (2005). Regulation of the polarity protein Par6 by TGFbeta receptors controls epithelial cell plasticity. Science. , 307, 1603-1609.

[27] Bhat, M. A, Izaddoost, S, Lu, Y, Cho, K. O, Choi, K. W, & Bellen, H. J. (1999). Discs Lost, a novel multi-PDZ domain protein, establishes and maintains epithelial polarity. Cell. , 96, 833-845.

[28] Varelas, X, Samavarchi-tehrani, P, Narimatsu, M, Weiss, A, Cockburn, K, Larsen, B. G, Rossant, J, & Wrana, J. L. (2010). The Crumbs complex couples cell density sensing to Hippo-dependent control of the TGF-β-SMAD pathway. Dev Cell. , 6, 831-44.

[29] Javier, R. T. (2008). Cell polarity proteins: common targets for tumorigenic human viruses'.Oncogene. , 27, 7031-7046.

[30] Thomas, M, Massimi, P, Navarro, C, Borg, J. P, & Banks, L. (2005). The hScrib/Dlg apico-basal control complex is differentially targeted by HPV-16 and HPV-18 E6 proteins.Oncogene. , 24, 6222-6230.

[31] Okajima, M, Takahashi, M, Higuchi, M, Ohsawa, T, Yoshida, S, Yoshida, Y, et al. (2008). Human T-cell leukemia virus type 1 Tax induces an aberrant clustering of the

tumor suppressor Scribble through the PDZ domain-binding motif dependent and independent interaction. Virus Genes. , 37, 231-240.

[32] Nakagawa, S, Yano, T, Nakagawa, K, Takizawa, S, Suzuki, Y, Yasugi, T, et al. (2004). Analysis of the expression and localisation of a LAP protein, human scribble, in the normal and neoplastic epithelium of uterine cervix. Br J Cancer. , 90, 194-199.

[33] Gardiol, D, Zacchi, A, Petrera, F, Stanta, G, & Banks, L. (2006). Human discs large and scrib are localized at the same regions in colon mucosa and changes in their expression patterns are correlated with loss of tissue architecture during malignant progression. Int J Cancer. , 119, 1285-1290.

[34] Ouyang, Z, Zhan, W, & Dan, L. (2010). hScrib, a human homolog of Drosophila neoplastic tumor suppressor, is involved in the progress of endometrial cancer. Oncol Res. , 18, 593-599.

[35] Pearson, H. B, Perez-mancera, P. A, Dow, L. E, Ryan, A, Tennstedt, P, Bogani, D, et al. (2011). SCRIB expression is deregulated in human prostate cancer and its deficiency in mice promotes prostate neoplasia. J Clin Invest. , 121, 4257-4267.

[36] Klezovitch, O, Fernandez, T. E, Tapscott, S. J, & Vasioukhin, V. (2004). Loss of cell polarity causes severe brain dysplasia in Lgl1 knockout mice. Genes Dev. , 18, 559-71.

[37] Debruin, L. S, & Harauz, G. (2007). White matter rafting- membrane microdomains in myelin.Neurochem Res. , 32, 213-228.

[38] Schipke, C. G, & Kettenmann, H. (2004). Astrocyte responses to neuronal activity. Glia. , 47, 226-232.

[39] Ridet, J. L, Malhotra, S. K, Privat, A, & Cage, F. H. (1997). Reactive astrocytes: cellular and molecular cues to biological function. Trends Neurosci, , 20, 570-577.

[40] Heasman, S. J, & Ridley, A. J. (2008). Mammalian Rho GTPases: new insights into their functions from in vivo studies. Nat Rev Mol Cell Biol. , 9, 690-701.

[41] Osmani, N, Vitale, N, Borg, J. P, & Etienne-manneville, S. (2006). Scrib controls Cdc42 localization and activity to promote cell polarization during astrocyte migration. Curr Biol, , 16, 2395-2405.

[42] Etienne-manneville, S, Manneville, J. B, Nicholls, S, Ferenczi, M, & Hall, A. (2005). Cdc42 and Par6-PKCζ regulate the spatially localized association of Dlg1 and APC to control cell polarization. J Cell Biol., 170, 895-901.

Chapter 12

Aquaporin, Midkine and Glioblastoma

Mine Ergüven

Additional information is available at the end of the chapter

http://dx.doi.org/10.5772/52429

1. Introduction

1.1. Glioblastoma

Glioblastoma (GBM) with their invasive and aggressive nature, are the most common primary brain tumours. GBM accounts for about 60% of all gliomas and 12–15% of all brain tumors, and it is per se the most frequent primary brain tumor [1,2]. Although advances in therapies, clinicians and researchers fail to arrive at overcoming poor prognosis with a median survival of only one year from the time of diagnosis. In Europe and North America, the incidence is three new cases per 100.000 inhabitants per year [3]. Although GBM can manifest itself at any age, it preferentially occurs in adults, with a wide peak age of incidence between 45 and 70 years [4].

GBMs arised from glial cells which are the building-block cells of the connective and supportive, tissues in the central nervous system. Diffuse gliomas defined as astrocytomas, oligodendrogliomas, and oligoastrocytomas are the common gliomas which infiltrate throughout the brain parenchyma. They are graded on a World Health Organization (WHO) classification system scale of I to IV according to their degree of malignancy based on different histological features and genetic alterations. Grade I tumors are pilocytic astrocytomas and they are benign and can be cured if they can be surgically resected; grade II tumors are low grade astrocytomas (LGAs) which are incurable with surgery because of their early diffuse infiltration of the surrounding brain, and long treatment regimens are needed to treat this disease completely; grade III tumors are anaplastic astrocytomas and they have increased anaplasia and proliferate over grade IV tumors and are more rapidly fatal; grade IV tumors are GBMs which possess advanced features of malignancy, and are resistant to radio/chemotherapy [5].

Important characteristics of GBMs are aberrant cellular proliferation, diffuse infiltration, prospensity for necrosis, robust angiogenesis, high resistance to apoptosis, and genomic instability. The intratumoral heterogenity combined with a putative cancer stem cell

(CSC) subpopulation and incomplete atlas of epigenetic lesions are the reasons of poor prognosis/high tumoral resistance against chemotherapeutics and recurrence [1,2,5-8]. Studies showing crosstalks between genetics and epigenetics in GBM are highlighted to solve mystery [5-7]. There are two types of GBM: Type 1 GBM typically shows inactivation of the TP53 tumor suppressor gene but no amplification of the EGFR oncogene. Mutations of p53, mostly associated with loss of heterozygosity (LOH) in the 17p chromosome region, can be observed in GBM originating from a less malignant glioma precursor. TP53 inactivation does not occur together with amplification of the EGFR oncogene, which is only identified in GBM without TP53 mutation More than 70% of malignant gliomas show a deregulated TP53 pathway not only by mutation of TP53 but also amplification of MDM2, homozygous deletion/mutation, or promoter hypermethylation-mediated silencing of CDKN2A. Type 2 GBM shows overexpression or amplification of the EGFR without mutations of TP53, and it appears de novo, that is, in patients without a less malignant precursor neoplasm such as grade II or III astrocytoma [6,7].

Two independent GBM pathways were also identified [9]. Moreover, epidermal growth factor receptor (EGFR) amplification is almost always consistent with LOH in chromosome region 10q [16]. The tumor suppressor gene Phosphatase and tensin homolog (PTEN), mapping the 10q23 region, is mutated in approximately 30% of type 2 GBM [6,10]. Mutations in this gene have been described only in malignant gliomas and are rarely associated with p53 mutations. Other frequent mutations in type 2 GBM affect the cyclin dependent kinase (CDK) cell-cycle-regulator genes. Amplification of CDK4 and CDK6 was observed in 15% of type 2 GBMs [6,7]. Mutations of the cell-cycle-regulator genes CDKN2A/CDKN2B have been observed in 40% of all GBM. Moreover, a functional loss of expression of the CDKN2A gene by promoter hypermethylation was found in 15% of GBM [6,7]. Mutations of the Isocitrate dehydrogenase 1 (IDH1) gene have been frequently observed in those GBM progressing from a less malignant precursor lesion, that is in type 1 GBM, mostly of them affecting young patients. Interestingly, these IDH1 mutations were associated with a better outcome [6]. In addition to type 1 and type 2 GBMs, there are other forms, whose molecular profiles do not identify them as belonging to either of the two classic pathways [6,7].

The methylation signature of gliomas is also rather associated with tumor lineage and malignancy grade. Thus, astrocytomas grades WHO II and III and GBM grade IV show different methylation status of several genes. Even though, primary and secondary GBMs were found to differ concerning methylation of genes which was associated with decreased mRNA levels. In this context, methylation of methyl guanine methyl transferase (MGMT) is more frequently observed in 75% of secondary GBM than in primary GBMs (36%). Moreover, MGMT methylation has been observed to be associated with TP53 mutations in secondary GBMs. Cellular pathways deregulated in gliomas and associated epigenetic events through promoter hypermethylation, CpGs hypomethylation, and histone alterations leading to modified chromatin states are Ras signaling (RASSF1A, RRP22, DIRAS3), Cell migration and adherence (NECL1, E-cadherin, SLIT2, EMP3, TIMP3), Wnt signaling (WIF1, FZD9, IGFBP-3, SFRP family, PEG3), Tyrosine kinase pathways (KIT, SYK, c-ROS),Transcription factors (SOX2, KLF4, GATA 6, ATOH1), Homeobox genes (HOXA 9, HOXA10, HOXA11), Sonic hedgehog signaling (PTCH1, Cyclin D2, Plakoglobin, PAX6, NKX2.2), Notch signaling (NEURL1, HES1, HEY1), bone morphogenic protein (BMP) developmental pathway (BMPR1B), Hypermutator pathways (hMLH1, hPMS2, MGMT,WRN), Apoptosis (TMS1, DAPK1, CASP8, DR4, DR5), TP53/cell cycle (HIC-1, CDKN2A, RB1, p16INK4a), MicroRNAs (miR-124a, miR-21, miR-7, miR-137, miR12) [6,7,11].

MGMT can be given for instance for these pathways MGMT, which has been observed to be hypermethylated in low-grade gliomas (grade II) further evolving to gliomas grade III and GBM [6,7]. Furthermore, this biomarker allows neurooncologists to predict patient's response to current chemotherapy with temozolomide [12]. Second instance can be microsatellite instability (MSI) which was observed to be more frequent in those GBMs evolving from less malignant gliomas grade II or III, which typically display TP53 mutations without EGFR amplification, as well as in relapse GBM [5,6]. Third instance can be given as epigenetic inactivation ofone of the apoptosis-related genes (TMS1/ASC and DAPK1, WIF-1, SFRP1 and CASP8) as proapoptotic gene CASP8 which is an epigenetic silenced during progression of primary-to-recurrent GBM. GBM can change its epigenetic profile quickly, therefore its adaptation (heterogenity) to novel therapies is big obstacle [6,7,11].

Because of incomplete atlas of genetic and epigenetic pathways, gene therapies and chemotherapies have limited efficacy and they are under investigation [6,7,13,14]. Researchers and clinicians are trying to fight this monster following products of these genes [15-17]. Many "Trojan horse" approaches, based on potential applications in the pharmacological therapy of GBMs which blood-brain barrier (BBB) represents an obstacle are being proposed day by day [18,19]. The passage of drugs across the BBB limits the efficacy of chemotherapy in brain tumors [18-21]. Many anti-neoplastic drugs evaluated as "magic bullets" that is effective against glioblastoma in vitro, has poor efficacy in vivo or has both efficacy in vitro and in vivo, has poor efficacy in clinic because it is extruded by P-glycoprotein (Pgp/ABCB1), multidrug resistance-related proteins (MRPs) and breast cancer resistance protein (BCRP/ABCG2) of BBB cells [20,21]. Although these proteins are commonly studied in order to overcome drug resistance for several decades, GBM attack with other weapons in order to win this war and it continues to surprise researchers and clinicians [20,21]. Other weapons of GBM can be defined as aquaporins (AQPs) [22,23].

2. AQPs

AQPs, water channels, have been proposed as novel targets in cancer and oedema and are associated with a surprising array of important processes in the brain and body, such as angiogenesis, cell migration, development and neuropathological diseases. In both cancer and brain oedema, current therapies are limited and new pharmacological approaches focused on AQPs offer exciting potential for clinical advances [23]. The expression of six isoforms of AQP protein (AQP1, 3, 4, 5, 8, 9) has been reported in the glial cells [in astrocytes (AQP1, 3, 4, 5, 8, 9), oligodendrocytes (AQP8), tanycytes (AQP9) and ependymal cells (AQP1, 4, 9) [24]. As astrocytes are the most numerous glial cell type and account for one third of brain mass [25] and they are involved in the maintenance of the blood–brain barrier (BBB), and as the GBM is the most malignant form astrocytic brain tumor [1,2], we focused on the AQPs on the astrocytes related to GBM. Previous reports showed that AQPs 1, 4, and 9 have significant roles in the pathogenesis of malignant brain tumours [24].

3. AQP1

AQP1 plays an important role in water transport in expressed in various organs and cells (microvascular endothelial cells, kidney, central nervous system, eye, lacrimal and salivary glands, respiratory apparatus, gastrointestinal tract, hepatobiliary compartments, female and male reproductive system, inner ear, skin) [26]. Previous reports sowed that brain astrocytes express AQP1 under pathologic conditions as the early stage of Alzheimer disease, subarachnoid hemorrhage, cerebral infarction [27-29]. Monzani and coworkers showed a role for AQPs in facilitating cell migration at the first time for AQP1 in human endothelial and melanoma cell lines in vivo [30].

Hypoxia stimulates astrocytic migration it is possible that hypoxic conditions after spinal cord injury (SCI) trigger AQP1 synthesis in astrocytes, as an attempt of injured spinal cords to facilitate astrocytic migration to the lesion site [31,32]. Hypoxic conditions may contribute to chronic accumulation of water within neurons and cytotoxic edema in chronically injured spinal cords [33]. AQP1 expression in spinal cord may have a role in axonal remodeling and plasticity, necessary for normal sensory processing [34]. Abreu-Rodríguez and coworkers showed that HIF-1α participates in the hypoxic induction of AQP1 in 9L glioma cells. They also demonstrated that the activation of AQP1 promoter by hypoxia is complex and multifactorial and suggested that in addition to HIF-1α other transcription factors might contribute to this regulatory process [35].

GBMs express increased aquaporin AQP1. AQPs may contribute to edema, cell motility, and shuttling of H_2O and H^+ from intracellular to extracellular space [36]. In comparison to normal brain, GBMs have different vascular structures and metabolic changes. GBM cells make higher aerobic glycolysis under hypoxia than under normoxia leading to invasion of cancer cell [37,38].

4. AQP4

AQP4, the most important water channel in the brain, is found in supporting cells as astrocytes (astrocyte endfeet abutting microvessels), ependyma and its also found in retina [39, 40]. AQP4 expression is polarized in astrocytes and AQP4 redistributes throughout the astrocyte cell membrane, suggesting that endothelial cells signal astrocytes to polarize AQP4 expression in the cell membrane [41]. Previous study showed that AQP4 is involved in the formation and resolution of brain and spinal cord edemas. In the absence of AQP4, brain edema is decreased and neurologic improvement following ischemic brain injury is increased [42].

AQP4 expression is commonly up-regulated in astrocytes associated with brain edema [42]. It was showed that an up-regulation and redistribution of AQP4 accompanied by a loss of its polarized expression pattern and so the evidence for a role of it in vasogenic edema formation in GBM [43, 44]. Altered expression levels of AQP4 and redistribution of the protein throughout the membranes of cells are found in GBM and this leads to development of the oedema often found surrounding the tumour mass. AQP4 also facilitates the elimination of excess brain water. Excess water is eliminated primarily through the glia limiting membranes into the CSF that vasogenic edema fluid is eliminated by an AQP4-dependent route. AQP4 pumps out excess fluid assembled in the brain parenchyma after BBB disruption [43,44]. Wang and coworkers suggested that HIF-1α plays a role in brain edema formation and BBB disruption via a molecular signaling pathway involving AQP4 and matrix metalloproteinase 9 (MMP-9) [45]. HIF-1α binds the promoter of AQP4 resulting in the increase in its' expression [46].

It was shown that in human immunodeficiency virus (HIV) infected patients, AQP4 expression was increased indicating the role of AQP4 in a protective and/or maladaptive response to CNS inflammation [47,48].

Recent study have found changes in astroglia Kir and AQP4 water channels in temporal lobe epilepsy specimens [49]. Dysregulation of AQP4 also occurs in hippocampal sclerosis and cortical dysplasia in patients with refractory partial epilepsy [50]. These are clue for both AQP4 and Kir4.1 participate in clearance of K^+ following neural activity. Othe report suggested that AQP4 and Kir4.1 may also act in concert in K^+ and H_2O regulation [51]. K^+ re-uptake into glial cells might be AQP4-dependent, as water influx coupled to K^+ influx is thought to underlie activity-induced glial cell swelling [52]. Further studies are required to clarify the expression and functional interaction of AQP4 and Kir4.1 in the hippocampus and their changes during epileptogenesis.

Recent reports have also suggested a role of AQP4 for neuroglial activation in autism and more studies are also needed as epileptogenesis to confirm its spesific role in autism [53].

AQP4 is highly expressed in the basolateral membrane of the ependyma and glia limitans. This meaning of this distribution feature can be evaluated that AQP4 provides a highly efficient pathway to transport the redundant water from parenchyma to ventricle system and subarachnoid space [42]. The highly polarized expression of AQP4 may be involved in the structural and functional integrity of the ependyma maintance [42,54,55]. AQP4 is highly related with the gap junction protein connexin43 (Cx43), which is the main gap-junction protein in astrocytes as well as ependymal cells [53,55].

Previous report showed that reactive microglial cells expresses AQP4 mRNA and protein in *in vivo* [56]. All cells which are expressing AQP4 in microglial cells may represent a molecular adaptation to maintain ion water homeostasis in the injured brain. Activated microglia is important in the clearance of K+ and restoration of osmotic equilibrium in absence of astrocytes. It is well known that glial cells play an important role in regulating the homeostasis to ensure an appropriate neuronal environment [24,56,57]. AQP4 seems to play an essential role because of the possible role of astrocytes in pomping out excess K^+ around active neuron [24,56,57].

5. AQP9

AQP9 transports glycerol, mannitol and urea. It was firstly found in human leukocytes, and it is also expressed in liver, testis, and brain [58,59]. In the brain, AQP9 is expressed in tanycytes (they possess no cilia). The tanycytes are found in circumventricular organs of the third ventricle lacking a BBB [60, 61]. More studies are needed to confirm AQP9 expression in the subset of ciliated ependymal cells [60]. AQP9 is also expressed in astrocytes and spinal cord of the glia limitans and white matter tracts. Its expression is throughout the astrocyte cell bodies and processes in the brain [62]. AQP9 may play a role in extracellular water homeostasis/ oedema and it also helps glycerol and monocarboxylate diffusion [63].

In addition, it is proposed that AQP9 plays a role in clearing lactate from the extracellular space in pathological ischemic conditions. Most glioma cells throughout the tumour revealed a strong AQP9 expression across the whole surface of the cells in human GBM. AQP9 expression is increased in all grades of human astrocytic tumours and this expression is increased from low-grade tumours to high-grade tumours [64]. The increase of AQP9 expression is essential for the clearance of glycerol and lactate from the extracellular space at the glioma-associated lactic acidosis [65]. AQP9 expression may account for GBM resistance to hypoxic and ischemic situations, by facilitating clearance of lactate and glycerol resulting from hypoxia and cellular damage, respectively [66-69]. HIF-1α binds AQP4 promoter, consequently it increases the expression of AQP4 [70].

It might, therefore, play a role in both the energy metabolism of normal brain tissue and provide increased tolerance for hypoxia under pathological conditions. AQP9 may play an important role in the malignant progression of brain tumours and it can be used as a biomarker for molecular diagnosis and as a new target for gene therapy.

6. AQPs 1,4,9 in stem cells

In the study of Fussdal and coworkers at biopsies from GBMs, they analyzed the expression of AQPs 1, 4, and 9 in isolated tumour stem cells grown in a tumoursphere assay and analyzed the progenitor and differentiated cells from these cultures. They compared these expressions to the situation in normal rat brain, its stem cells, and differentiated cells. They concluded that AQP 9 is markedly more highly expressed in the tumour progenitor population, whilst AQP4 is downregulated in tumour-derived differentiated cells. They proposed that AQP 9 may have a central role in the tumorigenesis of GBM [71].

7. Midkine

Midkine (MK) with the molecular weight of MK is 13 kDA is a heparin-binding growth factor/ an angiogenic factor with cytokine actions. MK binds to oversulfated structures in heparan sulfate and chondroitin sulfate. MK and pleiotrophin (known as PTN and HB-GAM) are belonging to same family [72]. MK is 50% homologous to PTN at the amino acid level and shares with PTN the genomic organization and predicted protein structure [72-73].

MK is mainly composed of two domains which are linked by disulfide bonds [74]. The C-domain has basic heparin-binding activity and this is responsible for the mechanism of action [75]. Each domain of MK has also homology to the thrombospondin Type I repeat [76]. Two domains are composed of three anti-parallel β-sheets [77]. The C-domain has two clusters of basic amino acids named as Cluster-1 and -2. These clusters are required for heparin-binding activity [78]. MK forms dimers via spontaneous association and transglutaminase stabilize dimers through crosslinking process. MK is seemed to require dimerization for its activity [79]. After dimerization, Cluster-2 forms a fused strong binding site [77].

MK was originally reported to be the product of a retinoic acid-responsive gene during embryogenesis [80]. its expression was high during embryogenesis, but interestingly, MK is not detectable in healthy adults and only re-appears in the body as a part of the pathogenesis of diseases [81]. MK promotes proliferation, migration, anti-apoptotic manner, mitogenesis, transforming, and angiogenesis various cells [82-87]. It has significant roles in reproduction, repair and in epidemiology of many diseases as rheumatoid arthritis, multiple sclerosis, hypertension and renal disease and cancer [88-90]. It's very important data that the expression of MK is increased in advanced tumors with high frequency [84, 91]. Previous reports showed that the blood MK level is frequently elevated with advance of human carcinomas, decreased after surgical removal of the tumors [91,92].

Human MK recognizes glycosaminoglycans through its C-domain as heparan sulfate trisulfated unit and chondroitin sulfate E unit is important in its mechanism of action. The component of the MK receptor is a chondroitin sulfate proteoglycan protein tyrosine phosphatase-z (PTPz). Low density lipoprotein receptor-related protein (LRP), $\alpha4\beta1$-integrin and $\alpha6\beta1$-integrin are also MK receptors [93,94].These proteins and PTPz form a receptor complex of MK. After the complex formation with PTPz and integrins, MK starts downstream signaling systems as Src family kinases and tyrosine phosphorylation,respectively. Increased tyrosine phosphorylation of paxillin leads to migration at osteoblast like cells and followed by suppression of caspases, activation of PI3 kinase and MAP kinase takes part in survival [83, 93, 95]. The previous report showed that when MK binds to a6b1-integrin and tetraspanin, and induces tyrosine phosphorylation of focal adhesion kinase (FAK) followed by activation of paxillin and signal transducer and activator of transcription (STAT) 1 alpha pathway, it increases migration and invasion at human head and neck squamous cell carcinoma cells in vitro [96]. Due to phosphorylation of STAT3 by MK, the proliferation of postconfluent 3T3-L1 cells are stimulated and this leads to adipogenesis [97]. Notch2 reserves an another receptor for MK and acting through the janus kinase 2 (Jak2)/STAT3 signalling pathway, MK leads to epithelial-mesenchymal transition (EMT) in immortalized keratinocytes. Both MK and PTN plays important role in EMT and neurogenesis during organogenesis process in embryonal development [96]. Previous reports proposed that anaplastic lymphoma kinase (ALK) can be included in the receptor group of MK [98]. Muramatsu and coworkers suggested that, ALK also involves in the MK complex with LRP and integrins that it is recruited to the receptor complex and plays roles in MK signaling [99]. After activation by MK, ALK phosphorylates insulin receptor substrate-1, activates MAP kinase and PI3 kinase leading to transcriptional activation of Nuclear Factor-KappaB (NF-κB) [98].

MK binds to nucleolin, a nuclear protein which is also located at the cell surface and functions as a shuttle to the nucleus [85]. A component of the MK receptor LRP has major function as endocytose and delivering its ligands to lysosomes for degradation or catabolism [100]. LRP takes part in internalization of MK [101]. MK is not internalized in LRP-deficient cells, whereas transfection of a LRP expression vector can restore MK internalization and subsequent nuclear translocation, suggesting that LRP binds to MK and mediates nuclear targeting by MK. After this internalization, nucleolin transfer cytoplasmic MK to the nucleus [101]. With respect to nuclear targeting by MK, laminin-binding protein precursor (LBP) binds to MK and is cotranslocated with MK into nuclei [102]. MK may use both nucleolin and LBP precursor as shuttle proteins, revealing a novel role of LRP in intracellular signaling by its ligand, and the importance of nucleolin and LBP in the process of nuclear target of MK. MK transferred to the nucleolus is involved in the synthesis of ribosomal RNA [85]. Muramatsu and coworkers observed, however didn't publish that translation initiation factor (eIF3) can be an MK-binding protein in the embryonic brain [31].

8. MK and GBM

In the central nervous system, MK is expressed by astrocytes in the fetal brain and its expression is developmentally regulated, decreasing progressively to an undetectable level as the fetus matures [103,104]. Previous reports showed that increased levels of MK expression correlate with the progression of human astrocytomas, MK mRNA and protein expression levels were higher in high-grade astrocytomas as anaplastic astrocytomas and GBMs than in low-grade astrocytomas (oligodendroglioma, ependioma, schwannoma, meningioma and pituitary adenoma) [105]. These reports conclude that MK correlates with the poor prognosis of GBM.

One of the report showed that MK activates PI3-kinase and MAP kinase signal transduction in U87MG human glioblastoma cells which express ALK protein [98]. In this report it was shown that MK is also unable to stimulate Akt phosphorylation upon reduction of ALK. In their report they revealed that in contrast with the diminished PTN and MK signals after reduction of ALK, Akt phosphorylation in the same cells via a different tyrosine kinase receptor, the platelet-derived growth factor receptor (PDGF-R), was not altered by the reduction of ALK levels [107]. Interestingly, in the U87MG cells MAPK is activated constitutively and remains unaffected by the ALK reduction or by MK addition. In contrast to other report showed that no mRNA levels of ALK and RPTP β/ς levels, but high mRNA levels of MK and PTN were determined in another human GBM cell lines named T98G [98, 107]. This condition is also same for human glioblastoma cell lines named G55T2. U118 GBM cells possess high mRNA levels of ALK, low mRNA levels of MK and RPTP β/ς but no mRNA levels of PTN are detected. All cell lines derived from human GBMs are different. Autophagy can both lead to cell death (autophagic cell death or apoptotic cell death) and cell survival (survival/recurrence/resistance). This means it becomes sometimes foe sometimes friend. Lorente and coworkers showed that activation of the tyrosine kinase receptor ALK by its ligand MK interferes with the signaling mechanism by which Δ9-tetrahydrocannabinol (THC) which is the main active component of marijuana, promotes cancer cell death via autophagy stimulation [108].

GBM has a complex tumor structure consisting of accumulating tumors cells, abnormal vessel and necrotic debris. The increasing tumor mass leads to increased capillary and venous collapse [109]. The new formed vessels are structurally and functionally abnormal, and leaky, leading to edema, and low oxygen tension [110]. High O2 tension degrades HIF-1α and consequently promotes differentiation or apoptosis, HIF-1α maintains at lower O_2 tension this augments signal transduction pathways leading to promote self-renewal [111]. Hypoxia induces MK expression through the binding of to a hypoxia responsive element in the MK promoter.

Notch2 has been suggested to lead embryonic brain tumor growth, however Notch3 has been implicated in choroid plexus tumors [112]. The frequency and the intensity of Notch2 expression is higher than that of Notch1 in GBM and in medulloblastoma [113]. As a consequence of local genomic amplifications at the Notch2 locus in both brain tumor types, this may also be linked to the later persistence of Notch2 expression in postnatal mouse brain [114]. Previous report showed that Notch1 regulates transcription of the epidermal growth factor receptor gene EGFR, known to be overexpressed or amplified in GBM, through TP53 [115]. Reports showed that there is a direct correlation between p53 and MK levels. Consistently, transcription of Notch signaling mediator genes are significantly overexpressed in the molecular subset of GBM with EGFR amplification [116]. Notch signaling pathway activates the major GBM signalling pathway. Glioma subsets with impaired Notch signaling have slower progression.

The most frequent genetic alteration occurring in GBM is genomic amplification of EGFR [117]. Consistently, EGF is the major proliferation pathway in GBM, mediated by activation of the RAS-RAF-MEK-ERK and the PI3K-AKT-mTOR cascades [58]. Interestingly, mTOR has recently been shown to activate Notch signaling in lung and kidney tumor cells through induction of the STAT3/p63/Jagged signaling cascade [118]. Lino and coworkers proposed this cross-talk for GBM that this suggests potential creation of a positive feedback loop between Notch and EGF signalling [119]. The most frequent GBM subset consists of the association of EGFR amplification, homozygous deletions at the cyclin dependent kinase 2A (CDKN2A) locus, and TP53 mutations [120]. Notch activates expression of EGFR via TP53 thus Notch is expected to stimulate the main GBM proliferation pathway [116]. In addition, Notch also transactivates the gene for the EGFR-related ERBB2 in a DTX1-dependent manner [121]. Notch-2 serves another receptor for MK and so cross-talk between MK and Notch-2 has been also shown to be a mediator of chemotherapy resistance to neighboring cells in GBM [122].

When a subset of cells overexpress drug transport proteins, possess receptor changes for the commitment of drug bounding and lack of ability to commit apoptosis, this situation leads to tumors resistance during chemotherapy. Mirkin and coworkers investigate the cytoprotective relationship between resistant and nonresistant cells in tumors which both accomplish to survive against drug cytotoxicity in human neuroblastoma and osteosarcoma [123]. They hypothized that drug-resistant cells may secrete in their culture medium factors able to protect sensitive cells from cytotoxicity of drug. They showed that expression of MK was only detected in drug resistant cells and MK-enriched fractions exert a significant cytoprotective effect against doxorubicin (DXR) in the wild-type drug-sensitive cells. In addition, they transfected these cells with MK gene resulting in decreased response to DXR due to activation of AKT pathway and supression of caspase pathway. They concluded that the existence of intercellular cytoprotective signals such as the one mediated by MK, originating from cells with acquired drug resistance to protect neighboring drug-sensitive cells and thus contribute to development of resistance to chemotherapy. They didn't show anything aout direct effect of MK on drug efflux transporters.

Report by Hu and coworkers showed that the possible effects of MK gene on the chemotherapeutic drugs efflux. They concluded that there was powerful drug efflux ability in lymphoblastic leukemia cells with high MK gene expression [124]. They proposed that MK gene expression regulates drug efflux upstream of the p-gp and the other transporter proteins in this cell line. Previous reports showed that the expression of MRP-1 is higher than expression of p-gp in T98G [125]. In our study, we investigated whether the combination of an antineoplastic imatinib mesylate (IM) and an antitussive noscapine (Nos) with new identified chemotherapeutic effects, can be an effective GBM treatment and the role of MK in this treatment by using T98G cells [126]. The lowest MRP-1 levels, but highest MK levels were detected in the combination group. The lowest MK levels were detected in IM group especially at the 72nd hr ($p<0.05$) but IM takes second place at MRP-1 inhibition. The highest and the lowest p-170 levels were detected at IM group ($p<0.05$) and Nos group ($p<0.05$), respectively. Thus, we can conclude that drug efflux ability was not correlated with MK levels in this experiment.

Suppression of PTN and ALK expression has already been employed as means to treat GBM, and promising results have been obtained in animal experiments [107].

9. MK and GBM stem cells

Previous publication showed that MK is expressed in mouse embryonic stem cells (mESCs), human embryonic stem cells (hESCs) and mouse embryonic fibroblasts (MEFs) [127]. In their study, MK promotes proliferation and self-renewal of both mESCs and hESCs. Another study showed that the promoted growth of mESCs by MK is occured through inhibiting apoptosis while accelerating the progression toward the S phase, and MK leads to enhancement of mESC self-renewal through PI3K/Akt signaling pathway. They concluded that MK plays profound roles in ESCs and MK/PTPzeta signaling pathway is a novel pathway in the signal network maintaining pluripotency of ESCs. Their results gives more detailed information about the pluripotency control of ESCs and the relationship between ESCs and cancers. Huang and coworkers showed that a highly tumorigenic subpopulation of cancer cells named GBM stem cells (GSCs) promotes therapeutic resistance [127]. In their study, they showed that GSCs stimulate tumor angiogenesis by expressing elevated levels of VEGF and contribute to tumor growth. In addition, cancer stem cells have been shown to promote metastasis. MK was found to be expressed in neural precursor cells, which consist of neural stem cells and the progenitor cells which has been translated into a useful therapeutic strategy in the treatment of recurrent or progressive GBMs [128].

10. MK and AQPs

Hypoxia is the intersection point for AQP and MK. Hypoxia increases all these protein levels as I mentioned above: their levels are all increased under hypoxic conditions. HIF-1α binds promoter of MK and AQP, then it increases its expression. In addition, HIF-1α serves as an upstream regulator of cerebral glycerol concentrations and brain edema via a molecular pathway involving AQP4 and AQP9 [70].

In our previous study published in Oncology Letter, we investigated the combination of imatinib (IM) and roscovitine (ROSC) to overcome resistance and whether or not MK had an effect on this combination in the treatment of GBM with other anti-apoptotic factors such as AQP4 in T98G human GBM cells. These cells are expressing high MK and AQP4 levels. In this study, all applications decreased the cell proliferation index and increased the apoptotic index, but ROSC was the most efficient drug and the second most efficient drug was IM to decrease cell proliferation and induce cell death. Combination therapy showed antagonist manner. Notably, ROSC increased AQP-4 levels, however it decreased MK levels. The combination group induced highest decrease in p170 levels ($p<0.05$), the second one was determined as the IM group ($p<0.05$). All drug applications decreased MRP-1 levels ($p<0.05$), but the highest decrease was determined in the combination group and the latter was IM ($p<0.05$). IM decreased AQP-4 levels, however the combination group and ROSC increased AQP4 levels in T98G GBM cells. This increase was higher in the combination group.

In our other study, we combined IM with lithium chloride (LiCl) in T98G cells [unpublished data]. This shows combination also showed antagonist effect. MRP-1 levels were decreased by LiCl, the combination group and IM, respectively. Firstly the combination group and secondly IM decreased p170 levels efficiently, but LiCl didn't make any change on these levels. Firstly LiCl and secondly the combination group induced highest decrease in AQP4 levels for 72 h. For MK levels, the decrease rate from highest to lowest were IM, LiCl and the combination group [unpublished data].

In this studies, you can see that we only searched for correlation between MK and AQP4 and there were no hypoxic conditions or no three dimensional cell culture model which hypoxic center is formed without hypoxic conditions. This means that we might have different results if 1) we used this model, 2) investigated other types of AQPs as AQP9, 3) use different GBM cell lines for these novel combinations.

Acknowledgement

This work was supported by Scientific Research Projects Coordination Unit of Istanbul University (Project number: T988/06102006) and Yeni Yüzyıl University. I would like to thank the investigators for their generous gifts and/or reagents.

Author details

Mine Ergüven

Aydin University Faculty of Health Sciences, Istanbul, Turkey

I declare that I have no competing interests.

References

[1] Krakstad, C, & Chekenya, M. Survival signalling and apoptosis resistance in glioblastomas: opportunities for targeted therapeutics. Mol Cancer. (2010).

[2] Ohgaki, H, Dessen, P, Jourde, B, Horstmann, S, & Nishikawa, T. Di Patre PL, Burkhard C, Schüler D, Probst-Hensch NM, Maiorka PC, Baeza N, Pisani P, Yonekawa Y, Yasargil MG, Lütolf UM, Kleihues P. Genetic pathways to glioblastoma: a population-based study. Cancer Res (2004). , 64(19), 6892-9.

[3] Central Brain Tumor Registry of the United States CBTRUS http://www.cbtrus.org/ accessed 08 July (2012).

[4] Aldape, K. D, Okcu, M. F, Bondy, M. L, & Wrensch, M. Molecular epidemiology of glioblastoma. Cancer J. (2003). , 9(2), 99-106.

[5] Nakazato, Y. The 4th Edition of WHO Classification of Tumours of the Central Nervous System published in 2007]. No Shinkei Geka. (2008). , 36(6), 473-91.

[6] Martínez, R. Beyond Genetics in Glioma Pathways: The Ever-Increasing Crosstalk between Epigenomic and Genomic Events. J Signal Transduct. (2012).

[7] Alelú-paz, R, Ashour, N, González-corpas, A, & Ropero, S. DNA Methylation, Histone Modifications, and Signal Transduction Pathways: A Close Relationship in Malignant Gliomas Pathophysiology. J Signal Transduct. (2012).

[8] Binda, E, Visioli, A, Reynolds, B, & Vescovi, A. L. Heterogeneity of cancer-initiating cells within glioblastoma. Front Biosci (Schol Ed). (2012). , 4, 1235-48.

[9] Von Deimling, A, Louis, D. N, & Wiestler, O. D. Molecular pathways in the formation of gliomas. Glia. (1995). , 15(3), 328-38.

[10] Boström, J, Cobbers, J. M, Wolter, M, Tabatabai, G, Weber, R. G, Lichter, P, Collins, V. P, & Reifenberger, G. Mutation of the PTEN (MMAC1) tumor suppressor gene in a subset of glioblastomas but not in meningiomas with loss of chromosome arm 10q. Cancer Res. (1998). , 58(1), 29-33.

[11] Uhlmann, K, Rohde, K, Zeller, C, Szymas, J, Vogel, S, Marczinek, K, Thiel, G, Nürnberg, P, & Laird, P. W. Distinct methylation profiles of glioma subtypes. Int J Cancer. (2003). , 106(1), 52-9.

[12] Gorlia, T. van den Bent MJ, Hegi ME, Mirimanoff RO, Weller M, Cairncross JG, Eisenhauer E, Belanger K, Brandes AA, Allgeier A, Lacombe D, Stupp R. Nomograms for predicting survival of patients with newly diagnosed glioblastoma: prognostic factor analysis of EORTC and NCIC trial 26981-22981/CE.3. Lancet Oncol. (2008). , 9(1), 29-38.

[13] Terzis, A. J, Niclou, S. P, Rajcevic, U, Danzeisen, C, & Bjerkvig, R. Cell therapies for glioblastoma. Expert Opin Biol Ther. (2006). , 6(8), 739-49.

[14] Johannessen, T. C, & Bjerkvig, R. Molecular mechanisms of temozolomide resistance in glioblastoma multiforme. Expert Rev Anticancer Ther. (2012). , 12(5), 635-42.

[15] Khaw, A. K, Yong, J. W, Kalthur, G, & Hande, M. P. Genistein induces growth arrest and suppresses telomerase activity in brain tumor cells. Genes Chromosomes Cancer. (2012). , 51(10), 961-74.

[16] Moreno Garcia VBasu B, Molife LR, Kaye SB. Combining antiangiogenics to overcome resistance: rationale and clinical experience. Clin Cancer Res. (2012). , 18(14), 3750-61.

[17] Eimer, S, Belaud-rotureau, M. A, Airiau, K, Jeanneteau, M, Laharanne, E, Véron, N, Vital, A, Loiseau, H, Merlio, J. P, & Belloc, F. Autophagy inhibition cooperates with erlotinib to induce glioblastoma cell death. Cancer Biol Ther. (2011). , 11(12), 1017-27.

[18] Pinzón-daza, M. L, Garzón, R, Couraud, P. O, Romero, I. A, Weksler, B, Ghigo, D, Bosia, A, & Riganti, C. The association of statins plus LDL receptor-targeted liposome-encapsulated doxorubicin increases the in vitro drug delivery across blood-brain barrier cells. Br J Pharmacol. (2012). Jul 12.

[19] Kanwar, J. R, Sriramoju, B, & Kanwar, R. K. Neurological disorders and therapeutics targeted to surmount the blood-brain barrier. Int J Nanomedicine. (2012). , 7, 3259-78.

[20] Gorter, J. A, & Potschka, H. Drug Resistance. In: Noebels JL, Avoli M, Rogawski MA, Olsen RW, Delgado-Escueta AV, editors. Jasper's Basic Mechanisms of the Epilepsies [Internet]. 4th edition. Bethesda (MD): National Center for Biotechnology Information (US); (2012). Available from http://www.ncbi.nlm.nih.gov/books/NBK98215

[21] Ohka, F, Natsume, A, & Wakabayashi, T. Current trends in targeted therapies for glioblastoma multiforme. Neurol Res Int. (2012).

[22] Yool, A. J, Brown, E. A, & Flynn, G. A. Roles for novel pharmacological blockers of aquaporins in the treatment of brain oedema and cancer. Clin Exp Pharmacol Physiol. (2010)., 37(4), 403 9.

[23] Zhao, W. J, Zhang, W, Li, G. L, Cui, Y, Shi, Z. F, & Yuan, F. Differential expression of MMP-9 and AQP4 in human glioma samples. Folia Neuropathol. (2012)., 50(2), 176-86.

[24] Albertini, R, & Bianchi, R. Aquaporins and glia. Curr Neuropharmacol. (2010)., 8(2), 84-91.

[25] Kandel, E. R. Nerve cell and behavior. In: Kandel ER, Schwartz JH, Jessel TM, editors. Principles of neural science. New York: Elsevier Science Publishing; (1991)., 18-32.

[26] Benga, G. The first discovered water channel protein, later called aquaporin 1: Molecular characteristics, functions and medical implications. Mol Aspects Med. (2012). Jun 15.

[27] Hoshi, A, Yamamoto, T, Shimizu, K, Ugawa, Y, Nishizawa, M, Takahashi, H, & Kakita, A. Characteristics of aquaporin expression surrounding senile plaques and cerebral amyloid angiopathy in Alzheimer disease. J Neuropathol Exp Neurol. (2012)., 71(8), 750-9.

[28] Badaut, J, Brunet, J. F, Grollimund, L, Hamou, M. F, Magistretti, P. J, Villemure, J. G, & Regli, L. Aquaporin 1 and aquaporin 4 expression in human brain after subarachnoid hemorrhage and in peritumoral tissue. Acta Neurochir Suppl. (2003)., 86, 495-8.

[29] Kim, J. H, Lee, Y. W, Park, K. A, Lee, W. T, & Lee, J. E. Agmatine attenuates brain edema through reducing the expression of aquaporin-1 after cerebral ischemia. J Cereb Blood Flow Metab. (2010)., 30(5), 943-9.

[30] Monzani, E, Bazzotti, R, & Perego, C. La Porta CA. AQP1 is not only a water channel: it contributes to cell migration through Lin7/beta-catenin. PLoS One. (2009). e6167.

[31] Xu, Q, Wang, S, Jiang, X, Zhao, Y, Gao, M, Zhang, Y, Wang, X, Tano, K, Kanehara, M, Zhang, W, & Ishida, T. Hypoxia-induced astrocytes promote the migration of neural progenitor cells via vascular endothelial factor, stem cell factor, stromal-derived factor-1alpha and monocyte chemoattractant protein-1 upregulation in vitro. Clin. Exp. Pharmacol. Physiol. (2007)., 34, 624-631.

[32] Badaut, J, Brunet, J. F, & Regli, L. Aquaporins in the brain: from aqueduct to "multi-duct". Metab Brain Dis. (2007).

[33] Nesic, O, Lee, J, Ye, Z, Unabia, G. C, Rafati, D, Hulsebosch, C. E, & Perez-polo, J. R. Acute and chronic changes in aquaporin 4 expression after spinal cord injury. Neuroscience. (2006)., 143(3), 779-92.

[34] Carulli, D, Buffo, A, & Strata, P. Reparative mechanisms in the cerebellar cortex. Prog Neurobiol. (2004)., 72(6), 373-98.

[35] Abreu-rodríguez, I. Sánchez Silva R, Martins AP, Soveral G, Toledo-Aral JJ, López-Barneo J, Echevarría M. Functional and transcriptional induction of aquaporin-1 gene by hypoxia; analysis of promoter and role of Hif-1α. PLoS One. (2011). e28385.

[36] Hayashi, Y, Edwards, N. A, Proescholdt, M. A, Oldfield, E. H, & Merrill, M. J. Regulation and function of aquaporin-1 in glioma cells. Neoplasia. (2007). , 9(9), 777-87.

[37] Gatenby, R. A, & Gillies, R. J. Glycolysis in cancer: a potential target for therapy. Int J Biochem Cell Biol. (2007).

[38] Kotliarova, S, & Fine, H. A. SnapShot: glioblastoma multiforme. Cancer Cell. (2012). e1., 21(5), 710-710.

[39] Mack, A. F, & Wolburg, H. A Novel Look at Astrocytes: Aquaporins, Ionic Homeostasis,nand the Role of the Microenvironment for Regeneration in the CNS. Neuroscientist. (2012). May 29.

[40] Hirrlinger, P. G, Pannicke, T, Winkler, U, Claudepierre, T, Varshney, S, Schulze, C, Reichenbach, A, Brunken, W. J, & Hirrlinger, J. Genetic deletion of laminin isoforms β2 and γ3 induces a reduction in Kir4.1 and aquaporin-4 expression and function in the retina. PLoS One. (2011). e16106.

[41] Tait, M. J, Saadoun, S, Bell, B. A, & Papadopoulos, M. C. Water movements in the brain: role of aquaporins. Trends Neurosci. (2008). , 31(1), 37-43.

[42] Saadoun, S, & Papadopoulos, M. C. Aquaporin-4 in brain and spinal cord oedema. Neuroscience. (2010). , 168(4), 1036-46.

[43] Steiner, E, Enzmann, G. U, Lin, S, Ghavampour, S, Hannocks, M. J, Zuber, B, Rüegg, M. A, Sorokin, L, & Engelhardt, B. Loss of astrocyte polarization upon transient focal brain ischemia as a possible mechanism to counteract early edema formation. Glia. (2012). Jul 10.

[44] Warth, A, Mittelbronn, M, & Wolburg, H. Redistribution of the water channel protein aquaporin-4 and the K+ channel protein Kir4.1 differs in low- and high-grade human brain tumors. Acta Neuropathol. (2005). , 109(4), 418-26.

[45] Wang, Z, Meng, C. J, Shen, X. M, Shu, Z, Ma, C, Zhu, G. Q, Liu, H. X, He, W. C, Sun, X. B, Huo, L, Zhang, J, & Chen, G. Potential Contribution of Hypoxia-Inducible Factor-1α, Aquaporin-4, and Matrix Metalloproteinase-9 to Blood-Brain Barrier Disruption and Brain Edema After Experimental Subarachnoid Hemorrhage. J Mol Neurosci. (2012). Apr 22.

[46] Krakstad, C, & Chekenya, M. Survival signalling and apoptosis resistance in glioblastomas: opportunities for targeted therapeutics. Mol Cancer. (2010).

[47] St Hillaire CVargas D, Pardo CA, Gincel D, Mann J, Rothstein JD, McArthur JC, Conant K. Aquaporin 4 is increased in association with human immunodeficiency virus dementia: implications for disease pathogenesis. J Neurovirol. (2005). , 11(6), 535-43.

[48] Aoki-yoshino, K, Uchihara, T, Duyckaerts, C, Nakamura, A, Hauw, J. J, & Wakayama, Y. Enhanced expression of aquaporin 4 in human brain with inflammatory diseases. Acta Neuropathol. (2005)., 110(3), 281-8.

[49] Binder, D. K, & Steinhäuser, C. Functional changes in astroglial cells in epilepsy. Glia. (2006)., 54, 358-368.

[50] Isoardo, G, Morra, I, Chiarle, G, Audrito, V, Deaglio, S, Melcarne, A, Junemann, C, Naddeo, M, Cogoni, M, Valentini, M. C, Limberti, A, Faccani, F, Malavasi, F, & Faccani, G. Different aquaporin-4 expression in glioblastoma multiforme patients with and without seizures. Mol Med. (2012). Jun 13

[51] Simard, M, & Nedergaard, M. The neurobiology of glia in the context of water and ion homeostasis. Neuroscience. (2004)., 129(4), 877-96.

[52] Walz, W. Mechanism of rapid K(+)-induced swelling of mouse astrocytes. Neurosci Lett. (1992)., 135(2), 243-6.

[53] Fatemi, S. H, Folsom, T. D, Reutiman, T. J, & Lee, S. Expression of astrocytic markers aquaporin 4 and connexin 43 is altered in brains of subjects with autism. Synapse. (2008). Jul;, 62(7), 501-7.

[54] Huang, X. N, Wang, W. Z, Fu, J, & Wang, H. B. The relationship between aquaporin-4 expression and blood-brain and spinal cord barrier permeability following experimental autoimmune encephalomyelitis in the rat. Anat Rec (Hoboken). (2011). , 294(1), 46-54.

[55] Li, X, Kong, H, Wu, W, Xiao, M, Sun, X, & Hu, G. Aquaporin-4 maintains ependymal integrity in adult mice. Neuroscience. (2009)., 162(1), 67-77.

[56] Tomás-camardiel, M, Venero, J. L, De Pablos, R. M, Rite, I, Machado, A, & Cano, J. In vivo expression of aquaporin-4 by reactive microglia. J Neurochem. (2004). , 91(4), 891-9.

[57] Newman, E. A. Glial cell regulation of extracellular potassium. In: Kettenmann H, Ransom BR, editors. Neuroglia. New York: Oxford University Press; (1995)., 717-731.

[58] Ishibashi, K, Kuwahara, M, Gu, Y, Tanaka, Y, Marumo, F, & Sasaki, S. Cloning and functional expression of a new aquaporin (AQP9) abundantly expressed in the peripheral leukocytes permeable to water and urea, but not to glycerol. Biochem. Biophys. Res. Commun. (1998)., 244, 268-274.

[59] Nagelhus, E. A, Veruki, M. L, Torp, R, Haug, F. M, Laake, J. H, Nielsen, S, Agre, P, & Ottersen, O. P. Aquaporin-4 water channel protein in the rat retina and optic nerve: polarized expression in Müller cells and fibrous astrocytes. J. Neurosci. (1998). , 18, 2506-2519.

[60] Elkjaer, M, Vajda, Z, Nejsum, L. N, Kwon, T, Jensen, U. B, Amiry-moghaddam, M, Frøkiaer, J, & Nielsen, S. Immunolocalization of AQP9 in liver, epididymis, testis, spleen, and brain. Biochem. Biophys. Res. Commun. (2000)., 276, 1118-1128.

[61] Nicchia, G. P, Frigeri, A, Nico, B, Ribatti, D, & Svelto, M. Tissue distribution and membrane localization of aquaporin-9 water channel: evidence for sex-linked differences in liver. J. Histochem. Cytochem. (2001). , 49, 1547-1556.

[62] Oshio, K, Binder, D. K, Yang, B, Schecter, S, Verkman, A. S, & Manley, G. T. Expression of aquaporin water channels in mouse spinal cord. Neuroscience. (2004). , 127, 685-693.

[63] Umenishi, F, & Schrier, R. W. Hypertonicity-induced aquaporin-1 (AQP1) expression is mediated by the activation of MAPK pathways and hypertonicity-responsive element in the AQP1 gene. J. Biol. Chem. (2003). , 278, 15765-15770.

[64] Tan, G, Sun, S. Q, & Yuan, D. L. Expression of the water channel protein aquaporin-9 in human astrocytic tumours: correlation with pathological grade. J. Int. Med. Res. (2008). , 36, 777-782.

[65] Warth, A, Mittelbronn, M, Hülper, P, Erdlenbruch, B, & Wolburg, H. Expression of the water channel protein aquaporin-9 in malignant brain tumors. Appl. Immunohistochem. Mol. Morphol. (2007). , 15, 193-198.

[66] Fischbarg, J, Kuang, K. Y, Vera, J. C, Arant, S, Silverstein, S. C, Loike, J, & Rosen, O. M. Glucose transporters serve as water channels. Proc. Natl. Acad. Sci. USA. (1990). , 87, 3244-3247.

[67] Gao, H, He, C, Fang, X, Hou, X, Feng, X, Yang, H, Zhao, X, & Ma, T. Localization of aquaporin-1 water channel in glial cells of the human peripheral nervous system. Glia. (2006). , 53, 783-787.

[68] Gatenby, R. A, & Gillies, R. J. Glycolysis in cancer: a potential target for therapy. Int. J. Biochem. Cell. Biol. (2007). , 39, 1358-1366.

[69] Hasegawa, H, Ma, T, Skach, W, Matthay, M. A, & Verkman, A. S. Molecular cloning of a mercurial-insensitive water channel expressed in selected water-transporting tissues. J. Biol. Chem. (1994). , 269, 5497-5500.

[70] Higashida, T, Peng, C, Li, J, & Dornbos, D. rd, Teng K, Li X, Kinni H, Guthikonda M, Ding Y. Hypoxia-inducible factor-1α contributes to brain edema after stroke by regulating aquaporins and glycerol distribution in brain. Curr Neurovasc Res. (2011). , 8(1), 44-51.

[71] Fossdal, G, Vik-mo, E. O, Sandberg, C, Varghese, M, Kaarbø, M, Telmo, E, Langmoen, I. A, & Murrell, W. Aqp 9 and brain tumour stem cells. ScientificWorldJournal. (2012).

[72] Rauvala, H, Peng, H. B, & Heparin-binding, H. B-G. A. M. growth-associated molecule) and heparin-type glycans in the development and plasticity of neuron-target contacts. Prog Neurobiol. (1997). , 52(2), 127-44.

[73] Sato, W, Kadomatsu, K, Yuzawa, Y, Muramatsu, H, Hotta, N, Matsuo, S, & Muramatsu, T. Midkine is involved in neutrophil infiltration into the tubulointerstitium in ischemic renal injury. J Immunol. (2001). , 167(6), 3463-9.

[74] Fabri, L, Maruta, H, Muramatsu, H, Muramatsu, T, Simpson, R. J, Burgess, A. W, & Nice, E. C. Structural characterisation of native and recombinant forms of the neurotrophic cytokine MK. J Chromatogr. (1993). , 646(1), 213-25.

[75] Muramatsu, H, Inui, T, Kimura, T, Sakakibara, S, Song, X. J, Maruta, H, & Muramatsu, T. Localization of heparin-binding, neurite outgrowth and antigenic regions in midkine molecule. Biochem Biophys Res Commun. (1994). , 203(2), 1131-9.

[76] Kilpelainen, I, Kaksonen, M, Kinnunen, T, Avikainen, H, Fath, M, Linhardt, R. J, Raulo, E, & Rauvala, H. Heparin-binding growth-associated molecule contains two heparin-binding beta-sheet domains that are homologous to the thrombospondin type I repeat. J Biol Chem. (2000). , 275(18), 13564-70.

[77] Iwasaki, W, Nagata, K, Hatanaka, H, Inui, T, Kimura, T, Muramatsu, T, Yoshida, K, Tasumi, M, & Inagaki, F. Solution structure of midkine, a new heparin-binding growth factor. EMBO J. (1997). , 16(23), 6936-46.

[78] Akhter, S, Ichihara-tanaka, K, Kojima, S, Muramatsu, H, Inui, T, Kimura, T, Kaneda, N, Talukder, A. H, Kadomatsu, K, Inagaki, F, & Muramatsu, T. Clusters of basic amino acids in midkine: roles in neurite-promoting activity and plasminogen activator-enhancing activity. J Biochem. (1998). , 123(6), 1127-36.

[79] Kojima, S, Inui, T, Muramatsu, H, Suzuki, Y, Kadomatsu, K, Yoshizawa, M, Hirose, S, Kimura, T, Sakakibara, S, & Muramatsu, T. Dimerization of midkine by tissue transglutaminase and its functional implication. J Biol Chem. (1997). , 272(14), 9410-6.

[80] Takei, Y, Kadomatsu, K, Matsuo, S, Itoh, H, Nakazawa, K, Kubota, S, & Muramatsu, T. Antisense oligodeoxynucleotide targeted to Midkine, a heparin-binding growth factor, suppresses tumorigenicity of mouse rectal carcinoma cells. Cancer Res. (2001). , 61(23), 8486-91.

[81] Muramatsu, T. Midkine, a heparin-binding cytokine with multiple roles in development, repair and diseases. Proc Jpn Acad Ser B Phys Biol Sci. (2010). , 86(4), 410-25.

[82] Muramatsu, H, Zou, P, Kurosawa, N, Ichihara-tanaka, K, Maruyama, K, Inoh, K, Sakai, T, Chen, L, Sato, M, & Muramatsu, T. Female infertility in mice deficient in midkine and pleiotrophin, which form a distinct family of growth factors. Genes Cells. (2006). , 11(12), 1405-17.

[83] Maeda, N, Ichihara-tanaka, K, Kimura, T, Kadomatsu, K, Muramatsu, T, & Noda, M. A receptor-like protein-tyrosine phosphatase PTPzeta/RPTPbeta binds a heparin-binding growth factor midkine. Involvement of arginine 78 of midkine in the high affinity binding to PTPzeta. J Biol Chem. (1999). Apr 30; , 274(18), 12474-9.

[84] Qin Li LHuang HL, Ping JL, Xu W, Li J, Dai LC. Expression of midkine and endoglin in breast carcinomas with different immunohistochemical profiles. APMIS. (2011). , 119(2), 103-10.

[85] Dai, L. C. Midkine translocated to nucleoli and involved in carcinogenesis. World J Gastroenterol. (2009). , 2009(15), 4-412.

[86] Nobata, S, Shinozawa, T, & Sakanishi, A. Truncated midkine induces transformation of cultured cells and short latency of tumorigenesis in nude mice. Cancer Lett.(2005). , 219(1), 83-9.

[87] Gustavsson, H, Jennbacken, K, Welén, K, & Damber, J. E. Altered expression of genes regulating angiogenesis in experimental androgen-independent prostate cancer. Prostate. (2008). , 68(2), 161-70.

[88] Maruyama, K, Muramatsu, H, Ishiguro, N, & Muramatsu, T. Midkine, a heparin-binding growth factor, is fundamentally involved in the pathogenesis of rheumatoid arthritis. Arthritis Rheum. (2004). , 50(5), 1420-9.

[89] Wang, J, Takeuchi, H, Sonobe, Y, Jin, S, Mizuno, T, Miyakawa, S, Fujiwara, M, Nakamura, Y, Kato, T, Muramatsu, H, Muramatsu, T, & Suzumura, A. Inhibition of midkine alleviates experimental autoimmune encephalomyelitis through the expansion of regulatory T cell population. Proc Natl Acad Sci U S A. (2008). , 105(10), 3915-20.

[90] Kadomatsu, K. Midkine regulation of the renin-angiotensin system. Curr Hypertens Rep. (2010). , 12(2), 74-9.

[91] Kemik, O, Sumer, A, Kemik, A. S, Hasirci, I, Purisa, S, Dulger, A. C, Demiriz, B, & Tuzun, S. The relationship among acute-phase response proteins, cytokines and hormones in cachectic patients with colon cancer. World J Surg Oncol. (2010).

[92] Lucas, S, Henze, G, Schnabel, D, Barthlen, W, Sakuma, S, Kurtz, A, & Driever, P. H. Serum levels of Midkine in children and adolescents without malignant disease. Pediatr Int. (2010). , 52(1), 75-9.

[93] Muramatsu, H, Zou, K, Sakaguchi, N, Ikematsu, S, Sakuma, S, & Muramatsu, T. LDL receptor-related protein as a component of the midkine receptor. Biochem Biophys Res Commun. (2000). , 270(3), 936-41.

[94] Muramatsu, H, Zou, P, Suzuki, H, Oda, Y, Chen, G. Y, Sakaguchi, N, Sakuma, S, Maeda, N, Noda, M, Takada, Y, & Muramatsu, T. alpha4betaand alpha6beta1-integrins are functional receptors for midkine, a heparin-binding growth factor. J Cell Sci. (2004). Pt 22):5405-15., 1.

[95] Ohuchida, T, Okamoto, K, Akahane, K, Higure, A, Todoroki, H, Abe, Y, Kikuchi, M, Ikematsu, S, Muramatsu, T, & Itoh, H. Midkine protects hepatocellular carcinoma cells against TRAIL-mediated apoptosis through down-regulation of caspase-3 activity. Cancer. (2004). , 100(11), 2430-6.

[96] Huang, Y, Sook-kim, M, & Ratovitski, E. Midkine promotes tetraspanin-integrin interaction and induces FAK-Stat1alpha pathway contributing to migration/invasiveness of human head and neck squamous cell carcinoma cells. Biochem Biophys Res Commun. (2008). , 377(2), 474-8.

[97] Cernkovich, E. R, Deng, J, Hua, K, & Harp, J. B. Midkine is an autocrine activator of signal transducer and activator of transcription 3 in 3T3-L1 cells. Endocrinology. (2007). , 148(4), 1598-604.

[98] Stoica, G. E, Kuo, A, Powers, C, Bowden, E. T, Sale, E. B, Riegel, A. T, & Wellstein, A. Midkine binds to anaplastic lymphoma kinase (ALK) and acts as a growth factor for different cell types. J Biol Chem. (2002). , 277(39), 35990-8.

[99] Muramatsu, T. Midkine, a heparin-binding cytokine with multiple roles in development, repair and diseases. Proc Jpn Acad Ser B Phys Biol Sci.(2010). , 86(4), 410-25.

[100] Hussain, M. M, Strickland, D. K, & Bakillah, A. The mammalian low-density lipoprotein receptor family. Annu Rev Nutr. (1999). , 19, 141-72.

[101] Shibata, Y, Muramatsu, T, Hirai, M, Inui, T, Kimura, T, Saito, H, Mccormick, L. M, Bu, G, & Kadomatsu, K. Nuclear targeting by the growth factor midkine. Mol Cell Biol. (2002). , 22(19), 6788-96.

[102] Owada, K, Sanjo, N, Kobayashi, T, Mizusawa, H, Muramatsu, H, Muramatsu, T, & Michikawa, M. Midkine inhibits caspase-dependent apoptosis via the activation of mitogen-activated protein kinase and phosphatidylinositol 3-kinase in cultured neurons. J Neurochem. (1999). , 73(5), 2084-2092.

[103] Satoh, J, Muramatsu, H, Moretto, G, Muramatsu, T, Chang, H. J, Kim, S. T, Cho, J. M, & Kim, S. U. Midkine that promotes survival of fetal human neurons is produced by fetal human astrocytes in culture. Brain Res Dev Brain Res. (1993). , 75(2), 201-205.

[104] Mitsiadis, T. A, Salmivirta, M, Muramatsu, T, Muramatsu, H, Rauvala, H, Lehtonen, E, Jalkanen, M, & Thesleff, I. Expression of the heparin-binding cytokines, midkine (MK) and HB-GAM (pleiotrophin) is associated with epithelial-mesenchymal interactions during fetal development and organogenesis. Development. (1995). , 121(1), 37-51.

[105] Mishima, K, Asai, A, Kadomatsu, K, Ino, Y, Nomura, K, Narita, Y, Muramatsu, T, & Kirino, T. Increased expression of midkine during the progression of human astrocytomas. Neurosci Lett. (1997). , 233(1), 29-32.

[106] Powers, C, Aigner, A, Stoica, G. E, Mcdonnell, K, & Wellstein, A. Pleiotrophin signaling through anaplastic lymphoma kinase is rate-limiting for glioblastoma growth. J Biol Chem. (2002). , 277(16), 14153-8.

[107] Grzelinski, M, Steinberg, F, Martens, T, Czubayko, F, Lamszus, K, & Aigner, A. Enhanced antitumorigenic effects in glioblastoma on double targeting of pleiotrophin and its receptor ALK. Neoplasia. (2009). , 11(2), 145-56.

[108] Lorente, M, Torres, S, Salazar, M, Carracedo, A, Hernández-tiedra, S, Rodríguez-fornés, F, García-taboada, E, Meléndez, B, Mollejo, M, Campos-martín, Y, Lakatosh, S. A, Barcia, J, Guzmán, M, & Velasco, G. Stimulation of the midkine/ALK axis renders glioma cells resistant to cannabinoid antitumoral action. Cell Death Differ. (2011). Jun;, 18(6), 959-73.

[109] Merlo, A. Genes and pathways driving glioblastomas in humans and murine disease models. Neurosurg Rev. (2003). , 26(3), 145-58.

[110] Bani-yaghoub, M, Tremblay, R. G, Lei, J. X, Zhang, D, Zurakowski, B, Sandhu, J. K, Smith, B, Ribecco-lutkiewicz, M, Kennedy, J, Walker, P. R, & Sikorska, M. Role of Sox2 in the development of the mouse neocortex. Dev Biol. (2006). , 295(1), 52-66.

[111] Panchision, D. M. The role of oxygen in regulating neural stem cells in development and disease. J Cell Physiol. (2009). , 220(3), 562-8.

[112] Dang, L, Fan, X, Chaudhry, A, Wang, M, Gaiano, N, & Eberhart, C. G. Notch3 signaling initiates choroid plexus tumor formation. Oncogene. (2006). , 25(3), 487-91.

[113] Sivasankaran, B, Degen, M, Ghaffari, A, Hegi, M. E, Hamou, M. F, Ionescu, M. C, Zweifel, C, Tolnay, M, Wasner, M, Mergenthaler, S, Miserez, A. R, Kiss, R, Lino, M. M, Merlo, A, Chiquet-ehrismann, R, & Boulay, J. L. Tenascin-C is a novel RBPJkappa-induced target gene for Notch signaling in gliomas. Cancer Res. (2009). Jan 15; , 69(2), 458-65.

[114] Tanaka, M, Kadokawa, Y, Hamada, Y, & Marunouchi, T. Notch2 expression negatively correlates with glial differentiation in the postnatal mouse brain. J Neurobiol. (1999). , 41(4), 524-39.

[115] Purow, B. W, Sundaresan, T. K, Burdick, M. J, Kefas, B. A, Comeau, L. D, Hawkinson, M. P, Su, Q, Kotliarov, Y, Lee, J, Zhang, W, & Fine, H. A. Notch-1 regulates transcription of the epidermal growth factor receptor through Carcinogenesis. (2008). , 53.

[116] Brennan, C, Momota, H, Hambardzumyan, D, Ozawa, T, Tandon, A, Pedraza, A, & Holland, E. Glioblastoma subclasses can be defined by activity among signal transduction pathways and associated genomic alterations. PLoS One. (2009). e7752.

[117] Libermann, T. A, Nusbaum, H. R, Razon, N, Kris, R, Lax, I, Soreq, H, Whittle, N, Waterfield, M. D, Ullrich, A, & Schlessinger, J. Amplification and overexpression of the EGF receptor gene in primary human glioblastomas. J Cell Sci Suppl. (1985). , 3, 161-72.

[118] Ma, J, Meng, Y, Kwiatkowski, D. J, Chen, X, Peng, H, Sun, Q, Zha, X, Wang, F, Wang, Y, Jing, Y, Zhang, S, Chen, R, Wang, L, Wu, E, Cai, G, Malinowska-kolodziej, I, Liao, Q, Liu, Y, Zhao, Y, Sun, Q, Xu, K, Dai, J, Han, J, Wu, L, Zhao, R. C, Shen, H, & Zhang, H. Mammalian target of rapamycin regulates murine and human cell differentiation through STAT3/Jagged/Notch cascade. J Clin Invest. (2010). , 63.

[119] Lino, M. M, Merlo, A, & Boulay, J. L. Notch signaling in glioblastoma: a developmental drug target? BMC Med. (2010).

[120] Ohgaki, H, Dessen, P, Jourde, B, Horstmann, S, & Nishikawa, T. Di Patre PL, Burkhard C, Schüler D, Probst-Hensch NM, Maiorka PC, Baeza N, Pisani P, Yonekawa Y, Yasargil MG, Lütolf UM, Kleihues P. Genetic pathways to glioblastoma: a population-based study. Cancer Res. (2004). , 64(19), 6892-9.

[121] Patten, B. A, Sardi, S. P, Koirala, S, Nakafuku, M, & Corfas, G. Notch1 signaling regulates radial glia differentiation through multiple transcriptional mechanisms. J Neurosci. (2006). , 26(12), 3102-8.

[122] Ikushima, H, Todo, T, Ino, Y, Takahashi, M, Miyazawa, K, & Miyazono, K. Autocrine TGF-beta signaling maintains tumorigenicity of glioma-initiating cells through Sry-related HMG-box factors. Cell Stem Cell. 2009; Erratum in: Cell Stem Cell. (2009). , 5(5), 504-14.

[123] Mirkin, B. L, Clark, S, Zheng, X, Chu, F, White, B. D, Greene, M, & Rebbaa, A. Identification of midkine as a mediator for intercellular transfer of drug resistance. Oncogene. (2005). , 24(31), 4965-74.

[124] Hu, R, Yan, Y, Li, Q, Lin, Y, Jin, W, Li, H, Lu, Y, & Pang, T. Increased drug efflux along with midkine gene high expression in childhood B-lineage acute lymphoblastic leukemia cells. Int J Hematol. (2010). , 92(1), 105-10.

[125] Rosenbaum, C, Röhrs, S, Müller, O, & Waldmann, H. Modulation of MRP-1-mediated multidrug resistance by indomethacin analogues. J Med Chem. (2005). , 48(4), 1179-87.

[126] Erguven, M, Bilir, A, Yazihan, N, Ermis, E, Sabanci, A, Aktas, E, Aras, Y, & Alpman, V. Decreased therapeutic effects of noscapine combined with imatinib mesylate on human glioblastoma in vitro and the effect of midkine. Cancer Cell Int. (2011).

[127] Yao, X, Tan, Z, Gu, B, Wu, R. R, Liu, Y. K, Dai, L. C, & Zhang, M. Promotion of self-renewal of embryonic stem cells by midkine. Acta Pharmacol Sin. (2010). , 31(5), 629-37.

[128] Huang, Z, Cheng, L, Guryanova, O. A, Wu, Q, & Bao, S. Cancer stem cells in glioblastoma--molecular signaling and therapeutic targeting. Protein Cell. (2010). , 1(7), 638-55.

Chapter 13

Porphyrin Synthesis from 5-Aminolevulinic Acid in Patients with Glioma

Satoshi Utsuki, Hidehiro Oka, Kiyotaka Fujii,
Norio Miyoshi, Masahiro Ishizuka,
Kiwamu Takahashi and Katsushi Inoue

Additional information is available at the end of the chapter

http://dx.doi.org/10.5772/51482

1. Introduction

The molecule 5-aminolevulinic acid (5-ALA) is a substrate for a heme synthesized in cells using succinyl CoA and glycine. Initially, 5-ALA is converted to porphobilinogen (PBG), and the metabolism progresses by the action of PBG deaminase, and its product is incorporated into the mitochondria via uroporphyrinogen and coproporphyrinogen by an enzymatic reaction and transformed into protoporphyrin IX (PPIX). This PPIX is then converted to a heme by the action of ferrochelatase. These metabolic reactions are conducted in the liver and erythroblasts of normal human subjects [16]. It is thought that a larger amount of 5-ALA is incorporated by rapidly proliferating tumor cells as compared to normal cells, due to the active synthesis of heme [5, 20]. In the metabolic pathway of 5-ALA, it is reported that the rate limiting enzyme in normal cells is different from that in tumor cells [16]. PBG deaminase is the rate limiting enzyme in normal cells [3]. Large amounts of uroporphyrinogen, coproporphyrinogen, and PPIX are produced in tumor cells compared to normal cells because metabolism after the PBG is promoted by high PBG deaminase activity and low ferrochelatase activity [15]. The PPIX accumulates in tumor cells and produces a red fluorescent response to ultraviolet light. Intraoperative photodynamic diagnosis using this method is used for patients with glioma [21, 24, 26]. There are numerous reports concerning the PPIX concentration in the tumor tissue; however, reports concerning plasma titers and urinary excretion of uroporphyrinogen and coproporphyrinogen after 5-ALA administration are rare [25]. In this study, 5-ALA was administered to healthy adult volunteers, and changes in serum and urinary porphyrins were measured. Urinary excretion of porphyrins in volunteers and patients with brain tumors after the 5-ALA administration were compared and examined.

2. Materials and Methods

Healthy adult volunteers (n = 8) and 58 patients with glioma (12 benign gliomas (WHO grade II) and 46 glioblastomas) who were resected by intraoperative fluorescence diagnosis using 5-ALA were enrolled in the study. Eight adult volunteers were given 1 gram of 5-ALA orally, and blood sampling was done before administration, 2 hours, 4 hours, and 6 hours later. Blood samples were analyzed for plasma titers of 5-ALA, PPIX, coproporphyrin I (CPI), coproporphyrin III (CPIII), uroporphyrin I (UPI), and uroporphyrin III (UPIII). Urine collection was done before and 4 hours after 5-ALA administration, and the urinary excretion of 5-ALA, CPI, CPIII, UPI, and UPIII were measured. Fifty-eight patients with glioma were given 1 gram of 5-ALA orally 2 hours before anesthesia, and blood and urine samples were collected from these patients 4 hours later for analyses of plasma titers and urinary excretion of 5-ALA, PPIX, CPI, CPIII, UPI, and UPIII. Intraoperative fluorescence diagnosis for 58 patients with glioma was performed using a semiconductor laser device (VLD-V1 version 2: M & M Co., Ltd., Tokyo, Japan). The brain tumor was exposed to a laser light that had a peak wavelength of 405 nm and a light output of 120 mW by placing the optical fiber as close as possible. The spectra of the response light from tumors were analyzed by a personal computer for a fluorescent identification of PPIX and the measurement of the fluorescent objective strength. When fluorescence from PPIX was observed, a waveform with a peak at 636 nm was observed. When the intensity of the peak at 636 nm was ≥3000, the tumor was defined as a strong fluorescence tumor. In contrast, when the intensity of the peak at 636 nm was < 3000, the tumor was defined as a weak fluorescence tumor. Two groups distributed based on these spectra were examined for macroscopic findings; i.e., fluorescence for the strong PPIX group was observed macroscopically in all of the strong fluorescence tumors. When there was not a waveform peak at 636 nm, and the fluorescence of PPIX was not observed for a tumor, the tumor was considered to be a non-fluorescence tumor. The total urinary excretion products were adjusted for creatinine value. Testing for significant differences was done using analysis of variance (analysis of variance; ANOVA) or the PLSD (protected least significant difference) method of Fisher as a post-hoc test.

3. Results

The plasma 5-ALA concentration in volunteers reached a peak 2 hours after 5-ALA administration (Figure 1). The plasma titer peaks of protoporphyrin IX, CPI, and CPIII in volunteers were reached 2 hours after administration of 5-ALA. The plasma titer peaks of UPI and UPIII in volunteers were reached 4 hours after 5-ALA administration (Figure 2). The plasma titer and urinary excretion of CPI, CPIII, UPI, UPIII, and 5-ALA were not significantly different in volunteers and glioma patients prior to 5-ALA administration (data not shown). Urinary excretion CPI and CPIII 4 hours after 5-ALA administration were significantly higher in patients with glioma than in volunteers (Figures 3, 4) ($p < 0.0001$). Urinary excretion of UPI and UPIII 4 hours after 5-ALA administration in volunteers and glioma patients were not significantly different (Figures 5, 6). Urinary excretion of CPI, CPIII, UPI, UPIII, and 5-

ALA 4 hours after 5-ALA administration in patients with benign glioma was not significantly different compared to patients with glioblastoma. All of the glioblastomas were strong fluorescence tumors. Benign gliomas were comprised of 3 strong fluorescence tumors, 5 weak fluorescence tumors, and 4 non-fluorescence tumors. Urinary excretion of CPI, CPIII, UPI, UPIII, and 5-ALA 4 hours after 5-ALA administration was not significantly different when comparing strong fluorescence tumors, weak fluorescence tumors, and non-fluorescence tumors in benign glioma patients (data not shown).

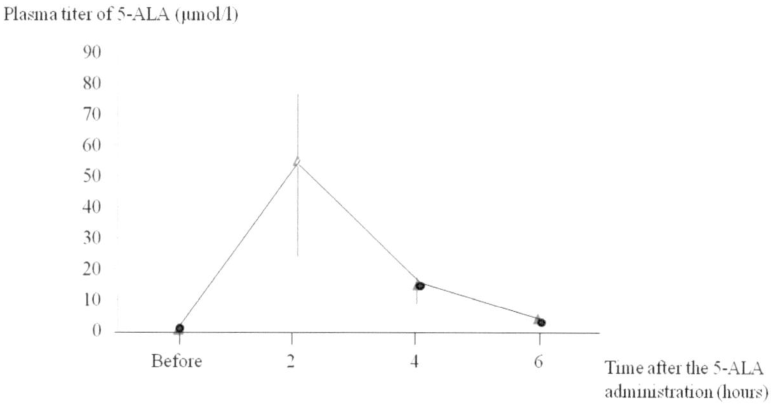

Figure 1. Graph shows the plasma titer of 5-ALA when 5-ALA was administered to volunteers. The peak concentration is reached 2 hours after administration of 5-ALA, and the concentration is ≤ 50% of the peak level 4 hours later. The concentration is ≤ 10% of the peak level 6 hours later.

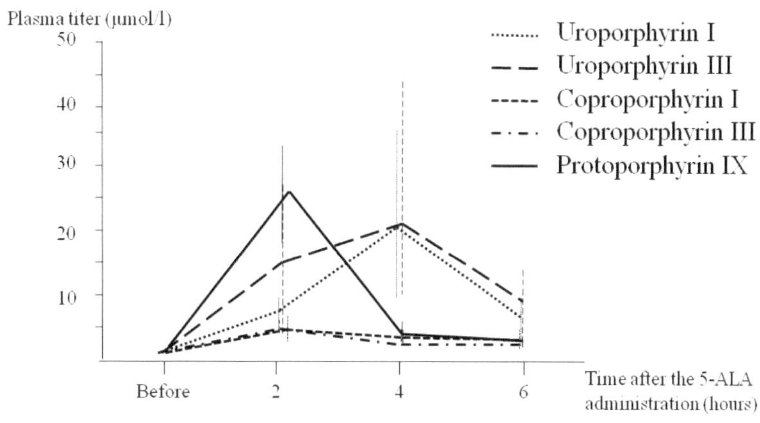

Figure 2. Graph shows various plasma titers of porphyrins when 5-ALA was administered to volunteers. The plasma titers of protoporphyrin IX, CPI, and CPIII reached maximal levels 2 hours following 5-ALA administration. The plasma titers of UPI and UPIII peaked at 4 hours after administration of 5-ALA.

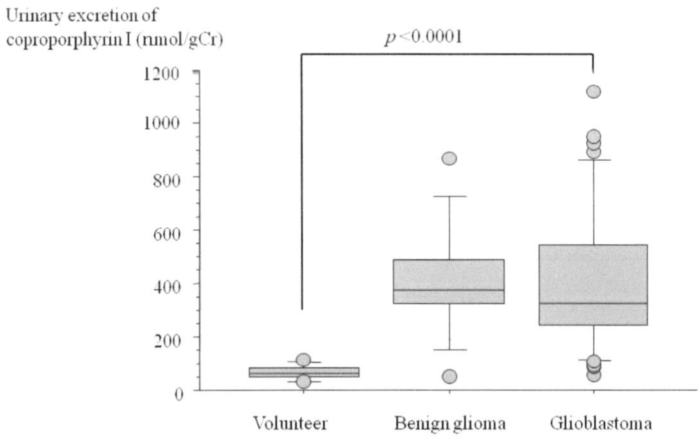

Figure 3. Graph shows urinary excretion of CPI 4 hours following administration of 5-ALA to normal volunteers, and patients with benign gliomas and glioblastomas. Urinary excretion of CPI in patients with benign gliomas and glioblastomas was significantly higher than in normal volunteers.

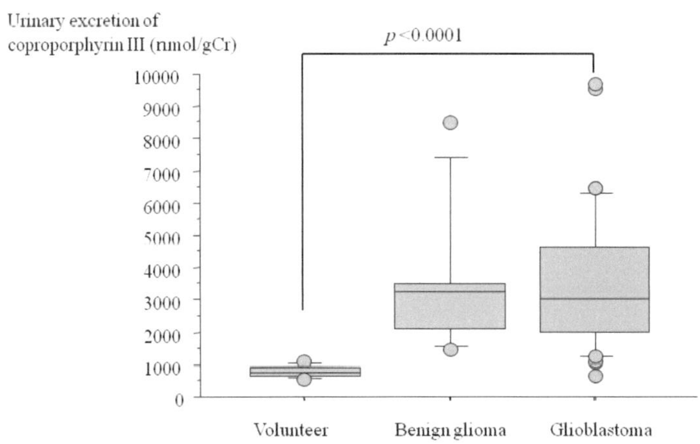

Figure 4. Graph shows urinary excretion of CPIII 4 hours after 5-ALA was administered to normal volunteers, and patients with benign gliomas and glioblastomas. Urinary excretion of CPIII in patients with benign gliomas and glioblastomas was significantly higher than in normal volunteers.

4. Discussion

It was reported that plasma titers and urinary excretion of porphyrins were increased when tumor-bearing mice were administered 5-ALA [8]. Also, it was reported that the plasma titers and urinary excretion of these porphyrins were increased when 5-ALA was administered to adult mice without malignant tumors [14]. The reason why these porphyrins increase in healthy volunteers after 5-ALA administration might be that those porphyrins leak as the intermediate product after being metabolized by the erythroblasts and liver [14]. When healthy volunteers were administered 5-ALA in our study, the plasma titers of 5-ALA, CPI, CPIII, UPI, UPIII, and PPIX reached maximum levels at 2-4 hours following 5-ALA administration. Therefore, it was thought that most of these porphyrins were done being excreted in the urine 4 hours after 5-ALA administration.

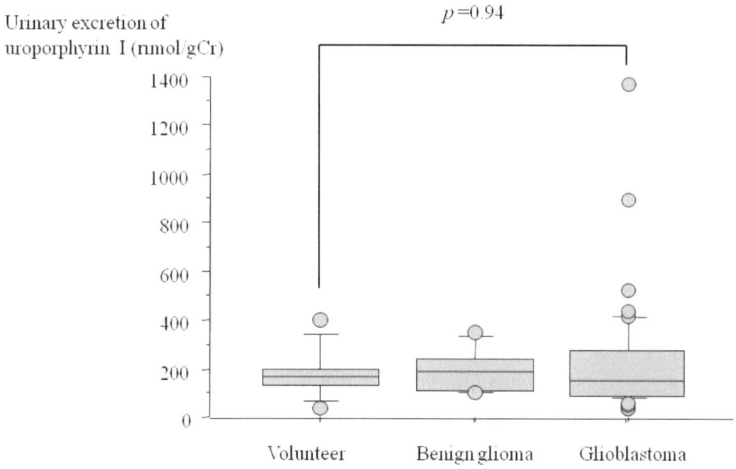

Figure 5. Graph shows urinary excretion of UPI 4 hours after 5-ALA was administered to normal volunteers, and patients with benign gliomas and glioblastomas. The urinary excretion of UPI showed no significant differences among subjects who were normal volunteers, and patients with benign gliomas and glioblastomas.

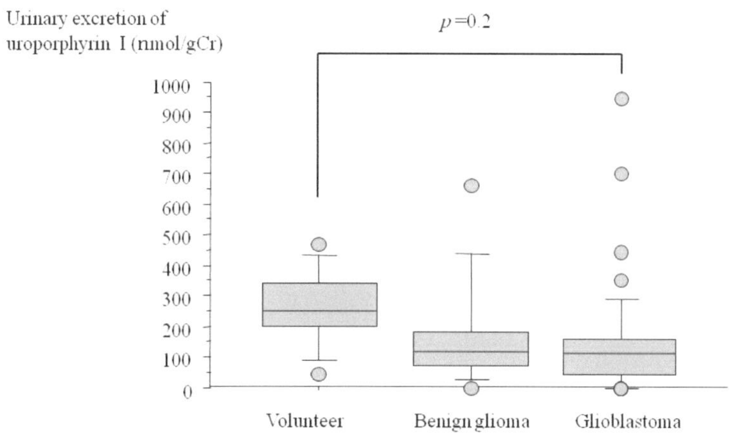

Figure 6. Graph shows urinary excretion of UPIII 4 hours after 5-ALA was administered to normal volunteers and patients with benign gliomas and the glioblastomas. The urinary excretion of UPIII showed no significant differences among subjects who were normal volunteers, and patients with benign gliomas and glioblastomas

If 5-ALA were not administered, there would be no difference in the metabolism of these porphyrins in volunteers and glioma patients, because plasma titers and urinary excretion of CPI, CPIII, UPI, UPIII, and 5-ALA were not significantly different in volunteers and glioma patients prior to 5-ALA administration. Also, there would not be the specific metabolic process in tumor cells for converting 5-ALA to uroporphyrin, because urinary excretion of UPI and UPIII was not different when comparing volunteers, patients with benign glioma, and patients with glioblastoma. However, the urinary excretion of CPI and CPIII 4 hours after 5-ALA administration significantly increased in patients with glioma as compared to volunteers. Therefore, it was thought that high levels of CPI and CPIII were being produced in tumor cells as compared to normal cells. Heme is rapidly synthesized in cells with accelerated metabolism, such as tumor cells, and 5-ALA is incorporated into tumor cells and metabolized. Consequently, large quantities of CPI and CPIII are produced as the metabolites, and it was thought that urinary excretion increased [11]. In the healthy adults without a tumor, PBG deaminase becomes the rate limiting enzyme even if 5-ALA is incorporated into cells, and extensive metabolism occurs prior to production of PBG. Therefore, CPI and CPIII, which are down-stream metabolites, will not be produced in large quantities [3].

It is known that ATP-binding cassette (ABC) transporters, such as ABCG2 and ABCB6, are associated with trafficking of these porphyrins. ABCG2 is expressed mainly in the cell membrane and serves as the active transporter for anticancer drugs present outside of cells [6]. ABCG2 drains excessive levels of porphyrin outside of cells while performing this function [13]. ABCB6 transports coproporphyrinogen from the cytoplasm into the mitochondria, and both. ABCG2 and ABCB6 are overexpressed in cancer cells [6, 12, 23]. ABCG2 is overexpressed in brain tumors [1, 9], and its presence is more common in malignant tumors [9]. CPI and CPIII that are produced in the cytoplasm of tumor cells are actively transported by ABCG2 overexpressed in brain tumor cells. This was considered the cause of higher urinary excretion of CPI and CPIII in patients with a brain tumor compared to normal volunteers. Similarly, it is reported that urinary excretion of porphyrins increases even in cancers other than brain tumors [7]. Therefore, these porphyrins may be used as a nonspecific marker in screening for tumors [25]. In other words, presence of hypermetabolic tumor cells may be suggested if urinary excretion measures of CPI and CPIII are elevated in a person orally administered orally 5-ALA. In such a case, it may be useful to investigate the whole body for the presence of a tumor.

The urinary excretion of CPI and CPIII were not different in benign glioma and glioblastoma patients, and the metabolism of 5-ALA to produce CPI and CPIII should not differ between benign gliomas and glioblastomas. Many of the benign gliomas were weak fluorescence or nonfluorescence tumors, whereas all glioblastomas were strong fluorescence tumors. In other words, high levels of PPIX had accumulated in the glioblastomas, while only low levels of PPIX accumulated in benign gliomas. Metabolic processes involved in the pathway leading from CPI and CP III to PPIX will be different in benign gliomas and glioblastomas. These differences will be due differences in the activity of ABCB6 which transports CPI and CPIII in mitochondria, or coproporphyrinogen oxidase, which converts CPI and CPIII into PPIX. Concerning these ABC transporters, it is reported in accordance with genetic polymorphism that the functions and levels of expression are different [23]. Therefore, the intracellular PPIX concentration will be higher for a tumor having higher levels of ABCB6 [12]. Also, the glioblastomas will have much higher levels of PPIX than benign gliomas, because the presence of coproporphyrinogen oxidase is common in a malignant tumor [22].

However, differences in PPIX accumulation (fluorescent strength) are not necessarily proportional to urinary excretion of these porphyrins after 5-ALA administration. The volume of a tumor (the total amount of PPIX) is one factor affecting results. The factors related to differences in accumulation of protoporphyrin IX have been investigated in various ways, and various factors such as ALA uptake by cells [2, 19], mitochondrial properties [18], molecules involved in PpIX metabolism including porphobilinogen deaminase [4], ferrochelatase [15], iron content [10], transferring receptor [17], and mRNA levels of the coproporphyrinogen oxidase (CPOX) gene [13] are thought to be associated with protoporphyrin IX accumulation. Due to the involvement of these multiple factors, differences in the accumulation of PPIX will occur [24].

5. Conclusion

Following administration of 5-ALA, patients with a brain tumor showed higher urinary excretion of CPI and CPIII than did healthy volunteers. This was due to the active production of porphyrins in metabolically active tumor cells. The urinary excretion of CPI and CPIII following administration of 5-ALAcould possibly be used as a screening assay for the presence or absence of a tumor. Differences in the presence of the ABC transporter may contribute to metabolic differences of the porphyrins in benign gliomas and glioblastomas.

Author details

Satoshi Utsuki[1*], Hidehiro Oka[1], Kiyotaka Fujii[1], Norio Miyoshi[2], Masahiro Ishizuka[3], Kiwamu Takahashi[3] and Katsushi Inoue[3]

1 Department of Neurosurgery, Kitasato University School of Medicine, Kitasato, Minami, Sagamihara, Kanagawa 228-0473 , Japan

2 Division of Tumor Pathology, Department of Pathological Sciences, Faculty of Medicine, University of Fukui, Matsuoka, Eiheiji, Fukui 910-1193 , Japan

3 SBI ALApromo Co, LTD, Roppongi, Minato-ku, Tokyo 106-6019, Japan

References

[1] Bleau, A. M., Huse, J. T., & Holland, E. C. (2009). The ABCG2 resistance network of glioblastoma. *Cell Cycle*, 8(18), 2936-2944.

[2] Doring, F., Walter, J., Will, J., Focking, M., Boll, M., Amasheh, S., Clauss, W., & Daniel, H. (1998). Delta-aminolevulinic acid transport by intestinal and renal peptide transporters and its physiological and clinical implications. *The Journal of Clinical Investigation*, 101(12), 2761-2767.

[3] Gibson, S. L., Cupriks, D. J., Havens, J. J., Nguyen, M. L., & Hilf, R. (1998). A regulatory role for porphobilinogen deaminase (PBGD) in delta-aminolaevulinic acid (delta-ALA)-induced photosensitization? *British Journal of Cancer*, 77(2), 235-242.

[4] Hinnen, P., de Rooij, F. W., Terlouw, E. M., Edixhoven, A., van Dekken, H., van Hillegersberg, R., Tilanus, H. W., Wilson, J. H., & Siersema, P. D. (2000). Porphyrin biosynthesis in human Barrett's oesophagus and adenocarcinoma after ingestion of 5-aminolaevulinic acid. *British Journal of Cancer*, 83(4), 539-543.

[5] Inoue, K., Karashima, T., Kamada, M., Shuin, T., Kurabayashi, A., Furihata, M., Fujita, H., Utsumi, K., & Sasaki, J. (2009). Regulation of 5-aminolevulinic acid-mediated protoporphyrin IX accumulation in human urothelial carcinomas. *Pathobiology*, 76(6), 303-314.

[6] Ishikawa, T., & Nakagawa, H. (2009). Human ABC transporter ABCG2 in cancer chemotherapy and pharmacogenomics. *Journal of Experimental Therapeutics Oncology*, 8(1), 5-24.

[7] Ishizuka, M., Abe, F., Sano, Y., Takahashi, K., Inoue, K., Nakajima, M., Kohda, T., Komatsu, N., Ogura, S. I., & Tanaka, T. (2011). Novel development of 5-aminolevurinic acid (ALA) in cancer diagnoses and therapy. *International Immunopharmacology*, 11(3), 358-365.

[8] Ishizuka, M., Hagiya, Y., Mizokami, Y., Honda, K., Tabata, K., Kamachi, T., Takahashi, K., Abe, F., Tanaka, T., Nakajima, M., Ogura, S., & Okura, I. (2011). Porphyrins in urine after administration of 5-aminolevulinic acid as a potential tumor marker. *Photodiagnosis and Photodynamic Therapy*, 8(4), 328-331.

[9] Jin, Y., Bin, Z. Q., Qiang, H., Liang, C., Hua, C., Jun, D., Dong, W. A., & Qing, L. (2009). ABCG2 is related with the grade of glioma and resistance to mitoxantone, a chemotherapeutic drug for glioma. *Journal of Cancer Research and Clinical Oncology*, 135(10), 1369-1376.

[10] Krieg, R. C., Fickweiler, S., Wolfbeis, O. S., & Knuechel, R. (2000). Cell-type specific protoporphyrin IX metabolism in human bladder cancer in vitro. *Photochemistry and Photobiology*, 72(2), 226-233.

[11] Krieg, R. C., Messmann, H., Rauch, J., Seeger, S., & Knuechel, R. (2002). Metabolic characterization of tumor cell-specific protoporphyrin IX accumulation after exposure to 5-aminolevulinic acid in human colonic cells. *Photochemistry and Photobiology*, 76(5), 518-525.

[12] Krishnamurthy, P. C., Du, G., Fukuda, Y., Sun, D., Sampath, J., Mercer, K. E., Wang, J., Sosa-Pineda, B., Murti, K. G., & Schuetz, J. D. (2006). Identification of a mammalian mitochondrial porphyrin transporter. *Nature*, 443(7111), 586-589.

[13] Krishnamurthy, P., & Schuetz, J. D. (2006). Role of ABCG2/BCRP in biology and medicine. *Annual Review of Pharmacology and Toxicology*, 46-381.

[14] Mustajoki, P., Timonen, K., Gorchein, A., Seppalainen, A. M., Matikainen, E., & Tenhunen, R. (1992). Sustained high plasma 5-aminolaevulinic acid concentration in a volunteer: no porphyric symptoms. *European Journal of Clinical Investigation*, 22(6), 407-411.

[15] Ohgari, Y., Nakayasu, Y., Kitajima, S., Sawamoto, M., Mori, H., Shimokawa, O., Matsui, H., & Taketani, S. (2005). Mechanisms involved in delta-aminolevulinic acid (ALA)-induced photosensitivity of tumor cells: relation of ferrochelatase and uptake of ALA to the accumulation of protoporphyrin. *Biochemical Pharmacology*.

[16] Peng, Q., Berg, K., Moan, J., Kongshaug, M., & Nesland, J. M. . (1997). Aminolevulinic acid-based photodynamic therapy: principles and experimental research. *Photochemistry and Photobiology*, 65(2), 235-251.

[17] Piccinelli, P., & Samuelsson, T. (2007). Evolution of the iron-responsive element. *RNA*, 13(7), 952-966.

[18] Rebeiz, N., Arkins, S., Kelley, K. W., & Rebeiz, C. A. (1996). Enhancement of coproporphyrinogen III transport into isolated transformed leukocyte mitochondria by ATP. *Archives of Biochemistry and Biophysics*, 333(2), 475-481.

[19] Rud, E., Gederaas, O., Hogset, A., & Berg, K. (2000). 5-aminolevulinic acid, but not 5-aminolevulinic acid esters, is transported into adenocarcinoma cells by system BETA transporters. *Photochemistry and Photobiology*, 71(5), 640-647.

[20] Stummer, W., Reulen, H. J., Novotny, A., Stepp, H., & Tonn, J. C. (2003). Fluorescence-guided resections of malignant gliomas--an overview. *Acta Neurochirurgica Supplement*, 88-9.

[21] Stummer, W., Stocker, S., Wagner, S., Stepp, H., Fritsch, C., Goetz, C., Goetz, A. E., Kiefmann, R., & Reulen, H. J. (1998). Intraoperative detection of malignant gliomas by 5-aminolevulinic acid-induced porphyrin fluorescence. *Neurosurgery*, 42(3), 518-526.

[22] Takahashi, K., Ikeda, N., Nonoguchi, N., Kajimoto, Y., Miyatake, S., Hagiya, Y., Ogura, S., Nakagawa, H., Ishikawa, T., & Kuroiwa, T. (2011). Enhanced expression of coproporphyrinogen oxidase in malignant brain tumors: CPOX expression and 5-ALA-induced fluorescence. *Neuro-oncology*, 13(11), 1234-1243.

[23] Tamura, A., Onishi, Y., An, R., Koshiba, S., Wakabayashi, K., Hoshijima, K., Priebe, W., Yoshida, T., Kometani, S., Matsubara, T., Mikuriya, K., & Ishikawa, T. (2007). In vitro evaluation of photosensitivity risk related to genetic polymorphisms of human

ABC transporter ABCG2 and inhibition by drugs. *Drug Metabolism and Pharmacokinetics*, 22(6), 428-440.

[24] Utsuki, S., Oka, H., & Fujii, K. (2011). Intraoperative photodynamic diagnosis of brain tumors using 5-aminolevulinic acid. In: Abujamra AL. (ed.) Diagnostic techniques and surgical management of brain tumors. *Brain tumor,* 4, Rijeka, InTech, 227-244, http://www.intechopen.com/books/diagnostic-techniques-and-surgical-management-of-brain-tumors/intraoperative-photodynamic-diagnosis-of-brain-tumors-using-5-aminolevulinic-acid.

[25] Utsuki, S., Oka, H., Fujii, K., Miyoshi, N., Ishizuka, M., Takahashi, K., & Inoue, K. (2011). Differential metabolism of 5-ALA in patients with brain tumors. *Miyoshi N, Pottier RH (eds.) In hope of going over the present Clinical PD and PDT.*, Nagoya: SANKEISHA, 160-173.

[26] Utsuki, S., Oka, H., Sato, S., Suzuki, S., Shimizu, S., Tanaka, S., & Fujii, K. (2006). Possibility of using laser spectroscopy for the intraoperative detection of nonfluorescing brain tumors and the boundaries of brain tumor infiltrates. Technical note. *Journal of Neurosurgery*, 104(4), 618-620.

Chapter 14

Mechanisms of Aggressiveness in Glioblastoma: Prognostic and Potential Therapeutic Insights

Céline S. Gonçalves, Tatiana Lourenço,
Ana Xavier-Magalhães, Marta Pojo and
Bruno M. Costa

Additional information is available at the end of the chapter

http://dx.doi.org/10.5772/52361

1. Introduction

1.1. Glioblastoma

Glioblastoma (GBM) is the most prevalent and most malignant (WHO grade IV) type of brain tumor in adults [1, 2]. In the United States, there are ~10,000 new cases diagnosed annually, and >50,000 patients living with the disease [2, 3]. The clinical responses of patients are particularly poor and vary greatly among individuals [4], and ~32% of all diagnosed cases survive less than a year [3]. This highly aggressive tumor develops either *de novo* (primary GBM), or as the result of the malignant progression from a lower-grade glioma (secondary GBM). In both cases, prognosis is very poor, and the median survival when radiotherapy and chemotherapy are combined is approximately 15 months [5]. Importantly, GBM is also characterized by extensive heterogeneity at the cellular and molecular levels. These tumors are highly diffuse, with extensive dissemination of tumor cells within the brain, which hinders complete surgical resection. These aggressive characteristics are associated with a remarkable resistance to therapies available today [6], which unfortunately are mostly palliative. In the context of their highest incidence of all malignant brain tumors in adults, their highly aggressive behavior and therapy-insensitive nature, which together account for a very poor prognosis of GBM patients, this chapter will focus specifically on GBM. In particular, it will review the different hypotheses of glioma/GBM-initiating cells, the major alterations at the levels of gene expression and signaling pathways found in GBM, as well as putative biomarkers of GBM prognosis, and current therapies currently available or under investigation for dealing with these tumors.

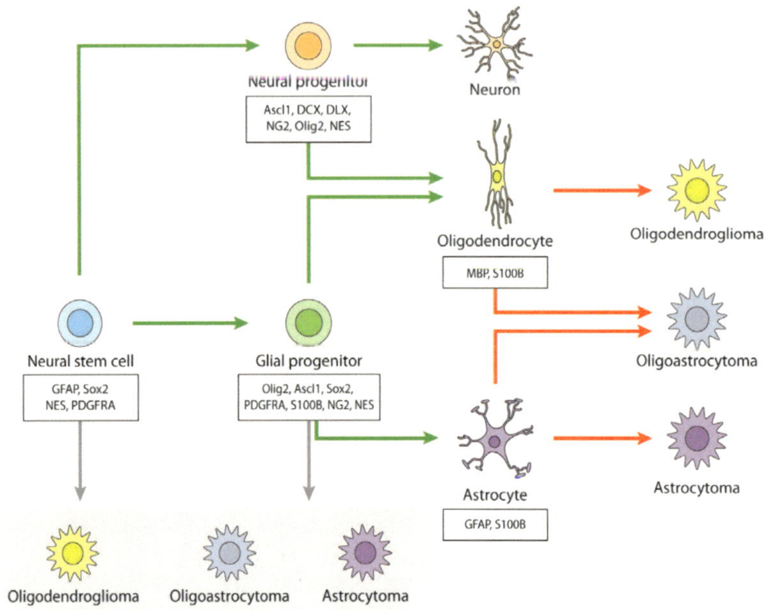

Figure 1. Schematic representation of the differentiation process of neural stem cells into different cell lineages of the CNS and putative cells of origin of gliomas. Protein markers for neural stem cells, progenitors cells, and differentiated cells are indicated in boxes. The normal differentiation process (green arrows) originates three main types of cells in the mature CNS, including neurons and glial cells (particularly oligodendrocytes and astrocytes; ependymal cells are not represented). The most classical hypothesis on the origin of glioma cells is represented by orange arrows (differentiated glial cells are malignantly transformed through a dedifferentiation process). The most recent hypothesis postulating that gliomas originate from the direct transformation of neural stem cells or glial progenitor cells is represented by grey arrows.

1.2. Glioma/GBM-Initiating cells

The true cellular origin of gliomas, including GBM, is still a debatable question. It is generally accepted that identifying such tumor-initiating cells may allow a better understanding of tumor biology, and ultimately help in designing improved therapies for GBM. All human tumors arise from a series of molecular alterations that occur in a small number, or even single, founder cells. These tumor cells present a clonal nature due to the sequential accumulation of multiple rare genetic and epigenetic events. The critical importance of the tumor microenvironment in influencing tumor cells behavior and evolution has been recently recognized [7]. Indeed, the tumor microenvironment has been associated with the generation and maintenance of tumor heterogeneity; thus, understanding not only the surrounding microenvironment but also tumor heterogeneity, as well as their relationships, may be crucial in understanding the biology of these tumors. In the case of the brain tissue, a highly complex microenvironment with extreme phenotypic and functional diversity, the multiplicity of putative brain tumor cells of origin, and the variety of niches in which the malignant cells may evolve, is even more challenging. Thus, understanding this complexity is crucial to provide firm evidence for the cellular origin of gliomas [8-10]. Two different hypotheses for the origin of glioma cells, or tumor cells in general, have been proposed (Figure 1), as detailed below.

One classical hypothesis postulates that cancer cells arise from the accumulation of alterations that occur in differentiated mature cells (glial cells in the case of glioma tumors, including GBM), which would result in a dedifferentiation of these cells along the carcinogenic process. This concept is supported, for instance, by the histological similarities between functional and differentiated glial cells and tumor cells from gliomas. In addition, before the experimental identification of the adult neural stem cells (NSCs), glial cells were the only known replication-competent population of cells in the adult brain, which further supported the idea that highly-proliferative glioma cells could derive from accumulated alterations in differentiated and proliferative glial cells. A landmark study supporting this theory showed that differentiated cells could be transformed into a pluripotent embryonic stem cell phenotype by using a cocktail of transcription factors [11]. However, this hypothesis has never been adequately tested, as there have been experimental limitations that preclude its validation, including: (i) the absence of good mature "astrocyte" markers in *in vivo* experiments [12], as it is now well known that the commonly used astrocyte marker GFAP is also expressed by adult NSCs; (ii) *in vitro*, the culture of mature astrocytes is particularly difficult; (iii) culturing astrocytes from neonatal mouse cortex has been described to contain also immature progenitor cells [13].

The second and most recent hypothesis assumes that cancer cells arise from the accumulation of alterations that occur directly in stem cells, or progenitor (multipotent) undifferentiated cells, that are present in different tissues throughout the entire lifetime (neural stem cells or glial progenitor cells in the case of brain gliomas). According to this rationale, the tumorigenic process would not be accompanied by a dedifferentiation mechanism, as the molecular alterations would accumulate directly in undifferentiated cells [7-9, 14]. In support of this hypothesis is the concept of cancer stem cells (CSCs), which is a subpopulation of cells in the tumor that displays self-renewal capacity, and which can give rise to heterogeneous cancer cells that constitute the tumor. However, it should be noted that the concepts of CSCs and tumor-initiating cells have been frequently confused. The term "tumor-initiating cells" refers to the cells of origin of the tumor, whose alterations support tumor establishment and progression; in contrast, CSCs would more accurately be referred to as tumor-propagating cells, with stem cell-like properties, which are not necessarily the cells of origin [8, 14, 15]. A study by Chen and colleagues (2010) may help to distinguish these different cell populations and their role on tumor development, particularly in GBM [16]. They demonstrated a hierarchical organization of brain tumor-initiating cells by identifying subpopulations of clonal and long-term proliferating cells in GBM specimens. These subpopulations were shown to be hierarchically organized and to give rise to tumors with different molecular and histopathological features [16]. There are specific and very well delimited regions in the brain where neural stem cells and progenitor cells exist, particularly the subventricular zone (SVZ) of the fore brain lateral ventricles, and the subgranular zone (SGZ) in the dentate gyrus of the hippocampus [8-10]. It has been hypothesized that these are favorable regions where the process of gliomagenesis may originate, as these regions present an attractive microenvironment that has been described as propitious for the growth of stem cells, namely in the SVZ [8-10]. There is increasing experimental evidence that the SVZ is one of the most important regions of origin for malignant gliomas [10] as it may present ideal conditions for gliomagenesis, like the exposure to a transcription factor cocktail ideal for their growth. When compared to any other brain regions, stem cell-containing compartments have been shown to be more susceptible to tumor transformation [10], which additionally may argue in favor of this hypothesis of tumors arising from changes in stem/progenitor cells. Additionally, while it may be coincidence, there is a great similarity between the SVZ stem/progenitor cells and glioma cells. For instance, malignant astrocytic tumors in the brain typically appear close to the lateral ventricles [9, 10].

In the recent years, the notable therapy resistance of gliomas, namely GBM, has been associated with the presence of glioma stem cells (GSCs). These cells present characteristics of stem cells, including: (i) self-renewal; (ii) multipotency, i.e., the capacity to differentiate into other cell lineages; and (iii) high replicative potential. GSCs are predicted to be difficult to target by anti-cancer therapeutics because they have a slow cell cycle, present high levels of proteins involved in drug efflux, and do not express or are dependent on particular oncoproteins for which targeted therapies are currently available [17]. GSCs were one of the first types of cancer stem cells isolated from solid tumors [18]. It was shown that as few as 100 GSCs could give rise to tumors that recapitulated the parental tumor when implanted in xenografted immunodeficient mice, whereas as many as 1,000,000 non-GSCs could not [18]. This suggests that neoplastic clones are maintained exclusively by a little fraction of cells with stem cell properties [18]. Of note, studies involving the use of GSCs face many difficulties, particularly in isolating such cells directly from biopsies, partly because of the high cellular heterogeneity composition of the specimen. On the other hand, currently there are no standardized methods available for cell sorting and assessment of "stemness" [8]. Indeed, there is a relevant discussion regarding the best methodology for culturing GSCs isolated from human GBM specimens. It has been argued by several authors that adherent monolayer cultures of glioma cells allow a more homogeneous exposure to the culture conditions (e.g., nutrients and oxygen levels) than nonadherent cultures, thus increasing the homogeneity of the cell population, reviewed in [8]. In contrast, the sphere-forming assay has been widely used for this purpose. The fidelity and benefits of these assays are still under debate. Thus, there is an exigency to standardize methods for identifying and isolating GSCs with unequivocal markers. It is believed that the use of NSCs markers is a good principle for identifying GSCs, as NSCs are now known to exist in very restricted areas of the brain, and can be unambiguously identified with specific markers [8]. Indeed, in the last decade, putative markers of GSCs have been identified, including Nestin, CD133, L1CAM, CD15, CD44, Id1, and integrin-α6 [8, 10, 14, 19-21]. Nonetheless, none of these markers is sufficient to, independently, identify specifically GSCs, implicating that a functional identification of GSCs (including their ability to (i) be tumorigenic in *in vivo* models, (ii) form neurospheres in culture; (iii) be multipotent) is still mandatory.

2. Gene expression and signaling in GBM

GBM, like other cancers, is a disease that presents several alterations, including DNA mutations, copy number aberrations, and chromosomal rearrangements, but also DNA and histones epigenetic modifications, ultimately resulting in alterations in the gene expression profiles [22]. Molecular studies from the last decades have identified critical genetic alterations that affect many key pathways involved in the regulation of typical cancer hallmarks, such as alterations in cell cycle, migration, proliferation, survival, angiogenesis, invasion and apoptosis [22]. While several alterations in signaling pathways occur in GBM, such as Wnt, Notch and Shh pathways (particularly relevant due to their associations with cancer stem-cells and resistance to radiochemotherapy) [23, 24], the most frequent aberrations in GBM occur in three critical signaling pathways: (i) retinoblastoma (RB), (ii) p53, and (iii) RTK/RAS/PI3K pathways [22, 25, 26], as detailed in Figure 2 and below.

2.1. Retinoblastoma (RB) pathway

Mutations in genes implicated in cell cycle regulation that allow cells to proliferate uncontrollably have been frequently identified in GBM, as in other human tumors [26-28]. The RB pathway, which is important in the G1/S transition, is aberrantly inactivated in GBM through the alteration of several genes and proteins [28].

In a normal condition, the RB protein (encoded by *RB1* gene, the first tumor suppressor gene described), a negative regulator of the cell cycle, is recruited to specific promoters through its interactions with E2F transcription factors. RB inhibits the transcription of genes by directly suppressing the transactivating function of E2F, and by recruiting factors that mediate transcriptional repression [27, 28]. E2F regulates the promoters' activity of several genes related to (i) cell cycle, such as Cyclin E (*CCNE*) and A (*CCNA*), (ii) DNA replication, such as minichromosome maintenance complex component 7 (MCM7) and cell division cycle 6 (*CDC6*), (iii) nucleotide byosynthesis, such as ribonucleotide reductase (*RRM*), (iv) mitotic progression, such as Cyclin B1 (*CCNB1*) and cyclin-dependent kinase 1 (*CDK1*), and (v) apoptosis activation, such as apoptotic peptidase activating factor 1 (*APAF-1*) and caspases, such as caspase 3 (*CASP3*) [27, 28]. The interaction between RB and E2F can be disrupted due to the phosphorylation of the RB protein by Cdk4/6 kinases [27, 28]. To be active, these kinases are dependent of Cyclin proteins, namely CCND2 that competes for the binding site with Ink4 proteins [27]. Thus, the function of Ink4 is to prevent the formation of the active kinase complex (CCND2/Cdk4/6) [27]. This process is ultimately regulated by external signals, such as growth factors, which induce the cell to progress to the S phase [27].

In GBM, the *RB1* gene is frequently mutated [26]. However, the loss of function of RB is also reported to be a consequence of the amplification of *CDK4* and *CDK6*, as well as by the inactivation of the INK4A/B (isoforms of CDKN2A/B) and INK4C (encoded by CDKN2C), which are inhibitors of Cdk4/6 [26]. Ultimately, these alterations lead to E2F accumulation and the consequent progression to S phase mediated by E2F-target genes [26, 27].

2.2. p53 Pathway

The *TP53* gene encodes a protein (p53) that also controls the cell cycle by regulating target genes involved in cell cycle arrest, apoptosis and senescence [27]. Moreover, p53 has been named as the "guardian of the genome" because it leads to the arrest of cells with DNA damage in G1 phase, in order to promote DNA repair processes [29]. On the other hand, if irreparable genetic injuries occur, p53 induces cell death by activating the apoptotic machinery [29]. In normal unstressed cycling cells, some proteins, such as the ubiquitin ligase Mdm2, bind to p53 to promote its degradation via the ubiquitin/proteasome pathway [29-31]. The p53-mediated upregulation of *MDM2* gene leads to a negative feedback that will maintain the levels of p53 very low in these cells [30, 31]. In this context, p53 loss of function may lead, for example, to uncontrolled growth and increased genetic instability. Its loss of function may be due to several reasons, including: (i) inactivating mutation [26], (ii) amplification of *MDM2* and *MDM4* [26, 31], and (iii) loss of function of ARF product encoded by *CDKN2A*, which interacts with and sequesters Mdm2 [26, 31, 32]. Unlike Mdm2, which degrades p53, Mdm4 inhibits p53 by binding to its transcriptional activation domain [31]. Moreover, Mdm4 also inhibits the degradation of Mdm2 [31].

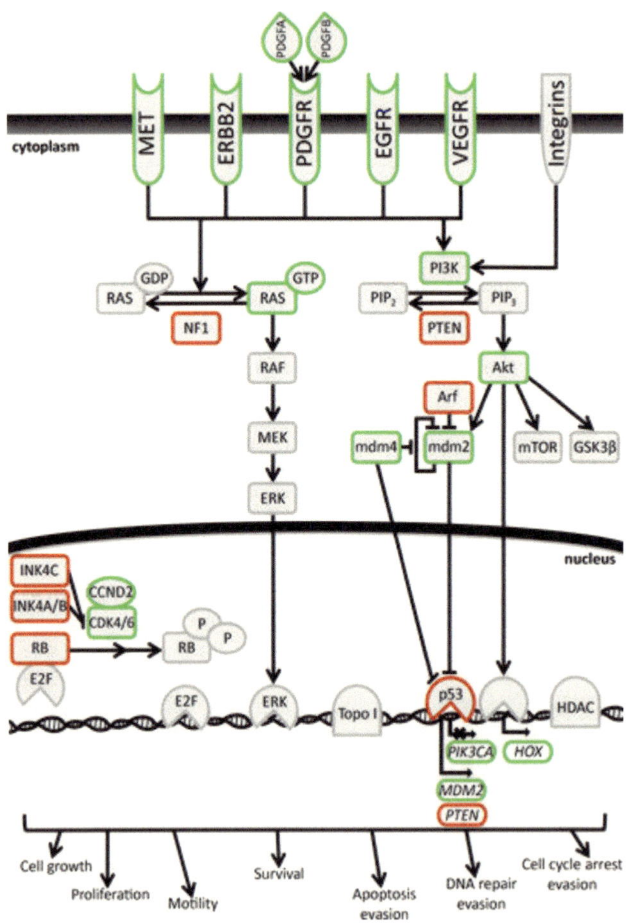

Figure 2 Common genetic alterations in GBM affect the RB, p53 and RTKs pathways. The aberrant deregulation of these pathways in GBM leads to alterations in cell cycle, migration, proliferation, angiogenesis, and apoptosis. Known proto-oncogenes or growth-promoting genes (shown in green), such as *EGFR*, *PIK3CA* (p110α) and *AKT*, are activated by mutations, overexpression and amplification, while tumor suppressor genes (show in red), such as PTEN, Arf and p53, are lost or inactivated by mutations, deletions, loss of heterozigosity, and epigenetic changes.

2.3. Receptor Tyrosine Kinase (RTK) pathways

GBM cells also commonly present a constitutive activation of cell growth signaling pathways by the overexpression of several mitogens and their specific membrane receptors [22, 24, 26, 33]. Glioma cells can also acquire mutations in the membrane receptors becoming independent of exogenous growth stimulation, increasing survival and motility [22, 24, 26, 33, 34]. In GBM, the deregulation of growth factor signaling occurs frequently by the amplification and/or activating mutations of RTKs [22, 26]. These play critical roles in several cellular processes, including cell growth, motility, survival and proliferation, and are tightly controlled by various physiological mechanisms (e.g., autocrine loops in which RTK ligands are produced in result of receptor activation) [26]. One of the most described RTK alteration in GBM is the deletion of exons 2-7 of epidermal growth factor receptor (*EGFR*) gene that results in the loss of the extracellular domain (EGFR-vIII mutant) [26]. Notwithstanding, other genetic alterations affecting *EGFR*, such as amplifications, activating point mutations that affect the extracellular domain, and other deletions in the region coding for the cytoplasmic domain, have also been described [26]. Moreover, alterations of other RTKs also occurs frequently in GBM, including: (i) overexpression of platelet-derived growth factor receptor (*PDGFR*) and its ligands *PDGFA* and *PDGFB*, suggesting an autocrine or paracrine loop activation, (ii) activating mutations in *ERBB2* (member of the EGFR family), and (iii) activating mutations in hepatocyte growth factor receptor (*MET)* [22, 26, 33, 34]. RTKs mediate its functions by downstream effectors, namely *phosphatidylinositol 3-kinase* (PI3K), *mitogen-activated protein kinase* (MAPK) and *signal transducer and activator of transcription* (STAT) signaling cascades [34]. Although genetic alterations in RTKs may potentially activate these pathways, they can also be specifically activated due to other aberrations. Among them, the PI3K pathway is the most described in GBM and is involved in cell growth, proliferation, differentiation, motility and survival [26, 34]. The most frequent alterations involve inactivating mutations and homozygous deletions of *PTEN* [26]. This gene encodes the enzyme phosphatidylinositol (3,4,5)-trisphosphate 3-phosphatase, which removes a phosphate from phosphatidylinositol-(3,4,5)-triphosphate (PIP_3), converting it to phosphatidylinositol-(4,5)-bisphosphate (PIP_2) [22]. Thus, PTEN counteracts the action of the PI3K, which catalyzes the addition of a phosphate to PIP_2 at the 3 position, converting it to PIP_3 [22]. The accumulation of PIP_3 recruits Akt to the plasma membrane. Here, Akt is activated by phosphorylation, promoting cell survival and proliferation [22]. The PI3K enzymatic complex is formed by 2 subunits, one regulatory protein (p85α), encoded by *PIK3R1*, and one catalytic protein (p110α), encoded by *PIK3CA* [22]. Note that other variants of this complex exist, but the referred subunits are the most expressed in GBM and the most widely-studied. Activating missense mutations and in-frame deletions have been detected in the *PIK3CA* [26]. One deletion was identified in the adaptor binding domain, raising the hypothesis that it may disrupt the normal interaction between p110α and its regulatory subunit, p85α [26]. Interestingly, in a few percentage of samples without activating mutations in the catalytic subunit, inactivating mutations were detected in the regulatory subunit [26]. This suggests a functional redundancy of these mutations as they individually activate PI3K. Again, the amplification of *AKT3* gene, which encodes one of the Akt proteins, was described recently in a small fraction of GBM samples [26]. Other known mutation that ultimately leads to activation of PI3K and MAPK is the activating mutation of *RAS* [26]. RAS is indirectly activated by RTKs through the dissociation of a GDP molecule and association to a GTP. However, in a normal condition, this activation is quickly reverted from RAS-GTP to RAS-GDP. This *RAS* mutation impedes the dissociation of GTP, remaining RAS constitutively active. Neurofibromin 1 (NF1), which negatively regulates RAS signaling, is also downregulated in GBM by *NF1* mutations or deletions, resulting in increased RAS signaling. Moreover, loss of expression of NF1 without evidence of genomic alteration was also observed [26]. In addition to its critical effects in cell growth, motility, and survival, the PI3K pathway seems to be also important in the activation of *HOX* genes, which were recently described to be important for the malignant phenotype of GBMs [35-37] (see section 3.3 for details).

2.4. Crosstalk between RB, p53, and RTK pathways in GBM

The development of new platforms of genome-scale screenings has allowed a more robust identification of the accumulation of genetic and epigenetic alterations. The Cancer Genome Atlas (TCGA) project, for example, was established with the aim of using genome-wide analysis technologies, which include DNA copy number, gene expression, DNA methylation, and nucleotide sequencing, to understand the molecular basis of cancer [26]. With this multiplatform profiling and using an integrative analysis, they identified a highly interconnected network of aberrations in GBM that include the pathways described above (RB, p53, RTKs and PI3K pathways) [26]. Interestingly, this integrative analysis showed a statistical tendency to mutual exclusivity for the specific alterations of components within each pathway. Nonetheless a great percentage of samples harbored aberrations in all signaling pathways [26], which is in agreement with the hypothesis that these pathways are a core prerequisite for GBM disease.

2.5. Other key alterations in GBM

In addition to the most common genetic alterations found in GBM, several other aberrations have been described. For example, mutations in *IDH1* and *IDH2* genes, which encode the metabolic enzymes isocitrate dehydrogenases were described. These reports suggest that these mutations lead to a new pro-oncogenic activity of IDH1/2 with the production of R(-)-2-hydroxyglutarate, an onco-metabolite [38, 39] (see section 3.2 for details). Other classes of proteins extremely important in GBM are DNA repair proteins, as they increase the probability of mutations. In fact, at least one of the MMR genes (*MLH1*, *MSH2*, *MSH6* or *PMS2*) is mutated in hypermutated GBM samples [26], decreasing DNA repair competencies in these cells.

2.6. Molecular subclasses of GBM

Using an unsupervised hierarchical clustering analysis, Verhaak *et al.* [40] used TCGA data to successfully classify GBM into four subtypes - classical, mesenchymal, proneural and neural - improving and validating previous classifications of GBM [37, 41-47].

The identity of the classical subtype was defined by displaying the most common genomic aberrations of GBM, with 93% of samples presenting amplifications in chromosome 7 paired with loss of chromosome 10, 95% showing high levels of *EGFR* amplification and/or expression, and *EGFR-vIII* activating point mutations. These amplifications of *EGFR* co-occurred with focal homozygous deletions targeting *CDKN2A,* which in turn was almost mutually exclusive with other alterations in RB pathway components, such as *RB1*, *CDK4* and *CCDN2*. However, this subtype does not present *TP53* mutations. Additionally, the Notch (*NOTCH3*, *JAG1*, *LFNG*) and Sonic hedgehog (*SMO*, *GAS1*, *GLI2*) signaling pathways, as well as the neural precursor and stem cell marker *NES*, were highly expressed in this subtype [40].

The mesenchymal subtype presents a focal hemizygous deletions of 17q11.2 region that contains the *NF1* gene. In fact, this deletion was associated with lower expression of *NF1* in most cases. However, *NF1* was also found to be mutated predominantly in this subtype, and sometimes this mutation co-occurred with *PTEN* inactivating mutations. Moreover, *TRADD*, *RELB* and *TNFRSF1A* genes, belonging to the tumor necrosis factor (*TNF*) superfamily, and genes encoding proteins from the NF-κB pathways, are highly expressed. Additionally, mesenchymal markers, such as *CHI3L1* and *MET*, were expressed [40].

The most relevant features of the proneural subtype were high levels of *PDGFRA* gene expression in combination with its focal amplification, and point mutations in *IDH1*. Importantly, these aberrations seem to be mutually exclusive. Loss of heterozygosity and inactivating mutations of *TP53* were frequent in this subtype. While less frequent than in classical GBM samples, half of proneural samples also manifested amplification in chromosome 7, paired with loss of chromosome 10. *PIK3CA* and *PIK3R1* activating and inactivating mutations, respectively, were observed mostly in samples without *PDGFRA* aberrations. Oligodendrocytic development genes, such as *PDGFRA*, *NKX2-2* and *OLIG2*, were highly expressed. Lower expression of *CDKN1A* was observed, probably due to *OLIG2* overexpression, which was described to be able to downregulate *CDKN1A*. Additionally, this subtype also presents the expression of proneural developmental genes, such as *SOX* genes, as well as *DCX*, *DLL3*, *ASCL1* and *TCF4* [40].

In what concerns the neural subtype, few characteristics were reported, and it was almost merely classified based on neuron markers expression, including neurofilament light chain polypeptide (NEFL), gamma-aminobutyric acid A receptor (GABRA1), synaptotagmin I (*STY1*), and solute carrier family 12 (SLC12A5) [40].

3. Molecular prognostic factors of GBM

It is widely recognized that the molecular stratification of GBM patients may prove crucial in rationalizing treatment decisions, for which a set of molecular markers predictive of tumor response to specific therapies and/or patient outcome are required. The most well established prognostic factors in GBM patients include age, general performance status, tumor histological features and the extent of tumor resection [48]. Recently, several studies have identified biological and molecular features of GBMs that present prognostic value [37, 46, 49-58] and may help in therapeutic decisions. The work performed so far presents reasons for both optimism and caution regarding the improvements in the diagnosis and treatment of patients, but also demand validation in prospectively followed and in uniformly treated patients.

Therefore, the focus remains in the identification of biomarkers that truly foster patient distinction in ways that may improve therapeutic decisions. The current most relevant prognostic biomarkers for GBM are summarized in Table 1, of which the most promising are briefly discussed below.

Molecular Prognostic Marker	References
MGMT promoter methylation	[52]
IDH1 and *IDH2* mutations	[57]
Loss of chromosome 10	[56]
Activation of the PI3K/AKT pathway	[50, 58]
HOX genes signature	[36, 37]
HOXA9 overexpression	[35, 36]
CHI3L1 (*YKL40*) expression	[53, 56]
miRNA expression signatures	[59]
EGFR expression	[37]
EGFR mutation (EGFR-vIII)	[51, 55]
PTEN expression (wild-type)	[55]
Molecular signatures	[40, 46]
High expression of angiogenic genes	[46]
Stem-cell like gene expression signatures	[37, 49, 54]
Activation of MAPK members	[58]
PTEN and *DLL3* expression	[46]

Table 1. Selected molecular prognostic markers for glioblastoma.

3.1. *MGMT* promoter methylation

Many studies have shown that the methylation status of *MGMT* (O^6-methylguanine-DNA methyltransferase) gene is currently one of the most promising biomarkers of prognosis in GBM patients, although it has not yet reached broad clinical applicability [52, 60]. *MGMT* encodes a DNA-repair protein that removes alkyl groups from the O^6 position of guanine, an important site for DNA alkylation. When DNA is left unrepaired, the lesions induced by chemotherapy trigger apoptosis and cytotoxicity [61]. Hegi and co-workers [52] showed that the epigenetic silencing of *MGMT* by promoter methylation leads to the loss of *MGMT* expression and reduced DNA-repair activity, resulting in increased sensitivity of the tumor cells to temozolomide (TMZ) treatment. In fact, they reported that this increased sensitivity is translated into differences in patient survival, as the methylation of the *MGMT* promoter is associated with longer overall survival (OS) in patients with GBM. Indeed, patients whose *MGMT* promoter is methylated and are treated with TMZ have an increased OS (median of 21.7 months), as well as a higher 2-year survival rate (46%), in comparison to patients treated with TMZ but with unmethylated *MGMT* promoter (median survival of 12.7 months and 2-year survival of 13.8%), suggesting that GBM patients whose tumors present *MGMT* expression do not benefit from TMZ treatment [52]. These results suggest *MGMT* promoter methylation as an independent and favorable predictive factor to patients' response to TMZ therapy [52]. Despite these remarkable findings suggesting *MGMT* as a prognostic biomarker and as a specific predictor of response to TMZ-based chemotherapy, there is still a significant body of controversy surrounding them. Such controversy is mainly due to the heterogeneity of the patients enrolled in the study groups, as they present different glioma histologies, grades and treatment regimens, as well as the fact that different studies analyzed *MGMT* at different levels, including mRNA expression, methylation status and protein levels (as summarized in [62]). In an attempt to replicate Hegi's findings, Costa and co-workers [62] analyzed a set of 90 GBM patients treated with postoperative TMZ-based chemoradiation regarding *MGMT* methylation. Despite a trend for longer overall and progression-free survival in GBM patients with *MGMT* promoter methylation, the differences did not reach statistical significance [62]. Moreover, sample classification as methylated or unmethylated for a certain gene is still controversial, as the relationship between the overall CpG island methylation, CpG methylation at individual sites, and their effects on gene silencing, is highly dependent on the location within the gene [63]. In this sense, Bady and co-workers [64] evaluated the relationship between the specific location of CpG methylation, *MGMT* expression and the outcome of patient in a population homogenously treated with alkylating agents. They reported two regions of methylated CpG's that present strong association with patient longer survival, which negatively correlate with *MGMT* gene expression [64]. This is consistent with *MGMT* expression silencing via CpG methylation, resulting in sensitization to alkylating agents [64]. Similarly, Shah and colleagues also identified three regions of methylated CpGs on *MGMT*, associated with favorable patient progression-free survival, within a population of 44 GBM patients treated with radiotherapy and concomitant and adjuvant TMZ [65]. Nonetheless, the value of *MGMT* methylation status is also supported by a recent clinical trial that compares radiotherapy and TMZ treatment in elder patients, and reported an association between *MGMT* methylation and good outcome in the TMZ cohort, but not in the radiotherapy cohort [66]. Similarly, a meta-analysis performed by Olson and co-workers [67] that included 2018 patients from 20 different studies, showed that the silencing of *MGMT* was highly associated with improved OS in patients receiving chemotherapy as a part of the adjuvant treatment, a mild association in patients that received adjuvant radiotherapy, and no benefit in those submitted to surgery alone.

3.2. *IDH1* and *IDH2* mutations

Other important prognostic factors for GBM have been revealed by recent genomic studies and concern the presence of mutations in isocitrate dehydrogenase 1 and 2 genes

(*IDH1* and *IDH2*; *IDH* when referring to both) [26, 57, 68]. These are NADP-dependent enzymes that catalyze the oxidative decarboxylation of isocitrate to α-ketoglutarate, with the simultaneous production of NADPH [69]. The high throughput sequencing of GBM revealed that *IDH1* mutations occur in 12% of GBM, are somatic and heterozygous, and a consequence of the change of a guanine to an adenine at position 395 of the *IDH1* gene (G395A), leading to the replacement of an arginine with a histidine at amino acid residue 132 of the protein (R132H) [57]. Similarly, sequence evaluation of *IDH2* exons revealed a mutation in a histidine at amino acid residue 172 (R172), which is the exact analogue of the R132 residue in *IDH1* [68]. Overexpression of *IDH1* ^{R132H} reduces the formation of α-ketoglutarate and increases the levels of HIF-1α [70]. As stated above, a recent study suggested that mutant IDH1 reduces α-ketoglutarate to R(-)-2-hydroxyglutarate, while converting NADPH to NADP$^+$ [38, 39]. Even though the mechanism is yet to be clarified, it seems probable that the increased capacity to produce 2-hydroxyglutarate of cells presenting *IDH1* ^{R132H} mutation contributes to tumorigenesis [38]. *IDH* mutations are highly frequent in secondary GBM (up to 80%), but are rare in primary GBM (less than 10%) [68, 71]. *IDH* mutations are correlated with younger age at diagnosis, and with GBM patients' longer survival when compared to patients with *IDH* ^{wt} genes [68, 72]. Mutations in *IDH1* and *IDH2* are mutually exclusive, which indicates that they might independently confer a growth advantage to mutated cells [73]. Moreover, *IDH* mutations generally associate with specific genetic and clinical characteristics when compared to gliomas that have *IDH* ^{wt}. In particular, it was shown that *IDH* mutations and amplification of *EGFR* in GBM are mutually exclusive events [74], and that the methylation of the *MGMT* gene promoter is often associated with *IDH* mutations [74, 75]. However, this association is yet to be clarified as it may represent a direct consequence of the activity of the mutant IDH, or an alternative marker for epigenetic changes in tumors presenting *IDH* mutations (reviewed in [76]). So, the deep understanding of the link between *IDH* mutations and common genetic events in GBM might furnish insights into their roles on gliomagenesis [40, 68]. Furthermore, a recent study evaluated the response of a series of 86 secondary GBM to TMZ treatment, and correlated several markers of GBM (including *IDH* mutations, 1p19q co-deletion, *MGMT* promoter methylation status, and *TP53* expression) with progression-free survival and OS [77]. This study showed that *IDH* mutations were present in 73.4% of the analyzed patients, and that these mutations were associated with higher progression-free survival [77]. The authors also evaluated the response of patients presenting *IDH* mutations and *MGMT* promoter methylation, and found that patients presenting this combination had the best response to TMZ treatment, reporting also that IDH mutations seems to be a significant marker for positive chemosensitivity in secondary GBM [77].

3.3. Molecular subclasses and prognostic value

Strikingly, as stated above, mutations in *IDH1* have been included in a GBM signature that allowed the division of GBMs into subtypes according to their recurrent genomic alterations [40] (see section 2.6 for details). The importance in the division of GBM into subtypes lies on the possible application of different therapeutic approaches, as treatments efficacy differs per subtype [40]. Aggressive therapy significantly delayed mortality in classical and mesenchymal subtypes, and a tendency to longer outcome was observed for the neural subtype, yet patients whose GBM present proneural features, associated with younger age, do not seem to benefit from highly aggressive therapies although presenting longer survival [40]. In this sense, some of the genetic events underlying the different GBM subtypes could become part of the clinical routine to rationalize therapeutic decisions, and ultimately lead to more personalized therapies for groups of patients with GBM.

3.4. *HOX* genes signature

Recent evidences have been revealing a remarkable resemblance between tumorigenic and developmental processes, indicating the relevance of molecular regulatory mechanisms crucial on normal development and on the tumorigenic process. Homeobox (*HB*) genes encode transcription factors that primarily play a crucial role during normal development, and are divided into two classes: class I comprises clustered homeobox (*HOX*) genes, and class II includes non-*HOX* genes, which are dispersed through the genome, and mainly serve as cofactors for HOX proteins [78]. During embryonic development, *HOX* genes are sequentially expressed from 3′ to 5′ along the anterior-posterior axis contributing to the temporospatial development of limbs and organs [79]. The mechanisms underlying *HOX* genes control in normal development occur according to three main principles: spatial collinearity, posterior prevalence, and temporal collinearity [80]. These were found to be altered in cancer as a consequence of three major mechanisms proposed by Abate-Shen [81]: temporospatial deregulation, gene dominance and epigenetic regulation. Different groups have been reporting the deregulation of these mechanisms in different *HOX* genes, and in different tumors (reviewed in [80]).

The aberrant expression of *HOX* genes have been reported as crucial in several hallmarks of cancer, including increased proliferation, angiogenesis and invasion, and apoptosis resistance in leukemia and in several solid tumors [80, 82-85]. Interestingly, in recent years, *HOX* genes aberrant expression has been implicated in gliomagenesis. Abdel-Fattah and co-workers [86] evaluated the expression of all *HOX* genes in primary astrocytomas and in non-tumor brain specimens, reporting that some *HOX* genes are abnormally expressed in malignant astrocytomas. A subsequent report by Murat *et al.* [37] identified a *HOX*-dominated gene cluster, suggestive of a signature that displays srm cell-like self-renewal properties. These authors argue show that the expression of *HOXA10* gene in GBM neurospheres is consistent with a role of *HOX* genes in glioma stem-like cell compartments [37]. Interestingly, the *HOX*-dominated gene signature arises along malignant progression to GBM, and is an independent predictive factor of chemo-radiotherapy resistance in patients [37]. Later, Costa and co-workers [35] showed that *HOXA* genes are predominantly activated in GBM, as compared to lower-grade gliomas and normal brain tissue, suggesting they may be a useful component of a molecular classification of gliomas. By analyzing expression microarrays data from 100 GBMs, they identified tumors with abnormal chromosomal domains of transcriptional activation, which comprise the *HOXA* cluster, and is reversibly regulated by the PI3K pathway [35]. Of all *HOXA* genes, *HOXA9* expression was predictive of worse GBM patient outcome, and associated with pro-proliferative and anti-apoptotic functions, which may explain the unfavorable prognosis of GBM patients with *HOXA9* reactivation [35]. More recently, Gaspar *et al.* [36], showed pediatric GBM cell lines that are resistant to TMZ present the coordinated expression of several *HOX* genes, of which *HOXA9* and *HOXA10* were highlighted as crucial effectors in this resistance [36]. In line with Costa *et al.* [35] report, Gaspar suggested that the *HOX*-enriched signature is regulated by the PI3K pathway, and interestingly, is associated with resistance to TMZ in pediatric GBM cell lines [36]. Moreover, pediatric patients with high-grade gliomas that express *HOXA9* and *HOXA10* presented shorter survival [36].

3.5. *CHI3L1* (*YKL40*) expression

The molecular prognostic biomarkers currently available require the evaluation of tumor tissue in order to assess gene expression and promoter methylation levels. Moreover, tumor progression and treatment responses are monitored using imaging techniques, which do not distinguish the effects of treatment and tumor regrowth. In fact, patients who are submitted to magnetic resonance imaging (MRI) shortly after radiotherapy show increased volume of the tumor, which in up to 50% of the cases, is a consequence of the increased blood vessel permeability due to radiotherapy, an effect called pseudoprogession [87]. As it is difficult to distinguish between the therapeutic effects and real growth of the tumor [88], in addition to the impossibility of multiple tumor sampling during the course of the malignancy [89, 90], demand the establishment of less invasive prognostic and predictive markers. Serum markers that correlate with tumor biological properties might prove crucial in providing prognostic information and response to treatment, therefore allowing the proper adjustment of therapeutics, and improve care of patients with GBM. A study conducted by Tanwar [91] analyzed gene expression microarray data of tumor tissue from glioma patients, and showed that chitinase 3-like 1 (*CHI3L1* or *YKL40*) was the most highly expressed among 10000 genes, when comparing to normal brain tissue [91]. The function of YKL-40 in gliomas and other tumors is yet to be fully clarified; however, it is thought to be involved in increased cell proliferation, differentiation, angiogenesis, decreased apoptosis, and extracellular matrix remodeling [92-94]. Interestingly, YKL-40 is secreted both by tumor cells and by tumor-associated macrophages in the bloodstream, therefore allowing its quantification in the blood. YKL-40 was found to be increased in the serum of patients with several solid tumor types, as breast, colorectal, ovary, small cell lung cancer and GBM (reviewed in [93]). Particularly in GBM, YKL-40 serum concentrations seem to be a strong predictor of an aggressive phenotype [53, 91], as the increased expression of YKL-40 appears to be associated with glioma grade, resistance to radiotherapy, shorter time to progression, and worse patient OS [53, 95-97]. However, to establish YKL-40 serum levels as a prognostic marker, there is still the need to perform further prospective studies that concern repeated determinations of YKL-40 levels before and after surgery. As YKL-40 can be reproducibly measured in the serum, and this biomarker is already well established for routine use, its inclusion in the clinical practice should be relatively straightforward, and might provide crucial information on tumor progression.

In conclusion, the identification of molecular biomarkers that truly aid in the distinction of patients and therapeutic decisions still requires much effort. The integration of clinical and molecular data is becoming more frequent, and easier to perform and analyze, which will

http://dx.doi.org/10.5772/52361

probably lead to more targeted and effective treatments. Moreover, it seems probable that sets of molecular biomarkers for GBM will be established in the next few years, and will become part of the clinical routine, leading to tailored therapies for subgroups of GBM patients. Importantly, the timely identification of patients who are not likely to respond to a certain therapy would allow their integration in clinical trials with novel therapies, but also to avoid the possible adverse side effects of a therapy that may not prove beneficial. Equally interesting, the establishment of molecular biomarkers of tumor therapy resistance may lead to a more guided and rational design of novel therapeutic agents and clinical trials for GBM patients. In the search for GBM patient individualized therapy, the discovery of particular tumor molecular features, as the status of *MGMT* promoter methylation status, the mutation status of *IDH1* and *IDH2*, the expression of *HOXA* genes, and the serum levels of YKL-40, may prove crucial as initial building blocks of a panel of molecular biomarkers that may have real clinical implications. The challenge ahead is to discover further molecular markers of GBM, but also to integrate all the knowledge in an interdisciplinary way, considering different GBM subtypes, which altogether might allow a more rational and efficient fight against GBM.

4. New molecular targets and treatments

As described throughout this chapter, the molecular and cellular heterogeneity of GBM represents a major therapeutic challenge, but also offers a large number of opportunities to specific targeting of tumor cells' alterations. Furthermore, the unsatisfactory prognosis of GBM patients, independently of the used treatment approaches, and the absence of a cure or significant advances in the treatment of GBM, are the major drivers of GBM therapeutics research.

4.1. Classic therapeutics

The current standard therapy for the treatment of GBM includes maximal surgical resection, followed by radiotherapy (RT) with concomitant and adjuvant administration of alkylating agents [98]. Administration of RT is usually given after the surgical removal of the tumor in order to eliminate residual tumor cells [99]. Alkylating agents act by introducing methyl groups in different positions in the DNA, resulting in DNA damage and specific cytotoxicity, that ultimately leads to apoptosis and cell death [100]. Before 1999, only nitrosourea-based chemotherapeutics were approved for the treatment of GBM, which includes oral lomustine (CCNU) and intravenous carmustine (BCNU) [101]. In 1999, FDA approved Gliadel® that consists in a polymeric biodegradable wafer that is able to release carmustine during 2-3 weeks after implantation in the gap where the tumor was removed during surgery [101-103]. Furthermore, in this same year, FDA granted accelerated approval to the imidazole derivative of the second-generation class of alkylating agents, TMZ, mainly because of its efficient absorption after oral administration and its ability to easily cross the blood-brain barrier [101, 104].

TMZ was regularly approved by the FDA in 2005, and became the standard chemotherapeutic agent for the treatment of GBM [5]. The approval of TMZ was mainly due to the improvement in the OS of patients observed in a landmark study by Stupp *et al.* [5]. This clinical trial involving 573 patients with newly diagnosed GBM showed an increase in OS from 12.1 months to 14.6 months when patients were treated with RT plus TMZ comparing with RT alone [5]. In 2009, the 5-years retrospective analysis from this phase III clinical trial reported that, in addition to the improvement in OS, the 5-year survival rate was also higher in the group of patients treated with RT and TMZ, showing again the benefits of this treatment [105]. Nevertheless, some molecular mechanisms of resistance to this agent were identified, like the methylation status of the *MGMT* gene, which encodes a protein that repairs the damage induced by TMZ, and alkylating agents in general, resulting in chemoresistance [106].

Besides TMZ, bevacizumab (BVZ, also known as Avastin®) was also conceded accelerated approval by the FDA in 2009 as monotherapy for patients with progressive GBM that did not respond to standard care (TMZ + RT) [101, 107]. This drug is a monoclonal antibody that targets VEGF, which is involved in the formation of new blood vessels [99]. Since GBM are highly vascularized tumors, this drug presented an attractive way to target tumor-associated increased angiogenesis [108]. When BVZ was combined with TMZ + RT for the treatment of newly diagnosed GBM patients in a phase II clinical trial, an improvement in OS (19.6 vs. 14.6 months) and progression-free survival (PFS, 13.6 vs. 6.9 months) was reported, when compared to the control cohort of the European Organization for Research and Treatment of Cancer-National Cancer Institute of Canada (EORTC/NCIC), in which patients were treated only with RT and TMZ [109]. BVZ also showed good radiographic responses in patients with recurrent GBM (71% and 35%, according to Levin and Macdonald criteria, respectively) when used first as a single agent, and later combined with irinotecan (topoisomerase I inhibitor) in a phase II clinical trial [110]. Although some exciting clinical results were described, several *in vitro* and *in vivo* studies have been unmasking unpredictable consequences of BVZ treatment. The treatment of intracranial xenograft mouse models of GBM with this VEGF inhibitor showed a decrease in the vascular network and contrast enhancement in MRI, but also a 68% increase in the infiltration of tumor cells trough the brain parenchyma [111, 112]. Furthermore, BVZ treatment increased the hypoxic microenvironment which is also implicated in increased invasion ability of tumor cells [24, 112].

4.2. Novel molecular targeted therapeutics

Conceptually, the development of targeted therapies for the treatment of GBM represents a significant advance in the search for a cure for this devastating disease. First, the specificity of these therapies has the potential to reduce toxic side effects. Second, the direct blockade of altered oncogenic signaling cascades may allow the reduction of tumor cell proliferation [113]. This next part will review some of the most promising therapeutic molecular and targeting strategies, including membrane proteins and growth factor receptors (e.g. RTK), and intracellular signaling pathways.

4.2.1. Therapeutic targeting of membrane protein/growth factor receptors

RTKs represent attractive targets for this therapeutic approach, since they are associated with GBM oncogenesis, and the binding of growth factors to these receptors activate signaling pathways that drive GBM cells survival and proliferation [113, 114] (see section 2.3 for information). There are two kinds of inhibitors for RTKs: (i) inhibitors targeting the intracellular tyrosine kinase domain (TKD), and (ii) monoclonal antibodies that can block RTK activation or target the RTK-expressing cells [115].

a. EGFR

As stated above, *EGFR* amplification, overexpression and mutation are frequent events in GBM cells and increased EGFR signaling is known to increase tumor proliferation, invasion ability, angiogenesis and blocking apoptosis [22, 116]. Several small molecule inhibitors targeting EGFR have been developed and approved for the treatment of particular cancers, as erlotinib and gefitinib in the treatment of advanced metastatic non-small cell lung cancer [24, 117]. This RTK can be targeted with a large number of inhibitors, like lapatinib (EGFR2, ErbB2), vandetanib (EGFR, VEGFR-2), PF-00299804 (EGFR, ERBB2 and ERBB4), BIBW2992 (EGFR, ERBB2, ERBB4), AEE 788 (EGFR, ERBB2, VEGFR), and monoclonal antibodies, as cetuximab (EGFR) and nimotuzumab (EGFR) [98, 116]; however, this section focus on the most reviewed and clinically tested drugs for the treatment of GBM (erlotinib, gefitinib and cetuximab). Erlotinib and gefitinib although, extensively tested in clinical trials for GBM patients (either already completed or currently ongoing), have not shown a significant benefit, and thus failed to reach clinical applicability (Table 2) [118]. The chimerical monoclonal antibody cetuximab (Erbitux) can also inhibit EGFR, and was shown to inhibit the mutant EGFR-vIII in glioma cells [119, 120]. Furthermore, preclinical studies using GBM xenograft models suggest that cetuximab could be effective for the treatment of invasive GBM [121]. The clinical evaluation of the administration of cetuximab in phase II trials for recurrent GBM patients has shown mixed results. The combination of cetuximab with BVZ and irinotecan resulted in 5% complete responses (CR), 21% partial responses (PR) and 40% of the patients with stable disease (SD), with only 9% of the GBM patients presenting signs of progressive disease (PD); the 6 months progression-free survival (6-PFS) of 33% obtained in this trial was also surprising [108]. In another phase II clinical trial for recurrent GBM patients, treatment with cetuximab showed worse outcomes, with a median time-to-progression (TTP) of only 1.9 months, and only 7.3% of the patients being progression free at 6 months after treatment [122].

Most of the *EGFR* amplified GBMs also present expression of the mutant EGFR-vIII [116]. Since this mutated form of EGFR is absent in normal tissues, an immunotherapy-based approach to target EGFR-vIII was developed and is now under clinical trials (phase I, II and III) [118, 123]. This vaccine, called rindopepimut (CDX-110, PEPvIII) consists in a 14 aminoacids peptide that specifically recognizes EGFR-vIII, combined with an immunoadjuvant (keyhole limpet hemocyanin), that will potentiate an immune response against EGFR-vIII-positive tumor cells [124]. The clinical applicability of this vaccine was already tested in different clinical trials showing the benefits of this strategy (Table 2). Newly diagnosed GBM EGFR-vIII positive had a significant improvement in OS from 15.2 months (treated with TMZ + RT) to 23.2 months

(CDX-110 + granulocyte macrophage-colony stimulating factor, GM-CSF, and TMZ, after RT), consistent with the benefit of this vaccine alone in other studies (OS 26 months vs. 15 months) [124, 125].

b. PDGFR

As referred previously, *PDGFR* is also frequently overexpressed in GBM [114]. As described for other RTK, PDGFR can also be blocked with different pharmacological inhibitors, such as imatinib mesylate (PDGFR, c-KIT, BCR-ABL), sunitinib (PDGFR, VEGFR, c-KIT), sorafenib (PDGFR, VEGFR, RAF), tandutinib (PDGFR, FLT3, c-KIT), vatalanib (PDGFR, VEGFR, c-KIT), IMC3G3 (PDGRFα), pazopanib (PDGFR, c-KIT, EGFR) or dasatinib (PDGFRβ, Src, BCR/Abl, c-KIT, ephrin A2) [98, 116]. However, this part will focus on the best characterized PDGFR inhibitor, imatinib mesylate (Gleevec or Livec), already evaluated in phase I/II clinical trials with GBM patients, which was originally FDA approved for the treatment of acute myeloid leukemia [106, 126]. *In vitro* treatments of GBM cells with imatinib have already shown inhibitory effects on cell proliferation, as a result of cell cycle arrest, increase apoptotic population and decreased clonogenic ability [127]. Its administration in mice models of GBM also showed an improvement in survival [128]. In clinical studies, imatinib mesylate was usually combined with hydroxyurea (HU), a ribonucleotide reductase inhibitor that blocks DNA synthesis [126, 129]. Treatment of recurrent GBM in phase II clinical trials was mostly disappointing, with 6-months PFS (6-PFS) of only 3% and 16% [130, 131]. Combination with HU, although showing a mild increase in OS and 6-PFS rates, again showed a lack of efficacy as compared to RT + TMZ [126]. The best result using imatinib was achieved in a phase I clinical trial for recurrent malignant glioma (MG), where imatinib was combined with HU and vatalanib (VEGFR inhibitor), with 24% of GBM patients revealing a radiographic partial response, 49% showing signals of stable disease, however 27% of the patients had progressive disease [132] (Table 2).

c. VEGFR

The therapeutic targeting of GBM-associated angiogenesis is already an approved strategy through VEGF inhibition with BVZ, but can also be achieved through inhibition of VEGF receptors using specific inhibitors, like cediranib, sorafenib, sunitinib, pazopanib, vandetanib, CT-332 (all VEGFR), XL-184 (VEGFR2, Met, RET, c-KIT, Flt3, Tie-2), semaxanib or AEE 788 [98, 116, 133]. For instance, cediranib (AZD2171) inhibits all VEGFR subtypes and was explored in phase I, II and III clinical trials [116]. The outcomes of cediranib (AZD2171) treatment in GBM patients are described as similar to the ones observed for BVZ, although only one of the completed trials has published results (Table 2) [116]. As reported for BVZ, also cediranib was associated with infiltrative cells not visible with contrast-enhanced MRI [112, 134]. In orthotopic mouse models of GBM, this VEGFR inhibitor induced alterations in the permeability and diameter of blood vessels, alleviating edema and increasing the survival of the mice [135].

d. Met

Met is an RTK for hepatocyte growth factor (HGF) that activates a series of signaling pathways, as referred above in section 2.3, similar to what is observed for EGFR or PDGFR activation, which ultimately leads to proliferative and invasive behaviors of cancer cells [106, 136]. In a series of 62 GBM patient samples, Met was found to be overexpressed and associated with poor prognosis, and with an invasive phenotype, supported by invasive multifoci lesions and expression of metalloproteinases 2 and 9 [137]. Inhibitors targeting Met include tivantinib, and cabozantinib (XL184) a potent inhibitor of several kinases, cabozantinib (XL184), which hase shown significant inhibitory effect on GBM tumor growth [138]. Furthermore, three phase I and II clinical trials for the evaluation of cabozantinib on the treatment of newly diagnosed GBM (monotherapy or combined with RT + TMZ) and recurrent GBM (monotherapy) (NCT00960492, NCT00704288 and NCT01068782) are now ongoing [118]. Another therapeutic approach to target HGF/Met axis is the use of the monoclonal antibody against HGF, rilotumumab (AMG-102), which was already tested during a phase II [116] clinical trial for recurrent GBM (Table 2); a second phase II trial to test the combination of rilotumumab with Avastin in patients with recurrent MG is now recruiting patients (NCT01113398) [118].

e. Integrins

Therapeutic targeting of the cell adhesion receptors integrins, which are transmembrane glycoproteins that attach cells to extracellular matrix proteins of the basement membrane or to ligands on other cells, have also proved to be a valuable therapeutic strategy for the treatment of GBM, with several recent clinical trials testing the success of the integrin inhibitor cilengetide (EMD 121974) as a monotherapy or in combination with RT + TMZ (Table 2) [139]. Cilengitide is an RGD (Asp-Gly-Asp) synthetic peptide that inhibits integrins $\alpha V\beta 3$ and $\alpha V\beta 5$ by receptor binding competition [139]. *In vitro* studies have shown an anti-angiogenic effect of this inhibitor by inhibiting proliferation and differentiation of endothelial progenitor cells, without affecting apoptosis [140]. In GBM cells, cilengitide exerted only a moderate loss of viability and was unable to sensitize GBM cells to radiotherapy and TMZ treatment [141]. Clinical studies with this drug have shown limited toxicity, but also reduced beneficial effect, when administered in newly diagnosed patients of GBM with RT+ TMZ (Table 2).

4.2.2. Therapeutic targeting of intracellular signaling pathways

a. PI3K/AKT/mTOR pathway

As already mentioned the PI3K/Akt/mTOR pathway represents one of the most altered pathways in cancer, including GBM [113, 116]. Several inhibitors targeting different elements of this pathway are available and being tested both pre-clinically and at the clinical level. Enzastaurin is a specific inhibitor of protein kinase C (PKC) proteins, thus indirectly inhibiting Akt [104, 113, 142]. In preclinical studies, this inhibitor was able to suppress proliferation of GBM cells and tumor growth in GBM xenograft mice models [143]. In clinical studies, especially for recurrent GBM patients this drug failed to improve patient outcome, with PFS, OS and 6-PFS inferior to that of patients treated with lomustine in phase III clinical trials (Table 2) [144]. Inhibition of Akt can also be achieved using perifosine (KRX-0401), which affects the interaction of PIP_3 with the PH domain of Akt [24]. When this drug was compared to mTOR inhibition in *in vivo* models with differential expression of *PTEN*, the treatment with perifosine did not alter tumor volume; on the other hand, treatment with mTOR inhibitor resulted in decrease tumor volume [145]. Furthermore, only a clinical trial phase II for patients with recurrent MG is under evaluation and no results are available until now (NCT00590954) [118]. A HIV type I (HIV-1) protease inhibitor called nelfinavir with applications in HIV infections is also able to downregulate Akt, and was proposed as an Akt inhibitor [146, 147]. Preclinical studies showed that treating GBM cells and xenograft mouse models with nelfinavir is able to sensitize tumor cells to RT and TMZ treatment [148]. Furthermore, this protease inhibitor decreases VEGF levels and angiogenesis, as well as HIF-1 expression levels and can cause endoplasmic reticulum stress and autophagy [146, 149]. Three phase I clinical trials to assess the toxicity of this treatment combined with RT + TMZ in newly diagnosed GBM are currently recruiting patients or active and ongoing (NCT01020292, NCT00694837, NCT00915694) [118].

Several inhibitors of PI3K are also available, but the clinical evaluation of their efficacy is still very preliminary [150]. The class of pan-PI3K inhibitors (inhibit the catalytic p110 subunit) include LY294002, ZSTK474, and wortmannin. Derivatives of LY294002 and wortmannin, include SF1126 (LY294002 conjugated with an RGD peptide), PWT-458 and PX-866 (the first is a PEGylated derivate of wortmannin and the second is a wortmannin analog) [150]. From this group of specific PI3K inhibitors, only evaluation of PX-866 is proposed in a phase II clinical trial for the treatment of recurrent GBM patients, and is currently recruiting patients (NCT01259869) (Table 2) [118]. XL147 and GDC-0941 are also class I PI3K inhibitors, and IC877114 (targets p110δ) and TG100-115 (targets p110δ and p110γ) are PI3K isoform-specific inhibitors [150]. In turn, LY294002 was able to potentiate the citotoxicity of TMZ in glioma cells [151, 152]. Besides these agents that only target PI3K there are several dual PI3K/mTOR inhibitors, as PI-103, PI-540, PI-620, XL765, BEZ235 and BGT226 [150]. XL765 and XL147 were already tested in a phase I clinical trial with recurrent GBM patients (Table 2). Some preclinical studies support the theory of targeting these pathways in GBM therapeutics. Combination of LY294002 with the mTOR inhibitor rapamycin (or sirolimus) was able to diminish the self-renewal capacity of GBM cells and induce differentiation of cancer stem cell like cells (CSC); the same effect was achieved using a dual PI3K/mTOR inhibitor, NVP-BEZ235, which additionally reduced the ability of GBM CSLC to form tumors *in vivo* [153].

For specific targeting of mTOR, several inhibitors were developed and tested clinically, like sirolimus (rapamycin), everolimus (RAD001) and temsirolimus (CCI-779) [106, 133]. All of these agents were already evaluated for the treatment of GBM in phase I and II clinical trials, but no significant improvements were seen (Table 2). A preclinical study showed that the outcome of mTOR inhibitory treatments could be efficiently monitored by Positron Emission Tomography (PET) based only in glucose and thymidine metabolism, through the uptake of [^{18}F]FDG and [^{18}F]FLT [154]. Furthermore, combination with other kinase inhibitors like AEE788 (inhibits both EGFR and VEGFR2) also showed some preclinical promising results, since its combination with everolimus (RAD001) resulted in increased effect on cell cycle arrest, proliferation and apoptosis, and impact tumor growth and survival *in vivo* [155]. This combination was tested in a phase I/II trial in 2006 for the treatment of recurrent GBM (NCT00107237) [118]. One liability of these therapies is that they only target mTORC1, and although this is the best characterized mTOR isoform, it is also known that full activation of PI3K/AKT pathway also requires mTORC2 [156]. Consequently, it is argued that dual inhibition of mTOR complexes 1 and 2 will be more effi-

http://dx.doi.org/10.5772/52361

cient [156]. Preclinical studies have shown a significant decrease in tumor volume and growth in xenograft mouse models of GBM treated with PI3K/mTOR inhibitor AZD8055 [157]. Furthermore, there are three phase I clinical trials recruiting patients with MG (drug/trial reference: AZD8055/NCT01316809; CC-223/NCT01177397; OSI-027/ NCT00698243) to test this possibility [118].

b. RAS/RAF/MEK/ERK/MAPK pathway

Another important pathway contributing to the neoplastic process is the one mediated by RAS/RAF/MEK/MAPK [106]. Inhibitors targeting members of this pathway include the farnesil transferase inhibitors of RAS, such as tipifarnib (Zanestra or R115777) and lonafarnib (Sarasar or SCH 66336) or multiple kinases inhibitors that target this pathway, like sorafenib [98, 116]. Some of the more significant clinical results of tipifarnib are summarized in Table 2. A phase I clinical trial to test the effectiveness of combining tipifarnib with TMZ and RT for newly diagnosed GBM or gliosarcoma is now ongoing (NCT00049387) [118]. Sorafenib is described as an inhibitor of EGFR, PDGFR and RAF, that can block MEK activation and, in preclinical studies, was able to induce apoptosis, and decreased proliferation of GBM cells [98, 158]. At the clinical level, it has been extensively studied in 12 clinical trials with completed, ongoing or recruiting status [118]; however, the results have still been somewhat different, with good results for newly diagnosed GBM and recurrent GBM, but when combined with BVZ for the treatment of recurrent GBM, it failed to improve survival, showing a high percentage of patients with progressive disease (Table 2) [118].

c. Histone deacetylases (HDACs)

Epigenetic events are crucial during the carcinogenic process, in which the chromatin state and remodeling are important mediators. Histone deacetylases (HDAC) are responsible for chromatin condensation and repression of transcription [159, 160]. Mechanistically they catalyze the elimination of acetyl groups from lysine residues in N-terminal tails of histone proteins [161]. The use of specific HDAC inhibitors has been described as an attractive opportunity to alter cancer-related epigenetic modifications [159]. These inhibitors are also reported as being able to block angiogenesis and invasion, promote cell cycle arrest and apoptosis, and to act as immunomodulators [116, 159, 160]. Valproic acid (VPA) is a short chain fatty acid, class I and IIa HDAC inhibitor, used as an anticonvulsant drug and frequently administered to treat glioma-associated seizures [159, 162, 163]. So, when the results of the EORTC/NCIC TMZ trial were analyzed taking in consideration the anti-epileptic drugs used, an interesting result showing a benefit in OS of the patients treated with TMZ + RT that were under VPA treatment was observed, suggesting that this drug could enhance the effects of TMZ + RT treatment [162]. VPA in combination with TMZ *in vitro* showed an increase in TMZ cytotoxicity, even for TMZ resistant cell lines, through downregulation of MGMT [164-166]; *in vivo*, this combination had also a benefit in tumor growth inhibition [164]; and increased the effects of γ-radiation in glioma cells [165]. Clinically, the evaluation of VPA for the treatment of GBM is proposed in two clinical trials: a phase II trial to evaluate the efficacy of VPA + RT followed by combination of VPA + BVZ for the treatment of children with high-grade gliomas (HGG) (NCT00879437) and a phase II trial to test the combination of VPA with TMZ and RT in adult HGG (NCT00302159) [118]. Vorinostat is also an inhibitor of class I and II HDACs, tested in several clinical trials now recruiting patients (NCT01378481, NCT01266031, NCT00731731, NCT01110876, NCT00555399) [118, 163]. The results of some of the already completed clinical trials for HDAC inhibitors as GBM therapeutics are in some way disappointing, with no radiographic responses observed when recurrent GBM patients treated with romidepsin and vorinostat failing to improve survival outcomes in different combinatory strategies (Table 2).

Drug; Target(s)	Clinical Trials/Population/Results	Refs
Erlotinib (Tarceva®); EGFR	Phase I, and II clinical trials Acceptable toxicity and tolerable treatment with daily administrations of 150-200 mg/day dose Newly diagnosed GBM: combined with TMZ showed a PFS of 7.2 months and OS of 15.3 months; worse outcome for patients older than 70 years old; combined with standard care (RT + TMZ), the OS was 19.3 months, and correlated with *MGMT* promoter methylation and PTEN expression; combinations with other drugs are also under clinical trials (BVZ, administration after TMZ + RT, RT and erlotinib in younger patients) (NCT00124657, NCT00720356). Recurrent GBM: erlotinib as a single agent was not able to improve PFS compared to standard treatment (TMZ or carmustine + RT); combined with mTOR inhibitor sirolimus, treatment was well tolerated and OS was 33.8 weeks; combination with carboplatin showed a 30 weeks OS; Recurrent MG: combination with BVZ resulted in partial or total radiographic response for 48% of GBM patients and association with PFS; GBM tumors showing high levels of HIF-2α and VEGFR2 expression presented a worst prognosis. Recruiting or ongoing clinical trials combining erlotinib with isotretinoin, sirolimus and vorinostat, and also single agent administration for patients harboring the EGFR-vIII mutation (NCT01110876, NCT01103375, NCT01257594, NCT00509431). Nonprogressive GBM: as single agent, 1-year PFS was only 9% and less than 53% of 2 months, and less than 57% of the patients were alive after 1 year.	[118, 167-175]
Gefitinib (Iressa or ZD1839); EGFR	Phase I, and II clinical trials Recurrent GBM: as single agent, the treatment was well tolerated and resulted in OS of 39.4 weeks and PFS of 8.1 weeks. In a phase II study, OS did not overcome 8.8 months. Newly diagnosed GBM: 1-year OS (54.2%) and 1-year PFS (16.7%) were not significantly different from controls of other clinical trials.	[176-178]
Rindopepimut (CDX-110, PEP-3); EGFR-vIII	Phase I, II, and III clinical trials EGFR-vIII-positive newly diagnosed GBM: given with GM-CSF, TTP of 14.2 months (vs. 6.3 months of historical controls) and OS of 26 months (vs. 15 months of historical controls); administration with TMZ also improved TTP (15.2 months vs. 6.4 months) and OS (23.2	[118, 124]

Drug; Target(s)	Clinical Trials/Population/Results	Refs
	months vs. 15.2 months); phase III trial (recruiting status) is projected to test the efficacy of rindopepimut with TMZ (NCT01480479). Newly diagnosed GBM: TTP was 10.2 months and OS was 22.8 months (vaccine given with DC); Phase II clinical trial is recruiting patients with relapsed GBM EGFR-vIII positive to test the efficacy of rindopepimut with BVZ (NCT01498328).	
Imatinib mesylate; PDGFR, KIT, ABL	Phase I, II, and III clinical trials Newly diagnosed GBM: a phase II study with 20 patients showed a OS of 6.2 months. Recurrent GBM or MG: as single agent was well tolerated until doses of 800-1200 g/day, but very poor outcome with 6-PFS of 3%, only 2/34 patients with PR, and 6/34 with SD; when combined with HU, 6-PFS (27%) improved, but still very poor; combination with HU and vatalanib was well tolerated and resulted in OS of 48 weeks, PFS of 12 weeks and 6-PFS of 25%. In another phase II study the outcome of patients treated with imatinib as single agent was also (in newly diagnosed GBM) very poor (6-PFS: 16%); when combined with HU, imatinib also lacked efficacy. A phase III clinical trial showed no differences in TMZ resistant GBM patients treated with imatinbib + HU or HU alone (NCT00154375); phase II clinical trials combining imatinib with HU and Zactima were also performed but no results have been published (NCT00613054).	[118, 126, 129-132, 179, 180]
Cediranib (AZD2171); VEGFR	Phase I, II, and III clinical trials Recurrent GBM: as a single agent showed a PFS was 117 days and OS was 227 days (phase II); phase I trials to test cediranib + lomustine to treat GBM is already completed but without published results (NCT00503204); a phase III trial with the same combinatory approach for the treatment of recurrent GBM in currently ongoing (NCT00777153); recruiting trials include combination with gefitinib (NCT01310855) and with cilengitide (NCT00979862). Newly diagnosed GBM: all clinical trials are currently ongoing or recruiting – phase I and phase I/II cediranib + RT + TMZ (NCT01062425 and NCT00662506); phase I combination with BVZ (NCT00458731); phase I combination with gamma secretase inhibitor RO4929097 (NCT0130855).	[118, 181, 182]
Rilotumumab (AMG-102); HGF	Phase II clinical trial Recurrent GBM: when combined with prior BVZ treatment, did not affect PFS (4-4.1 weeks vs. 4.1-4.7 weeks), but OS was significantly different (3.4-3.6 months vs. 10.9-11.4 months).	[183]
PX-866; PI3K	Phase I, and II clinical trials Completed a phase I clinical study in patients with solid tumors (NCT00726583); Recruiting recurrent GBM patients for a phase II clinical trial (NCT01259869).	[118]
XL765; PI3K/mTOR	Phase I clinical trial Recurrent GBM: combination with a PI3K inhibitor XL147 already completed phase I trial (NCT0124460). Recruiting for a phase I trial for combination with TMZ to treat MG (NCT00704080).	[118]

Drug; Target(s)	Clinical Trials/Population/Results	Refs
Enzastaurin; PKCβ (indirect inhibition of Akt)	Phase I, II, and III clinical trials Recurrent or progressive MG: in recurrent HGG, monotherapy had no significant impact in 6-PFS (7%); when compared with lomustine in a phase III clinical trial, no improvement in OS or PFS was achieved.	[118, 142, 144, 184, 185]
Everolimus (RAD001); mTOR	Phase I, and II clinical trials Phase I clinical trials showed that everolimus was well tolerated even when combined with RT + TMZ, BVZ or erlotinib. Changes in metabolism detected with FDG positron emission tomography days after administration of everolimus. Newly diagnosed GBM: combination with TMZ + RT + BVZ followed by BVZ + everolimus in a phase II clinical trial resulted in 57% PR, 1 CR, 18-months OS of 44%, and 18-months PFS of 29%.	[186-188]
Temsirolimus (CCI779); mTOR	Phase I, and II clinical trials Phase I trial showed that temsirolimus combined with TMZ and RT increased the risk of infectious diseases (3/25 fatal infections). Recurrent GBM: it was well tolerated as a single agent, and 36% radiographic responses were observed; 6-PFS was 7.8%, and OS was 4.4 months (phase II).	[189, 190]
Sirolimus; mTOR	Phase I, and II clinical trials Recurrent GBM or MG: in tumors without PTEN, mTOR inhibition correlated with decreased proliferation of the tumors (phase I/II); combination with erlotinib (phase II) resulted in 47% SD, no CR or PR and 6-PFS of 3.1%; phase I/II trial combinatory treatment with erlotinib is currently ongoing (NCT00509431); phase I trial is recruiting patients to test combinatory treatment with vandetanib (NCT00821080). Recruiting patients with solid tumors to test combination with a vaccine (NCT01522820).	[118, 172, 191]
Tipifarnib (Zarnestra, R115777); RAS	Phase I, and II clinical trials Newly diagnosed GBM: combined with RT and with or without TMZ, this treatment was well tolerated until doses of 300 mg (4-week cycle) (phase I). Administration with RT well tolerated until 200 mg/day, OS of 12 months and 1/9 PR, 4/9 SD, and 3/9 rapid progression. No significant improvement in survival with tipifarnib before RT (OS of 7.7 months). Recurrent GBM: treatment well tolerated, but 6-PFS (11.9%) and PFS (8 weeks) very poor, although one GBM patient remained progression-free for 36 months.	[192-195]
Sorafenib; RAF, VEGFR, PDGFR	Phase I, and II clinical trials Newly diagnosed GBM: combination of TMZ and sorafenib after RT + TMZ showed 13% PR, 53% SD, and 28% PD. OS was 12 months, 1-year PFS was 16%, and PFS was 6 months (phase II); also tested in combination with erlotinib/tipifarnib/temsirolimus (NCT00335764). Recurrent GBM: combination with TMZ resulted in OS of 41.5 weeks, 1-year OS of 34.4%, PFS of 6.4 weeks (6-PFS: 9.4%); 3% of the patients had PR, 4.7% SD, and 50% PD (phase II); combination with BVZ was also tested (NCT00621686).	[118, 196, 197]

Drug; Target(s)	Clinical Trials/Population/Results	Refs
	Ongoing or recruiting clinical trials: NCT00734526 (phase I/II: sorafenib + RT + TMZ for the treatment of newly diagnosed GBM), NCT00884416 (phase I single agent HGG), NCT00329719 (phase I/II: combination with temsirolimus for recurrent GBM).	
Cilengitide (EMD 121974); Integrins	Phase I, II, and III clinical trials Well tolerated until doses of 2400 mg/m^2 Newly diagnosed GBM: when combined with RT + TMZ, the OS was 16.1 months and patients with *MGMT* promoter methylation tend to show a higher PFS and OS; clinical trials testing the efficacy of cilengitide with TMZ + RT in patients with or without *MGMT* methylation are now recruiting or ongoing (NCT00813943, NCT0068922). Recurrent GBM: as a single agent no complete responses were observed, but median OS was at least 6.5-9.9 months.	[118, 198-200]
Vorinostat; HDAC	Phase I, and II clinical trials Progressive or recurrent GBM/MG: combination with bortezomib in a phase II trial resulted in very poor results (6-PFS 0%, OS 3.2 months, TTP 1.5 months); phase II monotherapy showed a 6-PFS of 15.2%, TTP of 1.9 months, PFS of 11.2 months, and OS of 5.7 months; Ongoing trials: phase I/II combination with BVZ and TMZ for recurrent MG (NCT00939991), phase I combination with TMZ for MG (NCT00268385), phase I combination with BVZ and irinotecan for recurrent GBM (NCT00762255).	[118, 201, 202]
Romidepsin; HDAC	Phase II clinical trial Recurrent MG: no radiographic responses, 72% PD and 28% SD; 6-PFS of 3%, PFS of 8 weeks, and OS of 34 weeks; 83% of the patients stopped treatment due to tumor progression, and 11% due to treatment toxicity.	[203]

PFS (median Progression-Free Survival); OS (median Overall Survival); TTP (median Time-to-Progression); PR (Partial Response); SD (Stable Disease); PD (Progressive Disease); 6-PFS (6 month PFS); BVZ (Bevacizumab); RT (Radiotherapy); TMZ (Temozolomide); GM-GSF (granulocyte macrophage-colony stimulating factor); DC (Dendritic Cells); HU (Hydroxyurea); MG (Malignant Glioma); HGG (High Grade Glioma).

Table 2. Examples of clinical trials with molecularly targeted therapies directed to the most commonly altered signalling pathways in GBM.

4.3. Novel therapeutic approaches

As stated above, a small population of cells within the tumor, called cancer stem-cells, presents self-renewal capacity, ability to differentiate and initiate tumorigenesis, and express several markers of neural stem cells [24, 33, 116]. Furthermore, these cells are increasingly recognized as a niche of radiochemotherapy-resistant cells, making then attractive targets for new therapies [24, 49, 204]. There are several signaling pathways altered in cancer stem cells and that represent possible targets, such as PI3K, OLIG2, Shh, Wnt and Notch signaling pathways [24, 116].

Another novel therapeutic strategy to treat cancer-related diseases is gene therapy (GT). GT was proposed for a long time as a molecular strategy that may help circumvent the non-specific cytotoxicity of the current pharmacological inhibitors, through specific delivery of suicide, pro-apoptotic, *TP53*, and other genes to tumor cells that, ultimately, lead to cancer regression or cure [106, 205]. GT can be performed delivering conditional or toxic transgenes using viral or non-viral delivery systems, including exosomes and stem cells [205, 206]. In GBM, the delivery of the thymidine kinase (TK) gene, produced by the herpes simplex virus type 1 (HSV1), in combination with the prodrug ganciclovir (GCV), using both retrovirus and adenovirus, was already tested at clinical level. The advantage of using retroviruses to deliver viral vectors is the specificity, since they target only highly proliferating cells. On the other hand, adenoviruses infect both quiescent cells and rapidly dividing cells [207]. A retroviralmediated delivery was already applied to newly diagnosed GBM patients until phase III clinical trial, but it was rejected after failing to improve survival compared to RT + TMZ [208]. Another promising strategy is the combination of viral vectors with factors that stimulate the immune system, as, for example, the delivery of the suicide gene HSV1 *TK* gene, with the cytokine IL-2. This strategy was already tested in 12 patients with recurrent GBM, where it was proved to be safe and well tolerable [209]. However, in terms of outcome, there were no patients with complete response and the PFS and OS were only 4.5 and 7.5 months, respectively [209].

The induction of an immune response against tumor cells, called immunotherapy, is also a novel approach for the treatment of cancer, including GBM [210]. Immunotherapy can be performed with two different approaches: increasing the immune response to the tumor (active immunotherapy) with long term immunization, or delivering immune effectors to an immediate immune response (passive immunotherapy) [106]. Potent anti-tumor immunity is achieved through antigen-presenting cells, of which dendritic cells (DC) are the most promising [210, 211]. In a phase I clinical trial with 12 GBM patients (7 newly diagnosed GBM and 5 recurrent GBM) the administration of autologous DC vaccines showed that this treatment was well tolerated and minimally toxic. Additionally, it revealed promising outcome results, such as 2 long term-survivors (≥4 years) and OS of 23.4 months; however, the benefit in clinical outcomes were mainly observed in patients with stable disease and low levels of TGF-β2, who also had a higher number of infiltrating cytotoxic T-cells in the tumor bulk, suggesting that this treatment may favor particularly these patients [212]. In another phase I/II clinical trial with patients with recurrent GBM, it was found more beneficial the treatment with mature DC vs. non-mature DC, as well as intradermal and intratumoral administration of the DC pulsed with autologous tumor lysate, compared to intradermal approach alone [213]. The transfer of *ex vivo* maturated immune cells like effector T cells or lymphokine activated killer cells (LAK) is also under clinical evaluation for GBM immunotherapy [214].

4.4. Current challenges and future trends

As illustrated by the vast panoply of drugs and therapeutic strategies under investigation for the treatment of GBM, there is a major effort to develop more effective therapies to treat this highly malignant and therapy-insensitive disease. Unfortunately, the success of these new therapies has mostly been somewhat disappointing. Nevertheless, the efficacy of some of these approaches has yet to be determined. Of note, in addition to the strategies reviewed here, therapies targeting apoptotic elements (like Bcl-2, and inhibitor of apoptosis proteins), the mechanisms of resistance to TMZ (such as PARP and MGMT), or gene therapy to *TP53*, are also some examples of the search for an effective therapy for GBM [33]. Additionally, several developments were also made in helping surgeons with fluorescence-guided resection of the tumor and in radiotherapy [116]. In conclusion, the relevance of the effort to find a cure for GBM is unquestionable. However, despite the hard working search for a therapeutic strategy to reverse the poor outcomes of these patients, the standard treatment with TMZ and RT remains presently the best option. Future therapeutic trends for the treatment of GBM will have to: (i) include the new molecular classification of GBM; (ii) incorporate more efficient drug delivery systems to overcome blood-brain barrier restraints; and (iii) redirect the therapeutic choices to each patient, considering the specific molecular alterations of each tumor.

Author details

Céline S. Gonçalves[1,2], Tatiana Lourenço[1,2], Ana Xavier-Magalhães[1,2], Marta Pojo[1,2] and Bruno M. Costa[1,2*]

*Address all correspondence to: bfmcosta@ecsaude.uminho.pt

1 Life and Health Sciences Research Institute (ICVS), School of Health Sciences, University of Minho, Braga, Portugal

2 ICVS/3B's - PT Government Associate Laboratory, Braga/Guimarães, Portugal

References

[1] Ohgaki, H, & Kleihues, P. Genetic pathways to primary and secondary glioblastoma. The American journal of pathology. (2007). May; , 170(5), 1445-53.

[2] Porter, K. R, Mccarthy, B. J, Freels, S, Kim, Y, & Davis, F. G. Prevalence estimates for primary brain tumors in the United States by age, gender, behavior, and histology. Neuro Oncol. (2010). Jun; , 12(6), 520-7.

[3] CBTRUSPrimary Brain and Other Nervous System Tumors, Estimated Number of Cases Overall and by Behavior by State, (2012). Primary Malignant Brain and Other Nervous System Tumors, Estimated Number of Deaths by State, 2012. http:// wwwcbtrusorg/ html2012.

[4] Burnet, N. G, Jefferies, S. J, Benson, R. J, Hunt, D. P, & Treasure, F. P. Years of life lost (YLL) from cancer is an important measure of population burden--and should be

considered when allocating research funds. British journal of cancer. (2005). Jan 31; , 92(2), 241-5.

[5] Stupp, R, & Mason, W. P. van den Bent MJ, Weller M, Fisher B, Taphoorn MJ, et al. Radiotherapy plus concomitant and adjuvant temozolomide for glioblastoma. N Engl J Med. (2005). Mar 10; , 352(10), 987-96.

[6] Louis, D. N, Ohgaki, H, Wiestler, O. D, Cavenee, W. K, Burger, P. C, Jouvet, A, et al. The 2007 WHO classification of tumours of the central nervous system. Acta neuropathologica. (2007). Aug; , 114(2), 97-109.

[7] Nguyen, L. V, Vanner, R, Dirks, P, & Eaves, C. J. Cancer stem cells: an evolving concept. Nat Rev Cancer. (2012). Feb; , 12(2), 133-43.

[8] Dirks, P. B. Brain tumor stem cells: bringing order to the chaos of brain cancer. J Clin Oncol. (2008). Jun 10; , 26(17), 2916-24.

[9] Charles, N. A, Holland, E. C, Gilbertson, R, Glass, R, & Kettenmann, H. The brain tumor microenvironment. Glia. (2012). Mar; , 60(3), 502-14.

[10] Heywood, R. M, Marcus, H. J, Ryan, D. J, Piccirillo, S. G, Al-mayhani, T. M, & Watts, C. A review of the role of stem cells in the development and treatment of glioma. Acta Neurochir (Wien). (2012). Jun; discussion 69., 154(6), 951-69.

[11] Bachoo, R. M, Maher, E. A, Ligon, K. L, Sharpless, N. E, Chan, S. S, You, M. J, et al. Epidermal growth factor receptor and Ink4a/Arf: convergent mechanisms governing terminal differentiation and transformation along the neural stem cell to astrocyte axis. Cancer cell. (2002). Apr; , 1(3), 269-77.

[12] Doetsch, F, Caille, I, Lim, D. A, Garcia-verdugo, J. M, & Alvarez-buylla, A. Subventricular zone astrocytes are neural stem cells in the adult mammalian brain. Cell. (1999). Jun 11; , 97(6), 703-16.

[13] Laywell, E. D, Rakic, P, Kukekov, V. G, Holland, E. C, & Steindler, D. A. Identification of a multipotent astrocytic stem cell in the immature and adult mouse brain. Proc Natl Acad Sci U S A. (2000). Dec 5; , 97(25), 13883-8.

[14] Chen, J, Mckay, R. M, & Parada, L. F. Malignant glioma: lessons from genomics, mouse models, and stem cells. Cell. (2012). Mar 30; , 149(1), 36-47.

[15] Vescovi, A. L, Galli, R, & Reynolds, B. A. Brain tumour stem cells. Nat Rev Cancer. (2006). Jun; , 6(6), 425-36.

[16] Chen, R, Nishimura, M. C, Bumbaca, S. M, Kharbanda, S, Forrest, W. F, Kasman, I. M, et al. A hierarchy of self-renewing tumor-initiating cell types in glioblastoma. Cancer cell. (2010). Apr 13; , 17(4), 362-75.

[17] Stiles, C. D, & Rowitch, D. H. Glioma stem cells: a midterm exam. Neuron. (2008). Jun 26; , 58(6), 832-46.

[18] Singh, S. K, Hawkins, C, Clarke, I. D, Squire, J. A, Bayani, J, Hide, T, et al. Identification of human brain tumour initiating cells. Nature. (2004). Nov 18; , 432(7015), 396-401.

[19] Dirks, P. B. Brain tumor stem cells: the cancer stem cell hypothesis writ large. Molecular oncology. (2010). Oct; , 4(5), 420-30.

[20] Brescia, P, Richichi, C, & Pelicci, G. Current strategies for identification of glioma stem cells: adequate or unsatisfactory? Journal of oncology. (2012).

[21] Jhanwar-uniyal, M, Albert, L, Mckenna, E, Karsy, M, Rajdev, P, Braun, A, et al. Deciphering the signaling pathways of cancer stem cells of glioblastoma multiforme: role of Akt/mTOR and MAPK pathways. Advances in enzyme regulation. (2011). , 51(1), 164-70.

[22] Dunn, G. P, Rinne, M. L, Wykosky, J, Genovese, G, Quayle, S. N, Dunn, I. F, et al. Emerging insights into the molecular and cellular basis of glioblastoma. Genes Dev. (2012). Apr 15; , 26(8), 756-84.

[23] Cheng, L, Bao, S, & Rich, J. N. Potential therapeutic implications of cancer stem cells in glioblastoma. Biochem Pharmacol. (2010). Sep 1; , 80(5), 654-65.

[24] Ohka, F, Natsume, A, & Wakabayashi, T. Current trends in targeted therapies for glioblastoma multiforme. Neurol Res Int. (2012).

[25] Lim, S. K, Llaguno, S. R, Mckay, R. M, & Parada, L. F. Glioblastoma multiforme: a perspective on recent findings in human cancer and mouse models. BMB Rep. (2011). Mar; , 44(3), 158-64.

[26] TCGAComprehensive genomic characterization defines human glioblastoma genes and core pathway. Nature. 2008 23 October (2008). , 455(7216), 1061-8.

[27] Sherr, C. J, Mccormick, F, & The, R. B. and pathways in cancer. Cancer Cell. (2002). Aug;2(2):103-12., 53.

[28] Shapiro, G. I. Cyclin-dependent kinase pathways as targets for cancer treatment. J Clin Oncol. (2006). Apr 10; , 24(11), 1770-83.

[29] Mao, H, Lebrun, D. G, Yang, J, Zhu, V. F, & Li, M. Deregulated signaling pathways in glioblastoma multiforme: molecular mechanisms and therapeutic targets. Cancer Invest. (2012). Jan; , 30(1), 48-56.

[30] Deb, S. P. Cell cycle regulatory functions of the human oncoprotein MDM2. Mol Cancer Res. (2003). Dec; , 1(14), 1009-16.

[31] Iwakuma, T, & Lozano, G. MDM2, an introduction. Mol Cancer Res. (2003). Dec; , 1(14), 993-1000.

[32] Zhang, Y, Xiong, Y, & Yarbrough, W. G. ARF promotes MDM2 degradation and stabilizes ARF-INK4a locus deletion impairs both the Rb and p53 tumor suppression pathways. Cell. (1998). Mar 20;92(6):725-34., 53.

[33] Krakstad, C, & Chekenya, M. Survival signalling and apoptosis resistance in glioblastomas: opportunities for targeted therapeutics. Mol Cancer. (2010).

[34] Moscatello, D. K, Holgado-madruga, M, Emlet, D. R, Montgomery, R. B, & Wong, A. J. Constitutive activation of phosphatidylinositol 3-kinase by a naturally occurring mutant epidermal growth factor receptor. J Biol Chem. (1998). Jan 2; , 273(1), 200-6.

[35] Costa, B. M, Smith, J. S, Chen, Y, Chen, J, Phillips, H. S, Aldape, K. D, et al. Reversing HOXA9 oncogene activation by PI3K inhibition: epigenetic mechanism and prognostic significance in human glioblastoma. Cancer Res. (2010). Jan 15; , 70(2), 453-62.

[36] Gaspar, N, Marshall, L, Perryman, L, Bax, D. A, Little, S. E, Viana-pereira, M, et al. MGMT-independent temozolomide resistance in pediatric glioblastoma cells associated with a PI3-kinase-mediated HOX/stem cell gene signature. Cancer Res. (2010). Nov 15; , 70(22), 9243-52.

[37] Murat, A, Migliavacca, E, Gorlia, T, Lambiv, W. L, Shay, T, Hamou, M. F, et al. Stem cell-related "self-renewal" signature and high epidermal growth factor receptor expression associated with resistance to concomitant chemoradiotherapy in glioblastoma. J Clin Oncol. (2008). Jun 20; , 26(18), 3015-24.

[38] Dang, L, White, D. W, Gross, S, Bennett, B. D, Bittinger, M. A, Driggers, E. M, et al. Cancer-associated IDH1 mutations produce 2-hydroxyglutarate. Nature. (2009). Dec 10; , 462(7274), 739-44.

[39] Sasaki, M, Knobbe, C. B, Munger, J. C, Lind, E. F, Brenner, D, Brustle, A, et al. IDH1(R132H) mutation increases murine haematopoietic progenitors and alters epigenetics. Nature. (2012). Jul 4.

[40] Verhaak, R. G, Hoadley, K. A, Purdom, E, Wang, V, Qi, Y, Wilkerson, M. D, et al. Integrated genomic analysis identifies clinically relevant subtypes of glioblastoma characterized by abnormalities in PDGFRA, IDH1, EGFR, and NF1. Cancer Cell. (2010). Jan 19; , 17(1), 98-110.

[41] Liang, Y, Diehn, M, Watson, N, Bollen, A. W, Aldape, K. D, Nicholas, M. K, et al. Gene expression profiling reveals molecularly and clinically distinct subtypes of glioblastoma multiforme. Proc Natl Acad Sci U S A. (2005). Apr 19; , 102(16), 5814-9.

[42] Mischel, P. S, Shai, R, Shi, T, Horvath, S, Lu, K. V, Choe, G, et al. Identification of molecular subtypes of glioblastoma by gene expression profiling. Oncogene. (2003). Apr 17; , 22(15), 2361-73.

[43] Shai, R, Shi, T, Kremen, T. J, Horvath, S, Liau, L. M, Cloughesy, T. F, et al. Gene expression profiling identifies molecular subtypes of gliomas. Oncogene. (2003). Jul 31; , 22(31), 4918-23.

[44] Freije, W. A, Castro-vargas, F. E, Fang, Z, Horvath, S, Cloughesy, T, Liau, L. M, et al. Gene expression profiling of gliomas strongly predicts survival. Cancer Res. (2004). Sep 15; , 64(18), 6503-10.

[45] Nutt, C. L, Mani, D. R, Betensky, R. A, Tamayo, P, Cairncross, J. G, Ladd, C, et al. Gene expression-based classification of malignant gliomas correlates better with survival than histological classification. Cancer Res. (2003). Apr 1; , 63(7), 1602-7.

[46] Phillips, H. S, Kharbanda, S, Chen, R, Forrest, W. F, Soriano, R. H, Wu, T. D, et al. Molecular subclasses of high-grade glioma predict prognosis, delineate a pattern of disease progression, and resemble stages in neurogenesis. Cancer Cell. (2006). Mar; , 9(3), 157-73.

[47] Tso, C. L, Freije, W. A, Day, A, Chen, Z, Merriman, B, Perlina, A, et al. Distinct transcription profiles of primary and secondary glioblastoma subgroups. Cancer Res. (2006). Jan 1; , 66(1), 159-67.

[48] Curran, W. J. Jr., Scott CB, Horton J, Nelson JS, Weinstein AS, Fischbach AJ, et al. Recursive partitioning analysis of prognostic factors in three Radiation Therapy Oncology Group malignant glioma trials. J Natl Cancer Inst. (1993). May 5; , 85(9), 704-10.

[49] Bao, S, Wu, Q, Mclendon, R. E, Hao, Y, Shi, Q, Hjelmeland, A. B, et al. Glioma stem cells promote radioresistance by preferential activation of the DNA damage response. Nature. (2006). Dec 7; , 444(7120), 756-60.

[50] Chakravarti, A, Zhai, G, Suzuki, Y, Sarkesh, S, Black, P. M, Muzikansky, A, et al. The prognostic significance of phosphatidylinositol 3-kinase pathway activation in human gliomas. J Clin Oncol. (2004). May 15; , 22(10), 1926-33.

[51] Haas-kogan, D. A, Prados, M. D, Lamborn, K. R, Tihan, T, Berger, M. S, & Stokoe, D. Biomarkers to predict response to epidermal growth factor receptor inhibitors. Cell Cycle. (2005). Oct; , 4(10), 1369-72.

[52] Hegi, M. E, Diserens, A. C, Gorlia, T, Hamou, M. F, De Tribolet, N, Weller, M, et al. MGMT gene silencing and benefit from temozolomide in glioblastoma. N Engl J Med. (2005). Mar 10; , 352(10), 997-1003.

[53] Hormigo, A, Gu, B, Karimi, S, Riedel, E, Panageas, K. S, Edgar, M. A, et al. YKL-40 and matrix metalloproteinase-9 as potential serum biomarkers for patients with high-grade gliomas. Clin Cancer Res. (2006). Oct 1; , 12(19), 5698-704.

[54] Liu, G, Yuan, X, Zeng, Z, Tunici, P, Ng, H, Abdulkadir, I. R, et al. Analysis of gene expression and chemoresistance of CD133+ cancer stem cells in glioblastoma. Mol Cancer. (2006).

[55] Mellinghoff, I. K, Wang, M. Y, Vivanco, I, Haas-kogan, D. A, Zhu, S, Dia, E. Q, et al. Molecular determinants of the response of glioblastomas to EGFR kinase inhibitors. N Engl J Med. (2005). Nov 10; , 353(19), 2012-24.

[56] Nigro, J. M, Misra, A, Zhang, L, Smirnov, I, Colman, H, Griffin, C, et al. Integrated array-comparative genomic hybridization and expression array profiles identify clinically relevant molecular subtypes of glioblastoma. Cancer Res. (2005). Mar 1; , 65(5), 1678-86.

[57] Parsons, D. W, Jones, S, Zhang, X, Lin, J. C, Leary, R. J, Angenendt, P, et al. An integrated genomic analysis of human glioblastoma multiforme. Science. (2008). Sep 26; , 321(5897), 1807-12.

[58] Pelloski, C. E, Lin, E, Zhang, L, Yung, W. K, Colman, H, Liu, J. L, et al. Prognostic associations of activated mitogen-activated protein kinase and Akt pathways in glioblastoma. Clin Cancer Res. (2006). Jul 1; , 12(13), 3935-41.

[59] Srinivasan, S, Patric, I. R, & Somasundaram, K. A ten-microRNA expression signature predicts survival in glioblastoma. PLoS One. (2011). e17438.

[60] Colman, H, & Aldape, K. Molecular predictors in glioblastoma: toward personalized therapy. Arch Neurol. (2008). Jul; , 65(7), 877-83.

[61] Liu, L, Markowitz, S, & Gerson, S. L. Mismatch repair mutations override alkyltransferase in conferring resistance to temozolomide but not to 1,3-bis(2-chloroethyl)nitrosourea. Cancer Res. (1996). Dec 1; , 56(23), 5375-9.

[62] Costa, B. M, Caeiro, C, Guimaraes, I, Martinho, O, Jaraquemada, T, Augusto, I, et al. Prognostic value of MGMT promoter methylation in glioblastoma patients treated with temozolomide-based chemoradiation: a Portuguese multicentre study. Oncol Rep. (2010). Jun; , 23(6), 1655-62.

[63] Van Vlodrop, I. J, Niessen, H. E, Derks, S, Baldewijns, M. M, Van Criekinge, W, Herman, J. G, et al. Analysis of promoter CpG island hypermethylation in cancer: location, location, location! Clin Cancer Res. (2011). Jul 1; , 17(13), 4225-31.

[64] Bady, P, Sciuscio, D, Diserens, A. C, & Bloch, J. van den Bent MJ, Marosi C, et al. MGMT methylation analysis of glioblastoma on the Infinium methylation BeadChip identifies two distinct CpG regions associated with gene silencing and outcome, yielding a prediction model for comparisons across datasets, tumor grades, and CIMP-status. Acta Neuropathol. (2012). Jul 19.

[65] Shah, N, Lin, B, Sibenaller, Z, Ryken, T, Lee, H, Yoon, J. G, et al. Comprehensive analysis of MGMT promoter methylation: correlation with MGMT expression and clinical response in GBM. PLoS One. (2011). e16146.

[66] Wick, W, Platten, M, Meisner, C, Felsberg, J, Tabatabai, G, Simon, M, et al. Temozolomide chemotherapy alone versus radiotherapy alone for malignant astrocytoma in the elderly: the NOA-08 randomised, phase 3 trial. Lancet Oncol. (2012). Jul; , 13(7), 707-15.

[67] Olson, R. A, Brastianos, P. K, & Palma, D. A. Prognostic and predictive value of epigenetic silencing of MGMT in patients with high grade gliomas: a systematic review and meta-analysis. J Neurooncol. (2011). Nov; , 105(2), 325-35.

[68] Yan, H, Parsons, D. W, Jin, G, Mclendon, R, Rasheed, B. A, Yuan, W, et al. IDH1 and IDH2 mutations in gliomas. N Engl J Med. (2009). Feb 19; , 360(8), 765-73.

[69] Koshland, D. E. Jr., Walsh K, LaPorte DC. Sensitivity of metabolic fluxes to covalent control. Curr Top Cell Regul. (1985). , 27, 13-22.

[70] Zhao, S, Lin, Y, Xu, W, Jiang, W, Zha, Z, Wang, P, et al. Glioma-derived mutations in IDH1 dominantly inhibit IDH1 catalytic activity and induce HIF-1alpha. Science. (2009). Apr 10; , 324(5924), 261-5.

[71] Balss, J, Meyer, J, Mueller, W, Korshunov, A, Hartmann, C, & Von Deimling, A. Analysis of the IDH1 codon 132 mutation in brain tumors. Acta Neuropathol. (2008). Dec; , 116(6), 597-602.

[72] Ichimura, K, Pearson, D. M, Kocialkowski, S, Backlund, L. M, Chan, R, Jones, D. T, et al. IDH1 mutations are present in the majority of common adult gliomas but rare in primary glioblastomas. Neuro Oncol. (2009). Aug; , 11(4), 341-7.

[73] Hartmann, C, Meyer, J, Balss, J, Capper, D, Mueller, W, Christians, A, et al. Type and frequency of IDH1 and IDH2 mutations are related to astrocytic and oligodendroglial differentiation and age: a study of 1,010 diffuse gliomas. Acta Neuropathol. (2009). Oct; , 118(4), 469-74.

[74] Sanson, M, Marie, Y, Paris, S, Idbaih, A, Laffaire, J, Ducray, F, et al. Isocitrate dehydrogenase 1 codon 132 mutation is an important prognostic biomarker in gliomas. J Clin Oncol. (2009). Sep 1; , 27(25), 4150-4.

[75] Noushmehr, H, Weisenberger, D. J, Diefes, K, Phillips, H. S, Pujara, K, Berman, B. P, et al. Identification of a CpG island methylator phenotype that defines a distinct subgroup of glioma. Cancer Cell. (2010). May 18; , 17(5), 510-22.

[76] Yen, K. E, Bittinger, M. A, Su, S. M, & Fantin, V. R. Cancer-associated IDH mutations: biomarker and therapeutic opportunities. Oncogene. (2010). Dec 9; , 29(49), 6409-17.

[77] SongTao QLei Y, Si G, YanQing D, HuiXia H, XueLin Z, et al. IDH mutations predict longer survival and response to temozolomide in secondary glioblastoma. Cancer Sci. (2012). Feb; , 103(2), 269-73.

[78] Mcginnis, W, & Krumlauf, R. Homeobox genes and axial patterning. Cell. (1992). Jan 24; , 68(2), 283-302.

[79] Wellik, D. M. Hox genes and vertebrate axial pattern. Curr Top Dev Biol. (2009). , 88, 257-78.

[80] Shah, N, & Sukumar, S. The Hox genes and their roles in oncogenesis. Nat Rev Cancer. (2010). May; , 10(5), 361-71.

[81] Abate-shen, C. Deregulated homeobox gene expression in cancer: cause or consequence? Nat Rev Cancer. (2002). Oct; , 2(10), 777-85.

[82] Care, A, Felicetti, F, Meccia, E, Bottero, L, Parenza, M, Stoppacciaro, A, et al. HOXB7: a key factor for tumor-associated angiogenic switch. Cancer Res. (2001). Sep 1; , 61(17), 6532-9.

[83] Hu, Y. L, Fong, S, Ferrell, C, Largman, C, & Shen, W. F. HOXA9 modulates its oncogenic partner Meis1 to influence normal hematopoiesis. Mol Cell Biol. (2009). Sep; , 29(18), 5181-92.

[84] Raman, V, Martensen, S. A, Reisman, D, Evron, E, Odenwald, W. F, Jaffee, E, et al. Compromised HOXA5 function can limit expression in human breast tumours. Nature. (2000). Jun 22;405(6789):974-8., 53.

[85] Wu, X, Chen, H, Parker, B, Rubin, E, Zhu, T, Lee, J. S, et al. HOXB7, a homeodomain protein, is overexpressed in breast cancer and confers epithelial-mesenchymal transition. Cancer Res. (2006). Oct 1; , 66(19), 9527-34.

[86] Abdel-fattah, R, Xiao, A, Bomgardner, D, Pease, C. S, Lopes, M. B, & Hussaini, I. M. Differential expression of HOX genes in neoplastic and non-neoplastic human astrocytes. J Pathol. (2006). May; , 209(1), 15-24.

[87] Brandsma, D, Stalpers, L, Taal, W, & Sminia, P. van den Bent MJ. Clinical features, mechanisms, and management of pseudoprogression in malignant gliomas. Lancet Oncol. (2008). May; , 9(5), 453-61.

[88] Wen, P. Y, & Kesari, S. Malignant gliomas in adults. N Engl J Med. (2008). Jul 31; , 359(5), 492-507.

[89] Sorensen, A. G, Batchelor, T. T, Wen, P. Y, Zhang, W. T, & Jain, R. K. Response criteria for glioma. Nat Clin Pract Oncol. (2008). Nov; , 5(11), 634-44.

[90] van den Bent MJVogelbaum MA, Wen PY, Macdonald DR, Chang SM. End point assessment in gliomas: novel treatments limit usefulness of classical Macdonald's Criteria. J Clin Oncol. (2009). Jun 20; , 27(18), 2905-8.

[91] Tanwar, M. K, Gilbert, M. R, & Holland, E. C. Gene expression microarray analysis reveals YKL-40 to be a potential serum marker for malignant character in human glioma. Cancer Res. (2002). Aug 1; , 62(15), 4364-8.

[92] Bhat, K. P, Pelloski, C. E, Zhang, Y, & Kim, S. H. deLaCruz C, Rehli M, et al. Selective repression of YKL-40 by NF-kappaB in glioma cell lines involves recruitment of histone deacetylase-1 and-2. FEBS Lett. (2008). Sep 22;582(21-22):3193-200.

[93] Johansen, J. S, Schultz, N. A, & Jensen, B. V. Plasma YKL-40: a potential new cancer biomarker? Future Oncol. (2009). Sep; , 5(7), 1065-82.

[94] Shao, R, Hamel, K, Petersen, L, Cao, Q. J, Arenas, R. B, Bigelow, C, et al. YKL-40, a secreted glycoprotein, promotes tumor angiogenesis. Oncogene. (2009). Dec 17; , 28(50), 4456-68.

[95] Bernardi, D, Padoan, A, Ballin, A, Sartori, M, Manara, R, Scienza, R, et al. Serum YKL-40 following resection for cerebral glioblastoma. J Neurooncol. (2012). Apr; , 107(2), 299-305.

[96] Iwamoto, F. M, Hottinger, A. F, Karimi, S, Riedel, E, Dantis, J, Jahdi, M, et al. Serum YKL-40 is a marker of prognosis and disease status in high-grade gliomas. Neuro Oncol. (2011). Nov; , 13(11), 1244-51.

[97] Pelloski, C. E, Mahajan, A, Maor, M, Chang, E. L, Woo, S, Gilbert, M, et al. YKL-40 expression is associated with poorer response to radiation and shorter overall survival in glioblastoma. Clin Cancer Res. (2005). May 1; , 11(9), 3326-34.

[98] Bai, R. Y, Staedtke, V, & Riggins, G. J. Molecular targeting of glioblastoma: Drug discovery and therapies. Trends Mol Med. (2011). Jun; , 17(6), 301-12.

[99] Jones, T. S, & Holland, E. C. Standard of care therapy for malignant glioma and its effect on tumor and stromal cells. Oncogene. (2012). Apr 19; , 31(16), 1995-2006.

[100] Villano, J. L, Seery, T. E, & Bressler, L. R. Temozolomide in malignant gliomas: current use and future targets. Cancer Chemother Pharmacol. (2009). Sep; , 64(4), 647-55.

[101] Cohen, M. H, Shen, Y. L, Keegan, P, & Pazdur, R. FDA drug approval summary: bevacizumab (Avastin) as treatment of recurrent glioblastoma multiforme. The oncologist. (2009). Nov; , 14(11), 1131-8.

[102] Pan, E, Mitchell, S. B, & Tsai, J. S. A retrospective study of the safety of BCNU wafers with concurrent temozolomide and radiotherapy and adjuvant temozolomide for newly diagnosed glioblastoma patients. J Neurooncol. (2008). Jul; , 88(3), 353-7.

[103] Preusser, M, De Ribaupierre, S, Wohrer, A, Erridge, S. C, Hegi, M, Weller, M, et al. Current concepts and management of glioblastoma. Ann Neurol. (2011). Jul; , 70(1), 9-21.

[104] Mrugala, M. M, & Chamberlain, M. C. Mechanisms of disease: temozolomide and glioblastoma--look to the future. Nature clinical practice Oncology. (2008). Aug; , 5(8), 476-86.

[105] Stupp, R, Hegi, M. E, & Mason, W. P. van den Bent MJ, Taphoorn MJ, Janzer RC, et al. Effects of radiotherapy with concomitant and adjuvant temozolomide versus radiotherapy alone on survival in glioblastoma in a randomised phase III study: 5-year analysis of the EORTC-NCIC trial. Lancet Oncol. (2009). May; , 10(5), 459-66.

[106] Clarke, J, Butowski, N, & Chang, S. Recent advances in therapy for glioblastoma. Archives of neurology. (2010). Mar; , 67(3), 279-83.

[107] (FDA) USFaDABevacizumab Injection. [updated 03/08/(2012). Available from: http://www.fda.gov/AboutFDA/CentersOffices/OfficeofMedicalProductsandTobacco/CDER/ucm149364.htm.

[108] Hasselbalch, B, Lassen, U, Hansen, S, Holmberg, M, Sorensen, M, Kosteljanetz, M, et al. Cetuximab, bevacizumab, and irinotecan for patients with primary glioblastoma and progression after radiation therapy and temozolomide: a phase II trial. Neuro Oncol. (2010). May;, 12(5), 508-16.

[109] Lai, A, Tran, A, Nghiemphu, P. L, Pope, W. B, Solis, O. E, Selch, M, et al. Phase II study of bevacizumab plus temozolomide during and after radiation therapy for patients with newly diagnosed glioblastoma multiforme. J Clin Oncol. (2011). Jan 10; , 29(2), 142-8.

[110] Kreisl, T. N, Kim, L, Moore, K, Duic, P, Royce, C, Stroud, I, et al. Phase II trial of single-agent bevacizumab followed by bevacizumab plus irinotecan at tumor progression in recurrent glioblastoma. J Clin Oncol. (2009). Feb 10;, 27(5), 740-5.

[111] De Groot, J. F, Fuller, G, Kumar, A. J, Piao, Y, Eterovic, K, Ji, Y, et al. Tumor invasion after treatment of glioblastoma with bevacizumab: radiographic and pathologic correlation in humans and mice. Neuro Oncol. (2010). Mar;, 12(3), 233-42.

[112] Keunen, O, Johansson, M, Oudin, A, Sanzey, M, Rahim, S. A, Fack, F, et al. Anti-VEGF treatment reduces blood supply and increases tumor cell invasion in glioblastoma. Proc Natl Acad Sci U S A. (2011). Mar 1;, 108(9), 3749-54.

[113] Wick, W, Weller, M, Weiler, M, Batchelor, T, Yung, A. W, & Platten, M. Pathway inhibition: emerging molecular targets for treating glioblastoma. Neuro Oncol. (2011). Jun;, 13(6), 566-79.

[114] Kanu, O. O, Hughes, B, Di, C, Lin, N, Fu, J, Bigner, D. D, et al. Glioblastoma Multiforme Oncogenomics and Signaling Pathways. Clin Med Oncol. (2009). Apr 8; , 3, 39-52.

[115] Lemmon, M. A, & Schlessinger, J. Cell signaling by receptor tyrosine kinases. Cell. (2010). Jun 25;, 141(7), 1117-34.

[116] Van Meir, E. G, Hadjipanayis, C. G, Norden, A. D, Shu, H. K, Wen, P. Y, & Olson, J. J. Exciting new advances in neuro-oncology: the avenue to a cure for malignant glioma. CA Cancer J Clin. (2010). May-Jun;, 60(3), 166-93.

[117] Cohen, M. H, Johnson, J. R, Chen, Y. F, Sridhara, R, & Pazdur, R. FDA drug approval summary: erlotinib (Tarceva) tablets. The oncologist. (2005). Aug;, 10(7), 461-6.

[118] ClinicalTrialsgov- a service of the U.S. National Institutes of Health. [27 July (2012). Available from: www.clinicaltrials.gov.

[119] Polivka, J. Jr., Polivka J, Rohan V, Topolcan O, Ferda J. New molecularly targeted therapies for glioblastoma multiforme. Anticancer Res. (2012). Jul;, 32(7), 2935-46.

[120] Fukai, J, Nishio, K, Itakura, T, & Koizumi, F. Antitumor activity of cetuximab against malignant glioma cells overexpressing EGFR deletion mutant variant III. Cancer Sci. (2008). Oct; , 99(10), 2062-9.

[121] Martens, T, Laabs, Y, Gunther, H. S, Kemming, D, Zhu, Z, Witte, L, et al. Inhibition of glioblastoma growth in a highly invasive nude mouse model can be achieved by targeting epidermal growth factor receptor but not vascular endothelial growth factor receptor-2. Clin Cancer Res. (2008). Sep 1; , 14(17), 5447-58.

[122] Neyns, B, Sadones, J, Joosens, E, Bouttens, F, Verbeke, L, Baurain, J. F, et al. Stratified phase II trial of cetuximab in patients with recurrent high-grade glioma. Ann Oncol. (2009). Sep; , 20(9), 1596-603.

[123] Gan, H. K, Kaye, A. H, & Luwor, R. B. The EGFRvIII variant in glioblastoma multiforme. J Clin Neurosci. (2009). Jun; , 16(6), 748-54.

[124] Heimberger, A. B, & Sampson, J. H. The PEPvIII-KLH (CDX-110) vaccine in glioblastoma multiforme patients. Expert Opin Biol Ther. (2009). Aug; , 9(8), 1087-98.

[125] Sampson, J. H, Heimberger, A. B, Archer, G. E, Aldape, K. D, Friedman, A. H, Friedman, H. S, et al. Immunologic escape after prolonged progression-free survival with epidermal growth factor receptor variant III peptide vaccination in patients with newly diagnosed glioblastoma. J Clin Oncol. (2010). Nov 1; , 28(31), 4722-9.

[126] Reardon, D. A, Egorin, M. J, Quinn, J. A, Rich, J. N, Gururangan, S, Vredenburgh, J. J, et al. Phase II study of imatinib mesylate plus hydroxyurea in adults with recurrent glioblastoma multiforme. J Clin Oncol. (2005). Dec 20; , 23(36), 9359-68.

[127] Ranza, E, Mazzini, G, Facoetti, A, & Nano, R. In-vitro effects of the tyrosine kinase inhibitor imatinib on glioblastoma cell proliferation. J Neurooncol. (2010). Feb; , 96(3), 349-57.

[128] Kilic, T, Alberta, J. A, Zdunek, P. R, Acar, M, Iannarelli, P, & Reilly, O. T, et al. Intracranial inhibition of platelet-derived growth factor-mediated glioblastoma cell growth by an orally active kinase inhibitor of the 2-phenylaminopyrimidine class. Cancer Res. (2000). Sep 15; , 60(18), 5143-50.

[129] Reardon, D. A, Dresemann, G, Taillibert, S, & Campone, M. van den Bent M, Clement P, et al. Multicentre phase II studies evaluating imatinib plus hydroxyurea in patients with progressive glioblastoma. Br J Cancer. (2009). Dec 15; , 101(12), 1995-2004.

[130] Raymond, E, Brandes, A. A, Dittrich, C, Fumoleau, P, Coudert, B, Clement, P. M, et al. Phase II study of imatinib in patients with recurrent gliomas of various histologies: a European Organisation for Research and Treatment of Cancer Brain Tumor Group Study. J Clin Oncol. (2008). Oct 1; , 26(28), 4659-65.

[131] Wen, P. Y, Yung, W. K, Lamborn, K. R, Dahia, P. L, Wang, Y, Peng, B, et al. Phase I/II study of imatinib mesylate for recurrent malignant gliomas: North American Brain Tumor Consortium Study 99-08. Clin Cancer Res. (2006). Aug 15; , 12(16), 4899-907.

[132] Reardon, D. A, Egorin, M. J, Desjardins, A, Vredenburgh, J. J, Beumer, J. H, Lagattuta, T. F, et al. Phase I pharmacokinetic study of the vascular endothelial growth factor receptor tyrosine kinase inhibitor vatalanib (PTK787) plus imatinib and hydroxyurea for malignant glioma. Cancer. (2009). May 15; , 115(10), 2188-98.

[133] Agarwal, S, Sane, R, Oberoi, R, Ohlfest, J. R, & Elmquist, W. F. Delivery of molecularly targeted therapy to malignant glioma, a disease of the whole brain. Expert Rev Mol Med. (2011). e17.

[134] Gerstner, E. R, Chen, P. J, Wen, P. Y, Jain, R. K, Batchelor, T. T, & Sorensen, G. Infiltrative patterns of glioblastoma spread detected via diffusion MRI after treatment with cediranib. Neuro Oncol. (2010). May; , 12(5), 466-72.

[135] Kamoun, W. S, Ley, C. D, Farrar, C. T, Duyverman, A. M, Lahdenranta, J, Lacorre, D. A, et al. Edema control by cediranib, a vascular endothelial growth factor receptor-targeted kinase inhibitor, prolongs survival despite persistent brain tumor growth in mice. J Clin Oncol. (2009). May 20; , 27(15), 2542-52.

[136] Eder, J. P. Vande Woude GF, Boerner SA, LoRusso PM. Novel therapeutic inhibitors of the c-Met signaling pathway in cancer. Clin Cancer Res. (2009). Apr 1; , 15(7), 2207-14.

[137] Kong, D. S, Song, S. Y, Kim, D. H, Joo, K. M, Yoo, J. S, Koh, J. S, et al. Prognostic significance of c-Met expression in glioblastomas. Cancer. (2009). Jan 1; , 115(1), 140-8.

[138] De Bono, J. S. Yap TA. c-MET: an exciting new target for anticancer therapy. Ther Adv Med Oncol. (2011). Nov;3(1 Suppl):S , 3-5.

[139] Tabatabai, G, Weller, M, Nabors, B, Picard, M, Reardon, D, Mikkelsen, T, et al. Targeting integrins in malignant glioma. Target Oncol. (2010). Sep; , 5(3), 175-81.

[140] Loges, S, Butzal, M, Otten, J, Schweizer, M, Fischer, U, Bokemeyer, C, et al. Cilengitide inhibits proliferation and differentiation of human endothelial progenitor cells in vitro. Biochem Biophys Res Commun. (2007). Jun 15; , 357(4), 1016-20.

[141] Maurer, G. D, Tritschler, I, Adams, B, Tabatabai, G, Wick, W, Stupp, R, et al. Cilengitide modulates attachment and viability of human glioma cells, but not sensitivity to irradiation or temozolomide in vitro. Neuro Oncol. (2009). Dec; , 11(6), 747-56.

[142] Kreisl, T. N, Kim, L, Moore, K, Duic, P, Kotliarova, S, Walling, J, et al. A phase I trial of enzastaurin in patients with recurrent gliomas. Clin Cancer Res. (2009). May 15; , 15(10), 3617-23.

[143] Graff, J. R, Mcnulty, A. M, Hanna, K. R, Konicek, B. W, Lynch, R. L, Bailey, S. N, et al. The protein kinase Cbeta-selective inhibitor, Enzastaurin (LY317615.HCl), suppresses signaling through the AKT pathway, induces apoptosis, and suppresses growth of human colon cancer and glioblastoma xenografts. Cancer Res. (2005). Aug 15; , 65(16), 7462-9.

[144] Wick, W, Puduvalli, V. K, & Chamberlain, M. C. van den Bent MJ, Carpentier AF, Cher LM, et al. Phase III study of enzastaurin compared with lomustine in the treatment of recurrent intracranial glioblastoma. J Clin Oncol. (2010). Mar 1; , 28(7), 1168-74.

[145] Pitter, K. L, Galban, C. J, Galban, S, Tehrani, O. S, Li, F, Charles, N, et al. Perifosine and CCI 779 co-operate to induce cell death and decrease proliferation in PTEN-intact and PTEN-deficient PDGF-driven murine glioblastoma. PLoS One. (2011). e14545.

[146] Gills, J. J, Lopiccolo, J, & Dennis, P. A. Nelfinavir, a new anti-cancer drug with pleiotropic effects and many paths to autophagy. Autophagy. (2008). Jan; , 4(1), 107-9.

[147] Pyrko, P, Kardosh, A, Wang, W, Xiong, W, Schonthal, A. H, & Chen, T. C. HIV-1 protease inhibitors nelfinavir and atazanavir induce malignant glioma death by triggering endoplasmic reticulum stress. Cancer Res. (2007). Nov 15; , 67(22), 10920-8.

[148] Jiang, Z, Pore, N, Cerniglia, G. J, Mick, R, Georgescu, M. M, Bernhard, E. J, et al. Phosphatase and tensin homologue deficiency in glioblastoma confers resistance to radiation and temozolomide that is reversed by the protease inhibitor nelfinavir. Cancer Res. (2007). May 1; , 67(9), 4467-73.

[149] Pore, N, Gupta, A. K, Cerniglia, G. J, & Maity, A. HIV protease inhibitors decrease VEGF/HIF-1alpha expression and angiogenesis in glioblastoma cells. Neoplasia. (2006). Nov; , 8(11), 889-95.

[150] Yap, T. A, Garrett, M. D, Walton, M. I, Raynaud, F, De Bono, J. S, & Workman, P. Targeting the PI3K-AKT-mTOR pathway: progress, pitfalls, and promises. Curr Opin Pharmacol. (2008). Aug; , 8(4), 393-412.

[151] Han, L, Yang, Y, Yue, X, Huang, K, Liu, X, Pu, P, et al. Inactivation of PI3K/AKT signaling inhibits glioma cell growth through modulation of beta-catenin-mediated transcription. Brain Res. (2010). Dec 17; , 1366, 9-17.

[152] Chen, L, Han, L, Shi, Z, Zhang, K, Liu, Y, Zheng, Y, et al. LY294002 enhances cytotoxicity of temozolomide in glioma by down-regulation of the PI3K/Akt pathway. Mol Med Report. (2012). Feb; , 5(2), 575-9.

[153] Sunayama, J, Sato, A, Matsuda, K, Tachibana, K, Suzuki, K, Narita, Y, et al. Dual blocking of mTor and PI3K elicits a prodifferentiation effect on glioblastoma stem-like cells. Neuro Oncol. (2010). Dec; , 12(12), 1205-19.

[154] Wei, L. H, Su, H, Hildebrandt, I. J, Phelps, M. E, Czernin, J, & Weber, W. A. Changes in tumor metabolism as readout for Mammalian target of rapamycin kinase inhibition by rapamycin in glioblastoma. Clin Cancer Res. (2008). Jun 1; , 14(11), 3416-26.

[155] Goudar, R. K, Shi, Q, Hjelmeland, M. D, Keir, S. T, Mclendon, R. E, Wikstrand, C. J, et al. Combination therapy of inhibitors of epidermal growth factor receptor/vascular endothelial growth factor receptor 2 (AEE788) and the mammalian target of rapamy-

cin (RAD001) offers improved glioblastoma tumor growth inhibition. Mol Cancer Ther. (2005). Jan; , 4(1), 101-12.

[156] Liu, P, Cheng, H, Roberts, T. M, & Zhao, J. J. Targeting the phosphoinositide 3-kinase pathway in cancer. Nat Rev Drug Discov. (2009). Aug; , 8(8), 627-44.

[157] Chresta, C. M, Davies, B. R, Hickson, I, Harding, T, Cosulich, S, Critchlow, S. E, et al. AZD8055 is a potent, selective, and orally bioavailable ATP-competitive mammalian target of rapamycin kinase inhibitor with in vitro and in vivo antitumor activity. Cancer Res. (2010). Jan 1; , 70(1), 288-98.

[158] Yang, F, Brown, C, Buettner, R, Hedvat, M, Starr, R, Scuto, A, et al. Sorafenib induces growth arrest and apoptosis of human glioblastoma cells through the dephosphorylation of signal transducers and activators of transcription 3. Mol Cancer Ther. (2010). Apr; , 9(4), 953-62.

[159] Bolden, J. E, Peart, M. J, & Johnstone, R. W. Anticancer activities of histone deacetylase inhibitors. Nature reviews Drug discovery. (2006). Sep; , 5(9), 769-84.

[160] Xu, W. S, Parmigiani, R. B, & Marks, P. A. Histone deacetylase inhibitors: molecular mechanisms of action. Oncogene. (2007). Aug 13; , 26(37), 5541-52.

[161] Wagner, J. M, Hackanson, B, Lubbert, M, & Jung, M. Histone deacetylase (HDAC) inhibitors in recent clinical trials for cancer therapy. Clin Epigenetics. (2010). Dec;1(3-4): 117-36.

[162] Weller, M, Gorlia, T, & Cairncross, J. G. van den Bent MJ, Mason W, Belanger K, et al. Prolonged survival with valproic acid use in the EORTC/NCIC temozolomide trial for glioblastoma. Neurology. (2011). Sep 20; , 77(12), 1156-64.

[163] Dokmanovic, M, Clarke, C, & Marks, P. A. Histone deacetylase inhibitors: overview and perspectives. Mol Cancer Res. (2007). Oct; , 5(10), 981-9.

[164] Ryu, C. H, Yoon, W. S, Park, K. Y, Kim, S. M, Lim, J. Y, Woo, J. S, et al. Valproic Acid Downregulates the Expression of MGMT and Sensitizes Temozolomide-Resistant Glioma Cells. J Biomed Biotechnol. (2012).

[165] Van Nifterik, K. A. Van den Berg J, Slotman BJ, Lafleur MV, Sminia P, Stalpers LJ. Valproic acid sensitizes human glioma cells for temozolomide and gamma-radiation. J Neurooncol. (2012). Mar; , 107(1), 61-7.

[166] Chen, C. H, Chang, Y. J, Ku, M. S, Chung, K. T, & Yang, J. T. Enhancement of temozolomide-induced apoptosis by valproic acid in human glioma cell lines through redox regulation. J Mol Med (Berl). (2011). Mar; , 89(3), 303-15.

[167] Krishnan, S, Brown, P. D, Ballman, K. V, Fiveash, J. B, Uhm, J. H, Giannini, C, et al. Phase I trial of erlotinib with radiation therapy in patients with glioblastoma multiforme: results of North Central Cancer Treatment Group protocol N0177. Int J Radiat Oncol Biol Phys. (2006). Jul 15; , 65(4), 1192-9.

[168] De Groot, J. F, Gilbert, M. R, Aldape, K, Hess, K. R, Hanna, T. A, Ictech, S, et al. Phase II study of carboplatin and erlotinib (Tarceva, OSI-774) in patients with recurrent glioblastoma. J Neurooncol. (2008). Oct;, 90(1), 89-97.

[169] Prados, M. D, Chang, S. M, Butowski, N, Deboer, R, Parvataneni, R, Carliner, H, et al. Phase II study of erlotinib plus temozolomide during and after radiation therapy in patients with newly diagnosed glioblastoma multiforme or gliosarcoma. J Clin Oncol. (2009). Feb 1;, 27(4), 579-84.

[170] Raizer, J. J, Abrey, L. E, Lassman, A. B, Chang, S. M, Lamborn, K. R, Kuhn, J. G, et al. A phase II trial of erlotinib in patients with recurrent malignant gliomas and nonprogressive glioblastoma multiforme postradiation therapy. Neuro Oncol. (2010). Jan;, 12(1), 95-103.

[171] Raizer, J. J, Abrey, L. E, Lassman, A. B, Chang, S. M, Lamborn, K. R, Kuhn, J. G, et al. A phase I trial of erlotinib in patients with nonprogressive glioblastoma multiforme postradiation therapy, and recurrent malignant gliomas and meningiomas. Neuro Oncol. (2010). Jan;, 12(1), 87-94.

[172] Reardon, D. A, Desjardins, A, Vredenburgh, J. J, Gururangan, S, Friedman, A. H, Herndon, J. E, et al. Phase 2 trial of erlotinib plus sirolimus in adults with recurrent glioblastoma. J Neurooncol. (2010). Jan;, 96(2), 219-30.

[173] Sathornsumetee, S, Desjardins, A, Vredenburgh, J. J, Mclendon, R. E, Marcello, J, Herndon, J. E, et al. Phase II trial of bevacizumab and erlotinib in patients with recurrent malignant glioma. Neuro Oncol. (2010). Dec;, 12(12), 1300-10.

[174] van den Bent MJBrandes AA, Rampling R, Kouwenhoven MC, Kros JM, Carpentier AF, et al. Randomized phase II trial of erlotinib versus temozolomide or carmustine in recurrent glioblastoma: EORTC brain tumor group study 26034. J Clin Oncol. (2009). Mar 10;, 27(8), 1268-74.

[175] Brown, P. D, Krishnan, S, Sarkaria, J. N, Wu, W, Jaeckle, K. A, Uhm, J. H, et al. Phase I/II trial of erlotinib and temozolomide with radiation therapy in the treatment of newly diagnosed glioblastoma multiforme: North Central Cancer Treatment Group Study N0177. J Clin Oncol. (2008). Dec 1;, 26(34), 5603-9.

[176] Hegi, M. E, Diserens, A. C, Bady, P, Kamoshima, Y, Kouwenhoven, M. C, Delorenzi, M, et al. Pathway analysis of glioblastoma tissue after preoperative treatment with the EGFR tyrosine kinase inhibitor gefitinib--a phase II trial. Mol Cancer Ther. (2011). Jun;, 10(6), 1102-12.

[177] Rich, J. N, Reardon, D. A, Peery, T, Dowell, J. M, Quinn, J. A, Penne, K. L, et al. Phase II trial of gefitinib in recurrent glioblastoma. J Clin Oncol. (2004). Jan 1;, 22(1), 133-42.

[178] Uhm, J. H, Ballman, K. V, Wu, W, Giannini, C, Krauss, J. C, Buckner, J. C, et al. Phase II evaluation of gefitinib in patients with newly diagnosed Grade 4 astrocytoma:

Mayo/North Central Cancer Treatment Group Study N0074. Int J Radiat Oncol Biol Phys. (2011). Jun 1; , 80(2), 347-53.

[179] Razis, E, Selviaridis, P, Labropoulos, S, Norris, J. L, Zhu, M. J, Song, D. D, et al. Phase II study of neoadjuvant imatinib in glioblastoma: evaluation of clinical and molecular effects of the treatment. Clin Cancer Res. (2009). Oct 1; , 15(19), 6258-66.

[180] Dresemann, G, Weller, M, Rosenthal, M. A, Wedding, U, Wagner, W, Engel, E, et al. Imatinib in combination with hydroxyurea versus hydroxyurea alone as oral therapy in patients with progressive pretreated glioblastoma resistant to standard dose temozolomide. J Neurooncol. (2010). Feb; , 96(3), 393-402.

[181] Batchelor, T. T, & Duda, D. G. di Tomaso E, Ancukiewicz M, Plotkin SR, Gerstner E, et al. Phase II study of cediranib, an oral pan-vascular endothelial growth factor receptor tyrosine kinase inhibitor, in patients with recurrent glioblastoma. J Clin Oncol. (2010). Jun 10; , 28(17), 2817-23.

[182] Sorensen, A. G, Batchelor, T. T, Zhang, W. T, Chen, P. J, Yeo, P, Wang, M, et al. A "vascular normalization index" as potential mechanistic biomarker to predict survival after a single dose of cediranib in recurrent glioblastoma patients. Cancer Res. (2009). Jul 1; , 69(13), 5296-300.

[183] Wen, P. Y, Schiff, D, Cloughesy, T. F, Raizer, J. J, Laterra, J, Smitt, M, et al. A phase II study evaluating the efficacy and safety of AMG 102 (rilotumumab) in patients with recurrent glioblastoma. Neuro Oncol. (2011). Apr; , 13(4), 437-46.

[184] Butowski, N, Chang, S. M, Lamborn, K. R, Polley, M. Y, Pieper, R, Costello, J. F, et al. Phase II and pharmacogenomics study of enzastaurin plus temozolomide during and following radiation therapy in patients with newly diagnosed glioblastoma multiforme and gliosarcoma. Neuro Oncol. (2011). Dec; , 13(12), 1331-8.

[185] Kreisl, T. N, Kotliarova, S, Butman, J. A, Albert, P. S, Kim, L, Musib, L, et al. A phase I/II trial of enzastaurin in patients with recurrent high-grade gliomas. Neuro Oncol. (2010). Feb; , 12(2), 181-9.

[186] Hainsworth, J. D, Shih, K. C, Shepard, G. C, Tillinghast, G. W, Brinker, B. T, & Spigel, D. R. Phase II Study of Concurrent Radiation Therapy, Temozolomide, and Bevacizumab Followed by Bevacizumab/Everolimus as First-Line Treatment for Patients With Glioblastoma. Clin Adv Hematol Oncol. (2012). Apr; , 10(4), 240-6.

[187] Mason, W. P, Macneil, M, Kavan, P, Easaw, J, Macdonald, D, Thiessen, B, et al. A phase I study of temozolomide and everolimus (RAD001) in patients with newly diagnosed and progressive glioblastoma either receiving or not receiving enzyme-inducing anticonvulsants: an NCIC CTG study. Invest New Drugs. (2011). Dec 9.

[188] Sarkaria, J. N, Galanis, E, Wu, W, Peller, P. J, Giannini, C, Brown, P. D, et al. North Central Cancer Treatment Group Phase I trial N057K of everolimus (RAD001) and temozolomide in combination with radiation therapy in patients with newly diag-

nosed glioblastoma multiforme. Int J Radiat Oncol Biol Phys. (2011). Oct 1; , 81(2), 468-75.

[189] Galanis, E, Buckner, J. C, Maurer, M. J, Kreisberg, J. I, Ballman, K, Boni, J, et al. Phase II trial of temsirolimus (CCI-779) in recurrent glioblastoma multiforme: a North Central Cancer Treatment Group Study. J Clin Oncol. (2005). Aug 10; , 23(23), 5294-304.

[190] Sarkaria, J. N, Galanis, E, Wu, W, Dietz, A. B, Kaufmann, T. J, Gustafson, M. P, et al. Combination of temsirolimus (CCI-779) with chemoradiation in newly diagnosed glioblastoma multiforme (GBM) (NCCTG trial N027D) is associated with increased infectious risks. Clin Cancer Res. (2010). Nov 15; , 16(22), 5573-80.

[191] Cloughesy, T. F, Yoshimoto, K, Nghiemphu, P, Brown, K, Dang, J, Zhu, S, et al. Antitumor activity of rapamycin in a Phase I trial for patients with recurrent PTEN-deficient glioblastoma. PLoS Med. (2008). Jan 22;5(1):e8.

[192] Lustig, R, Mikkelsen, T, Lesser, G, Grossman, S, Ye, X, Desideri, S, et al. Phase II preradiation R115777 (tipifarnib) in newly diagnosed GBM with residual enhancing disease. Neuro Oncol. (2008). Dec; , 10(6), 1004-9.

[193] Nghiemphu, P. L, Wen, P. Y, Lamborn, K. R, Drappatz, J, Robins, H. I, Fink, K, et al. A phase I trial of tipifarnib with radiation therapy, with and without temozolomide, for patients with newly diagnosed glioblastoma. Int J Radiat Oncol Biol Phys. (2011). Dec 1; , 81(5), 1422-7.

[194] Cloughesy, T. F, Wen, P. Y, Robins, H. I, Chang, S. M, Groves, M. D, Fink, K. L, et al. Phase II trial of tipifarnib in patients with recurrent malignant glioma either receiving or not receiving enzyme-inducing antiepileptic drugs: a North American Brain Tumor Consortium Study. J Clin Oncol. (2006). Aug 1; , 24(22), 3651-6.

[195] Moyal, E. C, Laprie, A, Delannes, M, Poublanc, M, Catalaa, I, Dalenc, F, et al. Phase I trial of tipifarnib (R115777) concurrent with radiotherapy in patients with glioblastoma multiforme. Int J Radiat Oncol Biol Phys. (2007). Aug 1; , 68(5), 1396-401.

[196] Hainsworth, J. D, Ervin, T, Friedman, E, Priego, V, Murphy, P. B, Clark, B. L, et al. Concurrent radiotherapy and temozolomide followed by temozolomide and sorafenib in the first-line treatment of patients with glioblastoma multiforme. Cancer. (2010). Aug 1; , 116(15), 3663-9.

[197] Reardon, D. A, Vredenburgh, J. J, Desjardins, A, Peters, K, Gururangan, S, Sampson, J. H, et al. Effect of CYP3A-inducing anti-epileptics on sorafenib exposure: results of a phase II study of sorafenib plus daily temozolomide in adults with recurrent glioblastoma. J Neurooncol. (2011). Jan; , 101(1), 57-66.

[198] Nabors, L. B, Mikkelsen, T, Rosenfeld, S. S, Hochberg, F, Akella, N. S, Fisher, J. D, et al. Phase I and correlative biology study of cilengitide in patients with recurrent malignant glioma. J Clin Oncol. (2007). May 1; , 25(13), 1651-7.

[199] Reardon, D. A, Fink, K. L, Mikkelsen, T, Cloughesy, T. F, Neill, O, & Plotkin, A. S, et al. Randomized phase II study of cilengitide, an integrin-targeting arginine-glycine-

aspartic acid peptide, in recurrent glioblastoma multiforme. J Clin Oncol. (2008). Dec 1; , 26(34), 5610-7.

[200] Stupp, R, Hegi, M. E, Neyns, B, Goldbrunner, R, Schlegel, U, Clement, P. M, et al. Phase I/IIa study of cilengitide and temozolomide with concomitant radiotherapy followed by cilengitide and temozolomide maintenance therapy in patients with newly diagnosed glioblastoma. J Clin Oncol. (2010). Jun 1; , 28(16), 2712-8.

[201] Friday, B. B, Anderson, S. K, Buckner, J, Yu, C, Giannini, C, Geoffroy, F, et al. Phase II trial of vorinostat in combination with bortezomib in recurrent glioblastoma: a north central cancer treatment group study. Neuro Oncol. (2012). Feb; , 14(2), 215-21.

[202] Galanis, E, Jaeckle, K. A, Maurer, M. J, Reid, J. M, Ames, M. M, Hardwick, J. S, et al. Phase II trial of vorinostat in recurrent glioblastoma multiforme: a north central cancer treatment group study. J Clin Oncol. (2009). Apr 20; , 27(12), 2052-8.

[203] Iwamoto, F. M, Lamborn, K. R, Kuhn, J. G, Wen, P. Y, Yung, W. K, Gilbert, M. R, et al. A phase I/II trial of the histone deacetylase inhibitor romidepsin for adults with recurrent malignant glioma: North American Brain Tumor Consortium Study 03-03. Neuro Oncol. (2011). May; , 13(5), 509-16.

[204] Eramo, A, Ricci-vitiani, L, Zeuner, A, Pallini, R, Lotti, F, Sette, G, et al. Chemotherapy resistance of glioblastoma stem cells. Cell Death Differ. (2006). Jul; , 13(7), 1238-41.

[205] Verma, I. M, & Weitzman, M. D. Gene therapy: twenty-first century medicine. Annu Rev Biochem. (2005). , 74, 711-38.

[206] Kroeger, K. M, Muhammad, A. K, Baker, G. J, Assi, H, Wibowo, M. K, Xiong, W, et al. Gene therapy and virotherapy: novel therapeutic approaches for brain tumors. Discov Med. (2010). Oct; , 10(53), 293-304.

[207] Castro, M. G, Candolfi, M, Kroeger, K, King, G. D, Curtin, J. F, Yagiz, K, et al. Gene therapy and targeted toxins for glioma. Curr Gene Ther. (2011). Jun; , 11(3), 155-80.

[208] Lesniak, M. S. Gene therapy for malignant glioma. Expert Rev Neurother. (2006). Apr; , 6(4), 479-88.

[209] Colombo, F, Barzon, L, Franchin, E, Pacenti, M, Pinna, V, Danieli, D, et al. Combined HSV-TK/IL-2 gene therapy in patients with recurrent glioblastoma multiforme: biological and clinical results. Cancer Gene Ther. (2005). Oct; , 12(10), 835-48.

[210] Vanneman, M, & Dranoff, G. Combining immunotherapy and targeted therapies in cancer treatment. Nat Rev Cancer. (2012). Apr; , 12(4), 237-51.

[211] Yong, R. L, & Lonser, R. R. Immunotherapy trials for glioblastoma multiforme: promise and pitfalls. World Neurosurg. (2012). May;77(5-6):636-8.

[212] Liau, L. M, Prins, R. M, Kiertscher, S. M, Odesa, S. K, Kremen, T. J, Giovannone, A. J, et al. Dendritic cell vaccination in glioblastoma patients induces systemic and intra-

http://dx.doi.org/10.5772/52361

cranial T-cell responses modulated by the local central nervous system tumor microenvironment. Clin Cancer Res. (2005). Aug 1; , 11(15), 5515-25.

[213] Yamanaka, R, Homma, J, Yajima, N, Tsuchiya, N, Sano, M, Kobayashi, T, et al. Clinical evaluation of dendritic cell vaccination for patients with recurrent glioma: results of a clinical phase I/II trial. Clin Cancer Res. (2005). Jun 1; , 11(11), 4160-7.

[214] Jackson, C, Ruzevick, J, Phallen, J, Belcaid, Z, & Lim, M. Challenges in immunotherapy presented by the glioblastoma multiforme microenvironment. Clin Dev Immunol. 2011;(2011).

Section 4

Novel Anticancer Agents

Chapter 15

A Rational for Novel Anti-NeuroOncology Drugs

Lee Roy Morgan

Additional information is available at the end of the chapter

http://dx.doi.org/10.5772/53889

1. Introduction

Glioblastoma multiforme (GBM) is the most prevalent and lethal type of primary central nervous system tumors with a medium survival of 10-12 months, even with aggressive surgery, radiation and advanced chemotherapy [1]. Poor prognosis of patients with GBM has recently been connected with elevated expressions of a sphingosine kinase [2].

Although, GBM is an extremely lethal cancer, metastatic cancers to the brain from other organs are the most common intracranial tumors, out numbering GBM and other primary brain tumors by at least 10-fold [3]. Lung, breast and melanoma are the 1, 2, 3 most common cancers that metastasize to the brain [4]. The prognosis for these patients is worse than for primary CNS malignancies – 3.7 *vs.*10-12 months for GBM [5].

Intracranial tumors, primary as well as metastatic, are increasing at an alarming rate since many patients with excellent quality of life who appear to have 'beaten the odds' develop metastatic disease to the brain after years of remission from breast and other cancers [3-6]. The development of CNS metastasis results in progressive physical and cognitive impairment and culminates in death within a few months of diagnosis.

In the US alone, the incidence of brain metastasis is expected to exceed 200,000 cases in 2012 – more than 20 times the incidence of primary high grade brain tumors. The median survival time for metastatic cancer to the brain is 2-3 months and with aggressive therapy – maybe 4-12 months [6]!

Over the past 25 years, approximately 4-25 MM cancer patients have died with brain metastasis! These staggering facts strengthen a plea for developing new treatments for both primary and secondary cancers of the brain.

There are many reasons so few drugs are available to treat CNS cancers. Classically patients with brain metastasis have been excluded from clinical trials because of their poor prognosis; the FDA has always had concerns regarding patient safety during Phase I trials with unknown drugs that may cause CNS toxicity and finally once a new drug is identified to have activity in non CNS cancer involvement, few sponsors want to risk the potential hazards of toxicity that could result from treating patients with CNS involvement – primary or metastatic. Thus, there have been limited attempts to develop drugs for patients with brain metastasis, as well as primary brain tumors. The problem has been compounded by the lack of attention to CNS drug distribution and penetration of brain tumors, with reduction in toxicities.

Thus, there is a major need for the development of unique anticancer molecules that are able to cross the blood brain barrier (BBB), initiate anticancer activity in the CNS tumors and are non-neurotoxicity.

2. Landscape analysis of drugs available for brain tumors

- **Temodar** (temozolamide, TMZ (Schering-Plough,) is currently approved and marketed by Schering-Plough for the treatment of high-grade glioblastoma multiforme and refractory anaplastic astrocytoma in both in combination with radiation.
- **Gliadel** (BCNU wafer, Eisai) is an implantable wafer also used for the treatment of primary brain tumors.
- **Avastin** (bevacizumab, Genentech/Roche) is an anti-angiogenic inhibitor that is being combined with other agents that can penetrate the BBB. Combinations such as *Avastin* plus *Camptosar* (*irinotecan/CPT-11*) +/- *Temodar* are in trials.
- **Tarceva** (erlotinib, OSI Pharmaceuticals), was granted FDA orphan drug designation in August 2003 for patients with malignant gliomas, a recent study of Tarceva found 16% of patients with malignant gliomas who were given Tarciva alone or in combination with Temodar showed tumor shrinkage. The main side effect was an acne-like rash.
- **Iressa** (gefitinib, AstraZeneca) and has been approved for relapsing non-small cell lung cancer. A recent phase II trial of Iressa in patients with relapsed glioblastoma resulted in one of 52 patients achieving a partial response and 22 patients achieving stable disease. Side effects were limited to rash and diarrhea.
- **Zarnestra** (tipifarnib, Johnson & Johnson Pharmaceutical) is in early phase trials for brain tumors. The drug is also being studied in patients with leukemia and breast or lung cancers.
- **81C6** is a tenascin radioactive monoclonal antibody that is injected into a cavity created by the neurosurgeon after removal of the tumor. The antibodies deliver radiation to kill the tumor cells with less radiation to normal brain tissue than conventional radiotherapy. The product is under development at Duke Comprehensive Cancer Center.
- **BMS-247550** (Bristol Myers Squibb) is in Phase II/III @ Memorial Sloan-Kettering.

- **Ipilimumab** (yervoy, Bristol Myers Squibb) a monoclonal antibody to CTLA-4 has activity in melanoma with improved PFS.
- **Vemurafenib** (zelboraf, Genentech) is a BRAF inhibitor approved to treat melanoma, however, CNS mets were excluded in the trials, so the drug is being checked formally now.
- Cisplatin + etoposide, capecitabine (Xeloda), etc. – TTP/PFS - 3 mos max
- Dabrafenib and trametinib have delayed melanoma progression (GlaxoSmithKline)
- And others .... [7-9]

3. A new approach to new novel agents for – 1° and 2° brain tumors

The current trend to develop 'personalized therapy' based on the presence of specific phenotypic or genotypic pathways is an improved approach over the structure activity relationships (SAR) of the 20th century medicinal chemists [10]. However, the management of unresectable brain tumors has not improved. There is still a deficit in drugs that cross the blood brain barrier (BBB), are not recycled out of the brain, are effective anticancer agents in the CNS and do not require hepatic activation. Most of the 21st century *'personalized medicine'* drugs are large molecules that are given with other drugs and are ionizable chemicals that cannot penetrate the BBB and/or recycled out of the brain.

A suggested platform for new novel agents – that might be effective therapies for brain tumors comes from the earlier 20th century literature that focused on – *'the energy of cancer cells vs. normal cells'* [11-13].

Brain tumor biochemistry began in 1930 with Warburg's publication - *The Metabolism of Tumors* [12]. The fundamental finding of this publication was that embryonic and tumor tissues have in common a high glycolytic metabolism even under aerobic conditions; in contrast to most normal tissue where oxidative metabolism predominates. The oxidative metabolism in cells is generally 16 x more economical in respect to energy than the glycolytic pathway. The Embden-Meyerhof glycolytic pathway is phylogenetically the more primitive form [12]. *In rapidly growing de-differentiated tissue, this pathway prevails over oxidative metabolism.*

These concepts are of interest because the energy for a healthy cell is generated from glucose where 36 ATP molecules are produced from 1 glucose molecule. Hydrolysis of ATP results in a free energy change of ~ -16,000 cal/ATP molecule, depending on the conditions.

Classically cancer cells generate 2 ATP/1 glucose molecule *vs.* 36 ATP/1 glucose molecule (for healthy normal cells) – with the end product of pyruvate, rather than CO_2 and water as occurs in healthy cells [12]. Otto Warburg explained the latter as a result of the cancer cell's energy-transfer conversion to aerobic glycolysis, a major shift in energy available for cellular work [12].

Albert Szent-Gyorgyi referred to the energy differences of cancer cells *vs.* normal cells as – the *alpha* (α) state with $\uparrow\Delta S$ and $\downarrow\Delta F$ *vs.* the *beta* state (β), with $\downarrow\Delta S$ and $\uparrow\Delta F$), resp. [13].

The α state is the ground state of life! The most stable state of any system is with minimum ΔF and maximum ΔS. If the cellular organization becomes unstable, cells will return to an α state and remain there. The more complete the return – the harder it will be to reverse.

The β state is where there is a high degree of differentiation and potential for release of F if the cells react and initiate differentiation. Here the energy present allow cellular regulation and multicellular organisms replication; not a mass of undifferentiated cells – cancer.

[Where, S = entropy or potential (stored capacity) for a reaction to occur and F (free energy), a state of function depending only on the initial and final states of a system [14].

The importance of ΔF is that the value immediately provides quantitative information about the potential ability of a substance to undergo a chemical or physical transformation. A reaction may proceed spontaneously without external energy only if the ΔF is negative (energy dissipated) [14]. Chemical thermodynamics tells us that "*F needs to be a released in order for the cell to be productive and do work, not just replicate with a low productive reactivity*" [13].

We should view entropy as an index of a condition or character. It is an index of the capacity for spontaneous changes. By historical accident, the index was actually defined so that it *increased* as the capacity of an isolated system for spontaneous change *decreased*.

Hence, entropy is an index of exhaustion. The more a system has lost its capacity for spontaneous change, the greater is the entropy [14].

Yes, cancer cells represent a primitive, high random energy, low functional state with unbridled proliferation [13]. Cancer cells are not sick or weak, their vitality, as a wild type, may be even higher than that of a normal cell.

The cancer cell is unable to rebuild its beta state after it has completed its division and has to persist in the proliferative alpha state until death. In itself, the proliferative state would not be pathological – it is only its timing and irreversibility, which makes it so. *It is not pathological to be an infant, but it is pathological to be one and remain so x 50 years!*

Is cancer an outward manifestation resulting from depletion in cellular free energy within cells and increased entropy?

Although oxygen is considered essential for life, sulfur (S) and phosphorus (P) are the most common biological selections for energy transfer. The latter two elements are members of the Third Period of the Periodic Table and are capable of accepting an additional pair of electrons into unoccupied *3d* orbitals. This phenomenon is characteristic of the elements of the Third Period, which possess *d,* in addition to *s* and *p* orbitals, and thus have a place to hold electrons beyond the normal outer-shell octet. Molecules that possess P or S can store electrons (energy) and then release the energy during the transfer of shared electrons to other electron deficient molecules [15].

ATP (Fig. 1) is a unique example of how a 3rd Period element - 'P' participates in a key natural energy-rich compound, which upon hydrolysis generates ~ 8 kcal/mole upon hydrolysis with a +ΔF. When hydrolyzed in the presence of suitable transformers (transducing systems), the energy liberated may be used for cellular or tissue processes – cellular metabolism, nerve conduction, cell membrane transport, etc.

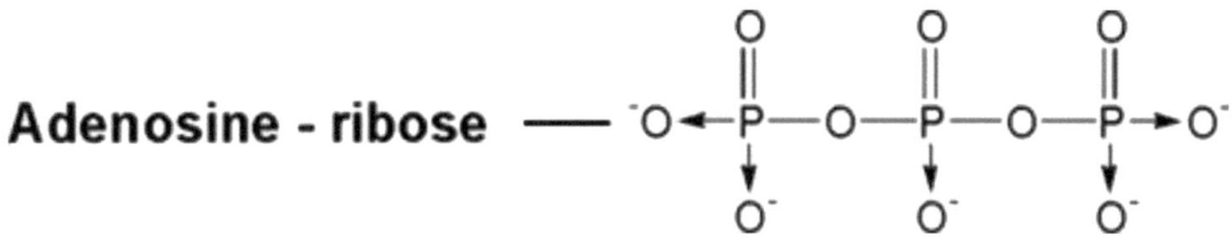

Figure 1. Adenosine triphosphate (ATP)

Energy rich phosphates usually possess either a second phosphoryl group or a resonating organic radical capable of entering into conjugation with the mobile electrons. This type of molecule usually contains a chain of at least three adjacent atoms, all bearing a net positive charge (deficient in π electrons), the chain sometimes extends over a five or even six atoms [Fig. 2], [16].

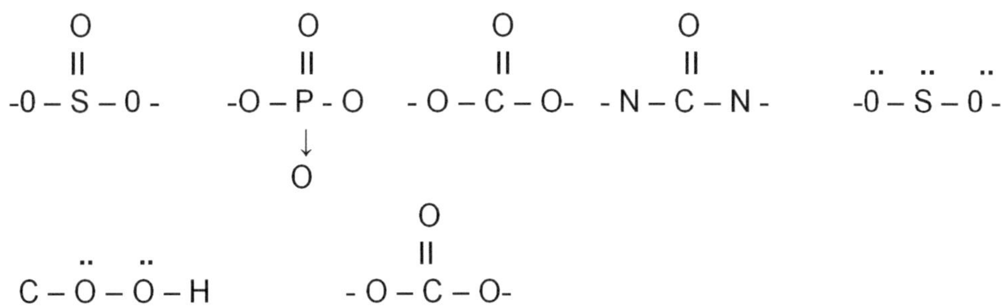

Figure 2. Examples of 3-atom high-energy moieties

Many of the small molecules used as anti-CNS cancer agents also possess 3-atom high energy moieties (in red) [3]

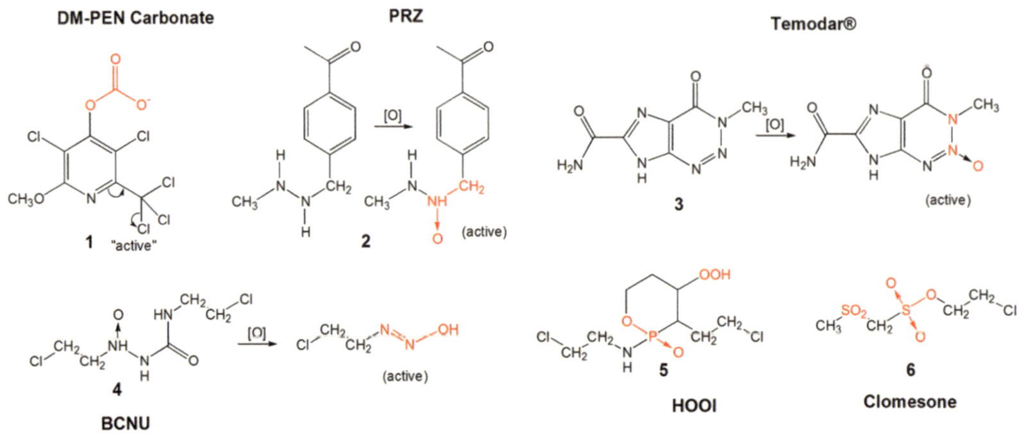

Figure 3. Small Molecules that are used to treat CNS cancer

Where: **DM-PEN carbonate**, 1 is a carbonate analog of 4-demethyl penclomedine; **PRZ**, 2 is dacarbazine; **Temodar®**, 3 is temozolamide (TMZ); **BCNU**, 4 is bis-(chloroethyl)nitrosourea; **HOOI**, 5 is 4-hydroperoxyifosfamide; **Clomesone**, 6 is a chloroethylating agent similar to BCNU – alkylates guanine-O^6 [17].

Compounds can be classified as "energy-rich" or "energy-poor" based on their ΔF. Energy poor compounds do not possess more than two adjacent atoms bearing a positive charge and poorly absorbed by the CNS.

Thus, the design of "high-energy molecules" that are lipophilic, energetic and absorbed into a low free energy (ΔF) and high entropy (ΔS) cancer environment are timely. The latter is a unique therapeutic target – *the result of inefficient energy of cancer cells* [14].

Life is controlled by the transfer of energy. All living systems obey the 1st law of thermodynamics – which states that the sum of all energies in an isolated system remains constant. Energy may be converted into another form but the quantity can be neither created nor destroyed [18].

A question to be answered – are high energy compounds really attracted to low energy highly utilized regions in the body?

4. Polyhalogenated pyridyl carbonates [16, 19-21]

The polyhalogenated pyridyl carbonates are neutral molecules that when coupled with lipids via high energy linkers – carbonates, phosphates, etc., fulfill the above requirements for novel high energy anticancer agents that could be attracted to and accumulate in CNS cancer tissue [16, 19-21]. The carbonate moiety like phosphate has the properties (resonance) of the high energy 3-atom moieties described in Fig. 3.

DEKK-TEC has designed a series of polychlorinated pyridyl carbonates (with 1 as a template, Fig. 3) that are linked with lipids and lipophilic moieties to promote CNS penetration [19]. DM-CHOC-PEN (4-demethyl-4-cholesteryloxycarbonylpenclomedine) is the most active and stable member of a large series of carbonates with improved activity vs. intracranially (IC) implanted human xenograft models – U251 and D54 glioblastoma and MX-1 breast cancer [Table 1] [19].

DM-CHOC-PEN is a unique molecule with several functional moieties that enable it to inhibit cancer replication. The structure contains the following moieties of interest:

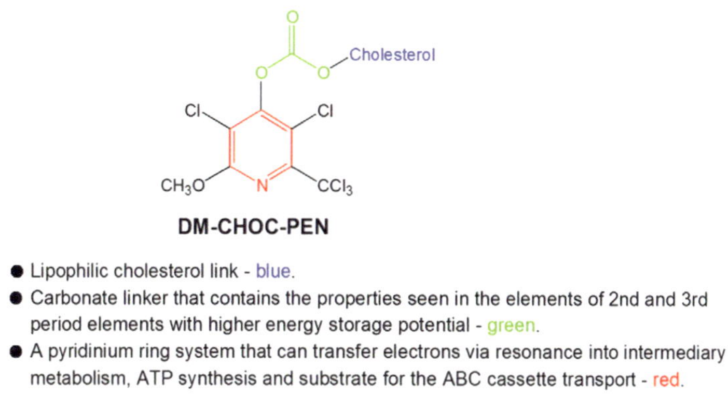

Figure 4. Lipophilic cholesterol link - blue. Carbonate linker that contains the properties seen in the elements of 2nd and 3rd period elements with higher energz storage potential - green. A pyridinium ring system that can transfer electrons via resonance into intermediary metabolism, ATP synthesis and substrate for the ABC cassette transport / red

The importance of the carbonate moiety is its internal energy and ability to transfer electrons through multiple structures (resonance) (see Fig. 5):

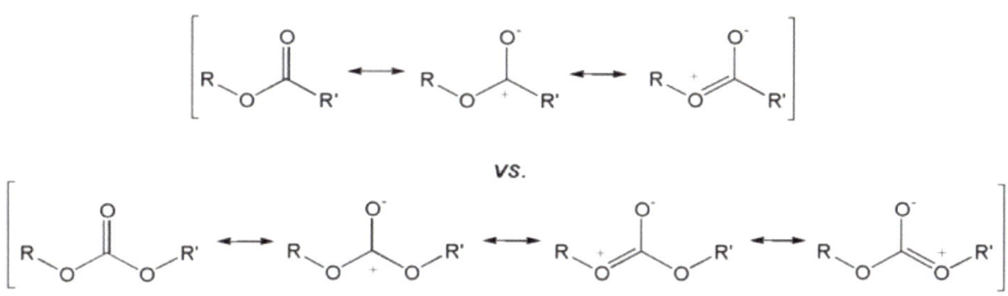

Figure 5. Mesomeric forms of the carbonate; where R = pyridyl group & R'=cholesterol

The additional oxygen in the carbonates [Fig. 5, lower structures] stabilizes the moiety and allows for distribution of charge through resonance (Fig. 5). This chemical property exists in the phosphates and other oxides of the 3rd period elements [see below] [15].

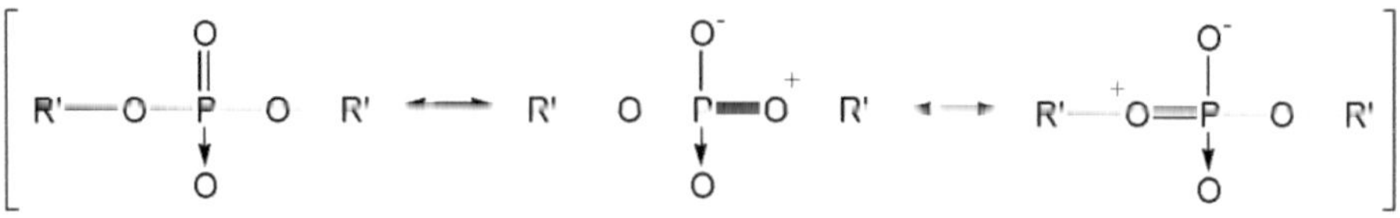

Scheme 1.

In contrast, esters lack the degree of resonance/electron distribution [Fig. 5, upper structures].

As indicated in Fig. 5, a carbonate is not isosteric with an acyl or ester group nor is it a direct extension of an ester group. The carbonate group is unique and when combined with cholesterol its CNS penetration properties are enhanced [Table 1] [16].

	DM-CHOC-PEN			BCNU			TMZ		
Tumor	*Dose	%ILS	%LTS	+Dose	%ILS	%LTS	#Dos	%ILS	%LTS
U251 Glioblastoma	135	+54	+20(1/5 CR)	9	52	+20(1/5 CR)	120	+54	+20(1/5 CR)
D54 Glioblastoma	200	+3	+20(1/5 CR)	NA	NA	NA	NA	NA	NA
MX-1 Breast Cancer	50 100	+20 Toxic	17(1/6 CR)	60	12	0/5	NA	NA	NA

Table 1. Activity of DM-CHOC-PEN vs. Intracerebrally Implanted Xenograft Tumors in Mice

Implant: 10^6 cells IC; Treatment Route: Intraperitoneal (- 5 days post IC implant); Schedule: *IV q1d x 5d; +IV q1d x 3d; #po 1d x 5d; Species: Athymic NCr/nu mice – female, Charles River; Dose: mg/kg; %ILS = % increased life span; %LTS = long term survival; all studies were terminated at 54 days

Based on the preclinical antitumor activities in Table 1, DM-CHOC-PEN produced a moderate increase in life span (% ILS); however it was comparable to that seen with BCNU and TMZ. DM-CHOC-PEN did yield long-term survivors that were healthy with no weight loss. Even the highly resistant IC implanted D54 glioma was sensitive to DM-CHOC-PEN. The drug has minimal toxicity and has encouraging potential [16, 19, 21].

An *in vivo* activation mechanism scheme is shown in Fig. 6, where DM-CHOC-PEN is proposed to be acting as a non-classical alkylating agent. The scheme describes a dual carbonium ion - DNA cross-linking mechanism (in a G-X-C sequence) with tumor DNA in the major groove via N^7- guanine [20]. A bi-molecular coupled product (*via* the trichloromethylene group) has been identified as the major microsomal metabolite of PEN

[20]. The trichloromethylene group is required, since the dichloromethylene analog of PEN is not active [does not react with 4-(*p*-nitrobenzyl) pyridine (NBP] (Struck, personnel communication).

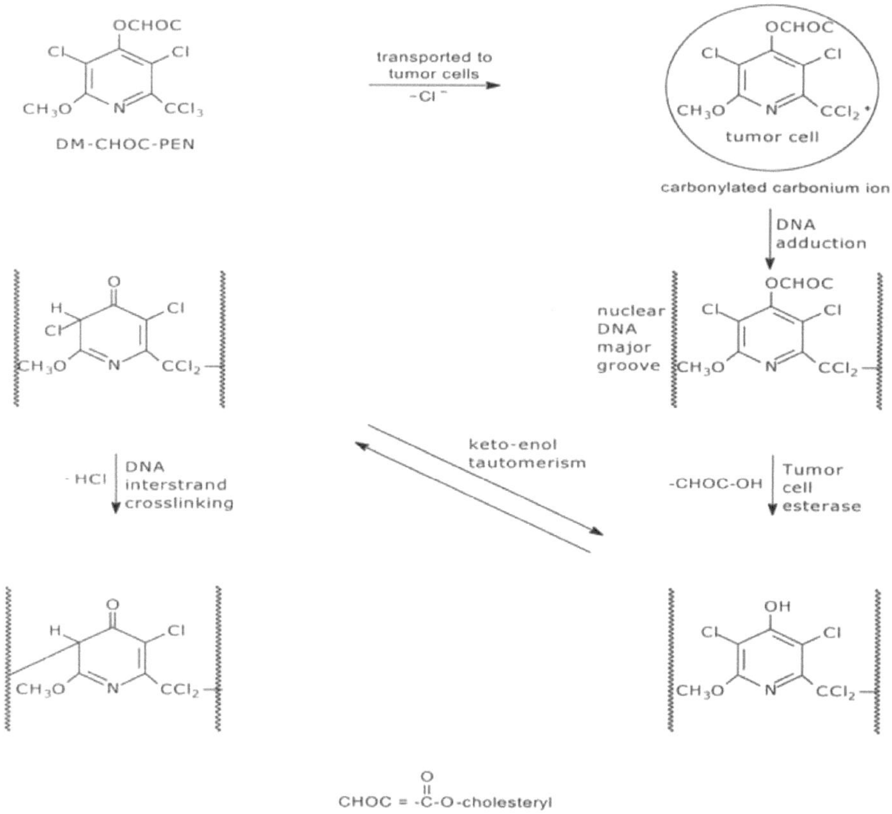

Figure 6. Proposed mechanism of action of 4 - demethyl - 4 - cholesterolyl - penclomedine (DM - CHOC - PEN)

Mice with IC growing U251 gliomas were treated with DM-CHOC-PEN, 135 mg/kg daily x 5-days and after 3-days the animals were sacrificed and the brains with tumors removed. The tumors were easily separated from the normal brain tissue. Each was homogenized in phosphate buffer, extracted with dichloromethane, and evaporated to dryness. The residues were assayed by HPLC and DM-CHOC-PEN, a guanine-N^7-CCl_2-adduct with DM-CHOC-PEN involving the $-CCl_3$ moiety and the DM-CHCO-PEN dimer-Cl_2C-CCl_2- were identified in the glioma tissue [16]. Neither DM-CHOC-PEN nor metabolites could be identified in the normal brain tissue.

Thus, DM-CHOC-PEN alkylates DNA with adducts at guanine-N^7 that could be quantitated in tumor tissue. The above MOA is in contrast to TMZ, BCNU and others, which alkylate guanine-O^6 [22].

The polyhalogenated pyridyl carbonates are unique structures that cross the BBB, accumulate in CNS tumor tissue, not normal brain tissue and are not recycled out of the CNS are cytotoxic *vs.* intracranially (IC) implanted human tumor xenografts in mouse models; fulfilling all of the criteria of the preceding paragraphs [23].

The combinations of responses in mouse xenograft tumor models, and a lack of neurotoxicity in rat and dog biopsychology studies, have allowed a Phase I trial to be conducted with DM- CHOC-PEN in patients with advanced cancer, including CNS involvement - IND 68,876 [24].

DEKK-TEC and its clinical investigators have satisfied the FDA that they are capable of treating patients with Phase I drugs and diagnosing physical and mental/cognitive alterations that may be associated with CNS tumor growth vs. toxicity secondary to drugs.

5. Phase I clinical trial with a high energy drug – DM-CHOC-PEN

Weiner, Ware, Friedlander, et al. reported preliminary data from a Phase I trial involving 18-patients treated with DM-CHOC-PEN in single IV doses of 39-87.5 mg/m^2 once every 21-days [25]. Six [6] patients had either CNS or spinal nervous system (SNS) involvement. Most patients had multiple treatments. The longest survivor (a sarcoma w/ SNS involvement) is 19+ months with NED [who also received doxorubicin at a later time] [25].

Support for DM-CHOC-PEN crossing the blood brain barrier in humans is provided from the above trial with reported observations for – GBM, CNS melanoma and breast cancer (BC) having PFS 4-13 mos., objective reductions in tumor sizes and no CNS toxicity.

One patient with pelvic sarcoma spread to the spinal cord required debulking surgery 21-days post treatment with DM-CHOC-PEN (39 mg/m^2). Tumor tissue was removed, assayed and DM-CHOC-PEN was quantitated in the spinal sarcoma tissue – 92 ng/g of tumor [25].

The only SLTs noted to date are hyperbilirubinemia in 2-patients with liver metastasis; patients with no liver pathology have not demonstrated SLTs. CNS toxicity has not been noted in any of the patients. Overall, the drug was reported as being tolerated very well [25].

6. CNS melanoma

Melanoma is the third most frequent cancer to metastasize to the brain. It is anticipated that there will be ~ 20,000 new cases of CNS stage melanoma diagnosed in 2012 [9]. Enrollment of these patients with CNS melanoma would be critical to appreciating the activity of the demethylpenclomedine carbonates in this stage of disease [9, 26]. Two of the patients enrolled and treated in the DM-CHOC-PEN Phase I trial had CNS melanoma; one patient had significant shrinkage of CNS lesions, the other stable (NC) disease [25].

To test the potential sensitivity of DM-CHOC-PEN as therapy for melanoma, the B-16 mouse melanoma was selected as a screening model and treated with DM-CHOC-PEN *in vitro* and *in vivo* [28].

7. Experimental methods

In Vitro – B-16 mouse melanoma cells [obtained from ATCC, Menassas, VA] were assayed in culture wells (10^4/mL) using a complete RPMI media containing 10% FBS with pen/strep and maintaining cells @ 36° C in a CO_2 incubator. Drugs (in 1 mL volumes; in conc. - 0.1-5 µg/mL) were added to the cells in a growth phase and removed after 8-12 h; cultures were washed with fresh medium. For florescent studies - cells in growth phase were incubated with dichlorofluorescein diacetate (DCFDA, 3 µg/mL RPMI) x 1-hr, washed and DM-CHOC-PEN added (1-5 µg/mL); incubation continued for an additional 5-hour. Cells were washed with fresh complete media and monitored with fluorescent microscopy. For the latter – RPMI without phenol red was used.

In Vivo – B-16 mouse melanoma cells (10^6) were implanted SC into the flank of adult female C57BL mice (age – 7-9 weeks, Harlan Labs.) and treatments with DM-CHOC-PEN, HOOI, and other drugs began were initiated when lesions were palpable - 3-5 days post implant.

Drugs – were dissolved in saline or in a soybean oil/egg yolk lecithin emulsion (2 mg/mL) and administer by IP injection. HOOI was administered as the L-lysine salt [27].

Results – B-16 cells were incubated with DM-CHOC-PEN and after ~ 6-8 hours became heavily melanotic, lost adherence and floated to the top of the wells. Isolation of the floating heavily pigmented melanotic cells that formed (Fig. 7b), followed by washing, extraction with dichloromethane, and HPLC assays revealed that the cells contained DM-CHOC-PEN in concentrations of 0.003-0.09 µg/mL of packed B-16 cells. Attached amelanotic cells contained 0-20 ng/mL of DM-CHOC-PEN (significant) [28].

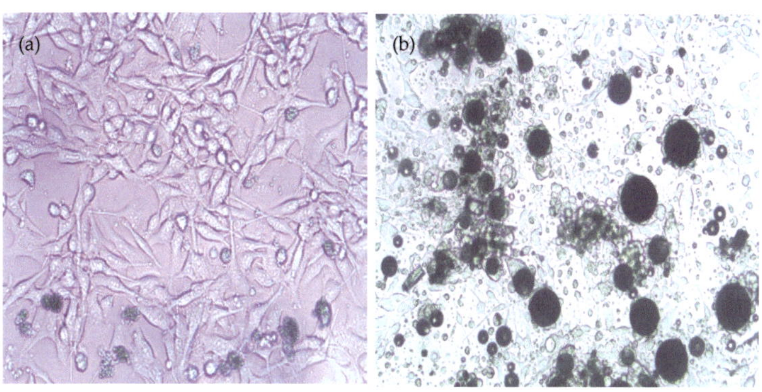

Figure 7. a) B-16 melanoma cells – untreated; b) After treatment with DM-CHOC-PEN

In comparison with other agents – DM-CHOC-PEN had an IC_{50} of 0.4 µg/mL and TMZ, BCNU, DOX and actinomycin D (Act D), HOOI – 0.5-0.9 µg/mL; *cis*-platinum (*cis*-platin) – 1.5 µg/mL resulted in IC_{50} cell death @ 36 hour post-intial exposure. With the exception of DM-CHOC-PEN, all treated cells died with ghosts remaining; excesive melanin formation only occurred with DM-CHOC-PEN; the terminal pathways were quite different for the other drugs.

Drug	IC_{50} (µg/mL)
DM CHOC-PEN	0.4 +/- 0.01
Actinomycin D	0.5 +/- 0.02
BCNU	0.9 +/- 0.1
cis-Platin	1.5 +/- 0.1
DOX	0.7 +/- 0.1
TMZ	"/>3.0
HOOI	0.8 +/- 0.2

Table 2. Drugs Responses vs. B-16 Melanoma (IC_{50})

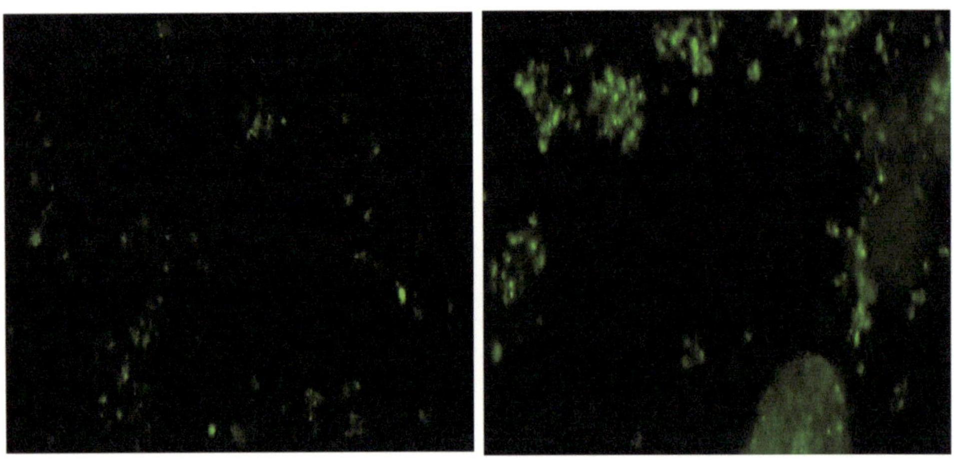

(a) (b)

Figure 8. a)B-16 cells + DCF-DA; b)B-26 cells plus DM-CHOC-PEN + DCF-DA

Viewed with florescent microscopy – green florescent cells are generating ROS and the DCF is florescent.

http://dx.doi.org/10.5772/53889

Melanoma cell death due to DM-CHOC-PEN could be a result of increased intracellular melanin, as well as DNA alkylation. Addition of DCF-DA (dichlorofluorescein diacetate) to the culture medium (10 μg/mL) documented the formation of radical oxygen species (ROS) in the DM- CHOC-PEN treated cultures; green labeled cells (Fig. 8b). ROS release was documented with DCF, which is due to the hydrolysis and oxidized of DCF-DA by ROS with the release of fluorescent DCF. The generation of ROS was not observed with B-16 melanoma cells treated with *cis*-platin or actinomycin D and cultured under similar conditions. There is some back ground florescence and secondary to melanin-associated ROS formation [16].

In Vivo Studies – Adult female C57BL mice in groups of 5-6 mice with palpable SC nodules were dosed IP daily (175 or 200 mg/kg) for 5-days with DM-CHOC-PEN and monitored daily until death (Fig. 9a).

Mice treated with DM-CHOC-PEN (200 mg/kg/d x 5 days, IP) alone demonstrated an ILS of 142% (Fig. 9a). No drug related toxicity was noted – weight gain occurred until tumor growth was obvious.

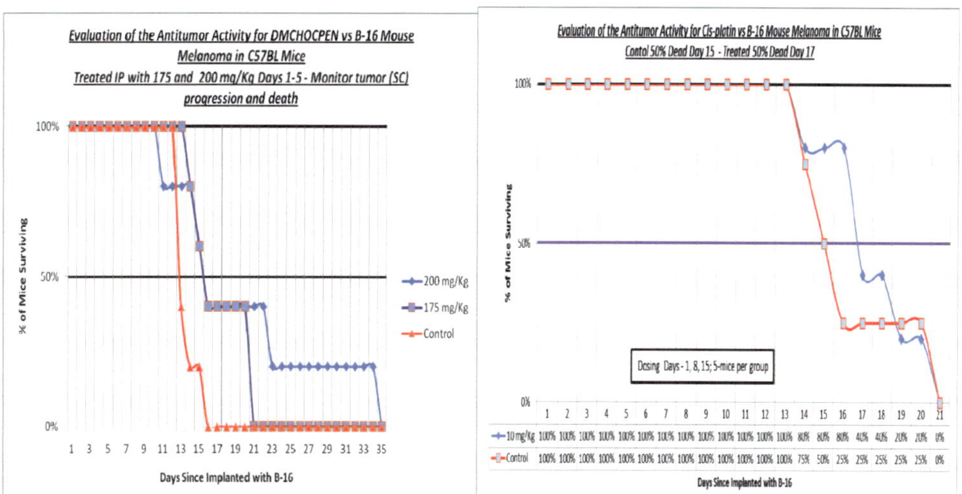

Figure 9. a)DM-CHOC-PEN treated; b)Cis-platin treated

Cis-platin was used as a drug control and administered (IP) once weekly x 3 (Fig. 9b); animals did not tolerate 3- or 5-day dosing schedules [28, 29]. Although active *in vitro, cis*-platin does not improve *in vivo* survival – as seen in Fig. 9b, although it is used in many melanoma clinical protocols [3].

Tumor histology of the DM-CHOC-PEN treated B-16 melanomas are reviewed in Fig. 10. On the left (a) is the saline control and right (b) the DM-CHOC-PEN treated – 200 mg/kg IP daily x 5 days. *Note* - the melanin deposits in the cells with vacuoles, similar to what was seen in culture [29].

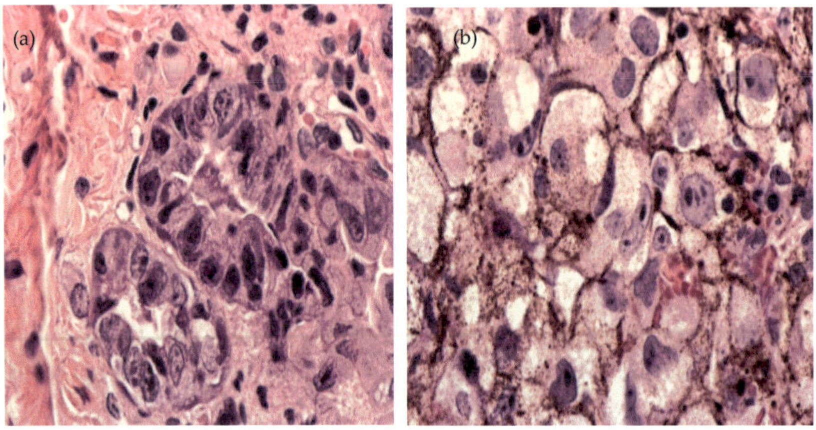

Figure 11. a)Histology of saline controls; b)Histology of DM-CHOC-PEN treated

Tumor tissue from the above DM-CHOC-PEN treated mice were assayed per cytoflorimetry using a BD FAC Scanner.

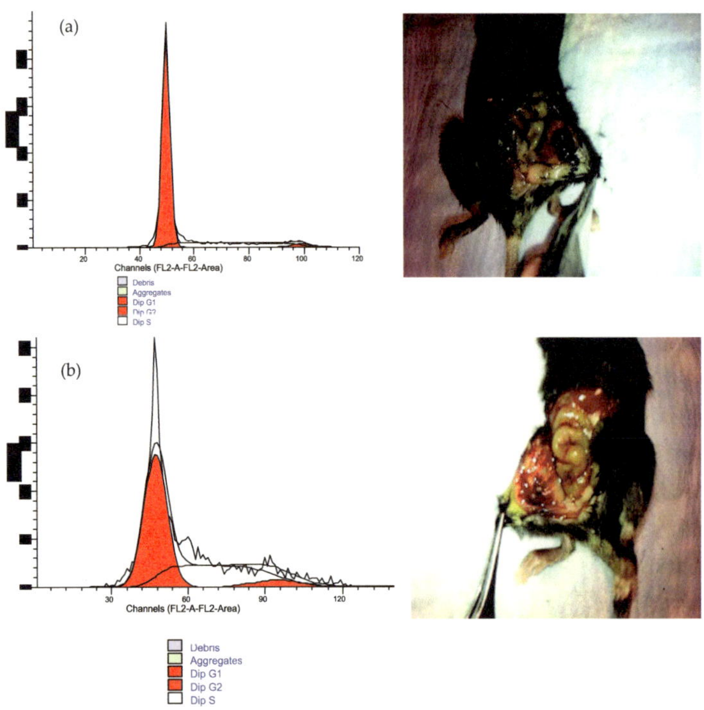

Figure 12. a) Mice bearing SC nodules – control animals. b) Mice bearing SC nodules dosed - 200 mg/kg; days 1-5 and sacrificed 3-days after the last treatment.

http://dx.doi.org/10.5772/53889

There were less viable cells available in the treated animals. DM-CHOC-PEN reduced the cellular concentration of the tumors and the cells accumulated in G_1 phase, with an inhibition in S-phase concentration of cells (Fig. 11b). Thus, more support for DM-CHOCPEN's potential use in melanoma. Unfortunately, there was a significant amount of debris present.

Discussion – Mice bearing B-16 melanoma, tolerated DM-CHOC-PEN well when administered IP daily x 5 days or days 1 & 5 with improved overall survival (OAS) for both schedules; the former was the superior.

Histological examinations of the melanoma tissue from animals that had been treated with DM-CHOC-PEN revealed tumor cells encompassed in extracellular melanin, very similar to what was seen in tissue culture (Fig. 7b). DM-CHOC-PEN was extracted in up to 92 ng/g tissue quantities from the melanoma tissue removed in Fig. 11b [16].

DM-CHOC-PEN is a pseudo-alkylator that binds to DNA's guanine-N^7 via the trichloromethyl moiety → dichloromethylene carbonium ion and can form DNA-guanine adducts and cell death [Fig. 6] [9]. However, the current observations in a melanoma model support DM-CHOC-PEN's additional ability to disrupt cellular metabolism with death via autooxidation of DOPA to melanin and superoxide formation – an additional MOA for consideration – Fig. 12 [28, 29].

Electronic modeling studies support DM-CHOC-PEN's ability to act as a pyridinium co-factor oxidized by the pyridine nucleotides (NAD, etc.) with red-ox transfer of electrons from 3,4-dihydroxyphenylalanine (DOPA) to the mitochondria and cytochrome C/cytochrome oxidase transport system (Fig. 13). This result is the formation of 5, 6-indolequinone and melanin with a trail of electrons that can enter the mitochondrion intermediary pool resulting in all the same type of lethal changes seen with electron beam therapy for cancer [30, 31].

The 'melanin balls' that were seen *in vitro* are spheres of extracellular melanin polymer encapsulating colonies of melanoma cells that could induce a hostile microenvironment through ROS formation with death via oxidative stress and apoptosis (Figs. 10) [30]. Clusters of melanin laden cells contained significantly elevated concentrations of DM-CHOC-PEN, as compared to the amelanotic variant; a possible storage site for the drug [31]. The initial DOPA → DOPA quinone transformation is catalyzed by tyrosinase (DOPA oxidase) intracellular [32-35]. However, the red-ox potential for DM-CHOC-PEN is sufficient to catalyze the conversion with excess melanin formation per the Rapier Scheme below [32].

Both malignant and benign melanocytes generate melanin pigment via the sequence of chemical reactions as depicted in the classical Rapier Scheme in Fig.12 [32].

Melanin is far from being an end-product of oxidation [34-37]. At a glance the existence of energy bands are obvious from the highly conjugated heterocyclic indole quinone structure for melanin (Fig. 12). The hypothesis has been proposed that non-localized empty molecular orbitals are associated with the copolymer chain of the indole quinoid units and that the melanin polymer acts as a one-dimensional semi-conductor/trap with bound protons producing electron traps in the system [36].

Thus, melanin is a polymer of indole-5, 6-quinone which is highly electrophilic due to its conjugated structure and capable of attracting, storing and/or transferring electrons as electrical energy [30, 31, 34]. DM-CHOC-PEN treatment induced ROS formation *via* the melanin system resulting in cancer cell death – an end point.

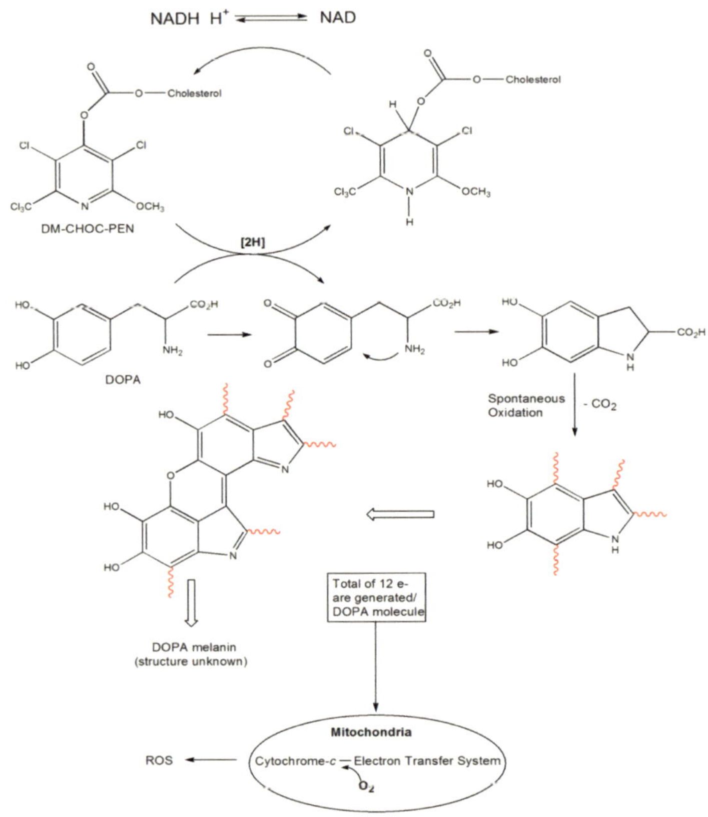

Figure 13. Interaction of DM-CHOC-PEN with Rapier melanin cell cycle and mitochondrion [32]

Melanin is potentially a storage deposit of electrons and/or for electron-rich molecules (reported by our group years ago) [31]. Due to the high redox potential between DOPA and DOPA quinone, +0.37v, a possible yield of -19.8 kcal/mole occurs upon the oxidation of 1 mole DOPA. A total of 12 e^- are generated per mole of DOPA oxidized to indole quinone which polymerize to melanin [Fig. 13 [31]. A field of melanin encompassing a colony of cancer cells could generate a hostile electrical microenvironment and inhibit cellular metabolism and replication [33].

Melanoma cells are a classical representation of cancer cells with a resting low free energy (ΔF) and high entropy (ΔS) – the *alpha state* [14]. The interactions of DM-CHOC-PEN and DOPA induced the formation of melanin and ROS which resulted in an increased environmental ΔF and a decrease in ΔS; a new resting high energy state – the *beta state*. The cells that are contained in the melanin balls are in a *beta state* - undergo apoptosis and die [28, 30, 31].

Thus, DM-CHOC-PEN is a new drug entity that crosses the BBB and couples two new targets – the melanin cycle and superoxide formation with apoptosis plus DNA guanine – N^7 adducts. DM-CHOC-PEN is a potential triple treat for CNS melanoma, the 3rd most common cancer that spreads to the CNS.

8. A 2nd High energy drug

Another high energy drug, 4-hydroperoxyifosfamide (HOOI) [Fig. 3, 14] and is a pre-activated form of ifosfamide (IFOS) which possesses the criteria for discussion [Fig. 14]. HOOI also contains a 3rd Period atom – 'P'; thus it has two centers of high energy – Fig 3, 14.

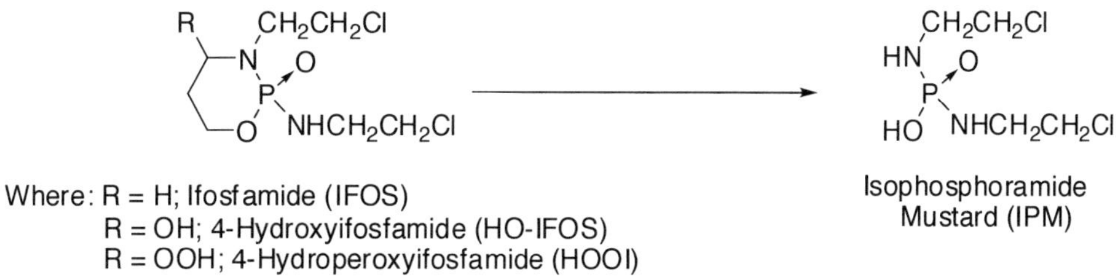

Figure 14. Ifosfamide and analogs

IFOS is a well-known anticancer agent that requires hepatic activation to 4-HO-IFOS which spontaneously undergoes hydrolysis with ring opening resulting in isophosphoramide mustard (IPM) [Fig. 14], the latter is the active cytotoxic form of IFOS [37-39]. As part of the IFOS activation process, hepatic metabolic dechloroethylation releases chloroacetaldehyde, which has been proposed to be the major cause of IFOS associated neurotoxicity [40]. Acrolein is also released and has been implicated in dose limiting toxicities - hemorrhagic cystitis and 2° tumor promotion [41-45].

In contrast, HOOI does not require hepatic microsomal activation, crosses the BBB and is readily absorbed by cancer cells where it releases IPM *in situ* [46, 47]. The former does not generate chloroacetaldehyde (neurotoxic) during its conversion to IPM, as does IFOS. Neither hemorrhagic cystitis nor renal toxicity has been observed with HOOI in animal toxicology models. Pulmonary damage that could occur with peroxides – pulmonary air emboli was not observed in the dog HOOI study [46]. Hematological toxicity (bone marrow depletion) was the dose limiting toxicity in the dog study [47].

The potential therapeutic usefulness of HOOI is supported by in vivo activity in human tumor xenografts and cyclophosphamide (CPA)-resistant murine tumor models plus reduced toxicities.

In vivo in comparison to CPA and IFOS in rodent and dog species [Table 3] [47], a potentially improved safety profile is anticipated – with reduced systemic formation of acrolein and the absence of chloroacetaldehyde during the conversion of HOOI to IPM – *in situ* [47].

Drug	Dose (mg/kg/day)	No of Mice	MX-1* T- C (Days)	ZR-75-1* T- C (Days)	U251 (%ILS)**	P388/CPA (% ILS)**
HOOI	90 (<LD_{10})	10	>28.8 9 (33% LTS)	>46.1 (83% CR)	+54 (1/5 CR)	+209+
DM-CHOC-PEN	135	10	>54 days (20% LTS) [Dose - 50]	NA	+54 (1/5 CR)	NA
IFOS	40 (MTD)++	10	8.6 (7% LTS)	>43.8 (17% CR)	50 (0/5 CR)	42
IPM	40 (MTD)++	10	2.1	NA	NA	+85
BCNU	9-15 (MTD)	5	12% LTS; 0 CR	NA	+52 (1/5 CR)	NA
TMZ	120 mg (MTD)	5	NA	NA	+54 (1/5 CR)	NA

Dose – qd x 5d (IP) – except TMZ – PO Q4D x 3; *human breast cancer – SC implanted, **human glioblastoma – IC implanted; ***CPA (cyclophosphamide) – resistant murine leukemia. For MX-1 – T-C (days) = difference in median times post implant for tumors of treated groups to attain an evaluation size compared to median of control group; +6-log cell kill; ++>40 mg/kg was too toxic; ***% ILS (increased length of survival – study terminated @ 54 days.

Table 3. Human Xenografts and Murine Tumors Growing in Mouse Models

HOOI possesses two [2] 3-high energy atom chains, thus the drug more than fits the criteria proposed earlier in this chapter (3). In addition, HOOI does not require activation by the liver and spontaneously undergoes conversion to IPM and cross-links with nuclear DNA via major groove alkylation – N^7-guanine, forming G-X-C adducts [39].

Of significance is that HOOI was curative (54% LTS, with 20% CR) *vs.* the human U251 glioblastoma implanted IC as well as the MX-1 breast cancer IC model (Table 3) [47]. It should also be noted that BCNU – the gold standard for years in the treatment of gliomas produced no CRs and TMZ the current standard produced identical responses to HOOI.

Like DM-CHOC-PEN, HOOI accumulates in U-251 glioma tissue in 50 ng/g tissue content when the drug is administered IP to animals bearing IC implanted tumors [47]. No CNS/behavioral alterations or toxicity have been noted for HOOI [48].

Unlike ifosfamide (IFOS), HOOI is more lipophilic, activated *in situ*, with less extracellular acrolein, no chloroacetaldehyde released and no IFOS associated CNS or GU toxicity [48]. In dogs the principal toxicity with HOOI was bone marrow suppression that reversed with time [47, 48].

An early study reported that SK-MEL-31 human melanoma cells were sensitive to HOOI, which prompted the comparison of the drug with DM-CHOC-PEN in the B-16 melanoma model [47].

In 2012, the incidence of new cases of melanoma in the US alone is estimated at 76,250, an increase of ~ 20% during the past 10 years [9]. Of these cases, ~ 25% will metastasize to the CNS; thus our interest in the drug [26].

Fig. 15 describes the impact on survival of B-16 mouse melanoma when HOOI is administered alone and with DM-CHOC-PEN [49].

DM-CHOC-PEN (200 mg/kg/d) was injected IP daily x 5-days followed by HOOI (90 mg/m^2) IP daily x 3 days (Day 6-8). The latter is a more classical mustard type agent with activity in the G_1 phase, as compared to DM-CHOC-PEN, which inhibited cell replication at the S phase – Fig. 12b [49].

The %LTS for the 2-drug combination was 173% vs. HOOI alone - 78%; for DM-CHOC-PEN alone - 142% (see Fig. 14).

No drug related toxicity was noted – weight gain continued until tumor growth was a burden and animals sacrificed. The use of 5-day dosing for HOOI was toxic and not considered [48].

Combination of the two -'high energy' agents selected for discussion as binary therapy has potential. It will be a while before these 2-drugs are administered together; however, other binary selections that incorporate DM-CHOC-PEN are in the planning stage for Phase II trials.

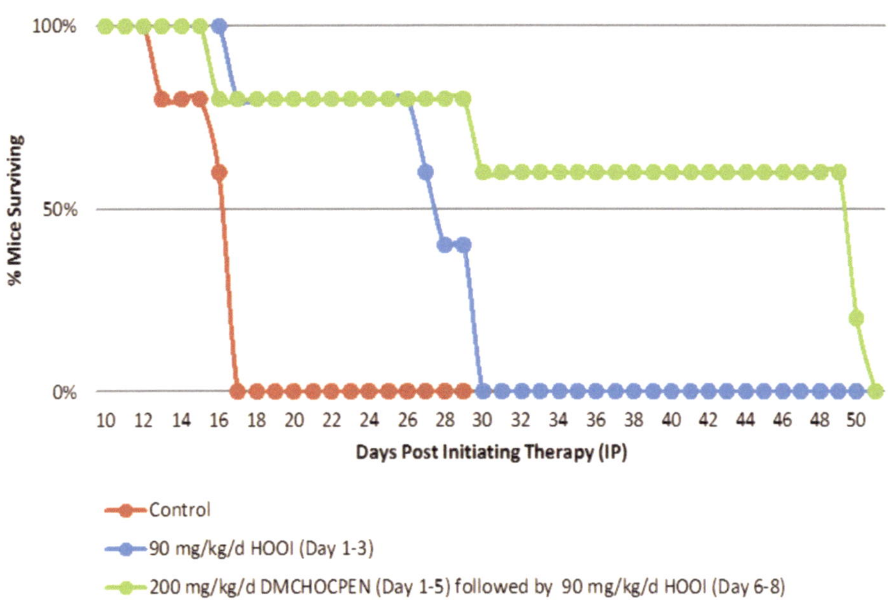

Figure 15. DM-CHOC-PEN plus HOOI in the Treatment of B-16 Mouse Melanoma

9. Conclusion

Melanoma cells, as seen in Fig. 7a represent classical cancer cells with a resting low free energy (ΔF) and high entropy (ΔS) – the *alpha state* [14]. The interaction of DM-CHOC-PEN and DOPA induced the formation of melanin – a high energy component/storage that resulted in an increase in environmental ΔF and a decrease in ΔS; a new resting high energy state – the *beta state* [14]. Cells that are encompassed in the 'melanin balls' (Fig. 7b) were converted to a well differentiated state and die. The addition of HOOI to DM-CHOC-PEN inhibited those cells that reversed to the *alpha state* – survive and continue to replicate. Thus, the binary combination improved %LTS vs. either drug alone; supporting the *in vitro* observations.

Although, only two patients with CNS melanoma have been treated with DM-CHOC-PEN in the Phase I trial, the report that one patient did demonstrate an interval response and one patent had a no change response, both with no neurotoxicity is encouragement for the potential use of the drug in the treatment of CNS melanoma [25]. HOOI has not been used in clinical trials as yet.

There are many novel drugs that fall in to the 'high-energy' category that should be evaluated or re-visited. In particular – clomesone [Fig. 3], a drug developed at Southern Research Institute, US had potential in animal studies, but produced hematological toxicity in Phase I trials and discontinued from studies [17, 50]. The drug has novel chloroethylating properties and like BCNU forms adducts with DNA guanine-O^6 [50]. In addition, the drug contains two - S - atoms which are a 3rd Period element and able to expand its 3d orbital – a real 'high-energy' molecule. However, only one of the latter groups has the ability to resonant with energy storage.

With the two sets of 3-atom chain as a point of interest (Fig. 3, 6), clomesone should be revisited with dose modifications; it has potential [52].

In summary, three 'high energy' drugs have been reviewed as support that a novel approach to the treatment of CNS malignancies could be through the inefficient energy system of brain tumors [11, 12]. Anticancer agents that have the appropriate structure, can penetrate the CNS, not be recycled out and inhibit cancer growth.

Over all, DM-CHOC-PEN has been well tolerated in Phase I studies with advanced –breast cancer, sarcoma, glioblastoma multiforme, melanoma, pancreas, esophageal, non-small cell lung cancer colorectal cancer and cervical cancer and will obviously enter Phase II trials alone or as binary therapy [25].

Furthermore, HOOI is being readied for Phase I clinical trials and the results should be equally interesting.

http://dx.doi.org/10.5772/53889

Acknowledgement

Grant support from NCI/SBIR R43/44CA85021 and R43CA132257 is appreciated.

The author wishes to thank Drs. Robert F. Struck, Branko S. Jursic, Roy S. Weiner, Marcus L. Ware, Barry Sartin, Philip Friedlander, Andrew Rodgers and Mr. Edmund Benes for their discussions, review and comments during the preparation of this manuscript.

Author details

Lee Roy Morgan*

Address all correspondence to: LRM1579@aol.com

CEO DEKK-TEC, Inc University of New Orleans New Orleans, LA, USA

References

[1] Maher, EA, Furnari, FB, Bachoo, RM, et al. Malignant glioblastoma: genetics and biology of a grave matter. Genes Dev., 15:1311-33, 2001.

[2] Van Brachlyn, JR, Jackson, CA, Pearl, DK, et al. Spingosine kinase -1 expression correlates with poor survival of patients with GBM: roles of spingosine kinase isoforms in glioblastoma cell lines. J. Neuropatol. Exp. Neurol, 64: 695-705, 2005.

[3] Patchell, RA. The management of brain metastasis. Cancer Treatment Rev. 29: 533-40.

[4] Johnson, JD, Young, B, Demographics of brain metastasis. Neurosurg. Clin. N. Am., 7: 337-44, 1996.

[5] Sampson, JH, Carter, JH, Friedman, AH, Seiger, HF. Demographics, prognosis and therapy in 702 patients with brain metastasis from malignant melanoma. J. Neurosurg., 88: 11-20, 1998.

[6] Eichler, AF, Loeffler, JS. Multidisciplinary management of brain metastasis. Oncologist 12: 884-98, 2007.

[7] Smit and Marshall. Editorial, Community Oncology, 9: 250-258, 2012.

[8] Villano, JL, Seery, TE, Bressler, LR. Temozolomide in malignant gliomas: current use and future targets. Cancer Chemotherapy and Pharmacology, 64: 647-655, 2009.

[9] Thompson, JA. Ten years of progress in melanoma. JNCCN, 10: 931-35, 2012.

[10] Genomics and Personalized Medicine Act of 2006; Bill of Congress 1093822.

[11] Wollemann, M. Biochemistry of brain tumours, University Park Press, Baltimore, 1974.

[12] Warburg, O. The Metabolism of tumours, Constable, London, 1930.

[13] Szent-Gyorgyi, A. The Living State and Cancer, New York, NY, Marcel Dekker, Inc. 1978, pp. 21-24.

[14] Klotz, IM, Rosenberg, RM. Introduction to chemical thermodynamics, WA Benjamin, Inc, Menlo Park, CA, 1964.

[15] Wald, G. Life in the second and third periods; or why phosphorus and sulfur for high energy bonds? In: Horizons in Biochemistry, Ed. Kasha, M, Pullman, Academic Press, New York, 1962, pp.127-142.

[16] Morgan, LR, Struck, RF, Rodgers, AH, Bastian, G, Jursic, BS, Papaginnis, C, Waud, W. Intracerebral metabolism and pharmacokinetics of 4-demethyl-4-cholesteryl-oxy-carbonylpenclomedine (DM-CHOC-PEN). Proc. Amer. Assoc. Res., 49: Abst. 3745, 2008.

[17] Shealy YF, Krauth CA, Laster WR. 2-Chloroethylmethylsulfonyl)methanesulfonate and related (methylsulfonyl)methanesulfonates. Antineoplastic activity in vivo. J Med. Chem. 27: 664-670, 1984; Dykes DJ, Waud WR, Harrison SD, Griswold DP, Shealy YF, Montgomery JA. Antitumor activity of 2-chloroethyl (ethylsulfonyl)methane-sulfonate (clomesone, NSC 33847) against selected tumor systems in mice. Cancer Res. 49: 1182-1186, 1989.

[18] Klotz, IM. Energy changes in biochemical reactions, Academic Press, New York, 1967.

[19] Morgan, LR, Struck, RF, Waud, WR, LeBlanc, B, Rodgers, AH, Jursic, BS. Carbonate and carbamate derivatives of 4-demethylpenclomedine as novel anticancer agents. Cancer Chemotherapy and Pharmacology, 64: 829-836, 2009.

[20] Morgan, LR, Rodgers, AH, Bastian, G, Struck, RF, Waud, WR. Comparative pharmacokinetics and intermediary metabolism of 4-demethyl-4-cholesteryl- oxycarbonylpenclomedine (DM-CHOC-PEN), EORTC/AACR/NCI, 567, 2010.

[21] Morgan, LR, Struck, RF, Rodgers, AH, Serota, DG. Preclinical Toxicity of 4- Demethyl-4-cholestryloxyl-carbonylpenclomedine (DM-CHOC-PEN). Proc. Amer. Assoc. Res., 48: abst. 5614, 2007.

[22] Pletsas, D, Wheelhouse, RT, Pletsa, V, Nicolaou, A, Jenkins, TC, Bibby, MC, Kytopoulas, SA. Polar, Functionalized guanine-O^6 derivatives resistant to repair by O^6-alkylguanine-DNA alkyltransferase: implications for the design of DNA-modifying drugs, Eur. J. Med Chem., 11: 1-10, 2006.

[23] Morgan, LR. Demethylpenclomedine analogs and their use as anti-cancer agents. US Patent 8,124,596, 2012.

[24] Morgan, LR IND 0688876 DM-CHOC-PEN- Study May Proceed, FDA September 24, 2010.

[25] Weiner, RS, Friedlander, P, Gordon, C, Ware, ML, Bastian, G, Rodgers, AH, Urien, S, Morgan, LR. Comparative Pharmacokinetics of 4-Demethyl-4-cholesteryloxycarbonylpenclomedine (DM-CHOC-PEN) in Humans, Proc. Amer. Assoc. Cancer Res., 53: 758, 2012.

[26] Philip Friedlander, Personnel communication.

[27] Morgan, LR. Complexes of 4-hydroperoxyifosfamide as antitumor agents, EU Patent 107060956, 2012.

[28] Morgan, LR, Benes, E, Rodgers, AH, Jursic, BS, Struck, BF, Waud, WR, Weiner, RS, Ware, M, Friedlander, P. Interaction of 4-Demethyl-4-cholesteryloxycarbonyl penclomedine (DM-CHOC-PEN) with Melanoma Melanin Metabolism and Cell Death, EC-CO, Abst. 457, 2011.

[29] Morgan, LR, Rodgers, AH, Bastian, G, Papagiannis, C, Krietlow, D, Struck, RF, Waud, WR. Comparative pharmacokinetics and intermediary metabolism of 4-demethyl-4-cholesteryloxycarbonylpenclomedine (DM-CHOC-PEN), EORTC/AACR/NCI, Abstr. 458, 2010.

[30] Morgan, LR, Singh, R. Cytochrome oxidase-succinic dehydrogenase activities and the melanin pigment cycle in poikilothermic vertebrates. Comp. Biochem. Physiol., 28: 83-94, 1969.

[31] Morgan, LR, Singh, R, Sylvest, V, Weimort, D. Oxidation of o-phenols by mouse and human melanoma dihydroxyphenyl alanine oxidase and dihydroxyphenyl alanine. Cancer Res. 27: 2395-2407, 1967.

[32] Rapier, HS. The aerobic oxidation. Physiol. Revs. 245-288, 1928.

[33] Mason, HS. Structure of Melanins, In: Pigment Cell Biology, Ed. Gordon, M. Academic Press Inc, Publishers, New York, 1959, pp. 563-582.

[34] Van Woert, HH, Nicholson, A, Cotzias, GC. Functional similarities between the cytoplasmic organelles of melanocytes and mitochondria of hepatocytes. Nature, 208, 810-811, 1965.

[35] Traub, EF, Spoor, HJ. Melanin and tyrosinase in skin pigmentation. In: Pigment Cell Growth, 3rd Conference on Biology of Normal and Atypical Pigment Cell Growth. Ed.: Myron Gordon, pp. 211-219, 1953, NYNY Academic Press.

[36] Pullmans, A and Pullman, B. The band structure of melanin. Biochem. Biophys. Acta, 54, 384-485, 1961.

[37] Zolwyski, M., and Baker, L.H. Ifosfamide. J. Natl. Cancer Inst. 80:556-566, 1988.

[38] Norpoth, K. Studies on the metabolism of isophosphamide in man. Cancer Treat. Rep. 60:437-443, 1976.

[39] Struck, RF, Dykes, DJ, Corbett, TH, Suling, WJ, MW. Isophosphoroamide mustard, a metabolite of ifosfamide with activity against murine tumors comparable to cyclophosphamide. Brit. J. Cancer 47:15-26, 1983.

[40] Goren, MP, Wright, RK, Pratt, CB, Pell, FE. Dechloroethylation of ifosfamide and neurotoxicity. Lancet 2:1219-1220, 1986.

[41] Cox, PJ. Cyclophosphamide cystitis – Identification of acrolein as the causativet. Biochem. Pharmacol. 28:2045-2049, 1979.

[42] Seo, IS, Clark, SA, McGovern, FD, Clark, DL, Johnson, EH. Leiomyosarcoma of the urinary bladder 13 years after cyclophosphamide therapy for Hodgkin's disease. Cancer 55:1597-1603, 1985.

[43] Colburn, KK, Cao, JD, Krick, EH, Mortensen, SE, Wong, LG. Hodgkins lymphoma in a patient treated for Wegeners granulomatosis with cyclophosphamide and azathioprine. J. Rheumatol. 12:599-602, 1985.

[44] Cuzick, J, Erskine, S, Edelman, D, Gelton, DAG. A comparison of the incidence of myelodyplastic syndrome and acute myeloid leukemia following melphalan and cyclophosphamide treatment for myelomatosis. Brit. J. Cancer 55:523-530, 1987.

[45] Durst, J., Ahrens, S., Paulussen, M., Rube, C., Winkelmann, W., Zoubek, A., Harms, D. and Jurgens, H. Second malignancies after treatment for Ewing's sarcoma: report of the CESS-studies. Int. J. Radiat. Oncol. Biol. Phys. 42:379-384, 1998.

[46] Narayanan, V. In vivo evaluation of 4-hydroperoxyifosfamide (NSC 207117 and 227114). Screening Data Summary, Dev. Ther. Program, Dir. Cancer Treat. NCI, Bethesda, MD 20205.

[47] Morgan, L.R, Struck, R.F. Rodgers, A.H., Jursic, B.S., Waud, W.S., Butera, D., Development of Clinical Products. NCI Translational Science Meeting, Washington, DC, 2008.

[48] Morgan, L.R., Struck, R.F., Rodgers, A.H., Jursic, B.S. Waud, W. R. Pre- clinical Pharmacology and Toxicology for 4-Hydeoperoxyifosfamide (HOOI) and its L-lysine Salt – A Novel Anticancer Agent. Amer. Assoc Cancer Res, 42, 3222, 2011; Cancer Chemotherapy Pharmacology, submitted.

[49] Morgan, LR, Benes, E, Rodgers, AH, Jursic, BS, Friedlander, P, Weiner, RS, Ware, ML, Struck, RF. 4-Demethyl-4-cholesterylcarbonylpenclomedine (DM-CHOC-PEN) and 4-Hydroperoxyifosfamide (HOOI) as Binary Therapy for Melanoma, EORTC/AACR/NCI, Abst, 703, 2011.

[50] Robert F. Struck, Personnel communication.

Chapter 16

DNA-PK is a Potential Molecular Therapeutic Target for Glioblastoma

P. O. Carminati, F. S. Donaires, P. R. D. V. Godoy,
A. P. Montaldi, J. A. Meador, A.S. Balajee,
G. A. Passos and E. T. Sakamoto-Hojo

Additional information is available at the end of the chapter

http://dx.doi.org/10.5772/53181

1. Introduction

Glioblastoma multiforme is one of the deadliest forms of brain tumor with a median survival of <12 months with a high rate of recurrence. Glioblastoma cells respond poorly to radiotherapy and chemotherapy due to elevated DNA repair efficiency coupled with anti-apoptotic mechanisms [1, 2]. Therefore, development of new therapeutic strategies is absolutely critical either to control or cure the disease. Since glioblastoma cells have inherently elevated levels of DNA damage response (DDR) and DNA repair efficiency, we sought to determine whether or not suppression of key DNA repair factor(s) might be effective in sensitizing the brain tumor cells to chemotherapy. To test our objective, a pair of isogenic glioblastoma cell lines that differ in the functional status of DNA dependent protein kinase (DNA-PK) has been chosen. DNA dependent protein kinase (DNA-PK) belongs to a super family of phosphatidylinositol-3 kinase like kinases (PIKK) which also includes the gene products of ataxia telangiectasia mutated (ATM) and ATM and Rad 3 related (ATR) kinases [3, 4]. DNA-PK is the main component of mammalian NHEJ (non-homologous end joining), and also plays a role as a sensor of DNA damage by phosphorylating several downstream targets [5]. Further, DNA-PK has been demonstrated to be an important component of nucleotide excision repair (NER) pathway, which is chiefly responsible for the repair of bulky and helix distorting lesions induced by ultraviolet radiation (UV) and chemotherapeutic drugs such as cisplatin. To determine whether or not DNA-PK is a potential molecular therapeutic target for glioblastoma, two agents with different modes of action have been chosen for our study: (1) Zebularine and (2) Cisplatin.

Many tumor cells have characteristic epigenetic alterations involving genome wide DNA hypo-methylation and gene specific hyper-methylation at CpG dinucleotide sequences leading to aberrant silencing of critical genes involved in DNA damage response, cell cycle and DNA metabolic processes. Recent studies [6-8] have demonstrated the usefulness of epigenetic targeting in treating many cancer cell types through inhibition of histone deacetylases (HDAC) or DNA methyl transferases (DNMTs). Zebularine is a potent inhibitor of DNMTs and is superior to 5-AzaCR in terms of lower cytotoxicity and increased stability in aqueous solutions [9]. While Zebularine is a DNA-demethylating agent, cisplatin is a DNA cross-linking agent that induces the formation of DNA inter- and intra-strand cross-links. These cross-links are removed preferentially by NER pathway and NER deficient tumor cells are often sensitized to cisplatin treatment. Since DNA-PK plays a critical role in genome surveillance and DNA repair mechanisms, we wished to evaluate the potential of DNA-PK as a molecular therapeutic target for glioblastoma.

2. DNA-PK deficient cells are sensitive to zebularine and cisplatin treatments

2.1. Zebularine sensitizes DNA–PK deficient glioblastoma cells

DNA-PK deficient (MO59J) and proficient (MO59K) glioblastoma cells were purchased from American Type Culture Collection (Rockville, MD, USA). Cells were routinely cultured in OPTI-MEM supplemented with 5% fetal bovine serum, vitamins and antibiotics. Zebularine [1-beta-D-ribofuranosyl)-1, 2-dihydropyrimidin-2-one] was purchased from EMD Biosciences (San Diego, CA, USA). Zebularine was dissolved in dimethyl sulfoxide (DMSO) at a stock concentration of 100 mM and stored at 4ºC. Clonogenic survival and proliferations assays were carried to determine the sensitivity of human gliomas (MO59J and MO59K) to different Zebularine concentrations (0-300 μM). The LC50 value for Zebularine was found to be 245 μM for DNA-PK deficient MO59J cells and at this concentration the survival of MO59K cells was reduced only by 20% [10]. This finding indicates that lack of DNA-PK potentiates the sensitization of gliomas to Zebularine. In contrast to MO59K cells, DNA-PK deficient cells (MO59J) showed a reduction in survival (20%) even at the lowest Zebularine concentration (10 μM). Further, an elevated frequency of polyploid cells observed specifically in MO59J cells after Zebularine treatment pointed out a mitotic checkpoint deficiency. Although depletion of DNMT1 by Zebularine occurred at similar levels in both glioblastoma cell lines, DNA-PK deficient MO59J cells displayed elevated DNA hypo-methylation detected both at genome overall and gene promoter levels. Consistent with increased sensitivity, deoxy-Zebularine adduct level, measured for the first time by us in the genomic DNA, was 3-6 fold higher in DNA-PK deficient MO59J cells relative MO59K cells. Elevated micronuclei frequency was also observed in MO59J cells indicating the impairment of DNA damage response and repair. Collectively, our study suggests that DNA-PK is a potentially useful molecular therapeutic target for gliomas.

2.2. DNA–PK deficient cells are sensitive to cisplatin treatment

The relationship between DNA-PK/Ku activity and cisplatin sensitivity has been observed earlier in gliomas. Gliomas with high expression level of DNA-PK are resistant to cisplatin [11]. In an earlier review, we suggested that DNA-PK inhibition may be a promising strategy for treating glioblastomas [for review see 12]. To determine the role of DNA-PK in conferring cisplatin resistance, MO59J and MO59K cells were treated with cisplatin (5-75 μM; Sigma Aldrich, USA) for 72 h and assayed for proliferation using a fluorescence based CyQuant assay (Invitrogen, USA). MO59J showed a greater sensitivity to cisplatin compared to MO59K, and displayed a dose dependent decrease in cell proliferation, being reduced to 20% relative to the vehicle (DMSO) treated control cells for the highest drug concentration (75 μM). In contrast, MO59K was sensitive to cisplatin only at high doses (>50 μM). These results clearly indicate that DNA-PK is a critical factor for cellular protection against cisplatin (Figure 1).

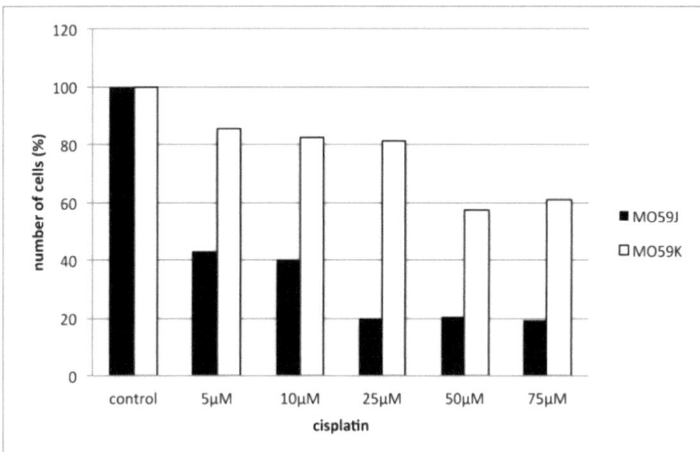

Figure 1. Cell proliferation assay using CyQuant (Invitrogen, USA) in MO59K and MO59J cells treated with cisplatin (5, 10, 25, 50, and 75 μM) for 72 h.

Cell cycle analysis was next performed to verify whether the enhanced cisplatin cytotoxicity of MO59J cells was due to defective cell cycle checkpoints. MO59K and MO59J cells in exponential growth phase were exposed to different concentrations (5 to 25 μM) of cisplatin and the cell cycle profile was analyzed by flow cytometry (24, 48 and 72 h after treatment). While DNA-PK proficient MO59K cells displayed an efficient accumulation of S-phase cells at all the concentrations of cisplatin exposure up to 72 h (Figure 2A), DNA-PK mutant MO59J cells exhibited only a modest S-phase accumulation after 24 h of drug treatment (25 μM cisplatin) (Figure 2B), which was alleviated at later time points (48 and 72 h).

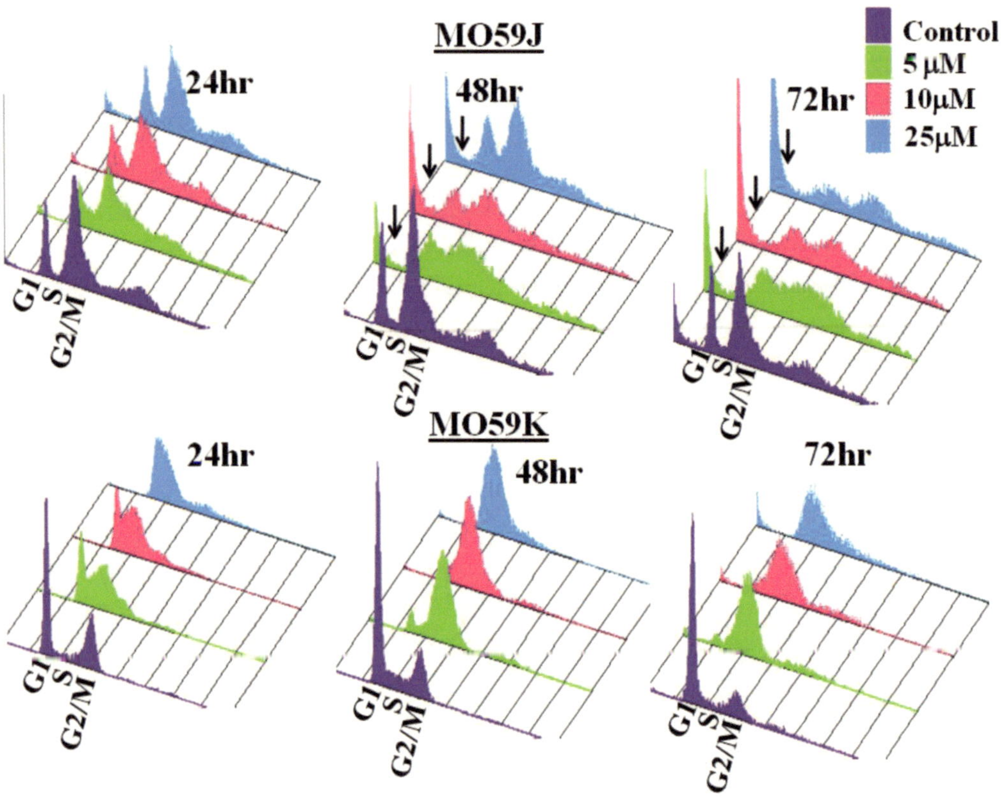

Figure 2. Cell cycle analysis for MO59K and MO59J cells treated with 5, 10 and 25 μM of cisplatin for 24, 48 and 72 h. DMSO was used as control.

Consistent with impaired cell cycle regulation, an increased frequency of apoptosis (43% for 25 μM cisplatin) was observed after cisplatin treatment in MO59J cells; in contrast to MO59K, DNA-PK deficient MO59J cells showed apoptotic death even at 5 μM of cisplatin (Figure 3A,B).

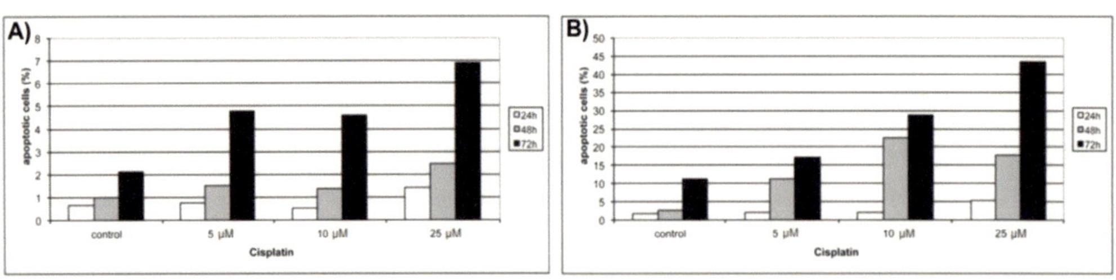

Figure 3. Frequency of apoptotic MO59K (A) and MO59J (B) cells detected by flow cytometry as a subG1 population after exposure to different concentrations of cisplatin (5, 10 and 25 μM). The results were obtained at 24, 48 and 72 h after treatment. 10,000 events were analyzed for each experiment.

Proliferating cell nuclear antigen (PCNA) is recruited to chromatin rapidly after DNA damage and the kinetics of disassembly from the chromatin is considered to reflect the DNA repair efficiency [13, 14]. PCNA expression was evaluated by Western blot in cisplatin- treated MO59K and MO59J cells. The expression of PCNA was increased in a dose-dependent manner in MO59K cells after 24 h of drug treatment, while a constant level of PCNA expression was observed in MO59J cells indicating the lack of S-phase specific PCNA accumulation (Figure 4). Our results from MO59K and MO59J cell lines indicate that DNA-PK is a critical determinant of cell survival after cisplatin treatment and the lack of S-phase arrest (as seen in MO59J cells) is presumably responsible for the increased cell death after drug treatment.

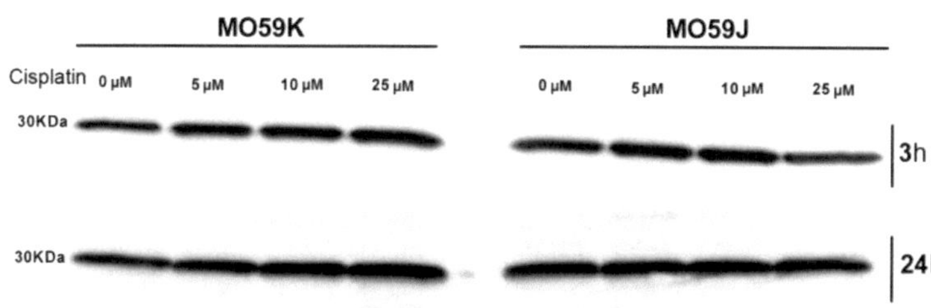

Figure 4. Expression of PCNA protein (30 KDa) analyzed by Western blot using specific antibody. MO59K and MO59J cells were treated with 5, 10 and 25 µM of cisplatin for 3 and 24 h. β-actin was used as control.

Therefore, DNA-PK may be an important molecule conferring cisplatin resistance in glioblastoma cells, with potential use as a molecular target, and we also observed that the combined effect of cisplatin and LY294002 (an inhibitor of DNA-PK) caused a significant decrease in cell proliferation and an increase in apoptotic cell death in glioma cell lines [15]. Our studies thus far performed indicate that the specific targeting of DNA-PK by small molecule inhibitors may be an effective strategy for the treatment of gliomas.

3. *In silico* analysis of transcription factors associated with differentially expressed genes in GBM cells

3.1. Introduction

Transcription factors (TFs) regulate gene expression by binding to specific DNA sequences of gene promoter regions. Their expression can be deregulated under certain pathological conditions, such as cancer. Therefore, studies on regulatory elements of the transcription machinery are essential for understanding the mechanisms involved in the regulation of oncogenes and tumor suppressor genes. Additionally, knowledge of the essential functions of TFs, may lead to strategic development of novel chemotherapy regimen for selectively killing cancer cells.

TFs play a critical role in various cellular processes through regulation of genes involved in cell cycle, proliferation, cell differentiation, and apoptosis. It has been suggested that TFs can be potential therapeutic targets for treating the patients with prostate [16] and breast cancer [17]. Recently, *in silico* prediction for regulation of TFs has been effectively utilized for diagnostics and therapeutics of breast cancer [17]. Identification and characterization of activated transcription regulatory elements hold a great promise not only in providing information on neoplastic mechanisms, but also in predicting targets for therapeutic intervention [18]. Although enormous amount of data exist for genes that are differentially expressed in tumor cells, knowledge of TFs associated with these genes is rather limited. Information on TFs may enable us to understand how differentially expressed genes in tumor cells respond to anticancer drugs, as a single or combined treatment with DNA repair inhibitors, which targets DNA repair proteins.

DNA-PK, one of the key components of mammalian NHEJ (non-homologous end joining) repair process, belongs to PI3K-related protein kinase (PIKK) family [19]. Recent studies have projected DNA-PK as a potential molecular target for cancer treatment. Many known PI3K inhibitors such as LY294002, wortmannin and PI-103, inhibit DNA-PK activity with a comparable potency to that observed for PI3K inhibition [20]. LY294002 is a PI3K (phosphatidylinositol-3 kinase) inhibitor, well recognized by its antitumor and pro-apoptotic properties in several cancer cell lines [21]. Although LY294002 alone can inhibit cell proliferation or induce apoptosis in cancer cells, its cytotoxic effects can be further enhanced when combined with radio- or chemotherapy [12, 22]. Consequently, PI3K inhibitors including LY294002 have been investigated as a possible adjuvant for cancer therapy in many tumor models [23-25], and its synergistic effects with other anti-tumoral drugs deserve to be investigated in cancer cells.

Our recent study demonstrated that a combined treatment of cisplatin (5-50μM) and LY294002 (50μM) for 24 h reduced the survival of U343 GBM cells with elevated apoptotic death at 72 h [15]. In this study, gene expression analysis was also performed using a glass slide microarray containing 4,300 cDNA clones from the human IMAGE Consortium cDNA library [http://image.llnl.gov/image/] essentially following the procedures published earlier [26]. Statistical analysis of the results [27] showed that 25μM cisplatin alone caused significant changes in the expression of 108 genes (28 up- and 80 down-regulated), while LY294002 alone altered the expression of 33 genes (6 up- and 27 down-regulated); additionally, 274 genes (97 up- and 177 down-regulated) were modulated by the combined treatment of cisplatin and LY294002. The complete gene lists are available at http//www.rge.fmrp.usp.br/passos/cislygbm/. The drug combination induced 2.6-fold higher numbers of modulated genes, relative to cisplatin alone, and these genes participate in several biological processes, such as DNA repair, cell death, and cell cycle control/proliferation, metabolism, transcription regulation, and cellular adhesion.

Using the gene sets obtained in the above-mentioned study, we performed an *in silico* analysis of TFs for the differentially expressed genes obtained in the following comparisons: 25μM cisplatin *versus* control, and 25μM cisplatin plus 50μM LY294002 *versus* control; these lists contained 108 and 274 differentially expressed genes (SAM analysis, FDR ≤ 0.05), respectively. Among the 274 genes, 97 (35.4%) genes were up-regulated and 177 (64.6%) genes were down-regulated. Both up- and down-regulated genes were submitted separately to *in silico* analysis through the FatiGO tool, Babelomics v3.2 [28]. For comparisons, the entire list of genes present in the microarray was subjected to analysis (4,300 transcripts).The data were analyzed by the two-tailed Fisher's exact test, with significance threshold for the p-values set at 0.05. Similar procedures were performed for the list of 108 genes (set of differentially expressed genes under 25μM cisplatin treatment). Information regarding the biological functions was obtained at SOURCE (http://smd.stanford.edu/cgi-bin/source/sourceSearch), and NCBI AceView (http://www.ncbi.nlm.nih.gov/IEB/Research/Acembly/).

3.2. TFs associated with up–regulated genes

Among the predicted TFs associated with up-regulated genes after treatment with cisplatin alone, the most significant ones are AHR (p = 9.9E–3, 7.7% of associated genes), HNF4 (p = 9.6E–3, 81% of associated genes), NFkappaB (p = 5.8E–3, 11.5% of associated genes), MRF2 (p = 1.9E–3, 53.8%), and SOX5 (p = 1.6E–2, 7.7% of associated genes). These TFs have been linked with distinct biological functions, including differentiation, homeostasis, cell growth, senescence and apoptosis. AHR regulates an array of physiological responses including xenobiotic metabolism, vasculature development, immunosuppression, T-cell differentiation, reproduction, and cell cycle progression [29]. Most genes known to be controlled by HNF4α are involved in lipid, carbohydrate or amino acid transport and metabolism, indicating a central role in energy homeostasis [30]. MRF2 (ARID5B) plays a vital role in regulating embryonic development, cell growth and differentiation through tissue-specific repression of differentiation-specific gene expression [31, 32]. Aberrant *ARID5B* expression in developing fetus could halt B-lymphocyte maturation and contribute to leukemogenesis [33]. SOX5 is involved in gene regulation and maintenance of chromatin structure during diverse developmental processes. Recently, SOX5 has been found associated with induced acute cellular senescence [34], while NFkappaB is related to apoptosis evasion in GBM cells [35, 36].

Term	Percentage with term		Enrichment index	p-value
	List #1	List #2		
GATA-3	30.1	16.3	1.85	1.7E–3
FOXP3	60.2	46.0	1.31	8.0E–3
FOXJ2	46.2	32.6	1.42	9.5E–3
C/EBP	18.3	9.8	1.87	1.5E–2
LXR, PXR, CAR COUP, RAR	62.4	54.6	1.14	1.6E–2

Table 1. Transcription factors (Term) associated with up-regulated genes in cisplatin and LY294002 treated U343 cells. "Percentage with term" corresponds to the amount of genes that was associated to each TF in each list: List #1 represents up-regulated genes obtained by statistical analysis, and List #2 represents all the genes present in the microarray slide. "Enrichment index" was calculated for each Term by dividing the percentage in the List #1 by that in the List #2.

For the combined treatment (cisplatin and LY294002), the predicted TFs associated with up-regulated genes showed different TFs (Table 1), indicating that the drug combination induced quantitative and qualitative differences in transcript expression profiles displayed by GBM treated cells.

All the TFs that were associated with up-regulated genes showed enrichment indexes greater than 1 (in the range of 1.14 to 1.87), indicating that these TFs were more specifically associated with the up-regulated genes as compared to the entire array of genes (Table 1). Biological functions of the predicted TFs associated with up- and down-regulated genes after the combined treatment (cisplatin and LY294002) in U343 cells are described below:

GATA-3 (*Trans-acting T-cell-specific transcription factor*) gene encodes a protein, which belongs to the GATA family of transcription factors. The protein contains two GATA-type zinc fingers and is an important regulator of T-cell development and plays an important role in endothelial cell biology; *GATA-3* is essential in the embryonic development of the parathyroid, auditory system and kidneys, and defects in this gene cause HDR syndrome (hypoparathyroidism with sensorineural deafness and renal dysplasia) [37]. *GATA-3* analysis and the phenotypic spectrum obtained for nine Japanese families with the HDR syndrome suggest that this syndrome is primarily caused by *GATA-3* haploinsufficiency [38]. This TF plays a dual role in transcription regulation in a positive and negative manner. In accordance with this, we found the association of GATA-3 with up-regulated genes (EI = 1.85) after drug treatment in U343 cells.

Another TF, FOXP3 (*Forkhead box P3*), a positive regulator of transcription, plays a critical role in the control of immune response. This TF was associated with up-regulated genes (EI = 1.31) in drug-treated U343 cells. Defects in this gene lead to X-linked autoimmunity-immunodeficiency syndrome [39]. In several neoplasias, such as breast [40], ovarian [41], skin [42] and stomach, FOXP3 was found over-expressed [43], or mutated in prostate cancer [44]. It is well established that tumor cells acquire molecular and biochemical changes which make them potentially vulnerable to the immune system [45]. Alterations in the immune system can be applied for cancer detection and therapies [46]. Interestingly, [47] demonstrated a dependency on functional TP53 for DNA damage induced activation of *FOXP3* in human breast and colon carcinoma cells. However, the precise role of *FOXP3* in drug responses is still unknown.

FOXJ2 (*Forkhead box J2*) was also associated with up-regulated genes (EI = 1.42); this TF is often described as a positive regulator of transcription [48] and is a member of Forkhead Box TFs, many of which have been reported to participate in tumor migration and invasion. Wang et al. [49] showed that the expression of *FOXJ2* was high in primary breast cancer tissues without lymph nodes metastases; moreover, *FOXJ2* may play a role in maintenance and survival of developing and adult neurons, but its function in the central nervous system is still unclear. Knockdown of this TF in cultured primary astrocytes by siRNA showed that *FOXJ2* played an important role in lipopolysaccharide-induced inflammatory responses [50]. Nonetheless, there is no information in the literature about its function in relation to chemotherapeutic drugs.

C/EBP (*CCAAT/enhancer-binding protein*) family plays important roles in many processes such as cell differentiation, metabolism, and development. *C/EBP* (CEBPA) gene, CCAAT/enhancer binding protein alpha, involved in cell cycle arrest [51], and also plays a role in DNA damage response dependent on TP53 [52]. The protein acts as a dominant-negative inhibitor by forming hetero-dimers with other C/EBP members, such as C/EBP and LAP (*liver activator protein*), and preventing their DNA binding activity. Another member, GADD153 (CHOP), is a critical initiator of ER stress-induced apoptosis, and its knockdown prevents perturbations in the *AKT* (*protein kinase B*)/*FOXO3a* (*forkhead box, class O, 3a*) pathway in response to ER stress [53]. C/EBP β, a member of a subfamily of basic leucine zipper (bZIP) protein family, play a potential role in the proliferation and invasion of glioma, being considered as a novel molecular target for therapy, as well as a predictive marker for survival of patients with glioma [54]. In the present study, C/EBP showed an association with up-regulated genes (EI = 1.87), suggesting a possible role in DNA damage responses under drug treatment, and most probably, via AKT pathway, which is a target for LY294002.

Three TFs (*LXR*, *PXR* and *CAR*) were related to the same percentage (62.4%) of up-regulated genes, presenting EI = 1.14. The *liver X receptors* (*LXR*), *LXRA* and *LXRB*, comprise a subfamily of the nuclear receptor superfamily and are key regulators of macrophage function, controlling transcriptional programs involved in lipid homeostasis and inflammation. Polymorphism of *LXR* gene is associated with obesity since this gene is involved in cellular lipid metabolic process [55]. *PXR*, also named *NR1I2* (*Nuclear receptor subfamily 1, group I, member 2*) is a TF that acts in both positive and negative regulation of transcription, as well as in xenobiotic transport and metabolic process, in addition to exogenous drug catabolic process; this gene seems to be also implicated in breast cancer development [56, 57]. Similarly to *PXR*, *CAR* (*NR1I3*, *Nuclear receptor subfamily 1, group I, member 3*) is also a key regulator of xenobiotic and endobiotic metabolism [58]. Identification of TFs related to liver and xenobiotic metabolism regulating the over-expressed genes suggests that these genes may play a role in drug responses. However, this interesting possibility needs further validation.

The foregoing account demonstrates that all the TFs that are associated with up-regulated genes after combined treatment (cisplatin and LY294002) are regulators of important biological processes, such as cell differentiation, metabolism, development, and immune response, but the literature is still scarce regarding the role of above mentioned TFs in cellular response mechanisms to chemotherapeutic drugs. In spite of this, the increment observed in the number of associated genes (in terms of EI index, which ranged from 1.14 to 1.87) tends to suggest the involvement of these TFs in the outcome of cellular response to combined treatment.

3.3. TFs associated with down–regulated genes

Similar to the prediction of TFs associated with up-regulated genes, we performed the same kind of analysis for determining the TFs associated with down-regulated genes. None of the TF was found associated with down-regulated genes after treatment with cisplatin alone. However, for the combined treatment (cisplatin and LY294002), six TFs were predicted (Table 2). All TFs displayed enrichment indexes greater than 1 (ranging from 1.10 to 1.80), indicating that the enrichment was greater in the list of down-regulated genes (list #1) in comparison to all the genes (list #2) included in the array.

Term	Percentage with term		Enrichment index	p-value
	List #1	List #2		
GATA-3	23.6	16.3	1.45	2.2E–2
Evi-1	50	38.1	1.31	3.9E–2
HNF-1	90.2	84.0	1.10	4.8E–2
USF1	26.4	20.1	1.31	5.1E–2
CDX	82.2	67.3	1.22	5.6E–2
AP-1	27.6	15.5	1.80	5.6E–2

Table 2. Transcription factors (Term) associated to down-regulated genes in treated U343 cells (cisplatin combined to LY294002) vs. control. "Percentage with term" corresponds to the amount of genes that was associated to each TF in each list: list #1 represents the down-regulated genes obtained in the statistical analysis, and list #2 represents all genes present in the microarray slide. An "Enrichment index" was calculated for each Term by dividing the percentage in the list #1 by that in the list #2.

GATA-3, as already described above, was found associated with both up- and down-regulated genes. This could be due to the dual activity of this TF, which acts as a positive or negative regulator of transcription. *GATA-3* also participates in the negative regulation of cell proliferation process, which can be triggered as a response to drug treatments. Accordingly, we found GATA-3 association with down-regulated genes (EI = 1.45) after drug treatment in U343 cells.

EVI-1, also known as *RUNX1* (*Runt-related transcription factor 1*), is a positive regulator of transcription related to peripheral nervous system, neuron development, hematopoietic stem cell proliferation, and angiogenesis, among other functions. Due to its role in hematopoietic and nervous systems, deregulation of this TF results in hematological disorders [59-62] and central nervous system diseases [63]. Recently, Satoh et al. [64] reported that the C-terminal deletion of RUNX1 attenuates DNA-damage repair responses in hematopoietic stem/progenitor cells, and additionally, they found that *RUNX1* directly regulates the transcription of *GADD45A* gene, which is involved in cell cycle arrest. Association of EVI-1 with down-regulated genes (EI = 1.31) presumably indicates an impaired function of this TF in U343 cells, since it is expected to positively regulate the gene targets.

HNF-1 is also named *HNF1A* (*Hepatocyte Nuclear Factor 1 Alpha*) and *TCF-1* (*Transcription Factor 1*). This TF, previously related to diseases such as diabetes and neoplasias [65-70], encodes a protein involved in the WNT signaling pathway [71]. The activation of this pathway has been pointed as one of the main causes of colon cancer; in addition, it has been reported that *HNF1A* plays an important role in transduction of this pathway in the intestine [72]. Furthermore, Roth et al. [73] demonstrated alterations in the regulation of WNT signaling pathway in glioma cells. Inhibition of genes participating in the WNT pathway promote blockage of tumor growth [74].This is compatible with reduction in cell survival after drug treatment in GBM cells which may be most likely due to down-regulation of several genes regulated by *HNF1A*.

USF1 (*Upstream transcription factor 1*), another TF predicted in our analysis, is a gene with known functions in cellular responses under stress conditions, such as UV and hypoxia. In breast tumors, a role for *USF1* in regulating the expression of *estrogen receptor alpha* (*ERalpha*) has been demonstrated [75]. Recently, Baron et al. [76] demonstrated a role for USF-1 in maintaining genome integrity in response to UV-induced DNA photolesions. Additionally, using a mouse knock out model, the authors showed that the loss of USF-1 compromises DNA repair, suggesting that USF-1 may play a similar role in human cells. However, in the present study, USF1 was found associated with down-regulated genes (EI = 1.31) in U343 and the role of USF1 remains to be investigated in tumor cells.

CDX represents a gene family of *caudal-related homeobox* TFs, composed of the following members: *CDX1*, *CDX2*, and *CDX4*. All these members participate in the regulation of intestine-specific gene expression, and also in anterior-posterior pattern specification and blood vessel development. These TFs have been found associated with several neoplasias, including esophageal [77, 78], gallbladder [79], liver [80], colorectal [81-83], and pancreatic [84], but their role in drug responses is still unknown.

AP-1 (presented EI = 1.8) is a TF complex formed by proteins of the JUN family dimerized with members of the *FOS* gene family, which consists of 4 members (*FOS*, *FOSB*, *FOSL1*, and *FOSL2*) that encode leucine zipper proteins. All these genes are oncogenes with established roles in neoplastic cell transformation [85-87], prostatic [88], colorectal [89, 90], liver [91, 92], stomach [93], and breast cancers [94]. Interestingly, Hamdi et al. [95] demonstrated the roles of AP-1 components, ATF3 and FRA1 (FOSL1), in JNK- and ERK-dependent cell cycle arrest and apoptosis after cisplatin or UV-light treatments, by activating both JNK and ERK pathways in human glioblastoma cells lacking functional TP53. Recently, Meise et al. [96] showed that *FOSL1* (*FRA1*) was up-regulated in glioblastoma cells following nimustine (ACNU) treatment. Thus, it becomes apparent that the AP-1 complex also participates in drug responses, and could be activated by combined treatment of cisplatin and LY294002 in GBM cells.

Therefore, TFs associated with down-regulated genes are critical participants in several biological processes such as neuron development, WNT signaling pathway, cellular response under stress conditions, and neoplastic cell transformation. It seems that all these TFs work in a concerted manner to regulate several genes leading to initiation of cellular responses after the combined treatment of cisplatin and LY294002 in GBM cells. Since most of the TFs predicted by us were not included in the gene arrays, expression of these TFS after drug treatment could not be verified. Further experiments are certainly warranted to understand their concerted roles in understanding the cellular response mechanisms to cisplatin and LY294002.

TFs and cis-regulatory elements are considered key components for transcription regulation [97]. Specific TFs can be involved in the control of co-expressed genes [98], and these genes tend to participate in related pathways, for example, cell cycle control and apoptosis [99, 100]. Thus, search for the common TFs that control the transcription of a specific group of genes such as those involved in DNA repair or replication may provide biomarkers, which can be potential targets for therapeutic intervention [101]. Interestingly, some of the predicted TFs were recently reported to be associated with DNA repair/DNA damage responses in human cells, but few were reported in GBM. Nevertheless, the TFs predicted by *in silico* analysis described above may be useful for understanding how the transcription machinery responds to chemotherapeutic agents in GBM cells. Further studies are required to get insights regarding the role of TFs identified by us in modulating the drug response of GBM cells.

3.4. Signaling pathways involved in drug responses

In addition, data obtained on differentially expressed genes between treated (cisplatin combined to LY294002) and control U343 cells were submitted to a pathway analysis, using tools available in the Database for Annotation, Visualization and Integrated Discovery (DAVID) v6.7 [102]. The KEGG pathway analysis was selected and pathways presenting p-values ≤ 0.05 were chosen.

Signaling pathway analysis was performed by means of tools available in DAVID, as previously described. This analysis allowed the identification of common biological pathways mapped in the KEGG pathway database, in which the up-regulated genes in treated U343 cells are involved. Three pathways were significantly associated with up regulated genes (Table 3), among which two are related to the inositol molecule (inositol phosphate metabolism and phosphatidylinositol signaling system); three genes (*PIK3C3, PIP5K1B, OCRL)* were included as participants of both pathways. The *TP53* signaling pathway was also associated which included three important genes: *ATR, CCNG1* and *SESN1*. These results are consistent with earlier studies demonstrating the activation of these signaling pathways under drug treatments [103-105].

KEGG term	Genes*	p-value
hsa00562: Inositol phosphate metabolism	*PIK3C3, PIP5K1B, OCRL*	3.3E–2
hsa04115: TP53 signaling pathway	*ATR, CCNG1, SESN1*	5.0E–2
hsa04070: Phosphatidylinositol signaling system	*PIK3C3, PIP5K1B, OCRL*	5.0E–2

* Genes participating in each pathway

Table 3. Cellular signaling pathways associated with up-regulated genes in treated U343 cells (cisplatin combined to LY294002), as analyzed by tools available in DAVID.

The *PIK3C3* gene (*Phosphoinositide-3-kinase, class 3*) participates in the innate immune response and cell cycle. This gene also plays an essential role in regulating functional autophagy and is crucial for normal liver and heart function [106]. *PIP5K1B* (*Phosphatidylinositol-4-phosphate 5-kinase, type I, beta*) is involved in the biosynthesis of phosphatidylinositol 4,5-bisphosphate. The *OCRL* gene (*Oculocerebrorenal syndrome of Lowe*) encodes a phosphatase enzyme with a demonstrated role in actin polymerization, and it is an important participant in the trans-Golgi network. Mutations in this gene cause oculocerebrorenal syndrome of Lowe and also Dent disease [107].

The protein encoded by the *ATR* gene (*Ataxia telangiectasia and Rad3 related*) act in the cell cycle checkpoint and is required for cell cycle arrest and DNA damage repair in response to DNA damage. The *ATR* gene belongs to the PI3/PI4-kinase family, as well as ATM and DNA-PK, and is known as playing an important role in cellular response to cisplatin [108-110]. The aberrantly activated antiapoptotic phospatidyl-3-inositol-kinase (PI3K)/Akt signaling is induced by cisplatin and restricts the efficiency of chemotherapy [49]. The *CCNG1* gene (*cyclin G1*) plays a role in cell cycle and growth, brain development and G2/M checkpoint, acting in the negative regulation of apoptotic process. Altered regulation of this gene was observed in breast cancer [111], and leukemia [112]. *SESN1* (*Sestrin 1*) is responsible for the negative regulation of cell proliferation, acting in cell cycle arrest in response to DNA damage stimulus. This gene was found differentially induced by genotoxic stress (UV, gamma-irradiation and cytotoxic drugs) in a TP53-dependent manner, presenting properties common to the GADD family of growth arrest and DNA damage-inducible stress-response genes [113].

Therefore, we found relevant pathways related to TP53 (cell cycle arrest and DNA repair) in response to DNA damage, as well as to the inositol phosphate metabolism and signaling. Furthermore, several predicted TFs associated with modulated genes participate in "basal vital processes", and these processes include the inositol metabolism and signaling, highlighting the importance of these pathways in cellular response mechanisms after drug treatment. However, it is not known whether the observed sensitivity of GBM to cisplatin and LY294002 is due to disruption of some of the above-mentioned vital processes through inhibition of PI3K dependent signaling pathways. A likely possibility that needs consideration is that several sub-pathways can be inactivated/activated due to loss of major tumor suppressor genes such as PTEN, which negatively regulates PI3K/AKT pathways [114] in TP53 proficient U343 GBM cell line. [115]. Furthermore, TP53 pathway, which has been extensively studied in cancer, was also involved in U343 cell line after drug exposure.

3.5. Conclusion

Identification of TFs associated with a set of differentially expressed genes is an interesting approach that may allow to interpret mechanisms triggered in a cellular milieu after a given treatment condition. In the context of cancer research, differential expression of genes and pathways in response to drug treatment may either result in tumor growth reduction or cell killing.

Beside the relevance of our findings, some methodological limitations should be mentioned regarding *in silico* prediction of TFs. Numerous TF binding sites exist for each of the gene targets and it is hard to predict which binding site is critical for transcriptional regulation. It is possible that a considerable fraction of these binding sites are nonfunctional and may constitute biological noise [116]. Other choices, such as ChIP experiments, may overcome this concern by detecting indirect TF-DNA interactions through protein/protein interaction [117]. Even though most of the predicted TFs we identified in our study have not been specifically shown to be associated with GBM in previous studies, they can be considered as potential predictors for evaluating the effectiveness of drug response in GBM. Further verification and validation of the TFs involved in GBM may provide useful information for developing novel therapeutic strategies for brain tumors.

Author details

P. O. Carminati[1], F. S. Donaires[1], P. R. D. V. Godoy[1], A. P. Montaldi[1], J. A. Meador[2], A.S. Balajee[2], G. A. Passos[3] and E. T. Sakamoto-Hojo[1,4]

1 Department of Genetics, Faculty of Medicine of Ribeirão Preto, São Paulo University (USP), Ribeirão Preto, SP, Brazil

2 Center for Radiological Research, Department of Radiation Oncology, College of Physicians and Surgeons, Columbia University, New York, NY, USA

3 Department of Genetics, Faculty of Medicine and Faculty of Dentistry, University of São Paulo, Ribeirão Preto, SP, Brazil.

4 Department of Biology, Faculty of Philosophy, Sciences and Letters of Ribeirão Preto, São Paulo University (USP), Ribeirão Preto, SP, Brazil

References

[1] Bao, S, Q Wu, RE McLendon, et al., Glioma stem cells promote radioresistance by preferential activation of the DNA damage response. Nature, 2006. 444(7120): p. 756-60.

[2] Johannessen, TC, R Bjerkvig, and BB Tysnes, DNA repair and cancer stem-like cells--potential partners in glioma drug resistance? Cancer Treat Rev, 2008. 34(6): p. 558-67.

[3] Durocher, D and SP Jackson, DNA-PK, ATM and ATR as sensors of DNA damage: variations on a theme? Curr Opin Cell Biol, 2001. 13(2): p. 225-31.

[4] Falck, J, J Coates, and SP Jackson, Conserved modes of recruitment of ATM, ATR and DNA-PKcs to sites of DNA damage. Nature, 2005. 434(7033): p. 605-11.

[5] Collis, SJ, TL DeWeese, PA Jeggo, et al., The life and death of DNA-PK. Oncogene, 2005. 24(6): p. 949-61.

[6] Jones, PA and SB Baylin, The fundamental role of epigenetic events in cancer. Nat Rev Genet, 2002. 3(6): p. 415-28.

[7] Jones, PA and SB Baylin, The epigenomics of cancer. Cell, 2007. 128(4): p. 683-92.

[8] Karagiannis, TC and A El-Osta, Clinical potential of histone deacetylase inhibitors as stand alone therapeutics and in combination with other chemotherapeutics or radiotherapy for cancer. Epigenetics, 2006. 1(3): p. 121-6.

[9] Cheng, JC, DJ Weisenberger, FA Gonzales, et al., Continuous zebularine treatment effectively sustains demethylation in human bladder cancer cells. Mol Cell Biol, 2004. 24(3): p. 1270-8.

[10] Meador, JA, Y Su, JL Ravanat, et al., DNA-dependent protein kinase (DNA-PK)-deficient human glioblastoma cells are preferentially sensitized by Zebularine. Carcinogenesis, 2010. 31(2): p. 184-91.

[11] Shao, CJ, J Fu, HL Shi, et al., Activities of DNA-PK and Ku86, but not Ku70, may predict sensitivity to cisplatin in human gliomas. J Neurooncol, 2008. 89(1): p. 27-35.

[12] Sakamoto-Hojo, ET and AS Balajee, Targeting poly (ADP) ribose polymerase I (PARP-1) and PARP-1 interacting proteins for cancer treatment. Anticancer Agents Med Chem, 2008. 8(4): p. 402-16.

[13] Balajee, AS, I Dianova, and VA Bohr, Oxidative damage-induced PCNA complex formation is efficient in xeroderma pigmentosum group A but reduced in Cockayne syndrome group B cells. Nucleic Acids Res, 1999. 27(22): p. 4476-82.

[14] Balajee, AS and CR Geard, Chromatin-bound PCNA complex formation triggered by DNA damage occurs independent of the ATM gene product in human cells. Nucleic Acids Res, 2001. 29(6): p. 1341-51.

[15] Carminati, PO, FS Donaires, MM Marques, et al., Cisplatin associated with LY294002 increases cytotoxicity and induces changes in transcript profiles of glioblastoma cells. manuscript in preparation, 2012.

[16] Sankpal, UT, S Goodison, M Abdelrahim, et al., Targeting Sp1 transcription factors in prostate cancer therapy. Med Chem, 2011. 7(5): p. 518-25.

[17] Liu, LY, LY Chang, WH Kuo, et al., In Silico Prediction for Regulation of Transcription Factors onTheir Shared Target Genes Indicates Relevant Clinical Implications in a Breast Cancer Population. Cancer Inform, 2012. 11: p. 113-37.

[18] Rhodes, DR, S Kalyana-Sundaram, V Mahavisno, et al., Mining for regulatory programs in the cancer transcriptome. Nat Genet, 2005. 37(6): p. 579-83.

[19] Anderson, CW and SP Lees-Miller, The nuclear serine/threonine protein kinase DNA-PK. Crit Rev Eukaryot Gene Expr, 1992. 2(4): p. 283-314.

[20] Kong, D, S Yaguchi, and T Yamori, Effect of ZSTK474, a novel phosphatidylinositol 3-kinase inhibitor, on DNA-dependent protein kinase. Biol Pharm Bull, 2009. 32(2): p. 297-300.

[21] Yamaguchi, K, SH Lee, JS Kim, et al., Activating transcription factor 3 and early growth response 1 are the novel targets of LY294002 in a phosphatidylinositol 3-kinase-independent pathway. Cancer Res, 2006. 66(4): p. 2376-84.

[22] Ohta, T, M Ohmichi, T Hayasaka, et al., Inhibition of phosphatidylinositol 3-kinase increases efficacy of cisplatin in in vivo ovarian cancer models. Endocrinology, 2006. 147(4): p. 1761-9.

[23] Kong, D and T Yamori, Phosphatidylinositol 3-kinase inhibitors: promising drug candidates for cancer therapy. Cancer Sci, 2008. 99(9): p. 1734-40.

[24] Prevo, R, E Deutsch, O Sampson, et al., Class I PI3 kinase inhibition by the pyridinylfuranopyrimidine inhibitor PI-103 enhances tumor radiosensitivity. Cancer Res, 2008. 68(14): p. 5915-23.

[25] Westhoff, MA, JA Kandenwein, S Karl, et al., The pyridinylfuranopyrimidine inhibitor, PI-103, chemosensitizes glioblastoma cells for apoptosis by inhibiting DNA repair. Oncogene, 2009. 28(40): p. 3586-96.

[26] Fachin, AL, SS Mello, P Sandrin-Garcia, et al., Gene expression profiles in human lymphocytes irradiated in vitro with low doses of gamma rays. Radiat Res, 2007. 168(6): p. 650-65.

[27] Tusher, VG, R Tibshirani, and G Chu, Significance analysis of microarrays applied to the ionizing radiation response. Proc Natl Acad Sci U S A, 2001. 98(9): p. 5116-21.

[28] Al-Shahrour, F, P Minguez, JM Vaquerizas, et al., BABELOMICS: a suite of web tools for functional annotation and analysis of groups of genes in high-throughput experiments. Nucleic Acids Res, 2005. 33(Web Server issue): p. W460-4.

[29] Bock, KW and C Kohle, Ah receptor: dioxin-mediated toxic responses as hints to deregulated physiologic functions. Biochem Pharmacol, 2006. 72(4): p. 393-404.

[30] Hayhurst, GP, H Strick-Marchand, C Mulet, et al., Morphogenetic competence of HNF4 alpha-deficient mouse hepatic cells. J Hepatol, 2008. 49(3): p. 384-95.

[31] Huang, TH, T Oka, T Asai, et al., Repression by a differentiation-specific factor of the human cytomegalovirus enhancer. Nucleic Acids Res, 1996. 24(9): p. 1695-701.

[32] Wilsker, D, A Patsialou, PB Dallas, et al., ARID proteins: a diverse family of DNA binding proteins implicated in the control of cell growth, differentiation, and development. Cell Growth Differ, 2002. 13(3): p. 95-106.

[33] Healy, J, C Richer, M Bourgey, et al., Replication analysis confirms the association of ARID5B with childhood B-cell acute lymphoblastic leukemia. Haematologica, 2010. 95(9): p. 1608-11.

[34] Tchougounova, E, Y Jiang, D Brasater, et al., Sox5 can suppress platelet-derived growth factor B-induced glioma development in Ink4a-deficient mice through induction of acute cellular senescence. Oncogene, 2009. 28(12): p. 1537-48.

[35] Honda, N, K Yagi, GR Ding, et al., Radiosensitization by overexpression of the non-phosphorylation form of IkappaB-alpha in human glioma cells. J Radiat Res, 2002. 43(3): p. 283-92.

[36] Yamagishi, N, J Miyakoshi, and H Takebe, Enhanced radiosensitivity by inhibition of nuclear factor kappa B activation in human malignant glioma cells. Int J Radiat Biol, 1997. 72(2): p. 157-62.

[37] Van Esch, H, P Groenen, MA Nesbit, et al., GATA3 haplo-insufficiency causes human HDR syndrome. Nature, 2000. 406(6794): p. 419-22.

[38] Muroya, K, T Hasegawa, Y Ito, et al., GATA3 abnormalities and the phenotypic spectrum of HDR syndrome. J Med Genet, 2001. 38(6): p. 374-80.

[39] van der Vliet, HJ and EE Nieuwenhuis, IPEX as a result of mutations in FOXP3. Clin Dev Immunol, 2007. 2007: p. 89017.

[40] Matsuura, K, Y Yamaguchi, A Osaki, et al., FOXP3 expression of micrometastasis-positive sentinel nodes in breast cancer patients. Oncol Rep, 2009. 22(5): p. 1181-7.

[41] Wolf, D, AM Wolf, H Rumpold, et al., The expression of the regulatory T cell-specific forkhead box transcription factor FoxP3 is associated with poor prognosis in ovarian cancer. Clin Cancer Res, 2005. 11(23): p. 8326-31.

[42] Klemke, CD, B Fritzsching, B Franz, et al., Paucity of FOXP3+ cells in skin and peripheral blood distinguishes Sézary syndrome from other cutaneous T-cell lymphomas. Leukemia, 2006. 20(6): p. 1123-9.

[43] Yuan, XL, L Chen, MX Li, et al., Elevated expression of Foxp3 in tumor-infiltrating Treg cells suppresses T-cell proliferation and contributes to gastric cancer progression in a COX-2-dependent manner. Clin Immunol, 2010. 134(3): p. 277-88.

[44] Wang, L, R Liu, W Li, et al., Somatic single hits inactivate the X-linked tumor suppressor FOXP3 in the prostate. Cancer Cell, 2009. 16(4): p. 336-46.

[45] Steer, HJ, RA Lake, AK Nowak, et al., Harnessing the immune response to treat cancer. Oncogene, 2010. 29(48): p. 6301-13.

[46] Hanash, S, Harnessing the immune response for cancer detection. Cancer Epidemiol Biomarkers Prev, 2011. 20(4): p. 569-70.

[47] Jung, DJ, DH Jin, SW Hong, et al., Foxp3 expression in p53-dependent DNA damage responses. J Biol Chem, 2010. 285(11): p. 7995-8002.

[48] Pérez-Sánchez, C, C Arias-de-la-Fuente, MA Gómez-Ferrería, et al., FHX.L and FHX.S, two isoforms of the human fork-head factor FHX (FOXJ2) with differential activity. J Mol Biol, 2000. 301(4): p. 795-806.

[49] Wang, L, P Wang, Y Liu, et al., Regulation of cellular growth, apoptosis, and Akt activity in human U251 glioma cells by a combination of cisplatin with CRM197. Anticancer Drugs, 2012. 23(1): p. 81-9.

[50] Chen, X, X Cao, G Tao, et al., FOXJ2 expression in rat spinal cord after injury and its role in inflammation. J Mol Neurosci, 2012. 47(1): p. 158-65.

[51] Wang, H, P Iakova, M Wilde, et al., C/EBPalpha arrests cell proliferation through direct inhibition of Cdk2 and Cdk4. Mol Cell, 2001. 8(4): p. 817-28.

[52] Yoon, K and RC Smart, C/EBPalpha is a DNA damage-inducible p53-regulated mediator of the G1 checkpoint in keratinocytes. Mol Cell Biol, 2004. 24(24): p. 10650-60.

[53] Ghosh, AP, BJ Klocke, ME Ballestas, et al., CHOP Potentially Co-Operates with FOXO3a in Neuronal Cells to Regulate PUMA and BIM Expression in Response to ER Stress. PLoS ONE, 2012. 7(6): p. e39586.

[54] Homma, J, R Yamanaka, N Yajima, et al., Increased expression of CCAAT/enhancer binding protein beta correlates with prognosis in glioma patients. Oncol Rep, 2006. 15(3): p. 595-601.

[55] Dahlman, I, M Nilsson, H Jiao, et al., Liver X receptor gene polymorphisms and adipose tissue expression levels in obesity. Pharmacogenet Genomics, 2006. 16(12): p. 881-9.

[56] Chen, Y, Y Tang, S Chen, et al., Regulation of drug resistance by human pregnane X receptor in breast cancer. Cancer Biol Ther, 2009. 8(13): p. 1265-72.

[57] Dotzlaw, H, E Leygue, P Watson, et al., The human orphan receptor PXR messenger RNA is expressed in both normal and neoplastic breast tissue. Clin Cancer Res, 1999. 5(8): p. 2103-7.

[58] Urquhart, BL, RG Tirona, and RB Kim, Nuclear receptors and the regulation of drug-metabolizing enzymes and drug transporters: implications for interindividual variability in response to drugs. J Clin Pharmacol, 2007. 47(5): p. 566-78.

[59] Ding, Y, Y Harada, J Imagawa, et al., AML1/RUNX1 point mutation possibly promotes leukemic transformation in myeloproliferative neoplasms. Blood, 2009. 114(25): p. 5201-5.

[60] Yanagida, M, M Osato, N Yamashita, et al., Increased dosage of Runx1/AML1 acts as a positive modulator of myeloid leukemogenesis in BXH2 mice. Oncogene, 2005. 24(28): p. 4477-85.

[61] Asou, N, The role of a Runt domain transcription factor AML1/RUNX1 in leukemogenesis and its clinical implications. Crit Rev Oncol Hematol, 2003. 45(2): p. 129-50.

[62] Hart, SM and L Foroni, Core binding factor genes and human leukemia. Haematologica, 2002. 87(12): p. 1307-23.

[63] Wang, Q, T Stacy, M Binder, et al., Disruption of the Cbfa2 gene causes necrosis and hemorrhaging in the central nervous system and blocks definitive hematopoiesis. Proc Natl Acad Sci U S A, 1996. 93(8): p. 3444-9.

[64] Satoh, Y, I Matsumura, H Tanaka, et al., C-terminal mutation of RUNX1 attenuates the DNA-damage repair response in hematopoietic stem cells. Leukemia, 2012. 26(2): p. 303-11.

[65] Umeyama, K, M Watanabe, H Saito, et al., Dominant-negative mutant hepatocyte nuclear factor 1alpha induces diabetes in transgenic-cloned pigs. Transgenic Res, 2009. 18(5): p. 697-706.

[66] Pal, A, AJ Farmer, C Dudley, et al., Evaluation of serum 1,5 anhydroglucitol levels as a clinical test to differentiate subtypes of diabetes. Diabetes Care, 2010. 33(2): p. 252-7.

[67] Pinés Corrales, PJ, MP López Garrido, S Aznar Rodríguez, et al., Clinical differences between patients with MODY-3, MODY-2 and type 2 diabetes mellitus with I27L polymorphism in the HNF1alpha gene. Endocrinol Nutr, 2010. 57(1): p. 4-8.

[68] Rebouissou, S, C Rosty, F Lecuru, et al., Mutation of TCF1 encoding hepatocyte nuclear factor 1alpha in gynecological cancer. Oncogene, 2004. 23(45): p. 7588-92.

[69] Bélanger, AS, J Tojcic, M Harvey, et al., Regulation of UGT1A1 and HNF1 transcription factor gene expression by DNA methylation in colon cancer cells. BMC Mol Biol, 2010. 11: p. 9.

[70] Piessen, G, N Jonckheere, A Vincent, et al., Regulation of the human mucin MUC4 by taurodeoxycholic and taurochenodeoxycholic bile acids in oesophageal cancer cells is mediated by hepatocyte nuclear factor 1alpha. Biochem J, 2007. 402(1): p. 81-91.

[71] Thierry-Mieg, D and J Thierry-Mieg, AceView: a comprehensive cDNA-supported gene and transcripts annotation. Genome Biol, 2006. 7 Suppl 1: p. S12.1-14.

[72] Najdi, R, A Syed, L Arce, et al., A Wnt kinase network alters nuclear localization of TCF-1 in colon cancer. Oncogene, 2009. 28(47): p. 4133-46.

[73] Roth, W, C Wild-Bode, M Platten, et al., Secreted Frizzled-related proteins inhibit motility and promote growth of human malignant glioma cells. Oncogene, 2000. 19(37): p. 4210-20.

[74] DeAlmeida, VI, L Miao, JA Ernst, et al., The soluble wnt receptor Frizzled8CRD-hFc inhibits the growth of teratocarcinomas in vivo. Cancer Res, 2007. 67(11): p. 5371-9.

[75] deGraffenried, LA, TA Hopp, AJ Valente, et al., Regulation of the estrogen receptor alpha minimal promoter by Sp1, USF-1 and ERalpha. Breast Cancer Res Treat, 2004. 85(2): p. 111-20.

[76] Baron, Y, S Corre, N Mouchet, et al., USF-1 is critical for maintaining genome integrity in response to UV-induced DNA photolesions. PLoS Genet, 2012. 8(1): p. e1002470.

[77] Vaninetti, N, L Williams, L Geldenhuys, et al., Regulation of CDX2 expression in esophageal adenocarcinoma. Mol Carcinog, 2009. 48(10): p. 965-74.

[78] Lord, RV, J Brabender, K Wickramasinghe, et al., Increased CDX2 and decreased PITX1 homeobox gene expression in Barrett's esophagus and Barrett's-associated adenocarcinoma. Surgery, 2005. 138(5): p. 924-31.

[79] Wu, XS, Y Akiyama, T Igari, et al., Expression of homeodomain protein CDX2 in gallbladder carcinomas. J Cancer Res Clin Oncol, 2005. 131(5): p. 271-8.

[80] Ishikawa, A, M Sasaki, S Ohira, et al., Aberrant expression of CDX2 is closely related to the intestinal metaplasia and MUC2 expression in intraductal papillary neoplasm of the liver in hepatolithiasis. Lab Invest, 2004. 84(5): p. 629-38.

[81] Wong, NA, MP Britton, GS Choi, et al., Loss of CDX1 expression in colorectal carcinoma: promoter methylation, mutation, and loss of heterozygosity analyses of 37 cell lines. Proc Natl Acad Sci U S A, 2004. 101(2): p. 574-9.

[82] Suh, ER, CS Ha, EB Rankin, et al., DNA methylation down-regulates CDX1 gene expression in colorectal cancer cell lines. J Biol Chem, 2002. 277(39): p. 35795-800.

[83] Mallo, GV, H Rechreche, JM Frigerio, et al., Molecular cloning, sequencing and expression of the mRNA encoding human Cdx1 and Cdx2 homeobox. Down-regulation of Cdx1 and Cdx2 mRNA expression during colorectal carcinogenesis. Int J Cancer, 1997. 74(1): p. 35-44.

[84] Yeh, TS, YP Ho, CT Chiu, et al., Aberrant expression of cdx2 homeobox gene in intraductal papillary-mucinous neoplasm of the pancreas but not in pancreatic ductal adenocarcinoma. Pancreas, 2005. 30(3): p. 233-8.

[85] Ekstrand, AJ and L Zech, Human c-fos proto-oncogene mapped to chromosome 14, band q24.3-q31. Possibilities for oncogene activation by chromosomal rearrangements in human neoplasms. Exp Cell Res, 1987. 169(1): p. 262-6.

[86] Verma, IM, J Deschamps, C Van Beveren, et al., Human fos gene. Cold Spring Harb Symp Quant Biol, 1986. 51 Pt 2: p. 949-58.

[87] Kalogeropoulou, M, A Voulgari, V Kostourou, et al., TAF4b and Jun/activating protein-1 collaborate to regulate the expression of integrin alpha6 and cancer cell migration properties. Mol Cancer Res, 2010. 8(4): p. 554-68.

[88] Sato, N, MD Sadar, N Bruchovsky, et al., Androgenic induction of prostate-specific antigen gene is repressed by protein-protein interaction between the androgen receptor and AP-1/c-Jun in the human prostate cancer cell line LNCaP. J Biol Chem, 1997. 272(28): p. 17485-94.

[89] Wang, L, Y Sun, M Jiang, et al., FOS proliferating network construction in early colorectal cancer (CRC) based on integrative significant function cluster and inferring analysis. Cancer Invest, 2009. 27(8): p. 816-24.

[90] Liu, G, W Ding, X Liu, et al., c-Fos is required for TGFbeta1 production and the associated paracrine migratory effects of human colon carcinoma cells. Mol Carcinog, 2006. 45(8): p. 582-93.

[91] Konsman, JP and A Blomqvist, Forebrain patterns of c-Fos and FosB induction during cancer-associated anorexia-cachexia in rat. Eur J Neurosci, 2005. 21(10): p. 2752-66.

[92] Endo, M, K Yasui, T Nakajima, et al., Infrequent amplification of JUN in hepatocellular carcinoma. Anticancer Res, 2009. 29(12): p. 4989-94.

[93] Myllykangas, S, O Monni, B Nagy, et al., Helicobacter pylori infection activates FOS and stress-response genes and alters expression of genes in gastric cancer-specific loci. Genes Chromosomes Cancer, 2004. 40(4): p. 334-41.

[94] Dahlman-Wright, K, Y Qiao, P Jonsson, et al., Interplay between AP-1 and estrogen receptor α in regulating gene expression and proliferation networks in breast cancer cells. Carcinogenesis, 2012.

[95] Hamdi, M, HE Popeijus, F Carlotti, et al., ATF3 and Fra1 have opposite functions in JNK- and ERK-dependent DNA damage responses. DNA Repair (Amst), 2008.

[96] Meise, R, MT Tomicic, B Kaina, et al., The chloroethylating anticancer drug ACNU induces FRA1 that is involved in drug resistance of glioma cells. Biochim Biophys Acta, 2012. 1823(7): p. 1199-207.

[97] Choi, D, SM Sharma, S Pasadhika, et al., Application of Biostatistics and Bioinformatics Tools to Identify Putative Transcription Factor-Gene Regulatory Network of Ankylosing Spondylitis and Sarcoidosis. Commun Stat Theory Methods, 2009. 38(18): p. 3326-3338.

[98] Eisen, MB, PT Spellman, PO Brown, et al., Cluster analysis and display of genome wide expression patterns. Proc Natl Acad Sci U S A, 1998. 95(25): p. 14863-8.

[99] Lee, HK, AK Hsu, J Sajdak, et al., Coexpression analysis of human genes across many microarray data sets. Genome Res, 2004. 14(6): p. 1085-94.

[100] Stuart, JM, E Segal, D Koller, et al., A gene-coexpression network for global discovery of conserved genetic modules. Science, 2003. 302(5643): p. 249-55.

[101] Mees, C, J Nemunaitis, and N Senzer, Transcription factors: their potential as targets for an individualized therapeutic approach to cancer. Cancer Gene Ther, 2009. 16(2): p. 103-12.

[102] Huang da, W, BT Sherman, and RA Lempicki, Systematic and integrative analysis of large gene lists using DAVID bioinformatics resources. Nat Protoc, 2009. 4(1): p. 44-57.

[103] Brabec, V and J Kasparkova, Modifications of DNA by platinum complexes. Relation to resistance of tumors to platinum antitumor drugs. Drug Resist Updat, 2005. 8(3): p. 131-46.

[104] Torigoe, T, H Izumi, H Ishiguchi, et al., Cisplatin resistance and transcription factors. Curr Med Chem Anticancer Agents, 2005. 5(1): p. 15-27.

[105] Zhang, P, Z Zhang, X Zhou, et al., Identification of genes associated with cisplatin resistance in human oral squamous cell carcinoma cell line. BMC Cancer, 2006. 6: p. 224.

[106] Jaber, N, Z Dou, JS Chen, et al., Class III PI3K Vps34 plays an essential role in autophagy and in heart and liver function. Proc Natl Acad Sci U S A, 2012. 109(6): p. 2003-8.

[107] Attree, O, IM Olivos, I Okabe, et al., The Lowe's oculocerebrorenal syndrome gene encodes a protein highly homologous to inositol polyphosphate-5-phosphatase. Nature, 1992. 358(6383): p. 239-42.

[108] Damia, G, L Filiberti, F Vikhanskaya, et al., Cisplatinum and taxol induce different patterns of p53 phosphorylation. Neoplasia, 2001. 3(1): p. 10-6.

[109] Yazlovitskaya, EM and DL Persons, Inhibition of cisplatin-induced ATR activity and enhanced sensitivity to cisplatin. Anticancer Res, 2003. 23(3B): p. 2275-9.

[110] Pabla, N, S Huang, QS Mi, et al., ATR-Chk2 signaling in p53 activation and DNA damage response during cisplatin-induced apoptosis. J Biol Chem, 2008. 283(10): p. 6572-83.

[111] Reimer, CL, AM Borras, SK Kurdistani, et al., Altered regulation of cyclin G in human breast cancer and its specific localization at replication foci in response to DNA damage in p53+/+ cells. J Biol Chem, 1999. 274(16): p. 11022-9.

[112] Kato, MV, The mechanisms of death of an erythroleukemic cell line by p53: involvement of the microtubule and mitochondria. Leuk Lymphoma, 1999. 33(1-2): p. 181-6.

[113] Velasco-Miguel, S, L Buckbinder, P Jean, et al., PA26, a novel target of the p53 tumor suppressor and member of the GADD family of DNA damage and growth arrest inducible genes. Oncogene, 1999. 18(1): p. 127-37.

[114] Konopka, G and A Bonni, Signaling pathways regulating gliomagenesis. Curr Mol Med, 2003. 3(1): p. 73-84.

[115] Ishii, N, D Maier, A Merlo, et al., Frequent co-alterations of TP53, p16/CDKN2A, p14ARF, PTEN tumor suppressor genes in human glioma cell lines. Brain Pathol, 1999. 9(3): p. 469-79.

[116] Struhl, K, Gene regulation. A paradigm for precision. Science, 2001. 293(5532): p. 1054-5.

[117] Chen, J, RM McKay, and LF Parada, Malignant glioma: lessons from genomics, mouse models, and stem cells. Cell, 2012. 149(1): p. 36-47.

Section 5

MicroRNAs

Chapter 17

Evolvement of microRNAs as Therapeutic Targets for Malignant Gliomas

Sihan Wu, Wenbo Zhu and Guangmei Yan

Additional information is available at the end of the chapter

http://dx.doi.org/10.5772/52672

1. Introduction

Malignant glioma (MG), consisting of anaplastic glioma (AA, WHO grade III) and glioblastomamultiforme (GBM, WHO grade IV, 60-70%), is the most common and destructive brain tumor [1]. Despite systemic treatment, surgical resection followed by radiotherapy and chemotherapy, the prognosis of patients with GBM remains poor with a median survival of 12 to 15 months and a 5-year survival rate of 9.8% [2, 3]. The dismal outcome fuels the need to understand the molecular basis of gliomagenesis and identify novel therapeutic targets for MG treatment.

With a developing understanding of core aberrant signaling pathways in MG, molecular targeted therapy has shown certain promise as a more rational strategy. Established targets, including receptor tyrosine kinases (RTK) such as EGFR, PDGFR and VEGFR, as well as mTOR, farnesyl transferase and PI3K, have drawn particular interests both in fundamental and clinical research. However, single targeted agents so far have not displayed desirable clinical outcomes as expected, with response rates of 0 to 15% and no prolongation of 6-month progression-free survival [4–6]. This disappointing outcome is primarily due to the nature of cancer with multi-genetic abnormality and inter/intra-tumor heterogeneity. Therefore, multiple targeting strategies are essential to achieve better clinical benefits.

MicroRNA (miRNA), a type of endogenous small non-coding RNA which negatively modulates gene expression in post-transcriptional level, has rapidly become a topical issue since it was firstly discovered in *C. elegans* two decades ago[7]. Increasing researches have reported that dysregulation of miRNA is closely associated with tumorigenesis and tumor progression. In gliomas, a group of miRNAs have been characterized as oncogenic and tumor-suppressive molecules. With a unique feature of multi-targeting, miRNA may become a new powerful weapon fighting against MG. Although much remains to be learned about formulating miRNAs as nucleic acid drugs, we feel that identification of miRNAs as therapeutic targets for gliomas is now within sight.

In this chapter, we will critically review issues relevant to contemporary researches on miRNAs and MG. Based upon other teams' and our data, this review will present findings on oncogenic and tumor-suppressive properties of miRNA in MG, focusing on the mechanisms of dysregulation, the involvement with core pathways of MG and the functional heterogeneity in different context. Besides, we will formulate evidences for miRNA-based clinical application in diagnosis and therapeutics of MG. The developing cognition of miRNAs will ultimately lead to innovative clinical approaches for MG.

2. Oncogenic and tumor-suppressive miRNAs in malignant gliomas

The very first oncogenic miRNA indentified in GBM is miR-21 as early as 2005 [8], although whose target genes were not fully understood at that time. In 2008, another group identified a set of targets of this miRNA which constitute a tumor-suppressive network including TGF-β, p53 and mitochondrial-apoptotic pathways [9]. This is one of the examples showing the multi-targeting nature of miRNAs in oncology. Beyond multi-targeting, these findings also prompt a hypothesis that miRNAs may have pathway preference in some cases.

Coincidently, also in 2005, S.A. Ciafre*et al.* firstly described that brain-enriched miR-128 and miR-181 family were frequently down-regulated in primary GBMs and cell lines [10], whose tumor-suppressive roles of these miRNAs were subsequently validated in the next few years [11–14].

In 2008, a milestone has been made in glioma research, accomplished by The Cancer Genome Atlas (TCGA) Research Network. Through integrative analysis of DNA copy number, gene expression and DNA methylation aberrations, TCGA defined three major pathways in GBM, which are RTK, p53 and RB signaling pathways, as shown in Figure 1 [15]. These pathways cannot be more familiar to every oncologist: frequently activated RTK signaling in cancer supports cell proliferation and survival, whereas p53 and RB signaling monitor cell cycle transition and couple to apoptosis and senescence pathways, which are commonly suppressed in cancer. To date, increasing oncogenic and tumor-suppressive miRNAs in MGs have been uncovered. In combination with genomic sketch of GBM described by TCGA, we have a deeper insight into the interactions within the core pathways of MG, which are controlled in coding and non-coding levels (Figure 1).

Here we do not pay our attention to the detail of each single miRNA, since several reviews have provided considerable details about their expression and function [16–18]. In this paper, we prefer to focus on how these miRNAs become aberrant, and which malignant phenotypes they contribute to.

As well as every protein coding gene, non-coding miRNA genes may similarly undergo over or lost expression, amplification, deletion, insertion, translocation and mutation, which lead to aberration of miRNAs. The mechanisms of miRNA aberration have not yet been extensively studied. Nevertheless, there have been some clues showing that transcriptional activity, single nucleotide polymorphism (SNP) and chromosome deletion contribute to aberrant genotype and malignant phenotype of MG.

The most interesting research addressing miRNA transcriptional regulation machinery in MGs is the *TP53* and miR-25/32 feedback circuitry [19]. Carlo M. Croce's and co-workers found that miR-25 and miR-32 are negatively regulated by *TP53* via repressing their transcriptional factors *MYC* and *E2F1*. Intriguingly, by directly targeting *MDM2* and *TSC1*, these miRNAs help stabilize P53 protein and suppress tumorigenicity in U87 GBM cells. Thus, a fine tuned recurrent autoregulatory circuit form. However, in the non-functional mutant *TP53* context, miR-25/32 support cell proliferation *per contra*. These findings not only provide insights into the interaction between miRNAs and *TP53* tumor-suppressive pathway, but also hint that a given miRNA may have distinct function in different genetic and biochemical status.

It is unexpected that miRNA genes rarely exhibit SNP or mutation within the major mature sequence segment, although which can be commonly found in the precursor (including the minor mature sequence which is formerly called the star sequence) and primary miRNA segments. Through mining human SNP database, Peng Jin's group identified a G>U polymorphism located in the eighth nucleotide of the mature miR-125a-5p. The U allele blocks the processing from pri-miRNA to miRNA precursor by altering the secondary structure, and impairs miRNA-mediated translational suppression [20]. MiR-125s have been demonstrated to be tumor-suppressive in GBM [21–23]. However, such nucleotide alteration has not yet been described in glioma clinical data. The rs11614913 SNP, which locates in the segment producing minor mature miR-196a-3p (termed miR-196a* previously), was firstly found to be associated with the risk of glioma in Chinese population [24]. Recent clinical study indicates that the rs2910164 in segment containing minor mature miR-146a-3p sequence is also relative to the risk and prognosis in adult glioma [25]. These findings improve our understandings of miRNA-related pathogenesis and diagnostics in gliomas. Further research is required to fully comprehend the exact mechanisms underlying the relationship between miRNA gene SNPs and clinical outcomes, which may have huge clinical potential.

Chromosome alteration undoubtedly contributes to miRNA aberration. Particularly in diffuse astrocytoma (DA, WHO II) and AA, chromosome 7q32 is a hotspot that frequently amplifies. This region embraces eight miRNAs: miR-593, miR-129-1,miR-335, miR-182, miR-96, miR-183, miR-29a and miR-29b-1. Among these miRNAs, our group recently reported that miR-335 is the most striking target in AA [26]. We have demonstrated that miR-335 confers invasive and proliferative malignant phenotype on astrocytoma via targeting *DAAM1*. Disrupting miR-335 by cholesterylated miRNA inhibitor abrogates invasion and elicits apoptosis both *in vitro* and *in vivo*. Chromosome amplification in cancer often creates abnormal high level of coding and non-coding products that subsequently infests the well-balanced signaling. Currently, drug screening and discovery in oncology specifically focus on over-expressed protein and over-activated kinase. We believe that miRNA, such as miR-335, may also be the target for drug development in the future.

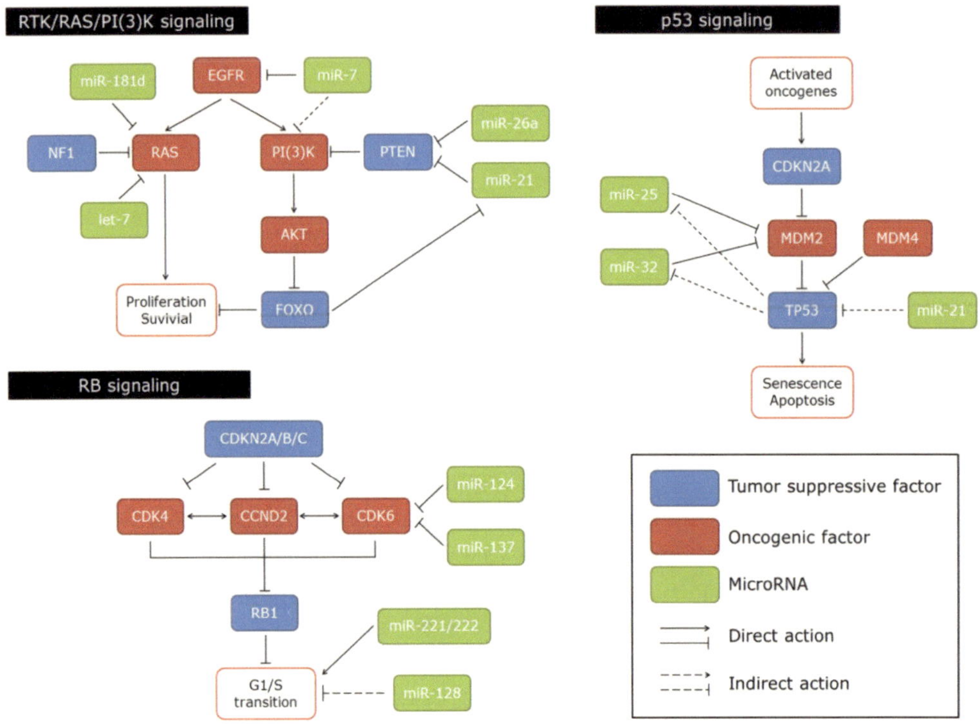

Figure 1. Interaction between microRNAs and core pathways in malignant gliomas.

3. Dual scripts for a miRNA

In the last session we have mentioned that miR-25/32 functions differently depended on *TP53* status in GBM. It is not the sole evidence that a given miRNA plays distinct roles in respective models. In fact, miRNAs show complicated functional heterogeneity.

One of the examples is miR-135a/b. Remco Nagel *et al.* found increased expression levels of miR-135a and miR-135b during colorectal cancer progression, which target the tumor suppressor gene Adenomatous Polyposis Coli (*APC*)[27]. The oncogenic role of miR-135a was further confirmed by BR Zetter's group. They demonstrated that paclitaxel resistance is associated with up-regulation of miR-135a in multiple solid tumor cell lines. Knocking-down of miR-135a acquires susceptibility to paclitaxel[28]. However, in classic Hodgkin lymphoma (cHL), miR-135a directly regulates *JAK2,* thus suppressing the expression of *BCL2L1* (also known as *BCL-XL*) and inducing apoptosis. Furthermore, higher level of miR-135a indicates better disease-free survival in cHL patients [29]. Likewise our group has also characterized that miR-135a functions as a selective killer of MG. We have reported that glial cell-enriched miR-135a is frequently down-regulated in MG and negatively correlates with the pathological grading of gliomas. Ectopic delivery of miR-135a selectively triggers mitochondrial dependent apoptosis in MG *in vitro* and *in vivo*. Interestingly, this lethal effect is neutral in normal glial cells and neurons [30].

MiR-335 gives us another example of the dual role nature of miRNAs. An early study identified that miR-335 suppresses breast cancer metastasis and migration through targeting *SOX4* and *TNC* [31]. However, as mentioned above, our recent research found that this miRNA promotes invasion and proliferation in AA [26]. In this way, miRNAs seems to have cell-type-dependent functional heterogeneity. The definition of "tumor-suppressive" and "oncogenic" should be carefully employed depended on the cell types and diseases.

Even within the same cell type, the functional behavior of a given miRNA can also be diverse. Previously we have reported that activation of cAMP/PKA pathway, manipulated by Cholera toxin, induces cellular differentiation of MG, showing malignant phenotype reversion and potent GFAP (glial fibrillary acidic protein) expression [32]. As it has been well characterized, we found that IL-6/JAK2/STAT3 contributes to GFAP expression in this model [33]. Notably, epigenetic mechanism is also involved. In this context, the so-called oncogenic miR-335 in MG induced by Cholera toxin enhances GFAP expression in MG cell lines and primary cultures [34]. Multi-targeting is one of the natures of miRNAs. Signaling networks composed of target genes and their relative molecules may both contribute to tumor-suppressive and oncogenic function. It seems that the oncogenic functions of miR-335 are hindered under a high endogenous level of cAMP, rewiring to pro-differentiation pathways.

To sum up, the role of a given miRNA depends on the script which is assigned by the cell type, the genomic context and in part the cellular biochemical status. These observations remind that disease state as well as the genomic subclass of MGs should be considered in the preclinical study especially for drug discovery involved miRNAs.

4. Involvement of miRNAs as novel biomarkers in malignant gliomas

Biomarkers are distinctive biological indicators that serve for diagnosis, prognosis and medication. Traditional biomarkers include mRNAs, proteins and metabolites. At present, miRNAs are emerging as novel and practical biomarkers in oncology. Due to their surprising stability, miRNAs can not only be detected in fresh and frozen tissues, but also in body fluids and even formalin-fixed paraffin-embedded samples. In the study of Roland Schroers, miR-15b and miR-21 are found in cerebrospinal fluid and demonstrated to be markers of glioma [35]. Although much remains to be studied, *e.g.* to discover more accurate and specific markers for respective glioma types, this finding provides a new opportunity to develop less invasive and early diagnostic approach for gliomas.

Besides diagnosis, miRNAs may be promising biomarkers for prognosis. Jun Li's group has reported that miR-182 is markedly up-regulated in various glioma cell lines and primary glioma specimens. Furthermore, higher level of miR-182 is associated with poor overall survival of patients with malignant glioma [36]. A more comprehensive study was recently carried out by Sujaya Srinivasan, *et al.* They analyzed miRNA expression profile of GBM patients (n = 222) from TCGA database and found a ten-miRNA expression signature that predicts survival for GBM. In detail, three miRNAs (miR-20a, miR-106a and miR-17-5p) were identified as protective markers and seven miRNAs (hsa-miR-31, hsa-miR-222, hsa-miR-148a, hsa-miR-221, hsa-miR-146b, hsa-miR-200b and hsa-miR-193a) were risky [37].

Recent studies have raised a possibility that miRNAs may function as predictive markers for therapeutics. Temozolomide (TMZ) is a well-known alkylating agent against gliomas, which methylates guanines in the O-6 position. Accumulating O-6 methyl guanines lead to DNA mismatch during replication and ultimately result in cell death. Although *MGMT* (methyl-guanine methyl transferase) promoter methylation has been proved to be a strongest marker to predict the TMZ response in low-grade and high-grade gliomas [38–40], it may not be the only indicator. Recent research indicates that miR-181b/c, miR-195, miR-455-3p and miR-10a-3p, rather than MGMT promoter methylation, predict response to concomitant chemoradiotherapy and acquired TMZ resistance in GBM cell line and patients [41, 42]. In addition, increasing evidences indicate that miRNAs also contribute to other drug response. For instance, up-regulated miR-21 confers teniposide and paclitaxel resistance on GBM cells [43, 44]. Various highly efficient MGMT inhibitors have been developed for sensitizing tumor to TMZ [45]. The emerging roles of miRNAs in drug resistance of TMZ and other antineoplastic agents give us a novel angle to include miRNAs as therapeutic targets.

5. Perspectives on miRNAs as nucleic acid drugs in malignant gliomas

5.1. MiRNAs replacement therapy and suppressive therapy

Human body has an extremely complicated internal environment, relying on balance and stability of which human keep their health. Once the homeostasis is disrupted by down-regulation or up-regulation of some important molecules including miRNAs, human will suffer from all kinds of diseases. Based on the disequilibrium status, the ideal protocols to cure diseases are believed to replace what is lost and to repress what is excessive, which are respectively called replacement therapy and suppressive therapy. For the former, estrogen replacement therapy is the most representative example, which is generally used in menopausal women with menopausal syndrome caused by ovarian hormones loss and has shown a positive effect [46]. For the latter, a typical case is a famous anti-angiogenesis drug Avastin, the humanized anti-vascular endothelial growth factor (VEGF) monoclonal antibody for cancer therapy [47]. Besides, Gefitinib and Glivec specially inhibiting EGFR tyrosine kinase, have both achieved high clinical benefit rates in treating cancer especially lung carcinoma and chronic myelocytic leukemia[48,49], further indicating the efficacy of suppressive therapy via targeting core molecules in tumorigenesis.

Notably, increasing evidences demonstrated that gliomagenesis is also closely associated with deregulation of miRNAs, such as up-regulation of oncogenic miRNAs and down-regulation of tumor suppressive miRNAs. Therefore, targeting these aberrant miRNAs has tremendous potential as a therapeutic strategy by down- or up-regulating altered genes.

Specially, miRNA mimics can be synthesized to replace lessened ones critical in gliomagenesis, and miRNA inhibitors can be designed to suppress the function of up-regulated oncogenic miRNAs. Just less than two decades after discovering the role of miRNAs in oncology, the replacement and suppressive therapies of miRNA are already being used in preclinical researches. We have proved that artificially rectification of abnormally expressed miRNAs inhibited growth of glioma xenografts in mice and prolonged the median survival of rat with orthotopic glioma[26,30], opening a new sight for glioma treatment.

5.2. MiRNA-targeting cocktail therapy

Glioma is a complicated disease of altered genes. TCGA has reported multiple chromosomal aberrations, nucleotide substitutions and epigenetic modifications that construct three core pathways (as shown in Figure 1] [15]. Furthermore, glioma is a disease of altered miRNAs. A genome-wide expression profiling of 26 GBMs, 13 AAs and 7 normal brain samples identifies multiple deregulated miRNAs in MGs [50]. In addition, large scale of sequencing analysis of GBMs has identified extensive genetic heterogeneity between GBM samples from different patients [51], implying the possibility of miRNA's heterogeneity. The multiplicity of deregulated miRNAs and the heterogeneity of deregulated miRNAs expression profiling may foster therapeutic failure and tumor adaptation to solo miRNA-targeting therapy.

To date, researchers just verified the efficiency of targeting solo miRNA as if by prior agreement. What will happen if target several pivotal miRNAs simultaneously? Given the multiplicity of deregulated miRNAs in glioma, a cocktail consisting of special miRNA mimics and/or inhibitors may kill multiple birds with one stone. In another word, components in cocktail may have an additive effect or even a synergistic effect against MGs. Furthermore, considering individual differences, one cocktail may not fit for each patient with MGs. If we can design a specific miRNA cocktail based on individual deregulated miRNAs, miRNA individualized treatment will be within our sights. Certainly, additional preliminary evidences are needed to verify the feasibility and availability of miRNA-targeting cocktail therapeutics.

5.3. Engineering miRNA

Engineering miRNA (emiRNA) is artificially designed in sequence, endowed with functional similarity to natural miRNA and functional specificity according to human's will. In a sense, emiRNA is a branch of small interfering RNA (siRNA) that possesses multi-targeting power just as natural miRNA.

Leastwise, there are two strategies to design emiRNA: (a) adjustment based on the natural miRNA sequence; (b) *de novo* design.

In the sessions above, we have discussed the fact that a given miRNA may play distinct role in different models, *e.g.* different genetic background, different cell type and different second messenger level. Even in a "conclusive"circumstance that a certain miRNA strongly kills a type of cancer cell, we still need to evaluate its pharmacodynamics in the cancer tissue and toxic side effect to the normal tissue before clinical application. If a natural sequence miRNA shows remarkable antitumor effect but exhibits unsatisfying selectivity, does it mean we should totally abandon this target? The problem may be solved by emiRNA technology. Different dominant target genes and their roles in different models determine the functional heterogeneity of a given miRNA. If we are able to find out the undesired targets that lead to unsatisfying selectivity, perhaps by keeping the seed region of the miRNA and adjusting its 3′ nucleotide sequence, we could either avoid the interaction between the miRNA and the undesired target genes, or enhance the binding to our goal targets.

In broader context, we could design an artificial miRNA in a *de nove* way. Cancers are known as a type of multigenic disease. By comprehensive sequencing, RTK/RAS/PI[3]K, p53 and RBsignalings are characterized as the core pathways in GBM [15]. In virtue of bioinformatics, it is possible to design a miRNA that contemporaneously targets the key components of two or more pathways by carefully examining their mutual microRNA recognition elements (MREs).

However, numbers of scientific problems need to be addressed before putting emiRNA into practice. We still have limited knowledge about the details of miRNA biogenesis and the MRE language passing on along evolution. Someday the secret will be unlocked and emiRNA may be a practical weapon against cancers.

5.4. MiRNA formulation

Another attractive issue of translating miRNA into clinical application is formulation. Although whose length is quite short in the RNA world, miRNA as well as siRNA is a type of high molecular weight drug in pharmaceutical point of view. Additionally, electric charge contributed by phosphate groups of the nucleic acid backbone make it inadequate for CNS delivery. Fortunately, new technical progress brings miRNA formulation within sight.

In the earlier period, viral vector including retrovirus, adenovirus, herpes simplex virus and adeno-associated virus were broadly used due to their high efficiency for both gene delivery and expression. However, limitations associated with safety, genomic stability and immunogenicity motivate scientists to focus on non-viral systems. At present, remarkable achievements have been made in chemical modifications and conjugations of small RNA. For example, locked nucleic acid (LNA) technology not only increases melting temperature of RNA-RNA duplex thus enhancing the binding affinity between small RNA and target transcript, but also improves the half-life of small RNA in serum, which is critical for therapeutic use [52]. Cholesterylation, *viz.* modification with cholesteryl functionality, which improves the cellular uptake of small RNA, is now extensively used for miRNA mimics/inhibitors and siRNA in preclinical research [53]. Two reviews have provided clear and comprehensive introduction of the progress on chemical small RNA encapsulation [54, 55]. Particularly, a recent study from Paula Hammond and colleagues reported a self-assembled microsponges of small RNA hairpin polymersin corporated more than half a million copies of siRNA in a single nanoparticle [56]. This novel technology allow one thousand times lower concentration to achieve same degree of gene silencing efficiency as conventional strategies, showing great clinical application potential. In the near future, small RNA formulation will further benefit from evolution of nanotechnology and biomaterial technology.

6. Concluding remark

Glioma is not the type of high incidence disease; however the depressive clinical outcomes still threaten human health. Special location, rapid proliferation, invasive growth and massive angiogenesis are the key issues that limit treatment for MG. In addition, extremely complicated histopathological and genomic classifications perplex fundamental and clinical research.

With the evolution of new generation high through-put sequencing technology, clearer insights of driver mutations and core pathways in various cancers are gradually revealed in the recent period [57–59]. According to these cancer genomic studies, we realize that not only aberrant coding genes lead to cancers, but also non-coding components underneath the iceberg. Twenty-year's research on miRNA opens a new world of genetics and oncology. More and more groups are dedicated to study the role of miRNA in cancer including glioma. Albeit fragmentary, accumulating data will offer deeper insights of glioma with more systematic considerations.

Compared with other non-coding protagonists, *e.g.* histone modification and DNA methylation, miRNA is the easiest role to be specifically manipulated, either by over-expression or inhibition, which determines miRNA to be the star with enormous clinical potential. Although we have not drawn an elaborate picture of miRNA biogenesis, especially how primary sequence and intra-cellular microenvironment influence secondary structure and eventually contribute to processing and maturation, as well as the communication principles between miRNA and MRE, we believe that technologies nowadays are poised to uncover the law of miRNA in oncology. We envision that this intrinsic biomolecule will be the therapeutic target for cancer.

Author details

Sihan Wu, Wenbo Zhu and Guangmei Yan

Zhongshan School of Medicine, Sun Yat-sen University, People's Republic of China

References

[1] Louis, D.N., Ohgaki, H., Wiestler, O.D., Cavenee WK. WHO Classification of Tumours of the Central Nervous System. IARC Press; 2007.

[2] Meyer M a. Malignant Gliomas in Adults. New England Journal of Medicine. 2008 Oct 23;359(17):1850–1850.

[3] Wirth T, Samaranayake H, Pikkarainen J, Määttä A-M, Ylä-Herttuala S. Clinical trials for glioblastomamultiforme using adenoviral vectors. Current opinion in molecular therapeutics. 2009 Oct;11(5):485–92.

[4] Sathornsumetee S, Rich JN, Reardon DA. Diagnosis and treatment of high-grade astrocytoma. Neurologic clinics. 2007 Nov;25(4):1111–39, x.

[5] Chi AS, Wen PY. Inhibiting kinases in malignant gliomas. Expert opinion on therapeutic targets. 2007 Apr;11(4):473–96.

[6] Sathornsumetee S, Reardon DA, Desjardins A, Quinn JA, Vredenburgh JJ, Rich JN. Molecularly targeted therapy for malignant glioma. Cancer. 2007 Jul 1;110(1):13–24.

[7] Lee RC, Feinbaum RL, Ambros V. The C. elegansheterochronic gene lin-4 encodes small RNAs with antisense complementarity to lin-14. Cell. 1993 Dec;75(5):843–54.

[8] Chan J a, Krichevsky AM, Kosik KS. MicroRNA-21 is an antiapoptotic factor in human glioblastoma cells. Cancer research. 2005 Jul 15;65(14):6029–33.

[9] Papagiannakopoulos T, Shapiro A, Kosik KS. MicroRNA-21 targets a network of key tumor-suppressive pathways in glioblastoma cells. Cancer research. 2008 Oct 1;68(19):8164–72.

[10] Ciafrè SA, Galardi S, Mangiola a, Ferracin M, Liu C-G, Sabatino G, et al. Extensive modulation of a set of microRNAs in primary glioblastoma. Biochemical and biophysical research communications. 2005 Sep 9;334(4):1351–8.

[11] Godlewski J, Nowicki MO, Bronisz A, Williams S, Otsuki A, Nuovo G, et al. Targeting of the Bmi-1 oncogene/stem cell renewal factor by microRNA-128 inhibits glioma proliferation and self-renewal. Cancer research. 2008 Nov 15;68(22):9125–30.

[12] Zhang Y, Chao T, Li R, Liu W, Chen Y, Yan X, et al. MicroRNA-128 inhibits glioma cells proliferation by targeting transcription factor E2F3a. Journal of molecular medicine (Berlin, Germany). 2009 Jan;87(1):43–51.

[13] Shi L, Cheng Z, Zhang J, Li R, Zhao P, Fu Z, et al. hsa-mir-181a and hsa-mir-181b function as tumor suppressors in human glioma cells. Brain research. 2008 Oct 21;1236:185–93.

[14] Wang X-F, Shi Z-M, Wang X-R, Cao L, Wang Y-Y, Zhang J-X, et al. MiR-181d acts as a tumor suppressor in glioma by targeting K-ras and Bcl-2. Journal of cancer research and clinical oncology. 2012 Apr;138(4):573–84.

[15] Cancer T, Atlas G, Information S. Comprehensive genomic characterization defines human glioblastoma genes and core pathways. Nature. 2008 Oct 23;455(7216):1061–8.

[16] Zhang Y, Dutta A. The role of microRNAs in glioma initiation and progression. Frontiers in Bioscience. 2012;700–12.

[17] Pang JC, Kwok WK, Chen Z, Ng H-K. Oncogenic role of microRNAs in brain tumors. Actaneuropathologica. 2009 Jul;117(6):599–611.

[18] Silber J, James CD, Hodgson JG. microRNAs in gliomas: small regulators of a big problem. Neuromolecular medicine. 2009 Jan;11(3):208–22.

[19] Suh S-S, Yoo JY, Nuovo GJ, Jeon Y-J, Kim S, Lee TJ, et al. MicroRNAs/TP53 feedback circuitry in glioblastomamultiforme. Proceedings of the National Academy of Sciences of the United States of America. 2012 Apr 3;109(14):5316–21.

[20] Duan R, Pak C, Jin P. Single nucleotide polymorphism associated with mature miR-125a alters the processing of pri-miRNA. Human molecular genetics. 2007 May 1;16(9):1124–31.

[21] Xia H, He T, Liu C, Cui Y, Song P, Jin X, et al. Cellular Physiology Biochemistry and Biochemistr y MiR-125b Expression Affects the Proliferation and Apoptosis of Human Glioma Cells by Targeting Bmf. Cellular Physiology and Biochemistry. 2009;100081:347–58.

[22] Shi L, Zhang J, Pan T, Zhou J, Gong W, Liu N, et al. MiR-125b is critical for the suppression of human U251 glioma stem cell proliferation. Brain research. Elsevier B.V.; 2010 Feb 2;1312:120–6.

[23] Cortez MA, Nicoloso MS, Shimizu M, Rossi S, Gopisetty G, Molina JR, et al. miR-29b and miR-125a regulate podoplanin and suppress invasion in glioblastoma. Genes, chromosomes & cancer. 2010 Nov;49(11):981–90.

[24] Dou T, Wu Q, Chen X, Ribas J, Ni X, Tang C, et al. A polymorphism of microRNA196a genome region was associated with decreased risk of glioma in Chinese population. Journal of cancer research and clinical oncology. 2010 Dec;136(12):1853–9.

[25] Permuth-Wey J, Thompson RC, Burton Nabors L, Olson JJ, Browning JE, Madden MH, et al. A functional polymorphism in the pre-miR-146a gene is associated with risk and prognosis in adult glioma. Journal of neuro-oncology. 2011 Dec;105(3):639–46.

[26] Shu M, Zheng X, Wu S, Lu H, Leng T, Zhu W, et al. Targeting oncogenic miR-335 inhibits growth and invasion of malignant astrocytoma cells. Molecular cancer. BioMed Central Ltd; 2011 Jan;10(1):59.

[27] Nagel R, le Sage C, Diosdado B, van der Waal M, Oude Vrielink J a F, Bolijn A, et al. Regulation of the adenomatous polyposis coli gene by the miR-135 family in colorectal cancer. Cancer research. 2008 Jul 15;68(14):5795–802.

[28] Holleman a, Chung I, Olsen RR, Kwak B, Mizokami a, Saijo N, et al. miR-135a contributes to paclitaxel resistance in tumor cells both in vitro and in vivo. Oncogene. Nature Publishing Group; 2011 May 9;(September 2010):1–13.

[29] Navarro A, Diaz T, Martinez A, Gaya A, Pons A, Gel B, et al. Regulation of JAK2 by miR-135a: prognostic impact in classic Hodgkin lymphoma. Blood. 2009 Oct 1;114(14):2945–51.

[30] Wu S, Lin Y, Xu D, Chen J, Shu M, Zhou Y, et al. MiR-135a functions as a selective killer of malignant glioma. Oncogene. 2011 Dec 5;31(34):3866–74.

[31] Tavazoie SF, Alarcón C, Oskarsson T, Padua D, Wang Q, Bos PD, et al. Endogenous human microRNAs that suppress breast cancer metastasis. Nature. 2008 Jan 10;451(7175):147–52.

[32] Li Y, Yin W, Wang X, Zhu W, Huang Y, Yan G. Cholera toxin induces malignant glioma cell differentiation via the PKA/CREB pathway. Proceedings of the National Academy of Sciences of the United States of America. 2007 Aug 14;104(33):13438–43.

[33] Shu M, Zhou Y, Zhu W, Wu S, Zheng X, Yan G. Activation of a pro-survival pathway IL-6/JAK2/STAT3 contributes to glial fibrillary acidic protein induction during the cholera toxin-induced differentiation of C6 malignant glioma cells. Molecular oncology. Elsevier B.V; 2011 Jun;5(3):265–72.

[34] Shu M, Zhou Y, Zhu W, Zhang H, Wu S, Chen J, et al. MicroRNA 335 is required for differentiation of malignant glioma cells induced by activation of cAMP/protein kinase A pathway. Molecular pharmacology. 2012 Mar;81(3):292–8.

[35] Baraniskin A, Kuhnhenn J, Schlegel U, Maghnouj A, Zöllner H, Schmiegel W, et al. Identification of microRNAs in the cerebrospinal fluid as biomarker for the diagnosis of glioma. Neuro-oncology. 2012 Jan;14(1):29–33.

[36] Jiang L, Mao P, Song L, Wu J, Huang J, Lin C, et al. miR-182 as a prognostic marker for glioma progression and patient survival. The American journal of pathology. 2010 Jul;177(1):29–38.

[37] Srinivasan S, Patric IRP, Somasundaram K. A ten-microRNA expression signature predicts survival in glioblastoma. PloS one. 2011 Jan;6(3):e17438.

[38] Everhard S, Kaloshi G, Crinière E, Benouaich-Amiel A, Lejeune J, Marie Y, et al. MGMT methylation: a marker of response to temozolomide in low-grade gliomas. Annals of neurology. 2006 Dec;60(6):740–3.

[39] Hegi ME, Diserens A-C, Gorlia T, Hamou M-F, de Tribolet N, Weller M, et al. MGMT gene silencing and benefit from temozolomide in glioblastoma. The New England journal of medicine. 2005 Mar 10;352(10):997–1003.

[40] Stupp R, Hegi ME, Mason WP, van den Bent MJ, Taphoorn MJB, Janzer RC, et al. Effects of radiotherapy with concomitant and adjuvant temozolomide versus radiotherapy alone on survival in glioblastoma in a randomised phase III study: 5-year analysis of the EORTC-NCIC trial. The lancet oncology. 2009 May;10(5):459–66.

[41] Ujifuku K, Mitsutake N, Takakura S, Matsuse M, Saenko V, Suzuki K, et al. miR-195, miR-455-3p and miR-10a(*) are implicated in acquired temozolomide resistance in glioblastomamultiforme cells. Cancer letters. 2010 Oct 28;296(2):241–8.

[42] Slaby O, Lakomy R, Fadrus P, Hrstka R, Kren L, Lzicarova E, et al. MicroRNA-181 family predicts response to concomitant chemoradiotherapy with temozolomide in glioblastoma patients. Neoplasma. 2010 Jan;57(3):264–9.

[43] Li Y, Li W, Yang Y, Lu Y, He C, Hu G, et al. MicroRNA-21 targets LRRFIP1 and contributes to VM-26 resistance in glioblastomamultiforme. Brain research. 2009 Aug 25;1286:13–8.

[44] Ren Y, Zhou X, Mei M, Yuan X-B, Han L, Wang G-X, et al. MicroRNA-21 inhibitor sensitizes human glioblastoma cells U251 (PTEN-mutant) and LN229 (PTEN-wild type) to taxol. BMC cancer. 2010 Jan;10:27.

[45] McElhinney RS, McMurry TBH, Margison GP. O6-alkylguanine-DNA alkyltransferase inactivation in cancer chemotherapy. Mini reviews in medicinal chemistry. 2003 Aug;3(5):471–85.

[46] Sullivan JM. Estrogen replacement therapy. The American Journal of Medicine. 1996 Oct;101(4):56S–60S.

[47] Ferrara N, Hillan KJ, Novotny W. Bevacizumab (Avastin), a humanized anti-VEGF monoclonal antibody for cancer therapy. Biochemical and biophysical research communications. 2005 Jul 29;333(2):328–35.

[48] Costanzo R, Piccirillo MC, Sandomenico C, Carillio G, Montanino A, Daniele G, et al. Gefitinib in non small cell lung cancer. Journal of biomedicine & biotechnology. 2011 Jan;2011:815269.

[49] Capdeville R, Buchdunger E, Zimmermann J, Matter A. Glivec (STI571, imatinib), a rationally developed, targeted anticancer drug. Nature reviews. Drug discovery. 2002 Jul;1(7):493–502.

[50] Rao SAM, Santosh V, Somasundaram K. Genome-wide expression profiling identifies deregulated miRNAs in malignant astrocytoma. Modern pathology®: an official journal of the United States and Canadian Academy of Pathology, Inc. 2010 Oct; 23(10):1404–17.

[51] Parsons DW, Jones S, Zhang X, Lin JC-H, Leary RJ, Angenendt P, et al. An integrated genomic analysis of human glioblastomamultiforme. Science (New York, N.Y.). 2008 Sep 26;321(5897):1807–12.

[52] Elmén J, Thonberg H, Ljungberg K, Frieden M, Westergaard M, Xu Y, et al. Locked nucleic acid (LNA) mediated improvements in siRNA stability and functionality. Nucleic acids research. 2005 Jan;33(1):439–47.

[53] Soutschek J, Akinc A, Bramlage B, Charisse K, Constien R, Donoghue M, et al. Therapeutic silencing of an endogenous gene by systemic administration of modified siRNAs. Nature. 2004 Nov 11;432(7014):173–8.

[54] Corey DR. Chemical modification: the key to clinical application of RNA interference? The Journal of clinical investigation. 2007 Dec;117(12):3615–22.

[55] Whitehead K a, Langer R, Anderson DG. Knocking down barriers: advances in siRNA delivery. Nature reviews. Drug discovery. 2009 Feb;8(2):129–38.

[56] Lee JB, Hong J, Bonner DK, Poon Z, Hammond PT. Self-assembled RNA interference microsponges for efficient siRNA delivery. Nature materials. 2012 Apr;11(4):316–22.

[57] Tao Y, Ruan J, Yeh S-H, Lu X, Wang Y, Zhai W, et al. Rapid growth of a hepatocellular carcinoma and the driving mutations revealed by cell-population genetic analysis of whole-genome data. Proceedings of the National Academy of Sciences of the United States of America. 2011 Jul 19;108(29):12042–7.

[58] Puente XS, Pinyol M, Quesada V, Conde L, Ordóñez GR, Villamor N, et al. Whole-genome sequencing identifies recurrent mutations in chronic lymphocytic leukaemia. Nature. 2011 Jul 7;475(7354):101–5.

[59] Stephens PJ, Tarpey PS, Davies H, Van Loo P, Greenman C, Wedge DC, et al. The landscape of cancer genes and mutational processes in breast cancer. Nature. 2012 Jun 21;486(7403):400–4.

Chapter 18

MicroRNAs Regulated Brain Tumor Cell Phenotype and Their Therapeutic Potential

Chunzhi Zhang, Budong Chen, Xiangying Xu,
Baolin Han, Guangshun Wang and Jinhuan Wang

Additional information is available at the end of the chapter

http://dx.doi.org/10.5772/52362

1. Introduction

MicroRNAs (miRNAs)are short 18–25 nucleotide small non-coding RNA molecules that function to silence gene expression via sophisticated post-transcriptional regulation[1]. Since their discovery in the early 1990s, these small molecules have been shown to play an important regulatory role in a wide range of biological and pathological processes. Over 30% of human messenger RNAs (mRNAs) are regulated by miRNAs[2]. miRNAs generated by the canonical biogenesis pathway are transcribed as precursor RNAs from intergenic, intronic or polycistronic genomic loci by RNA polymerase II (Pol II). The primary miRNA (pri-miRNA) transcript forms a stem–loop structure that is recognized and processed by the Drosha and DGCR8 RNase III complex or the spliceosome apparatus in the nucleus. In the non-canonical miRNA pathway, miRNAs are transcribed directly as endogenous short hairpin RNAs (endo-shRNAs) or derive directly through splicing from introns that can refold into hairpins (mirtrons). The trimmed precursor (pre-miRNA) hairpins from both canonical and non-canonical miRNA pathways are then transported by an exportin 5 and RAN-GTP-dependent process to the cytosol, where they are typically further processed by the Dicer and transactivation-response RNA-binding protein (TRBP) RNase III enzyme complex to form the mature double-stranded ~22-nucleotide miRNA. Argonaute proteins (for example, AGO2)

then unwind the miRNA duplex and facilitate incorporation of the miRNA-targeting strand (also known as the guide strand) into the AGO-containing RNA-induced silencing complex (RISC). The RISC– miRNA assembly is then guided to specific target sequences in mRNAs. The initial recognition of mRNAs by the RISC–miRNA complex is driven primarily by Watson–Crick base-pairing of nucleotides 2 to 8 in the mature miRNA (termed the seed sequence) with specific mRNA target sequences chiefly located in the 3′ untranslated region, and additional base-pairing affords greater affinity and targeting efficiency(Figure1)[3].

Given the pivotal regulatory role of miRNAs in a broad range of biological processes, it is not surprising that miRNAs play a role in human cancers, including brain tumor. First, about 50% of human miRNAs are located in cancer-associated genomic regions and fragile sites, suggesting that they might be the target genes underlying such aberrant intervals [5]. Second, the advent of high-throughput detection method has promoted expression profiling of miRNAs in normal and tumor tissues. Compared to normal tissues, anomalous levels of miRNA subsets have been found in almost all tumor types examined [6, 7]. Third, miRNAs with tumor-suppressive gene and oncogene-like properties have been described.

Since the first description of aberrant miRNA expression in glioblastomas and pituitary adenomas in 2005 [8, 9], there have been increasing reports each year about miRNA deregulation and function in various brain tumors. In this chapter, we summarize the current findings of miRNA study in brain cancers and discuss the diagnostic and therapeutic potential of miRNAs, mainly in glioma.

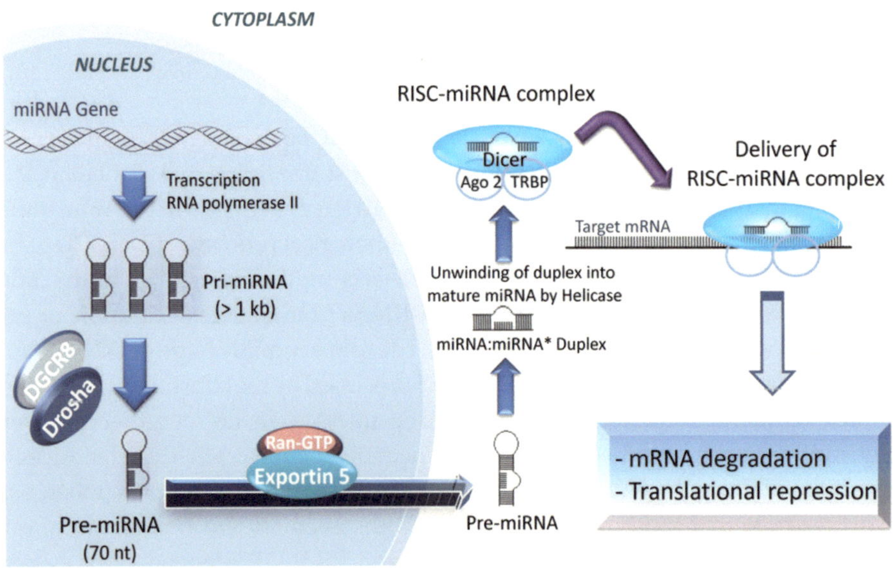

Figure 1. The miRNA biogenesis pathway[4]

2. MiRNAs profile in brain tumor

CBTRUS obtained incidence data from 48 population-based cancer registries that include cases of malignant and non–malignant (benign and uncertain) primary brain and central nervous system tumors in the United States in 2004-2007. The most frequently reported histology is the predominately non–malignant meningioma, which accounts for 34% of all tumors, followed by glioblastoma (17%). The predominately non-malignant pituitary and nerve sheath tumors account for 13% and 9% of all tumors, respectively. Acoustic neuromas (defined by ICD-O-3 site code C72.4 and histology code 9560) account for 63% of all nerve sheath tumors(Figure2).

Only recently, the miRNAs attracted increasing attention as potential diagnostic or even therapeutic tools in brain tumors. Profiling techniques to identify global expression patterns of miRNAs in brain tumors have been widely used to uncover aberrantly expressed micro-RNAs in tumor genomes. Ciafrè et al. found nine (miR-10b, miR-130a, miR-221, miR-125b-1, miR-125b-2, miR-9-2, miR-21, miR-25, miR-123) and four miRNAs (miR-128a, miR-181c, miR-181a, miR-181b), respectively, out of 245 miRNAs to be up-/down-regulated in human glioblastoma samples, and nine (miR-221, miR-23a, miR-24-2, miR-24-1, miR-23b, miR-21,miR-222-prec, miR-191, miR-220) and seven miRNAs(miR-181a, miR-181b, miR-128b, miR-197, miR-181c,miR-125b-2, miR-125b-1), respectively, to be up-/down-regulated in human glioblastoma cell lines[10]. Chan et al.[8] demonstrated five (miR-21, miR-138, miR-347, miR-291-5′, miR-135) and three miRNAs (miR-198, miR-188,miR-202), respectively, out of 180 miRNAs to be up- and downregulated in glioblastoma samples. Sasayama et al.[11] found miR-10b, miR-21, miR-183, miR-92b and miR-106b to be up-, and miR- 302c*, miR-379, miR-329, miR-134 and miR-369-3p to be downregulated in human glioblastoma samples. Other studies reported several miRNAs to be significantly deregulated in glioma samples of Chinese patients (including miR-34a, miR-15b, miR-200a and miR-146b) [12], or miR-29b, miR-125a and miR-149 to be downregulated in glioblastomas [13]. In an array study with 192 miRNAs, 13 miRNAs (miR-101, miR-128a, miR-132, miR-133a, miR-133b, miR-149, miR-153, miR-154*, miR-185, miR-29b, miR-323, miR-328, miR-330) were found to be downregulated and three miRNAs to be upregulated (miR-21, miR-155, miR-210) in glioblastoma multiforme [14]. Another micro-array study identified 55 miRNAs out of 756 miRNAs to be upregulated and 29miRNAs to be downregulated in malignant astrocytomas (primary and secondary glioblastoma and ana-plastic astrocytoma, respectively) compared to controls [15].

In additional to gliomas, miRNA profiling also had been discovered in some other brain tumors. Ferretti et al were the first to identify signatures of a set of 248 miRNAs in a panel of primary medulloblastomas and normal cerebellar controls using high throughput expression profiles. They showed different expression profiles between normal brain and tumor and between distinct tumor histotypes. In particular, they detected an upregulation of mir-21 and miR-17-92 cluster (miR-17-5p, miR-20a and miR-19a) and a downregulation of miR-128a/b, let-7, miR-124a, miR-103, miR-134, miR-138, miR-149, miR-181b, miR-9 and miR-125a, most of them previously reported to be dysregulated in other brain tumor cell lines or nervous system cancers [16]. Moreover, Recent microarray data reported a possible role of miRNAs in pituitary adenomas. The first connection between pituitary adenomas and miRNAs was established by Bottoni et al in 2005, that showed a downregulation of mir-15a and miR-16-1 in GH-secreting and in PRL-secreting adenomas compared to normal pituitary tissue[8]. In 2007 Bottoni et al explored the miRNAome of pituitary tumors by microarray. They found that 30 miRNAs are differentially expressed between normal pituitary gland and pituitary adenomas. Among them, miR-150, miR-152, miR-191, and miR-192 were found to be upregulated in pituitary

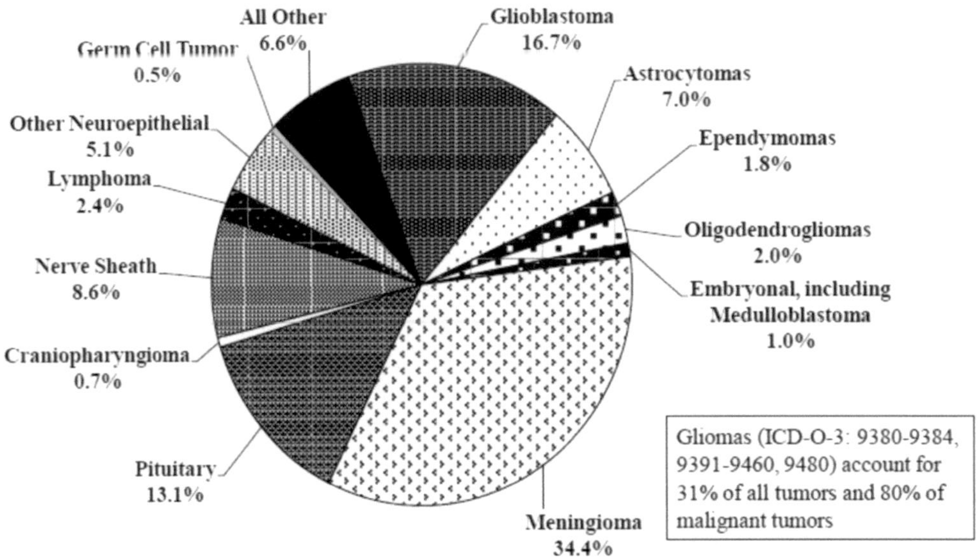

Figure 2. Distribution of All Primary Brain and CNS Tumors by Histology (N=226,791) CBTRUS Statistical Report: NPCR and SEER Data from 2004-2007

adenomas, and miR-132, miR-128a, miR-136, miR-16-1, and let-7 are downregulated[17]. As for meningioma, Feng Zhi et al found a list of 14 miRNAs that were differentially expressed in meningioma compared to normal adjacent tissue(NAT)samples. Twelve miRNAs, including miR-17-5p, miR-22-3p, miR-24-3p, miR-26b-5p, miR-27a-3p, miR-27b-3p, miR-96-5p, miR-146a-5p, miR-155-5p, miR-186-5p, miR-190a and miR-199a were shown to be upregulated by a factor greater than twofold, whereas two miRNAs, including miR-29c-3p and miR-219-5p, were significantly downregulated[18].

3. Abberant miRNAs as prognostic and/or diagnostic marker for brain tumor patients

The use of miRNAs as tumor biomarkers has gained growing interest in the last few years. Accumulating evidence indicates that miRNA expression can be used as a prognostic and/or diagnostic marker for brain tumor patients. Niyazi et al. separated 35 glioblastoma patients into long- and short-term survivors. Then, they found that some miRNAs were significantly different in two group, including miR-3163, miR-539, miR-1305, miR-1260 and let-7a. this is the first dataset defining a prognostic role of miRNA expression patterns in patients with glioblastoma[19]. Moreover, Ma also identified that MiR-196b is overexpressed and confers a poor prognosis via promoting cellular proliferation in glioblastoma patients[20]. Costa et al identified miRNAs that are over-expressed in ependymomas, such as miR-135a and miR-17-5p, and downregulated, such as miR-383 and miR-485-5p. We have also uncovered

http://dx.doi.org/10.5772/52362

associations between expression of specific miRNAs which portend a worse prognosis. For example, we have identified a cluster of miRNAs on human chromosome 14q32 that is associated with time to relapse. We also found that miR-203 is an independent marker for relapse compared to the parameters that are currently used. Additionally, we have identified three miRNAs (let-7d, miR-596 and miR-367) that strongly correlate to overall survival[21].

4. Deregulated miRNAs regulated brain tumor cell phenotype

Increasing evidence supports the supposition that miRNAs play an important role in different types of cancers and in various aspects of cancer biology. Abnormal miR levels in tumors have important pathogenetic consequences: miRNAs may act as oncogenes or suppressor genes[22]. For examples, Calin et al. [23] identified two clustered miRNAs (miR-15a and miR-16-1) on the minimal deletion region of chromosome 13q14 and showed that the levels of these miRNAs were significantly reduced in the majority (68%) of B-cell chronic lymphocytic leukemia (CLL). Both miRNAs target the anti-apoptotic gene BCL2, which is frequently overexpressed in CLL [24]. These findings indicate that downregulation of miR-15a and miR-16-1 elevates BCL2 level, contributing to CLL formation and suggesting a tumor-suppressive role for both miRNAs. In contrast, miR-17-92 showed marked upregulation in B-cell lymphomas. Enforced expression of miR-17-92 cluster acted with c-myc to accelerate the onset of B-cell lymphoma in a mouse model [25]. The data suggest that miR-17-92 cluster is a potential oncogene.

Recent evidence supports the ability of miRNAs to regulate brain tumor cell phenotype. We had done some work to identified that miR-221 and miR-222 regulated their target expression to co-modulated glioma cell phenotype, including proliferation, cell cycle, apoptosis and invasion(Figure3)[26-28], and so on.

MiRNAs also regulated radio- and chemo-resistence of glioma. Hierarchical clustering analysis of expression 1100 miRNAs in three glioma cell lines treated with clinically relevant doses of radiation (2Gy) revealed significant (3-4 fold) up-regulation of several miRNA that are implicated in stimulation of survival and proliferation of tumor cells [29]. The set of up-regulated miRNAs includes miR-1285, miR-151-5p, and miR-24-1 that display beneficial effects on tumors by inhibiting the core tumor suppressor p53 (miR-1285) and supporting migration, local metastasis (miR-151-5p), and antiapoptosis (miR-24-1) [30]. Overall, activation of these miRNAs might possibly increase tumor radioresistance in subsequent radiotherapy sessions and stimulate motility of cancer cells thereby at least partially explaining the evidence on enhanced migration of malignant glioma cells in response to radiotherapy [31]. The radiation treatment of glioma cell lines with normal capacity to repair radiation-induced double strand breaks (DSB) of DNA caused activation of let-7 [29], a family of miRNA that suppresses proliferation of gliomblastoma cells [30] (Fig. 4). In contrast, in the radiosensitive human glioma cell line M059J that is deficient in DNA-dependent protein kinase (DNA-PK) and has a low activity of ATM, two key members of the non-homologous end joining pathway of DNA-DSB repair, let-7 miRNA was down-regulated [30].

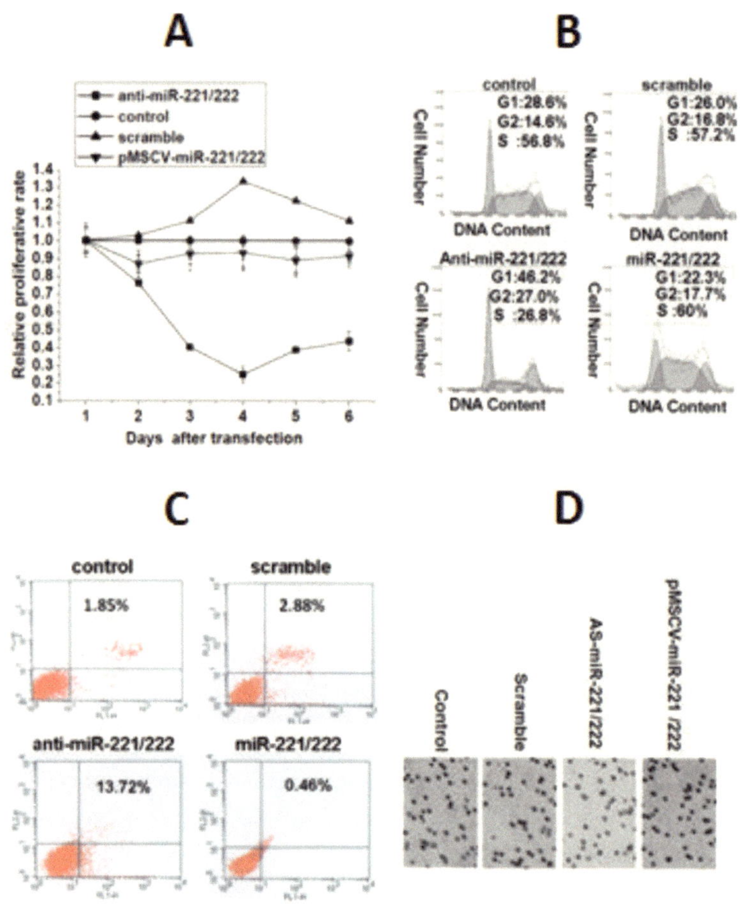

Figure 3. miR-221 and miR-222 regulated their target expression to co-modulated glioma cell phenotype. (A: MTT assay show that knockdown of miR-221/222 lowed proliferated rate of glioma cell; B: knockdown of miR-221/222 induce G1 arrest in glioma cell ;C: Annexin V analysis showed that knockdown of miR-221/222 significantly increased glioma cell apoptosis; D: The transwell assay revealed that knockdown of miR-221/222 significantly decreased glioma cell invasion.

Moreover, MiRNAs were shown to be also involved in the regulation of chemoresistence of glioma by modulating some relevant proteins that are involved in drug metabolism and drug transporter. MiRNAs also affect chemotherapeutic agents induced DNA damage repair (Fig. 4).

5. MiRNAs in gliomas and glioblastoma

MiRNAs affect biological character of varies cells by regulating their targets. So, deregulated miRNAs regulated brain tumor cell phenotype by regulating their targets, including proliferation, cell cycle, apoptosis, invasion, and so on.

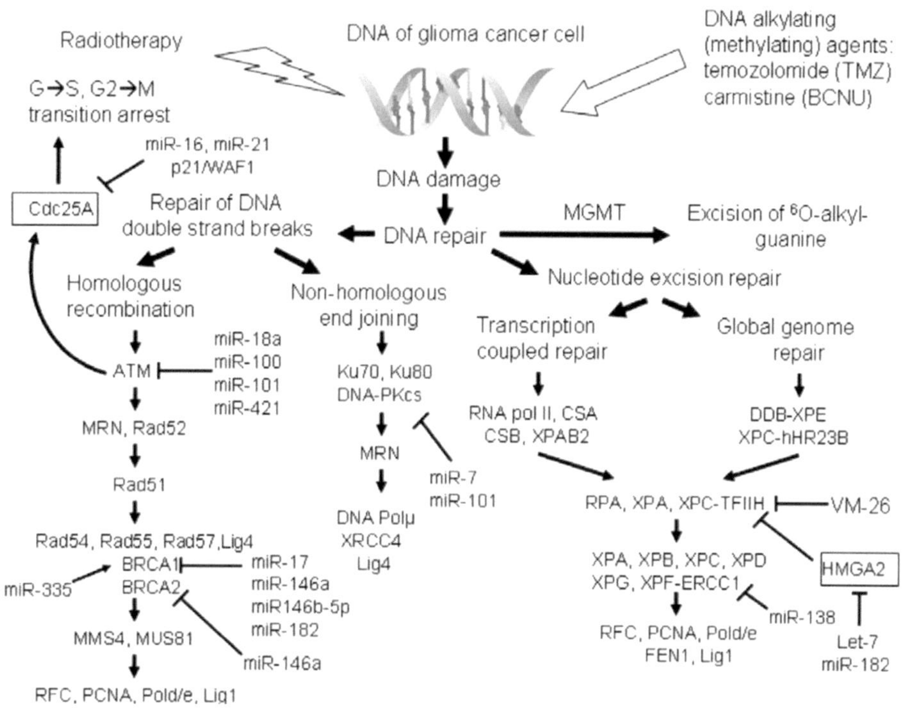

Figure 4. MicroRNAs are involved in the regulation of DNA repair in cancer cells after treatment with ionizing radiation (radiotherapy) and DNA alkylating drugs such as temozolomide and carmistine[30].

5.1. MiR-221 and miR-222

MiR-221 and miR-222 are both up-regulated in several glioma derived cell lines and in glioma samples [26-28]. They are clustered within a 1-kb genomic interval on chromosome X, so they could be generated from the same primary transcript [26].

Two members of the Kip/Cip family of CDK inhibitors and key negative regulators of the cell cycle, p57 and p27, have been identified as putative direct targets of these miRNAs. According to this theory, the 3'-UTR of p57 harbors one site expected to be recognized by both miR-221 and miR-222, whereas the 3'-UTR of p27 contains two sites for both miRNAs. Transfection of both miR-221 and miR-222 greatly reduce the levels of p57 and p27 proteins, while downregulation of either microRNA 221 or 222 in glioblastoma cells caused an increase in p27 levels and enhanced expression of the luciferase reporter gene fused to the p27 3'-UTR. These results suggest that miR-221 and miR-222 could promote cell proliferation and S-phase entry together with further cooperative events and that miRNA 221 and 222 inhibition may be a potential therapeutic target to reduce the aggressive growth of glioblastoma by restoring normal levels of their target proteins [32]. The inverse correlation between mir-221/222 and p27 levels, the impairment of growth potential and the G1 to S shift in the cell cycle of glioma cells after inhibition of mir-221/222, were later confirmed by Zhang et al. They extended their study to in vivo trials and showed that miR-221/222 knocked-down through antisense oligonucleotides strongly reduced glioma subcutaneous mice xenografts growth through up regulation of p27 [26] and enhanced radiosensitivity of glioblastoma cell lines [33]. Further evidence showed that knockdown of miR-221/222 induced a change of mitochondrial membrane potential and caspase-mediated apoptosis on glioblastoma cells. Indeed, mir-221/222 directly downregulate the proapoptotic protein PUMA, which leads in turn to decrease Bcl-2 and increase BAX. these results confirm the oncogenic role of mir-221/222 on glioblastoma [27]. Our recent studies identified that mir-221/222 increased cell invasion and reduced gap junction intercellular communication (GJIC) by regulating TIMP3 and Cx43[28,34].

5.2. MiR-21

Microarray profiling studies, further validated by Northern blotting qRT-PCR and real-time PCR analysis, showed that miRNA-21 is strongly elevated in glioma and glioblastoma tumor samples and glioma cell lines when compared to non-neoplastic control samples, and upregulation is particularly prominent in grade IV astrocytomas [35-37]. High expression of miR-21 was significantly associated with poor patient survival, suggesting that, in combination with other aberrant expressed miRNAs (low expression of miR-181b or miR-106a), miRNA-21 profiling has potential application as novel diagnostic and prognostic indicator [37].

Suppression of mir-21 in glioblastoma cells decreased the metabolic activity of cell culture and cell number, and was associated with a marked increase in apoptosis and caspase activation [35]. MiR-21 knockdown also leads to a considerable reduction of glioma volumes in mouse xenografts [38]. Knockdown mir-21 inhibited proliferation and cell invasion and induced apoptosis through the activation of caspase-3 and -9 in glioma cell lines, which may be related to a mir-21-dependent modulation of multiple potential target genes, such as TIMP3 [39,40].

From an in silico constructed study of miR-21 predicted targets and further pathway analysis of computer generated lists of the identified target genes, emerged that mir-21 targets multiple components of the p53, transforming growth factor-β (TGF-β) and mitochondrial apoptosis pathways, that contribute to its tumor promoting and antiapoptotic activity. The phenotypic effects observed upon downregulation of miR-21 in glioblastoma cells, reflect the repression of these pathways and result in significant increase in apoptotic cells, reduced growth and cell cycle arrest at G0-G1 [41]. Further bioinformatics analysis evidenced that multiple genes involved in apoptosis pathways (such as PDCD4, MTAP, and SOX5), carry putative miR-21 binding sites. PDCD4 mRNA is a direct functional target of miR-21 and its expression inversely correlates with mir-21 in a number of glioblastoma cell lines (T98G, A172, U87, and U251). Consistent with these observations, downregulation of mir-21 restored protein level of PDCD4 while, ectopic overexpression of mir-21, inhibits PDCD4-dependent apoptosis [42]. Mir-21 controls tumor invasiveness and microvascular proliferation by regulating the expression of two of the major inhibitors of matrix metalloproteinases (MMPs): RECK and TIMP3. Mir-21 knockdown decreases RECK and TIMP3 protein levels and MMPs activity both in vivo and in vitro leading to a reduction of glioma cell motility and invasion [43]. Although PTEN tumor suppressor gene has been validated as a miR-21 target by computational analysis, downregulation of mir-21 leads to an inhibition of tumor growth in glioblastoma cell lines and xenograft tumors independently of PTEN mutational status [44,45]. MiRNA expression profile scanning data after inhibition of miR-21, strongly indicated that BID, FAS, PRS6, and SOCS4 tumor suppressor genes were upregulated and evidenced a suppression of EGFR, activated Akt, cyclin D, and Bcl-2. This study highlighted that miR-21 targets multiple pathways responsible of inhibition of glioma growth in absence of PTEN [46].

Further findings strengthened the hypothesis that miR-21 represents a promising target to improve the efficacy of chemotherapy. In a recent study mir-21 was shown to play a key role in promoting human glioblastoma cells U87MG resistance against the antitumoral agent temozolomide (TMZ). Indeed, ectopic overexpression of mir-21 significantly reduced TMZ-induced apoptosis in this cell line through a suppression of Bax/Bcl-2 ratio and caspase-3 activity. These results confirm the hypothesis that mir-21 overexpression during glioma progression could be responsible of clinical resistance to chemotherapy with the promising alkylating agent TMZ [47]. Li et al demonstrated that mir-21 is also involved in glioblastoma cell chemoresistance to the chemotherapeutic agent VM-26, as shown by the observation that miR-21 knockdown sensitized GBM cells to VM-26. This is likely to happen because mir-21 regulates and inhibit LRRFIP1 gene expression by direct interaction [48]. This gene encodes a protein, also known as the TRAF-interacting protein (TRIP), that inhibits NF-κB signaling, a pathway that is known to be responsible for protection against apoptosis [49] and tumor chemoresistance [50]. Additionally, suppression of miRNA-21 expression in glioblastoma cell lines enhances sensitivity of cancer cells to antineoplastic cytotoxic therapy with neural precursor cells (NPC) expressing a secretable variant of the cytotoxic agent tumor necrosis factor related apoptosis inducing ligand (S-TRAIL). The synergistic effect was observed both in vitro, through an increased caspase associated cytotoxic death, and in vivo, where miR-21 knockdown and NPC-mediated S-TRAIL reduce cancer growth in tumor xenografts [38]. A recent study that evaluated the potential role of mir-21 as a therapeutic tool to enhance the cytotoxic effect of standard chemotherapy showed that co-delivery of miR-21 and 5-fluorouracil (5-FU) by using a poly(amidoamine) (PAMAM) dendrimer as a carrier, significantly improved the cytotoxicity of the antitumor agent leading to an higher apoptosis rate and a reduction of the migration ability of tumor cells [51]. Finally, downregulation of miR-21, contributes to the antitumor effects of IFN-β on glioma cell and intracranial tumor xenografts and the activation of the transcription factor STAT3 may have a key role in the IFN-β mediated suppression of mir-21 [52].

5.3. Mir-34a

Mir-34a, transcriptional target of p53 located within chromosome 1p36, has been proposed as a potential tumor suppressor. MiR-34a is also downregulated in glioblastoma tissues and cell lines compared to normal brain tissues and is markedly reduced in p53-mutant cells compared to cells expressing wild-type p53 [53,54].

MiR-34a possesses hundreds of predicted mRNA targets which could mediate its inhibitory effects on tumor growth. A few of these have been experimentally verified and include oncogenes such as MYC, CCND1, CDK6, SIRT1 [55] and c-Met [56]. It was shown to directly inhibit c-Met in glioma and medulloblastoma cells and Notch-1/Notch-2 in glioma cells and stem cells by binding to the 3'-UTRs of their mRNA. Furthermore, mir-34a inversely correlates with c-Met, Notch1, Notch2 and CDK6 protein expression in glioma cells. Transfection of microRNA34a in brain tumor cells strongly inhibits cell proliferation, cell cycle progression, cell survival, cell invasion, and in vivo glioma xenograft growth but do not affect cell cycle or death when transfected to human astrocytes, which showed normal expression levels of microRNA 34a. Restoration of c-Met or Notch-1 and Notch-2 expression by constructs lacking 3'-UTR regions partially reverted cell cycle arrest and apoptosis induced by miR-34a in glioma cells or stem cells, confirming the hypothesis that the antitumor effects of miR-34a are achieved via targeting of multiple oncogenes [53]. Interestingly, mir-34a also affect glioma stem cell differentiation and growth. Luan et al recently reported silent information regulator 1 (Sirt1) as a direct negative target of mir34a in glioma cell lines at a posttranscriptional level [54]. Sirt1 is a NAD-dependent deacetylase that regulates apoptosis in response to oxidative and genotoxic stress, and has recently been involved in tumorigenesis acting as an oncogene [57].

5.4. Mir-128

Mir-128, a brain enriched microRNA, is downregulated in glioma cell lines and tissue when compared to normal brain samples [58]. Mir-128 overexpression decreased glioma cell proliferation in vitro and glioma xenograft growth in vivo, and is inversely correlated to Bmi-1 expression. Mir-128 directly targets and downregulates Bmi-1 by binding its 3'-UTR region [59] and leads to a concomitant overexpression of p21CIP1 and a decrease in phosphorylated Akt [58]. Bmi-1 expression is a critical factor of normal stem cell maintenance and glioblastoma self-renewal and loss of Bmi-1-mediated self-renewal of neural stem cells has been shown to be associated with upregulation of p21CIP1 [60] and decreased Akt activation [61]. Consistently with these observations, miR-128 overexpression in human glioma neurosphere cultures possessing a glioma 'stem-like' cell phenotype, evidenced that miR-128 specifically blocked glioma self-renewal reducing neurosphere number and size. In conclusion, mir-128 downregulation is likely to enhance glioma tumorigenesis by promoting an undifferentiated phenotype and self renewing state through Bmi-1 increased expression [58]. By bioinformatical analysis, E2F3a, a transcription factor involved in cell cycle progression [62], has been identified as a direct target of this miRNA. Indeed, Mir-128 and E2F3a levels are negatively correlated and mir-128 overexpression has similar inhibitory effects on proliferation of glioma cell lines as E2F3a knocking down Ectopic overexpression of E2F3a partially reversed the effects of mir-128, suggesting that mir-128 could exert its antitumor effects at least partially by inhibiting E2F3a expression. Among its target genes angiopoietin-related protein 5 (ARP5) was identified with bioinformatical tools and then confirmed to be inversely correlated to mir-128 levels in glioblastoma cells and tissue and downregulated after ectopic overexpression of this miRNA [58]. ARP5 seems to be a key regulator of cell proliferation, remodeling and regeneration [63] and could be a member of a group of genes regulated by mir-128 that coordinately contribute to glioma and GBM pathology [59].

5.5. Mir-451

Mir-451 was found to be upregulated in glioma samples compared to normal brain on microarray-based miRNAome profiling [64]. MiR-451 showed a striking spatial distribution, with groups of positive cells concentrated around a subset of blood vessels. Moreover, high levels of mir-451 are correlated to a poor prognosis in glioma patients. Mir-451 could regulate the balance of proliferation and migration in glioma cells in response to changes in glucose levels and metabolic stress. It regulates 5'-adenosine monophosphate activated protein kinase (AMPK) pathway in response to glucose levels in glioma cells, through the modulation of the activity of its upstream activator LKB1 [65]. Activation of LKB1 is a potent anti-proliferative signal, and also influences cell polarity, a process known to affect cell motility [66].

MiR-451 regulates LKB1 activity by directly targeting CAB39, a component of the active LKB1complex, leading to a downregulation of CAB39 protein levels. Down-regulation of mir-451 levels in response to glucose deprivation leads to intense activation of LKB1 and downstream pathways, allowing cells to survive metabolic stress and promoting cancer cell migration. Conversely, when glucose is sufficient, elevated miR-451 levels lead to reduced LKB1/AMPK pathway activation. This facilitates cell proliferation but makes cells more sensitive to glucose deprivation. Thus mir-451 could be a key regulator of adaptive response of cancer cells to altered energy availability [65].

In partial contrast with these studies a recent report found mir-451 to be downregulated in glioma cell lines. Transfection of mir-451 to glioma cell lines was able to inhibit cell growth, induced G0/G1 phase arrest, increased cell apoptosis and most notably diminished the invasive capacity of these cells as evidenced by transwell invasion assay. These tumor suppressive effects may be due to modulated expression of a panel of proteins including CyclinD1, p27, MMP 2/9 and Bcl-2, probably via regulation of the PI3K/AKT signaling pathway. Indeed, expression of Akt1 protein decreased after mir-451 transfection [67].

5.6. Mir-7

Mir-7, a miRNA modulated during neural differentiation of embryonic stem cells is a putative tumor suppressor gene in glioblastoma. It inhibits EGFR gene expression by directly binding its mRNA at 3'-UTR. Furthermore, miRNA-7 suppresses the activation of Akt pathway and reduces phospho-Akt levels by directly targeting its upstream regulators IRS-1 and IRS-2 [68]. They also identified Raf1 as a direct target of miR-7 by microarray analysis, Western blot and luciferase reporter assays of glioblastoma cells transfected with miR-7 [69]. Inhibition of Akt activation seems to occur independently of mir-7-mediated repression of EGFR pathway. Consistenly with these findings miRNA-7 was markedly downregulated in glioblastoma tissue when compared to normal brain. The proposed mechanism that explains the lower expression of this miRNA is a processing defect in generating pre-miR-7 from pri-miR-7 in glioblastoma. Pre-miRNA-7 transfection decreased viability and invasiveness of glioblastoma lines and glioblastoma derived stem cells and led to an increase in the sub-G0 apoptotic fraction, a decrease in the S fraction and determined a G2-M arrest, most likely by affecting EGFR and Akt pathways, which have an established key role in gliomagenesis [68]. Indeed, EGFR is frequently amplified and highly expressed in glioblastomas [26]. In a recent report mir-7 was also shown to directly inhibit p21-activated kinase 1 (Pak1) in non-brain cancer cells [70]. Pak1 is a widely upregulated signaling kinase in multiple human cancers, and it is involved in the regulation of many signaling pathways, including EGFR and Akt, thus interfering with cell motility, proliferation, and apoptosis [71]. Furthermore, in glioblastomas, PAK1 upregulation is a negative prognostic marker and its knockdown results in impaired cell invasion [72]. These preliminary results suggest mir-7 could have a potential and prom ising therapeutic role in brain tumors.

5.7. Mir-181

Mir-181a and mir-181b are well known brain-enriched miRNAs [73]. Downregulation of mir-181a and mir-181b was detected in both glioma samples and cell lines [74]. Transfection of both these miRNAs on glioma cell lines results in cell growth inhibition, invasion reduction and apoptosis induction, miR-181b being more effective than miR-181a [74]. In a recent miRNA expression profiling conducted on a set of 124 astrocytoma samples and 60 normal adjacent tissue samples by qRT-PCR, Zhi et al found that downregulation of miR-181b is significantly associated with poor patient survival independently of other clinicopathological factors. Thus, mir-181b has a great potential for being used as a diagnostic and prognostic marker and to better select patients for adjuvant therapy [39].

In a recent study MiR-181b and miR-181c downregulation was found to be significantly associated to a positive response to concomitant chemoradiotherapy with temozolomide in glioblastoma patients, suggesting they could be used as predictive factors for therapy efficacy [75].

5.8. Mir-124/137

MiRNA-124 and miRNA-137 are downregulated in anaplastic astrocytomas and glioblastoma multiforme relative to non-neoplastic brain tissue [9-10]. Consequently, growth factor signaling could promote brain tumor formation through suppression of miR-124 and/or miR-137 expression and inhibition of neural stem cells/tumor stem cell differentiation. Transfection of mir-124 and mir-137 to neural stem cells and tumor-derived stem cells leads to induction of cellular markers of differentiation, G1 cell cycle arrest and reductions of the expression of the cell cycle regulator CDK6, a direct target of both miRNAs. These changes are accompanied by reduced self-renewal and tumorigenicity. Overexpression of miR-124 or miR-137 also reduced the expression of phosphorylated RB, a downstream target of CDK6 [76]. These results suggest that ectopic expression of miRNA-124 and miRNA-137 could represent a valid therapy for glioblastoma multiforme treatment inducing differentiation of tumor cells and cell cycle arrest.

5.9. MiR-125

Mir-125b downregulated in glioma cell lines after treatment with ATRA (all-trans-retinoic acid), a regulator of neural differentiation and proliferation. Ectopic overexpression of mir-125b stimulated glioma cell proliferation, partially recovering the cell growth inhibition induced by ATRA treatment, while mir-125b knockdown promoted ATRA-mediated cell apoptosis. Furthermore, Bmf was identified as a direct target of miR-125b, and they are inversely correlated [77]. Bmf interacts with the prosurvival Bcl-2 proteins, regulating cellular apoptotic pathways [78]. Indeed, transfection with miR-125b increase BCL-2 levels in glioma cells, and expression of BCL-2 was significantly decreased when cells were transfected with miR-125b inhibitor. Thus, Bmf may play an important role in the process of miR-125b influencing cell apoptosis [77].

Recently, Cortez et al identified that mir-125a downregulated in glioblastomas and particulary in glioma stem cells CD133+. Overexpression of mir-125a inhibits invasion properties of glioblastomas, probably through a direct downregulation of podoplanin (PDPN), a membrane sialo-glycoprotein related to invasion and malignancy [79].

5.10. MiR-326

Kefas et al evidenced a feedback loop between miRNA-326 and Notch pathway, frequently deregulated in gliomas. Notch-1 knockdown induced mir-326 upregulation in glioma stem cells, and ectopic overexpression of mir-326 decreased Notch pathway members level and activity. Forced expression of mir-326 also inhibited cell proliferation, viability and invasiveness and induced apoptosis in both established and stem cell-like glioma lines, these effects are at least partially explained through downregulation of the Notch pathway. Moreover, it reduced tumorigenicity in mouse glioma xenografts. Together with the observation that mir-326 is downregulated in glioblastomas, these findings suggest that miR-326 is a potential tumor suppressor in glioma cells and that reversing Notch/miR-326 axis toward miR-326 prevalence appears to be a potential therapy for brain tumors [80].

5.11. Mir-26a

Mir-26a up-regulated in high-grade gliomas. MiR-26a is a direct negative regulator of PTEN and significantly represses PTEN expression. MiR-26a overexpression was attributed to the amplification of miR-26a-2 locus (chromosome 12q), one of the two miR-26a loci present in the human genome (mir-26a-1 and miR-26a-2) and is correlated with monoallelic PTEN deletion. It was suggested a temporal sequence to the molecular evolution of miR-26a-amplified gliomas, with PTEN loss most likely preceding miR-26a-2 amplification and, concordantly, miR-26a overexpression in genetically engineered PTEN+/- mice precluded loss of their remaining PTEN allele. Amplification of mir-26a is likely to promote the silencing of the remaing PTEN transcript in PTEN+/- tumors, event analogous to a loss of heterozygosity. Furthermore, in a murine glioma model, PTEN repression mediated by overexpression of miR-26a, enhanced de novo tumor formation. Akt pathway activation and suppression of its negative regulator PTEN are particularly important and frequently occur in glioma development. These observations document a new epigenetic mechanism for PTEN regulation in gliomagenesis, further highlighting that dysregulation of Akt signaling is crucial to the glioma development and could be modulated through manipulation of miRNA expression [64]. Moreover, MiR-26a is a frequent target of the 12q13.3-14.1 amplicon that also contain CDK4 and CENTG1, two oncogenes that regulate the RB1 and PI3 kinase/AKT pathways, respectively. The presence of this amplification is negatively correlated to patient survival. PTEN, RB1, and MAP3K2/MEKK2 were detected as functional targets of mir-26a in glioblastoma. Ectopic overexpression of miR-26a increased GBM cell growth, decreased apoptosis and enhanced gliomagenesis in vivo. Thus, miR-26a decreases PTEN expression, activates AKT, and promotes tumor growth. Using human U87 GBM cells that lack functional PTEN, mir-26a overexpression increased cell growth and decreased apoptosis despite the absence of PTEN, most probably by downregulating RB1 and MAP3K2, a gene that encodes MEKK2[81]. MEKK2 is a mitogen-activated protein kinase kinase involved in JNK activation pathway that promote apoptosis in GBM cells [82].

5.12. Mir-10b

Mir-10b is upregulated in glioma samples and glioma cell lines compared to non-neoplastic brain tissues. RhoC and urokinasetype plasminogen activator receptor (uPAR), which are known to contribute to glioma invasion and migration, were correlated with mir-10b expression in gliomas, probably via inhibition of the translation of the mRNA encoding homeobox D10 (HOXD10], which in turn represses the expression of these genes [83]. These results suggest that mir-10 could be involved in regulation of the invasion and migration abilities of gliomas.

5.13. Mir-15b

Mir-15b was shown to be elevated in a panel of glioma cell lines. Transfection of glioma cells with miR-15b significantly increased G0/G1 cells and decreased the percentage of cells in S phase, while inhibition of mir-15b increased G0/G1 cell amount. Thus, miR-15b regulates cell cycle progression in glioma cells by targeting cell cycle-related factors as CCNE1 (cyclin E1], a validated downstream target of mir-15b [84].

5.14. Mir-146b

Mir-146b, a miRNA found to be downregulated in human glioma tissue, could exert an antitumor activity by reducing the expression of a matrix metalloproteinase gene, MMP16, one of its direct downstream targets. Indeed, transfection of U373 glioma cells with miR-146b precursor decreased tumor cell migration and invasion, while inhibition of miR-146b by LNA modified anti-miR-146b produced the opposite effect, without affecting cell proliferation [85].

5.15. Mir-296

Recent studies support a role of mir-296 in promoting angiogenesis in gliomas. When brain microvascular endothelial cells were co-cultured with U87 glioma cells or when vascular endothelial growth factor (VEGF) was added to cultured human brain microvascular endothelial cells, miR-296 was upregulated. Moreover, mir-296 levels were higher in endothelial cells isolated from human brain tumors compared to normal brain endothelial cells. Downregulation of miR-296 in endothelial cells resulted in the inhibition of morphologic characteristics associated with angiogenesis and reduced angiogenesis in glioma xenografts in vivo. This probably happens through the downregulation of the hepatocyte growth factor-regulated tyrosine kinase substrate (HGS), a validated target of mir-296, thus leading to a reduced HGS-mediated degradation of the platelet derived growth factor receptor (PDGFR) and vascular endothelial growth factor receptor (VEGFR). This result points out an interesting feedback loop, where VEGF induces miR-296 expression, which in turn increases cell response to VEGF. Consequently, manipulating mir-296 expression, could enable to control a key step in cancer angiogenesis [86].

5.16. Mir-29

Mir-29b was found to be significantly downregulated in glioblastoma samples and cells and CD133+ tumor stem cells. Forced overexpression of this miRNA inhibited invasion and proliferation and induced apoptosis in glioblastoma cells. Mir-29b as well mir-125a directly targets podoplanin (PDPN), a putative marker of neural stem cells, related to invasion and malignancy in glioblastoma [13].

5.17. MiR-17-92 cluster

MiR-17-92 cluster, located within the locus 13q31-q32, encloses five miRNAs (miR-92-1, miR-19a, miR-20a, miR-19b, miR-17-5p), which have been frequently involved in tumorigenesis [87]. This cluster was detected to be amplified in glioblastoma samples. Furthermore, expression of miR-17-92 cluster is downregulated upon induction of differentiation of GBM spheroid cultures by using ATRA. Induction of differentiation leads to deregulation of most of the key pathways associated with self-renewal such as insulin-like growth factor 1 signaling, vitamin D receptor/retinoic acid X receptor activation, Wnt/β-catenin signaling and retinoic acid receptor activation. Inhibition of miR-17-92 cluster leads to decreased cell viability and decreased cell proliferation probably through a de-repression of CDKN1, E2F1, PTEN and CTGF which are upregulated. Particularly, connective tissue growth factor (CTGF) gene was shown to be a direct target of miR-17-92 in glioblastoma spheroids by luciferase reporter assays [88]. CTGF binds vascular endothelial growth factor (VEGFA), which is a central mediator of angiogenesis [89], and inhibits VEGFA-induced angiogenesis [90]. Conversely, VEGFA was shown to inhibit MiR-17-92 [91], thus explaining the concomitant downregulation of VEGFA and miR-17-92 upon induction of differentiation. In conclusion, the interaction between CTGF, VEGFA and miR-17-92 might have a key role in gliomagenesis by targeting multiple regulatory pathways [88].

5.18. Let-7

Let-7 expression is not downregulated in human glioblastoma tissues and cell lines, let-7 ectopic overexpression by transfection on U251 and U87 human glioblastoma cells, reduced in vitro proliferation and migration and also in vivo tumor growth after xenotransplantation into nude mice. Furthermore, let-7 miRNA reduced the expression of total RAS, N-RAS, and K-RAS in glioblastoma cells [92]. These results suggest that let-7 miRNA is able to impair glioblastoma growth and cellular migration via RAS inhibition.

6. MicroRNAs and tumor stem cells

Glioma stem cells (GSCs) have been recently identified [93]. They express common neural stem cell (NSC) markers (CD133, Nestin, Musashi, and Sox2) and display multiple-lineage differentiation potential and a greater tumorigenic activity in rodent xenografts. GSCs also show an increased angiogenic potential through a higher expression of vascular endothelial growth factor (VEGF). GSCs are strongly resistant to radiation [94]and chemotherapy [95].

A recent study by Lavon et al showed a similar expression pattern of mir-21, mir-124, and mir-137 in gliomas and stem cells. Among them we mention the miR-17 family cluster that contains 3 miRNAs upregulated in gliomas and NPCs (mir-17-92, mir-106b-25, mir-106a); the mir-183-182 cluster, also upregulated in gliomas and NPCs; the large 7+46 bipartite miRNA cluster on chromosome 14, as most of miRNAs located within this region have been shown to be downregulated in the same samples [96]. This latter cluster is located within a region which shows a frequent loss of heterozygosity in glioblastomas [97]. Finally, mir302-367 cluster on chromosome 4q25 and mir371-373 cluster on chromosome 19q13, are upregulated in gliomas and NPCs. These data confirm the hypothesis that brain cancers arise from multipotent GSCs, thus explaining the phenotypic heterogeneity of tumors.

Many groups investigated the role of miRNAs in GSCs so far: in a first report Silber et al found that mir-124 and mir-137 are reduced in grade III and IV gliomas compared to normal brain. Besides, transfection of these two miRNAs in neural stem cells and glioma cancer cell lines leads to induction of cellular markers of differentiation, G1 cell cycle arrest and reductions of CDK6, thus indicating a hypothetical tumor suppressor role of micro-124 and microRNA-137 in GSCs [29]. As previously mentioned in this review, mir-128 was identified as a negative regulator of glioma self renewal when ectopically overexpressed on human glioma neurosphere cultures [58].

A recent analysis showed that mir-451 is significantly downregulated in CD133+cells. Transfection of miR-451 inhibits proliferation and neurosphere formation in GSCs, highlighting that it can act as a tumor suppressor: two target sites for SMAD protein in the upstream promoter region of miR-451 have been found, leading to draw the conclusion that this miRNA is activated by SMAD pathway. Transfection of SMAD in GBM cells inhibited their growth, suggesting it could induce differentiation of glioma CD133+stem cells through up-regulation of miR-451, thus reducing their tumorigenicity [98].In conclusion, a stable and selective delivery of these miRNAs to GSCs could represent a great advance for brain tumor therapy.

MiR -125b is required for stem cell fission, allowing them to bypass the G1/S checkpoint and making them insensitive to chemotherapy [99]. It has been found to be significantly downregulated in CD133+glioma stem cells compared to CD133-ones, leading to the hypothesis that it may be involved in cell differentiation. As expected, transfection of mir-125b to CD133+cells, decreased the number of proliferating cells and induced G0-G1 arrest: this effect occurs through a mir-125b-dependent downregulation of CDC25A and CDK6, two cell cycle regulatory proteins [47]. Moreover, miR-29b and miR-125a, are under-expressed in glioblastoma CD133+cells compared with their counterpart CD133-cells (see above), suggesting a potential role for these microRNAs in regulation of signaling pathways related to maintenance of stem cell properties and self-renewal of cancer cells [79].

Some miRNAs could have a role in the regulation of key pathways of GSCs. We already mentioned above the existence of a regulatory feedback loop between the tumor suppressor mir-326 and Notch pathway, shifted towards a prevalence of Notch activity in brain tumor cells and GSCs [80] Recently, pyruvate kinase type M2 (PKM2) has been identified as a putative target of mir-326, as levels of PKM2 and mir-326 are inversely correlated in glioma cells. PKM2, highly expressed on cancer cells and GSCs, plays the role of mediator in mir-326 metabolic effects: experimental knockdown of this molecule led to an impairment of glioma invasiveness and clonogenicity and decreased ATP levels, suggesting that PKM2 could represent a valid target for glioma therapy [100].

Mir-34a downregulated in gliomas and GSCs. When transfected into GSCs, it decreased the expression of the stem cell markers CD133 and nestin and caused an higher immunostaining for astrocytes and oligodendrocytes markers, besides modestly inhibiting several malignancy end-points (migration, survival, proliferation, cell cycle progression). Remarkably, miR-34a levels in glioma stem cells are significantly lower than in differentiated wild-type p53 glioma cell lines, suggesting that restoration of miR-34a expression for therapeutic purposes could achieve strong anti-tumor effects not only by targeting differentiated glioma cells, but also by inducing glioma stem cell differentiation [56].

7. MicroRNAs in medulloblastoma

Medulloblastoma (MB) is the most common brain malignancy observed in childhood (WHO grade IV) [101]. Ferretti et al were the first showed that miRNAs profiles is different between primary medulloblastomas and normal cerebellar controls. These aberrant miRNAs have a potentially role in MB development: e.g., let-7 microRNAs has been shown to inhibit Ras oncogene expression [102], reported to be a key factor for MB metastatic behavior [103]; miR-17-92 cluster cooperates with myc, frequently overexpressed in MB, to induce neoplastic transformation [104]; miR-9 and miR-125a, both downregulated in MB, are involved in cell proliferation and, when transfected into MB cells, promote apoptosis and impair anchorage-independent growth by downregulating the truncated isoform of the neurotropin receptor TrkC (t-TrkC). T-TrkC expression levels are higher in MB, inversely correlate with miR-9 and miR-125a levels and are responsible of enhanced cell proliferation and worse prognosis. Mir-9 and mir-124 have a common molecular target, REST/NRSF (RE1 silencing transcription factor/neuron-restrictive silencer factor) complex [105]. These observations suggest that Mir-9 and mir-124 could play an important role in cerebellar tumorigenesis as REST inactivation has been reported to inhibit tumor growth [106] and is overexpressed in many MBs [107]. Consequently, a REST/mir-124 axis shifted towards a prevalence of REST activity, could block neuronal differen-tiation and promote neoplastic transformation [108].

Mir-124 also modulates medulloblastoma growth by targeting CDK6, a key pro-proliferative factor overexpressed in 30% of medulloblastomas, which represents an adverse prognostic marker for clinical outcome [109]. The role of mir-124 in MB development was later confirmed by Li et al who additionally demonstrated that ectopic expression of mir-124 in medulloblastoma cell lines inhibits cell growth by directly targeting SLC16A1, a protein upregulated in MBs, that serve as a carrier to export lactic acid extracellularly, thus maintaining homeostasis of tumor cells, where aerobic glycolysis is known to be accelerated [110].At the same time, downregulation of miR-218 could account for an overexpression of the pro-oncogene EGFR, which activates MAPK pathway and CTNND2, which in turn encodes the gene of β-catenin that activates the APC/Wnt signal transduction pathway and leads to tumor growth [111].

Hedgehog (Hh) patched (Ptch1) signalling pathway is a key regulator of the development of cerebellar granule cell progenitors and its constitutive activation makes cells susceptible of malignant transformation into medulloblastoma [112]. Hh is a secreted protein that binds to the transmembrane receptor Ptch1 transducing an intracellular signal through the protooncogene Smoothened (Smo) to the downstream transcription factors Gli1, Gli2, and Gli3 [113].

Ferretti et al found that miR-125b, miR-326 and miR-324-5p target and repress activator downstream components of the Hh signalling pathway (Smo and Gli1); consistent with these findings, 50% of MBs showed a downregulation of these miRNAs together with an overexpression of Gli1. Deletion of chromosome 17p, the most frequent mutation in medulloblastoma, could account for several genetic defects, including miR-324-5p, p53 and HIC1 tumor suppressors loss, which cooperate in Hh-dependent tumorigenesis: loss of these genes, together with other molecular events, contribute to a persistent hyperactivation of Hh signalling during cerebellar granule cell progenitors development, leading to higher proliferative activity and susceptibility to malignant MBs [114].

Recently, Hedgehog signalling pathway has been identified as a target of miR-17-92 cluster. Indeed, miRNAs from the miR-17-92 cluster are specifically overexpressed in mouse MB models with specific initiating mutations in Ptch1 and in human MB subgroups with an activated SHH signaling pathway. To evaluate its oncogenic potential, miR-17-92 was retrovirally transduced into mouse granule neuron progenitors cells (GNPs) before orthotopic transplantation into immunocompromised mice. Interestingly, only cells with an SHH signaling defect (Ptc+/-) developed MBs. Tumor cells from this model exhibited markers of activated SHH signaling as elevated Math1 and Gli1 mRNA levels, and lost expression of the wild-type Ptc allele, reinforcing the hypothesis of a functional link between the SHH pathway and this miRNA cluster [115]. Some studies showed that miR-17-92 is most highly expressed in SHH-driven medulloblastomas, and higher levels of miR-17-92 are also related to an overexpression of the oncogene MYC. Moreover, transfection of miR-17-92 maintains mouse CGNP cells in a proliferative state in the absence of SHH, and synergizes with SHH to promote cell growth, while treatment of the same cells with SHH results in upregulation of miR-17-92, confirming that this cooperation is crucial in MB tumorigenesis [116].

Notch pathway plays a key role in regulating granule-cell progenitor differentiation and an increased copy number of Notch-2 was detected in 15% of medulloblastomas [117]. Expression of the downstream effector of Notch, HES1, normally declines during neuronal differentiation, while persistent activation of this factor prevents differentiation of precursor cells [118]. Garzia et al identified mir-199-5p as capable of directly targeting and repress expression of HES1 in MB cell lines. Ectopic expression of this miRNA reduced MB cell proliferation, population expressing stem cell marker CD133 and xenograft tumor growth in mouse models. Their studies also suggest that the documented downregulation of miR-199b-5p in metastatic tumors may be related to epigenetic silencing [119].

http://dx.doi.org/10.5772/52362

Venkataraman et al recently showed that several miRNAs known to be involved in CNS development, are downregulated in medulloblastoma cell line cultures and tissues. A specific one, miR-128a, is able to decrease tumor growth and proliferation if ectopically re-expressed on MB cells. Bmi-1 has been identified as a putative target of miR-128a, a critical factor in cerebellar development frequently upregulated in MBs. MiR-128a seems to normally down-regulate Bmi-1 oncogene, leading to increased levels of p16, a cell cycle inhibitor. Furthermore, Bmi-1 could be involved in regulating reactive oxygen species by decreasing superoxide generation, thus leading to a lower redox state in cancer stem cells [120]; this event is known to be partially responsible of tumor resistance against common therapies [121].

Finally, mir-34a appeared to be a tumor suppressor gene also in medulloblastomas other than in glioblastomas. Indeed, transient transfection of miR-34a into medulloblastoma cell lines, strongly inhibited cell proliferation, cell cycle progression, cell survival and cell invasion most probably through a direct inhibition of c-Met [56].

8. MiRNAs in pituitary tumors

Pituitary adenomas are benign and frequent neoplasms, accounting for about 15% of primary intracranial tumors [122]. Bottoni et al found that 30 miRNAs are differentially expressed between normal pituitary gland and pituitary adenomas. Furthermore, their expression is inversely correlated with tumor size. They probably act through a negative regulation of RARS (arginyl-tRNA synthetase), which is in turn upregulated in pituitary adenomas and modulates the expression of factors influencing pituitary tumor growth [123]. Mir-15a and mir-16-1 are located within chromosome region 13q14. Interestingly, loss of 13q region of chromosome 13 was frequently detected in pituitary tumors, confirming that this region likely contains tumor suppressor genes [124].

These findings support the hypothesis that miRNA-16-1 plays a key role in tumor growth [195], most probably by interacting with BCL2 [125], which is overexpressed in about one third of pituitary adenomas [126]. MiRNAome could also function as a signature for specific histotypes of pituitary adenomas. Overexpression of miR-23a, miR-23b, and miR-24-2 and lower expression of mir-26b are more typical of GH-secreting and PRL-secreting adenomas, differentiating them from non-functioning adenomas (NFA), characterized by mir-26 upregulation and miRNA-24-2 downregulation. Moreover, NFA express higher concentration of miR-137 and lower of miR-127, miR-129, miR-203, and miR-134 compared to GH-secreting adenomas. Finally, ACTH-secreting adenomas are defined by a strong expression of mir-30 cluster (miR-30a, miR-30b, miR-30c, and miR-30d), supporting the hypothesis that miRNAs could be useful diagnostic markers to distinguish pituitary tumor histotypes [127].More recently, Amaral et al evaluated the expression of microRNAs in ACTH-secreting pituitary tumors: they found that let-7a, miR-21, miR-141, miR-143, miR-145, and miR-150, besides miR-15 and miR-16, are downregulated in corticotropinomas compared to normal pituitary tissue and that a lower expression of mir-141 is linked to a better chance of remission after surgery [128]. Moreover, downregulation of Mir-143 could be involved in tumorigenesis by activating MAPK pathway via ERK5 [129].

Quian et al showed that let-7 expression is decreased in more than one third of pituitary adenomas and is related to higher tumor grade, thus it may act as a tumor suppressor. Levels of let-7 were found to be inversely correlated to HMGA2 expression [130], confirming some previous studies which showed that HMGA2 is repressed by let-7 [131]. High levels of HMGA2 have been detected in most types of pituitary adenomas [132] and they are significantly associated with tumor grade, extent of invasion, tumor size and Ki-67 proliferation index, probably through regulation of E-cadherin, E2F1, cyclin A, and p53 expression. Accordingly, let-7 may be useful as a novel anticancer agent in the future [130]. A recent study on the role of miRNAs in NFAs and GH-secreting pituitary tumors was performed by Butz et al, showing that a group of miRNAs (miR-128a, miR-155, and miR-516a-3p) targets the 3'-untranslated region of Wee1, a nuclear protein kinase that acts as a tumor suppressor, and which was found to be significantly decreased in pituitary tumor samples [133].

9. Therapeutic potential of miRNAs

Current evidence indicates that miRNA deregulation is common in human cancers. The discovery of miRNAs with oncogenic or tumor-suppressive function raises the possibility of exploiting these RNA molecules for therapeutic intervention and the development of novel therapies. The oncogenic miRNAs can be downregulated using antisense miRNA oligonucleotides (AMOs or antagomirs) or miRNA sponges[134,135], whereas tumor-suppressive miRNAs may be targeted by replacement with miRNA mimetics.

AMOs are synthetic oligonucleotides with sequence complementary either to mature miRNA or its precursor and have been widely used to inhibit miRNA activities in vitro and in vivo[136]. A number of chemical modifications to AMOs have been developed to improve specific binding to target miRNAs and to resist nuclease degradation. These include modifications at the 20-hydroxyl position (20-O-methyl (20OMe), 20-Omethoxyethyl(20MOE), 20-fluoro (20F) and locked nucleic acids (LNA)), on the phosphorothioate backbone, and conjugation with cholesterol [137]. Of these modifications,LNA shows high stability, strong affinity for target miRNAs and low toxicity in biological system and has emerged as a strong candidate for targeting miRNAs in vivo. One clinical trial using LNA anti-miRNA in treating human disease has been initiated recently. Using LNA antimiR-21, Corsten et al. demonstrated that miR-21 knockdown in glioma cells led to an increase of apoptotic cell death and a significant reduction of glioma growth in vivo, suggesting that miR-21 is a potential therapeutic target. They further showed that combination of miR-21 suppression and the cytotoxic agent tumor necrosis factor-related apoptosis-inducing ligand (TRAIL) resulted in enhanced caspase activity and synergistic killing of glioma cells in vitro. When these treated glioma cells were implanted intracranially into nude mice, tumor cells were completely eradicated after day 6 of implantation, compared to reduced tumor volume with either treatment alone. This finding suggests that miR-21 knockdown sensitizes glioma cells to apoptosis agent, and that the combined treatment is a promising approach for glioma elimination [138].

Angiogenesis is a process essential for malignant glioma growth. By co-culturing glioma cells with microvascular endothelial cells, Wurdinger et al. showed that glioma cells could induce changes of miRNA expression in endothelial cells, with miR-296 being significantly upregulated. Enhanced expression of miR-296 was also observed in endothelial cells treated with glioma-conditioned medium or proangiogenic growth factor VEGF or EGF, as well as in endothelial cells isolated from glioma samples. These results suggested a role for miR-296 in angiogenesis. It was further demonstrated that miR-296 contributed to angiogenesis by targeting hepatocyte growth factor-regulated tyrosine kinase substrate (HGS), which controls the levels of growth factor receptors (VEGFR2 and PDGFRb) by directing these macromolecules to lysosomes for degradation. Importantly, intravenous administration of antimiR- 296 AMO significantly reduced angiogenesis in glioma xenografts in vivo[139]. These results suggest that inhibition of angiogenesis by targeting miR-296 in endothelial cells may represent an alternative approach in glioma therapy.

10. Conclusion

MiRNAs are an astonishing new class of gene regulators, and it had been demonstrated that these molecules play a crucial role in cancer development and progression in a variety of malignancies, including brain tumors. Most importantly, in a clinical context, there is first evidence that miRNAs might provide new options to improve diagnostics and therapy in the two most common malignant primary brain tumors in adults (glioblastoma) and children (medulloblastoma). In vitro and in vivo data suggest that miRNAs could be used to discriminate brain tumors from normal brain tissue, and to identify different astrocytoma grades. More important, clinico-pathological features seem to correlate with miRNA expression in these tumors. Furthermore, there is increasing evidence that miRNAs might help to generate targeted therapies and to overcome resistance to conventional anticancer strategies for example in glioblastomas. Of course, it has to be acknowledged at this stage that translation of these preliminary "in vitro data" into "hard clinical facts" is not feasible. But these findings provide a very promising basis for future studies to determine the effect of miRNA modulation on chemotherapy in "in vivo studies". Although therapeutic delivery of miRNAs is still a developing field, and there is much more work to be done before these molecules can be securely applied in clinical settings, miRNA modulation may one day have a therapeutic application in patients. In summary, the presented data supports the enormous clinical potential of miRNAs in brain tumors, and mandate further intensive investigations in this field.

Acknowledgements

Supported by China National Natural Scientific Found (30901772).

Author details

Chunzhi Zhang[1], Budong Chen[2], Xiangying Xu[3], Baolin Han[3], Guangshun Wang[3] and Jinhuan Wang[2]

1 Department of Radiation Oncology, Tianjin Huan Hu Hospital, Tianjin, China

2 Department of Neurosurgery, Tianjin Huan Hu Hospital, Tianjin, China

3 Department of Oncology, Tianjin Baodi Hospital, Tianjin, China

References

[1] Feng, W, & Feng, Y. MicroRNAs in neural cell development and brain diseases. Sci China Life Sci. (2011).

[2] Zen, K, & Zhang, C. Y. Circulating MicroRNAs: a novel class of biomarkers to diagnose and monitor human cancers. Med Res Rev. (2012).

[3] Rottiers, V, & Näär, A. M. MicroRNAs in metabolism and metabolic disorders. Nat Rev Mol Cell Biol. (2012).

[4] Babashah, S, & Soleimani, M. The oncogenic and tumour suppressive roles of microRNAs in cancer and apoptosis. Eur J Cancer. (2011).

[5] Calin, G. A, Sevignani, C, Dumitru, C. D, Hyslop, T, Noch, E, Yendamuri, S, Shimizu, M, Rattan, S, Bullrich, F, Negrini, M, & Croce, C. M. Human microRNA genes are frequently located at fragile sites and genomic regions involved in cancers. Proc Natl Acad Sci USA.(2004).

[6] Lu, J, Getz, G, Miska, E. A, Alvarez-saavedra, E, Lamb, J, Peck, D, Sweet-cordero, A, Ebert, B. L, Mak, R. H, Ferrando, A. A, Downing, J. R, Jacks, T, Horvitz, H. R, & Golub, T. R. MicroRNA expression profiles classify human cancers. Nature.(2005).

[7] Volinia, S, Calin, G. A, Liu, C. G, Ambs, S, Cimmino, A, Petrocca, F, Visone, R, Iorio, M, Roldo, C, Ferracin, M, Prueitt, R. L, Yanaihara, N, Lanza, G, Scarpa, A, Vecchione, A, Negrini, M, Harris, C. C, & Croce, C. M. A microRNA expression signature of human solid tumors defines cancer gene targets. Proc Natl Acad Sci USA.(2006).

[8] Bottoni, A, Piccin, D, Tagliati, F, Luchin, A, & Zatelli, M. C. degliUberti EC. miR-15a and miR-down-regulation in pituitary adenomas. J Cell Physiol.(2005). , 16-1.

[9] Chan, J. A, Krichevsky, A. M, & Kosik, K. S. MicroRNA-21 is an antiapoptotic factor in human glioblastoma cells. Cancer Res.(2005).

[10] Ciafrè, S. A, Galardi, S, Mangiola, A, Ferracin, M, Liu, C. G, Sabatino, G, Negrini, M, Maira, G, Croce, C. M, & Farace, M. G. Extensive modulation of a set of microRNAs in primary glioblastoma. Biochem Biophys Res Commun.(2005).

[11] Sasayama, T, Nishihara, M, Kondoh, T, Hosoda, K, & Kohmura, E. MicroRNA-10b is overexpressed in malignant glioma and associated with tumor invasive factors, uP-AR and RhoC. Int J Cancer.(2009).

[12] Xia, H, Qi, Y, Ng, S. S, Chen, X, Li, D, Chen, S, Ge, R, Jiang, S, Li, G, Chen, Y, He, M. L, Kung, H. F, Lai, L, & Lin, M. C. microRNA-146b inhibits glioma cell migration and invasion by targeting MMPs. Brain Res.(2009).

[13] Cortez, M. A, Nicoloso, M. S, Shimizu, M, Rossi, S, Gopisetty, G, & Molina, J. R. Carlotti C Jr, Tirapelli D, Neder L, Brassesco MS, Scrideli CA, Tone LG, Georgescu MM, Zhang W, Puduvalli V, Calin GA. miR-29b and miR-125a regulate podoplanin and suppress invasion in glioblastoma. Genes Chromosomes Cancer.(2010).

[14] Silber, J, Lim, DA, Petritsch, C, Persson, AI, Maunakea, AK, Yu, M, Vandenberg, SR, Ginzinger, DG, James, CD, Costello, JF, Bergers, G, Weiss, WA, Alvarez-Buylla, A, Hodgson, JG, & mi, . -137 inhibit proliferation of glioblastoma multiforme cells and induce differentiation of brain tumor stem cells. BMC Med.2008, 6:14

[15] Rao, S. A, Santosh, V, & Somasundaram, K. Genome-wide expression profiling identifies deregulated miRNAs in malignant astrocytoma. Mod Pathol. (2010).

[16] Ferretti, E, De Smaele, E, & Po, A. Di Marcotullio L, Tosi E, Espinola MS, Di Rocco C, Riccardi R, Giangaspero F, Farcomeni A, Nofroni I, Laneve P, Gioia U, Caffarelli E, Bozzoni I, Screpanti I, Gulino A. MicroRNA profiling in human medulloblastoma. Int J Cancer. (2009).

[17] Bottoni, A, Zatelli, M. C, Ferracin, M, Tagliati, F, Piccin, D, Vignali, C, Calin, G. A, Negrini, M, & Croce, C. M. Degli Uberti EC. Identification of differentially expressed microRNAs by microarray: a possible role for microRNA genes in pituitary adenomas. J Cell Physiol. (2007).

[18] Zhi, F, Zhou, G, Wang, S, Shi, Y, Peng, Y, Shao, N, Guan, W, Qu, H, Zhang, Y, Wang, Q, Yang, C, Wang, R, Wu, S, Xia, X, & Yang, Y. A microRNA expression signature predicts meningioma recurrence. Int J Cancer. (2012). doi:ijc.27658.

[19] Niyazi, M, Zehentmayr, F, Niemöller, O. M, Eigenbrod, S, Kretzschmar, H, Schulze-osthoff, K, Tonn, J. C, Atkinson, M, Mörtl, S, & Belka, C. MiRNA expression patterns predict survival in glioblastoma. Radiat Oncol. (2011).

[20] Ma, R, Yan, W, Zhang, G, Lv, H, Liu, Z, Fang, F, Zhang, W, Zhang, J, Tao, T, You, Y, Jiang, T, & Kang, X. Upregulation of miR-196b Confers a Poor Prognosis in Glioblastoma Patients via Inducing a Proliferative Phenotype. PLoS One. (2012). e38096.

[21] Costa, F. F, Bischof, J. M, Vanin, E. F, Lulla, R. R, Wang, M, Sredni, S. T, & Rajaram, V. Bonaldo Mde F, Wang D, Goldman S, Tomita T, Soares MB. Identification of microRNAs as potential prognostic markers in ependymoma. PLoS One. (2011). e25114.

[22] Liu, J, Zheng, M, Tang, Y. L, Liang, X. H, & Yang, Q. MicroRNAs, an active and versatile group in cancers. Int J Oral Sci. (2011).

[23] Calin, G. A, Dumitru, C. D, Shimizu, M, Bichi, R, Zupo, S, Noch, E, Aldler, H, Rattan, S, Keating, M, Rai, K, Rassenti, L, Kipps, T, Negrini, M, Bullrich, F, & Croce, C. M. Frequent deletions and down-regulation of micro- RNA genes miR15 and miR16 at 13q14 in chronic lymphocytic leukemia.Proc Natl Acad Sci U S A. (2002).

[24] Cimmino, A, Calin, GA, Fabbri, M, Iorio, MV, Ferracin, M, Shimizu, M, Wojcik, SE, Aqeilan, RI, Zupo, S, Dono, M, Rassenti, L, Alder, H, Volinia, S, Liu, CG, Kipps, TJ, Negrini, M, Croce, CM, & mi, . -16 induce apoptosis by targeting BCL2.Proc Natl Acad Sci U S A. 2005,102(39):13944-13949.

[25] Mu, P, Han, Y. C, Betel, D, Yao, E, Squatrito, M, Ogrodowski, P, De Stanchina, E, Andrea, D, Sander, A, & Ventura, C. A. Genetic dissection of the miR-17~92 cluster of microRNAs in Myc-induced B-cell lymphomas. Genes Dev. (2009).

[26] Zhang ChunzhiKang Chunsheng, You Yongpin, Pu Peiyu, Yang Weidong, Zhao Peng, Wang Guangxiu, Zhang Anling, Jia Zhifan, Han Lei and Jiang Hao. Co-suppression of miR-221/222 cluster suppresses human glioma cells growth by targeting in vitro and in vivo. International Journal of Oncology.(2009). , 27kip1.

[27] Chun-Zhi ZhangJun-Xia Zhang, An-Ling Zhang, Zhen-Dong Shi, Lei Han, Zhi-Fan Jia, Wei-Dong Yang, Guang-Xiu Wang, Tao Jiang, Yong-Ping You, Pei-Yu Pu, Jin-Quan Cheng, Chun-Sheng Kang. MiR-221 and miR-222 target PUMA to induce Cell suvivalI in glioblastoma. Molecular Cancer. (2010).

[28] Zhang, C, Zhang, J, Hao, J, Shi, Z, Wang, Y, Han, L, Yu, S, You, Y, Jiang, T, Wang, J, Liu, M, Pu, P, & Kang, C. High level of miR-221/222 confers increased cell invasion and poor prognosis in glioma. J Transl Med. (2012).

[29] Niemoeller, O. M, Niyazi, M, Corradini, S, Zehentmayr, F, Li, M, Lauber, K, & Belka, G. MicroRNA expression profiles in human cancer cells after ionizing radiation. Radiat. Oncol. (2011).

[30] Chistiakov, D. A, & Chekhonin, V. P. Contribution of microRNAs to radio- and chemoresistance of brain tumors and their therapeutic potential. Eur J Pharmacol. (2012).

[31] Wild-bode, C, Weller, M, Rimner, A, Dichgans, J, & Wick, W. Sublethal irradiation promotes migration and invasiveness of glioma cells: implications for radiotherapy of human glioblastoma. Cancer Res. (2001).

[32] Medina, R, Zaidi, S. K, Liu, C. G, Stein, J. L, Van Wijnen, A. J, Croce, C. M, & Stein, G. S. MicroRNAs 221 and 222 bypass quiescence and compromise cell survival. Cancer Res.(2008).

[33] Zhang, C, Kang, C, Wang, P, Cao, Y, Lv, Z, Yu, S, Wang, G, Zhang, A, Jia, Z, Han, L, Yang, C, Ishiyama, H, Teh, B. S, Xu, B, & Pu, P. MicroRNA-221/-222 regulate radiation sensitivity by targeting the PTEN pathway. Int J Radiat Oncol Biol Phys, (2011).

[34] Hao, J, Zhang, C, Zhang, A, Wang, K, Jia, Z, Wang, G, Han, L, Kang, C, Pu, P, & mi, . -221/222 is the regulator of Cx43 expression in human glioblastoma cells. Oncol Rep, 2012,27(5): 1504-1510.

[35] Chan, J. A, Krichevsky, A. M, & Kosik, K. S. MicroRNA-21 is an antiapoptotic factor in human glioblastoma cells. Cancer Res.(2005).

[36] Conti, A, & Aguennouz, M. La Torre D, Tomasello C, Cardali S, Angileri FF, Maio F, Cama A, Germanò A, Vita G and Tomasello F. miR-21 and 221 upregulation and miR-181b downregulation in human grade II-IV astrocytic tumors. J Neurooncol. (2009).

[37] Zhi, F, Chen, X, Wang, S, Xia, X, Shi, Y, Guan, W, Shao, N, Qu, H, Yang, C, Zhang, Y, Wang, Q, Wang, R, Zen, K, Zhang, C. Y, Zhang, J, & Yang, Y. The use of hsa-miR-21, hsa-miR-181b and hsa-miR-106a as prognostic indicators of astrocytoma. Eur J Cancer.(2010).

[38] Corsten, M. F, Miranda, R, Kasmieh, R, Krichevsky, A. M, Weissleder, R, & Shah, K. MicroRNA-21 knockdown disrupts glioma growth in vivo and displays synergistic cytotoxicity with neural precursor cell delivered S-TRAIL in human gliomas. Cancer Res.(2007).

[39] Zhou, X, Zhang, J, Jia, Q, Ren, Y, Wang, Y, Shi, L, Liu, N, Wang, G, Pu, P, You, Y, & Kang, C. Reduction of miR-21 induces glioma cell apoptosis via activating caspase 9 and 3. Oncol Rep.(2010).

[40] Shi, L, Cheng, Z, Zhang, J, Li, R, You, Y, & Fu, Z. The mechanism of apoptosis in human U87 glioma cells induced by miR-21 antisense oligonucleotide. Zhonghua Yi Xue Yi Chuan Xue Za Zhi.(2008).

[41] Papagiannakopoulos, T, Shapiro, A, & Kosik, K. S. MicroRNA-21 targets a network of key tumor-suppressive pathways in glioblastoma cells. Cancer Res.(2008).

[42] Chen, Y, Liu, W, Chao, T, Zhang, Y, Yan, X, Gong, Y, Qiang, B, Yuan, J, Sun, M, & Peng, X. MicroRNA-21 down-regulates the expression of tumor suppressor PDCD4 in human glioblastoma cell T98G. Cancer Lett.(2008).

[43] Gabriely, G, Wurdinger, T, Kesari, S, Esau, C. C, Burchard, J, Linsley, P. S, & Krichevsky, A. M. MicroRNA 21 promotes glioma invasion by targeting matrix metalloproteinase regulators. Mol Cell Biol.(2008).

[44] Endersby, R, & Baker, S. J. PTEN signaling in brain: neuropathology and tumorigenesis. Oncogene.(2008).

[45] Leslie, N. R, & Downes, C. P. PTEN: The down side of PI kinase signalling. Cell Signal.(2002). , 3.

[46] Zhou, X, Ren, Y, Moore, L, Mei, M, You, Y, Xu, P, Wang, B, Wang, G, Jia, Z, Pu, P, Zhang, W, & Kang, C. Downregulation of miR-21 inhibits EGFR pathway and suppresses the growth of human glioblastoma cells independent of PTEN status. Lab Invest.(2010).

[47] Shi, L, Chen, J, Yang, J, Pan, T, Zhang, S, Wang, Z, & Mi, . -21 protected human glioblastoma U87MG cells from chemotherapeutic drug temozolomide induced apoptosis by decreasing Bax/Bcl-2 ratio and caspase-3 activity. Brain Res.2010, 1352: 255-264.

[48] Li, Y, Li, W, Yang, Y, Lu, Y, He, C, Hu, G, Liu, H, Chen, J, He, J, & Yu, H. MicroRNA-21 targets LRRFIP1 and contributes to VM-26 resistance in glioblastoma multiforme. Brain Res.(2009).

[49] Lee, S. Y, Lee, S. Y, & Choi, Y. TRAF-interacting protein (TRIP): a novel component of the tumor necrosis factor receptor (TNFR)- and CDTRAF signaling complexes that inhibits TRAF2-mediated NF-kappaB activation. J Exp Med.(1997). , 30.

[50] Nakanishi, C, & Toi, M. Nuclear factor-kappaB inhibitors as sensitizers to anticancer drugs. Nat Rev Cancer. (2005).

[51] Ren, Y, Kang, C. S, Yuan, X. B, Zhou, X, Xu, P, Han, L, Wang, G. X, Jia, Z, Zhong, Y, Yu, S, Sheng, J, & Pu, P. Y. Co-delivery of as-miR-21 and FU by poly(amidoamine) dendrimer attenuates human glioma cell growth in vitro. J Biomater Sci Polym Ed. (2010). , 5.

[52] Ohno, M, Natsume, A, Kondo, Y, Iwamizu, H, Motomura, K, Toda, H, Ito, M, Kato, T, & Wakabayashi, T. The modulation of microRNAs by type I IFN through the activation of signal transducers and activators of transcription 3 in human glioma. Mol Cancer Res.(2009).

[53] Li, Y, Guessous, F, Zhang, Y, Dipierro, C, Kefas, B, Johnson, E, Marcinkiewicz, L, Jiang, J, Yang, Y, Schmittgen, T. D, Lopes, B, Schiff, D, Purow, B, & Abounader, R. MicroRNA-34a inhibits glioblastoma growth by targeting multiple oncogenes. Cancer Res.(2009).

[54] Luan, S, Sun, L, & Huang, F. MicroRNA-34a: a novel tumor suppressor in glioma cell line U251. Arch Med Res.(2010). , 53.

[55] Guessous, F, Zhang, Y, Kofman, A, Catania, A, Li, Y, Schiff, D, Purow, B, & Abounader, R. icroRNA-34a is tumor suppressive in brain tumors and glioma stem cells. Cell Cycle.(2010).

[56] Yan, D, Zhou, X, Chen, X, Hu, D. N, Dong, X. D, Wang, J, Lu, F, Tu, L, & Qu, J. MicroRNA-34a inhibits uveal melanoma cell proliferation and migration through downregulation of c-Met. Invest Ophthalmol Vis Sci.(2009).

[57] Huffman, D. M, Grizzle, W. E, Bamman, M. M, Kim, J. S, Eltoum, I. A, Elgavish, A, & Nagy, T. R. SIRT1 is significantly elevated in mouse and human prostate cancer. Cancer Res.(2007).

[58] Godlewski, J, Nowicki, M. O, Bronisz, A, Williams, S, Otsuki, A, Nuovo, G, Raychaudhury, A, Newton, H. B, Chiocca, E. A, & Lawler, S. Targeting of the Bmi-1 oncogene/stem cell renewal factor by microRNA-128 inhibits glioma proliferation and self-renewal. Cancer Res.(2008).

[59] Cui, J. G, Zhao, Y, Sethi, P, Li, Y. Y, Mahta, A, Culicchia, F, & Lukiw, W. J. MicroRNA-128 (miRNA-128) down-regulation in glioblastoma targets ARP5 (ANGPTL6), Bmi-1 and E2F-3a, key regulators of brain cell proliferation. J Neurooncol. (2010).

[60] Fasano, C. A, Dimos, J. T, Ivanova, N. B, Lowry, N, Lemischka, I. R, & Temple, S. shRNA knockdown of Bmi-1 reveals a critical role for pathway in NSC self-renewal during development. Cell Stem Cell. (2007). , 21.

[61] Guo, W. J, Zeng, M. S, Yadav, A, Song, L. B, Guo, B. H, Band, V, & Dimri, G. P. Mel-18 acts as a tumor suppressor by repressing Bmi-1 expression and down-regulating Akt activity in breast cancer cells. Cancer Res. (2007).

[62] Iaquinta, P. J, & Lees, J. A. Life and death decisions by the E2F transcription factors. Curr Opin Cell Biol. (2007).

[63] Oike, Y, Yasunaga, K, Ito, Y, Matsumoto, S, Maekawa, H, Morisada, T, Arai, F, Nakagata, N, Takeya, M, Masuho, Y, & Suda, T. Angiopoietin-related growth factor (AGF) promotes epidermal proliferation, remodeling, and regeneration. Proc Natl Acad Sci U S A. (2003).

[64] Huse, J. T, Brennan, C, Hambardzumyan, D, Wee, B, Pena, J, Rouhanifard, S. H, & Sohn-lee, C. Le Sage C, Agami R, Tuschl T and Holland EC. The PTEN-regulating microRNA miR-26a is amplified in high-grade glioma and facilitates gliomagenesis in vivo. Genes Dev. (2009).

[65] Godlewski, J, Nowicki, M. O, Bronisz, A, & Nuovo, G. Palatini JDe Lay M, Van Brocklyn J, Ostrowski MC, Chiocca EA andLawler SE. MicroRNA-451 regulates LKB1/AMPK signalingand allows adaptation to metabolic stress in glioma cells. Mol Cell. (2010).

[66] Alessi, D. R, Sakamoto, K, & Bayascas, J. R. LKB1-dependent signaling pathways. Annu Rev Biochem.(2006). , 75, 137-163.

[67] Nan, Y, Han, L, Zhang, A, Wang, G, Jia, Z, Yang, Y, Yue, X, Pu, P, Zhong, Y, & Kang, C. MiRNA-451 plays a role as tumor suppressor in human glioma cells. Brain Res. (2010).

[68] Kefas, B, Godlewski, J, Comeau, L, Li, Y, Abounader, R, Hawkinson, M, Lee, J, Fine, H, Chiocca, E. A, Lawler, S, & Purow, B. microRNA-7 inhibits the epidermal growth

factor receptor and the Akt pathway and is down-regulated in glioblastoma. Cancer Res. (2008).

[69] Webster, R. J, Giles, K. M, Price, K. J, Zhang, P. M, Mattick, J. S, & Leedman, P. J. Regulation of epidermal growth factor receptor signaling in human cancer cells by microRNA-7. J Biol Chem. (2009).

[70] Reddy, S. D, Ohshiro, K, Rayala, S. K, & Kumar, R. MicroRNA-7, a homeobox D10 target, inhibits kinase 1 and regulates its functions. Cancer Res. (2008). , 21.

[71] Kumar, R, Gururaj, A. E, & Barnes, C. J. p. activated kinases in cancer. Nat Rev Cancer. (2006). , 21.

[72] Aoki, H, Yokoyama, T, Fujiwara, K, Tari, A. M, Sawaya, R, Suki, D, Hess, K. R, Aldape, K. D, Kondo, S, Kumar, R, & Kondo, Y. Phosphorylated Pak1 level in the cytoplasm correlates with shorter survival time in patients with glioblastoma. Clin Cancer Res. (2007). Pt 1):6603-6609.

[73] Miska, E. A, Alvarez-saavedra, E, Townsend, M, Yoshii, A, Sestan, N, Rakic, P, Constantine-paton, M, & Horvitz, H. R. Microarray analysis of microRNA expression in the developing mammalian brain. Genome Biol. (2004). R68.

[74] Shi, L, Cheng, Z, Zhang, J, Li, R, Zhao, P, Fu, Z, You, Y, & Hsa-mir, a. and hsa-mir-181b function as tumor suppressors in human glioma cells. Brain Res. (2008).

[75] Slaby, O, Lakomy, R, Fadrus, P, Hrstka, R, Kren, L, Lzicarova, E, Smrcka, M, Svoboda, M, Dolezalova, H, Novakova, J, Valik, D, Vyzula, R, & Michalek, J. MicroRNA-181 family predicts response to concomitant chemoradiotherapy with temozolomide in glioblastoma patients. Neoplasma. (2010).

[76] Silber, J, Lim, DA, Petritsch, C, Persson, AI, Maunakea, AK, Yu, M, Vandenberg, SR, Ginzinger, DG, James, CD, Costello, JF, Bergers, G, Weiss, WA, Alvarez-Buylla, A, Hodgson, JG, & mi, . -137 inhibit proliferation of glioblastoma multiforme cells and induce differentiation of brain tumor stem cells. BMC Med. 2008,6:14.

[77] Xia, HF, He, TZ, Liu, CM, Cui, Y, Song, PP, Jin, XH, Ma, X, & Mi, . -125b expression affects the proliferation and apoptosis of human glioma cells by targeting Bmf. Cell Physiol Biochem. 2009;23(4-6):347-358.

[78] Puthalakath, H, Villunger, A, Reilly, O, Beaumont, L. A, Coultas, J. G, Cheney, L, Huang, R. E, Strasser, D. C, Bmf, A, & Proapoptotic, a. BHonly protein regulated by interaction with the myosin V actin motor complex, activated by anoikis. Science. (2001). , 3.

[79] Cortez, M. A, Nicoloso, M. S, Shimizu, M, Rossi, S, Gopisetty, G, & Molina, J. R. Carlotti C Jr, Tirapelli D, Neder L, Brassesco MS, Scrideli CA, Tone LG, Georgescu MM, Zhang W, Puduvalli V, Calin GA. miR-29b and miR-125a regulate podoplanin and suppress invasion in glioblastoma. Genes Chromosomes Cancer. (2010).

[80] Kefas, B, Comeau, L, Floyd, D. H, Seleverstov, O, Godlewski, J, Schmittgen, T, & Jiang, J. diPierro CG, Li Y, Chiocca EA, Lee J, Fine H, Abounader R, Lawler S, Purow B. The neuronal microRNA miR-326 acts in a feedback loop with notch and has therapeutic potential against brain tumors. J Neurosci. (2009).

[81] Kim, H, Huang, W, Jiang, X, Pennicooke, B, Park, P. J, & Johnson, M. D. Integrative genome analysis reveals an oncomir/oncogene cluster regulating glioblastoma survivorship. Proc Natl Acad Sci U S A. (2010).

[82] Su, B, Cheng, J, Yang, J, & Guo, Z. MEKK2 is required for T-cell receptor signals in JNK activation and interleukin-2 gene expression. J Biol Chem. (2001).

[83] Sasayama, T, Nishihara, M, Kondoh, T, Hosoda, K, & Kohmura, E. MicroRNA-10b is overexpressed in malignant glioma and associated with tumor invasive factors, uPAR and RhoC. Int J Cancer. (2009).

[84] Xia, H, Qi, Y, Ng, S. S, Chen, X, Chen, S, Fang, M, Li, D, Zhao, Y, Ge, R, Li, G, Chen, Y, He, M. L, Kung, H. F, Lai, L, & Lin, M. C. MicroRNA-15b regulates cell cycle progression by targeting cyclins in glioma cells. Biochem Biophys Res Commun. (2009).

[85] Xia, H, Qi, Y, Ng, S. S, Chen, X, Li, D, Chen, S, Ge, R, Jiang, S, Li, G, Chen, Y, He, M. L, Kung, H. F, Lai, L, & Lin, M. C. microRNA-146b inhibits glioma cell migration and invasion by targeting MMPs. Brain Res. (2009).

[86] Würdinger, T, Tannous, BA, Saydam, O, Skog, J, Grau, S, Soutschek, J, Weissleder, R, Breakefield, XO, Krichevsky, AM, & mi, . -296 regulates growth factor receptor overexpression in angiogenic endothelial cells. Cancer Cell. 2008,14(5):382-393.

[87] Navarro, A, Marrades, R. M, Viñolas, N, Quera, A, Agustí, C, Huerta, A, Ramirez, J, Torres, A, & Monzo, M. MicroRNAs expressed during lung cancer development are expressed in human pseudoglandular lung embryogenesis. Oncology. (2009).

[88] Ernst, A, Campos, B, Meier, J, Devens, F, Liesenberg, F, Wolter, M, Reifenberger, G, Herold-mende, C, Lichter, P, & Radlwimmer, B. De-repression of CTGF via the miR-cluster upon differentiation of human glioblastoma spheroid cultures. Oncogene. (2010). , 17-92.

[89] Ferrara, N. Role of vascular endothelial growth factor in physiologic and pathologic angiogenesis: therapeutic implications. Semin Oncol. (2002). Suppl 16):10-14.

[90] Inoki, I, Shiomi, T, Hashimoto, G, Enomoto, H, Nakamura, H, Makino, K, Ikeda, E, Takata, S, Kobayashi, K, & Okada, Y. Connective tissue growth factor binds vascular endothelial growth factor (VEGF) and inhibits VEGF-induced angiogenesis. FASEB J. (2002).

[91] Suárez, Y, Fernández-hernando, C, Yu, J, Gerber, S. A, Harrison, K. D, Pober, J. S, Iruela-arispe, M. L, Merkenschlager, M, & Sessa, W. C. Dicer-dependent endothelial microRNAs are necessary for postnatal angiogenesis. Proc Natl Acad Sci U S A. (2008).

[92] Lee, S. T, Chu, K, Oh, H. J, Im, W. S, Lim, J. Y, Kim, S. K, Park, C. K, Jung, K. H, Lee, S. K, Kim, M, & Roh, J. K. Let-7 microRNA inhibits the proliferation of human glioblastoma cells. J Neurooncol. (2011).

[93] Galli, R, Binda, E, Orfanelli, U, Cipelletti, B, Gritti, A, De Vitis, S, Fiocco, R, Foroni, C, Dimeco, F, & Vescovi, A. Isolation and characterization of tumorigenic, stem-like neural precursors from human glioblastoma. Cancer Res. (2004).

[94] Bao, S, Wu, Q, Mclendon, R. E, Hao, Y, Shi, Q, Hjelmeland, A. B, Dewhirst, M. W, & Bigner, D. D. and Rich JN: Glioma stem cells promote radioresistance by preferential activation of the DNA damage response. Nature.(2006).

[95] Johannessen, T. C, Wang, J, Skaftnesmo, K. O, Sakariassen, P. Ø, Enger, P. Ø, Petersen, K, Øyan, A. M, Kalland, K. H, & Bjerkvig, R. and Tysnes BB: Highly infltrative brain tumours show reduced chemosensitivity associated with a stem cell-like phenotype. Neuropathol Appl Neurobiol.(2009).

[96] Lavon, I, Zrihan, D, Granit, A, Einstein, O, Fainstein, N, Cohen, M. A, Cohen, M. A, Zelikovitch, B, Shoshan, Y, Spektor, S, Reubinoff, B. E, Felig, Y, Gerlitz, O, Ben-hur, T, Smith, Y, & Siegal, T. Gliomas display a microRNA expression profile reminiscent of neural precursor cells. Neurooncology.(2010).

[97] Felsberg, J, Yan, P. S, Huang, T. H, Milde, U, Schramm, J, Wiestler, O. D, Reifenberger, G, Pietsch, T, & Waha, A. DNA methylation and allelic losses on chromosome arm 14q in oligodendroglial tumours. Neuropathol Appl Neurobiol.(2006).

[98] Gal, H, Pandi, G, Kanner, A. A, Ram, Z, Lithwick-yanai, G, Amariglio, N, Rechavi, G, & Givol, D. MIR-451 and Imatinib mesylate inhibit tumor growth of Glioblastoma stem cells. Biochem Biophys Res Commun. (2008).

[99] Hatfield, S. D, Shcherbata, H. R, Fischer, K. A, Nakahara, K, Carthew, R. W, & Ruohola-baker, H. Stem cell division is regulated by the microRNA pathway. Nature. (2005).

[100] Kefas, B, Comeau, L, Erdle, N, Montgomery, E, Amos, S, & Purow, B. Pyruvate kinase M2 is a target of the tumor-suppressive microRNA-326 and regulates the survival of glioma cells. Neuro Oncol. (2010).

[101] Gajjar, A, Hernan, R, Kocak, M, Fuller, C, Lee, Y, Mckinnon, P. J, Wallace, D, Lau, C, Chintagumpala, M, Ashley, D. M, Kellie, S. J, & Kun, L. and Gilbertson RJ: Clinical, histopathologic, and molecular markers of prognosis: toward a new disease risk strati-fcation system for medulloblastoma. J Clin Oncol.(2004).

[102] Johnson, S. M, Grosshans, H, Shingara, J, Byrom, M, Jarvis, R, Cheng, A, Labourier, E, Reinert, K. L, Brown, D, & Slack, F. J. RAS is regulated by the let-7 microRNA family. Cell.(2005).

[103] MacDonald TJBrown KM, LaFleur B, Peterson K, Lawlor C, Chen Y, Packer RJ, Cogen P, Stephan DA. Expression profiling of medulloblastoma: PDGFRA and the RAS/MAPK pathway as therapeutic targets for metastatic disease.Nat Genet. (2001).

[104] Ferretti, E, De Smaele, E, & Po, A. Di Marcotullio L, Tosi E, Espinola MS, Di Rocco C, Riccardi R, Giangaspero F, Farcomeni A, Nofroni I, Laneve P, Gioia U, Caffarelli E, Bozzoni I, Screpanti I, Gulino A. MicroRNA profiling in human medulloblastoma. Int J Cancer. (2009).

[105] Visvanathan, J, Lee, S, Lee, B, Lee, J. W, & Lee, S. K. The microRNA miR-124 antagonizes the anti-neural REST/SCP1 pathway during embryonic CNS development. Genes Dev. (2007).

[106] Lawinger, P, Venugopal, R, Guo, Z. S, Immaneni, A, Sengupta, D, Lu, W, & Rastelli, L. Marin Dias Carneiro A, Levin V, Fuller GN, Echelard Y, Majumder S.The neuronal repressor REST/NRSF is an essential regulator in medulloblastoma cells. Nat Med. (2000).

[107] Fuller, G. N, Su, X, Price, R. E, Cohen, Z. R, Lang, F. F, Sawaya, R, & Majumder, S. Many human medulloblastoma tumors overexpress repressor element-1 silencing transcription (REST)/neuron-restrictive silencer factor, which can be functionally countered by REST-VP16. Mol Cancer Ther. (2005).

[108] Conaco, C, Otto, S, Han, J. J, & Mandel, G. Reciprocal actions of REST and a microRNA promote neuronal identity. Proc Natl Acad Sci U S A. (2006).

[109] Mendrzyk, F, Radlwimmer, B, Joos, S, Kokocinski, F, Benner, A, Stange, D. E, Neben, K, Fiegler, H, Carter, N. P, Reifenberger, G, Korshunov, A, & Lichter, P. Genomic and protein expression profiling identifies CDK6 as novel independent prognostic marker in medulloblastoma. J Clin Oncol. (2005).

[110] Li, KK, Pang, JC, Ching, AK, Wong, CK, Kong, X, Wang, Y, Zhou, L, Chen, Z, Ng, HK, & mi, . -124 is frequently down-regulated in medulloblastoma and is a negative regulator of SLC16A1. Hum Pathol. 2009,40(9):1234-1243.

[111] Liu, W, Gong, Y. H, Chao, T. F, Peng, X. Z, Yuan, J. G, Ma, Z. Y, Jia, G, & Zhao, J. Z. Identification of differentially expressed microRNAs by microarray: a possible role for microRNAs gene in medulloblastomas. Chin Med J (Engl). (2009).

[112] Ruiz i Altaba ASánchez P, Dahmane N. Gli and hedgehog in cancer: tumours, embryos and stem cells. Nat Rev Cancer. (2002).

[113] Kimura, H, Stephen, D, Joyner, A, & Curran, T. Gli1 is important for medulloblastoma formation in Ptc1+/- mice. Oncogene. (2005).

[114] Ferretti, E, De Smaele, E, Miele, E, Laneve, P, Po, A, Pelloni, M, & Paganelli, A. Di Marcotullio L, Caffarelli E, Screpanti I, Bozzoni I, Gulino A. Concerted microRNA control of Hedgehog signalling in cerebellar neuronal progenitor and tumour cells. EMBO J. (2008).

[115] Uziel, T, Karginov, F. V, Xie, S, Parker, J. S, Wang, Y. D, Gajjar, A, He, L, Ellison, D, Gilbertson, R. J, Hannon, G, & Roussel, M. F. The miR-17~92 cluster collaborates with the Sonic Hedgehog pathway in medulloblastoma. Proc Natl Acad Sci U S A. (2009).

[116] Northcott, P. A, Fernandez-l, A, Hagan, J. P, Ellison, D. W, Grajkowska, W, Gillespie, Y, Grundy, R, Van Meter, T, Rutka, J. T, Croce, C. M, Kenney, A. M, & Taylor, M. D. The miR-17/92 polycistron is up-regulated in sonic hedgehog-driven medulloblastomas and induced by N-myc in sonic hedgehog-treated cerebellar neural precursors. Cancer Res. (2009).

[117] Solecki, D. J, Liu, X. L, Tomoda, T, Fang, Y, & Hatten, M. E. Activated Notch2 signaling inhibits differentiation of cerebellar granule neuron precursors by maintaining proliferation. Neuron. (2001).

[118] Ishibashi, M, Moriyoshi, K, Sasai, Y, Shiota, K, Nakanishi, S, & Kageyama, R. Persistent expression of helix-loop-helix factor HES-1 prevents mammalian neural differentiation in the central nervous system. EMBO J. (1994).

[119] Garzia, L, Andolfo, I, Cusanelli, E, Marino, N, Petrosino, G, De Martino, D, Esposito, V, Galeone, A, Navas, L, Esposito, S, Gargiulo, S, Fattet, S, Donofrio, V, Cinalli, G, Brunetti, A, Vecchio, L. D, Northcott, P. A, Delattre, O, Taylor, M. D, Iolascon, A, & Zollo, M. MicroRNA-199b-5p impairs cancer stem cells through negative regulation of HES1 in medulloblastoma. PLoS One. (2009). e4998.

[120] Venkataraman, S, Alimova, I, Fan, R, Harris, P, Foreman, N, & Vibhakar, R. MicroRNA 128a increases intracellular ROS level by targeting Bmi-1 and inhibits medulloblastoma cancer cell growth by promoting senescence. PLoS One. (2010). e10748.

[121] Diehn, M, Cho, R. W, Lobo, N. A, Kalisky, T, Dorie, M. J, Kulp, A. N, Qian, D, Lam, J. S, Ailles, L. E, Wong, M, Joshua, B, Kaplan, M. J, Wapnir, I, Dirbas, F. M, Somlo, G, Garberoglio, C, Paz, B, Shen, J, Lau, S. K, Quake, S. R, Brown, J. M, Weissman, I. L, & Clarke, M. F. Association of reactive oxygen species levels and radioresistance in cancer stem cells. Nature. (2009).

[122] Vandeva, S, Jaffrain-rea, M. L, Daly, A. F, Tichomirowa, M, Zacharieva, S, & Beckers, A. The genetics of pituitary adenomas. Best Pract Res Clin Endocrinol Metab. (2010).

[123] Bottoni, A, Piccin, D, Tagliati, F, Luchin, A, & Zatelli, M. C. degli Uberti EC. miR-15a and miR-down-regulation in pituitary adenomas. J Cell Physiol. (2005). , 16-1.

[124] Fan, X, Paetau, A, Aalto, Y, Välimäki, M, Sane, T, Poranen, A, Castresana, J. S, & Knuutila, S. Gain of chromosome 3 and loss of 13q are frequent alterations in pituitary adenomas. Cancer Genet Cytogenet. (2001).

[125] Cimmino, A, Calin, GA, Fabbri, M, Iorio, MV, Ferracin, M, Shimizu, M, Wojcik, SE, Aqeilan, RI, Zupo, S, Dono, M, Rassenti, L, Alder, H, Volinia, S, Liu, CG, Kipps, TJ, Negrini, M, Croce, CM, & mi, . -16 induce apoptosis by targeting BCL2. Proc Natl Acad Sci U S A. 2005,102(39):13944-13949.

[126] Wang, D. G, Johnston, C. F, Atkinson, A. B, Heaney, A. P, Mirakhur, M, & Buchanan, K. D. Expression of bcl-2 oncoprotein in pituitary tumours: comparison with c-myc. J Clin Pathol. (1996).

[127] Bottoni, A, Zatelli, M. C, Ferracin, M, Tagliati, F, Piccin, D, Vignali, C, Calin, G. A, Negrini, M, & Croce, C. M. Degli Uberti EC. Identification of differentially expressed microRNAs by microarray: a possible role for microRNA genes in pituitary adenomas. J Cell Physiol. (2007).

[128] Amaral, F. C, Torres, N, Saggioro, F, Neder, L, & Machado, H. R. Silva WA Jr, Moreira AC, Castro M. MicroRNAs differentially expressed in ACTH-secreting pituitary tumors. J Clin Endocrinol Metab. (2009).

[129] Zhou, G, Bao, Z. Q, & Dixon, J. E. Components of a new human protein kinase signal transduction pathway. J Biol Chem. (1995).

[130] Qian, Z. R, Asa, S. L, Siomi, H, Siomi, M. C, Yoshimoto, K, Yamada, S, Wang, E. L, Rahman, M. M, Inoue, H, Itakura, M, Kudo, E, & Sano, T. Overexpression of HMGA2 relates to reduction of the let-7 and its relationship to clinicopathological features in pituitary adenomas. Mod Pathol. (2009).

[131] Lee, Y. S, & Dutta, A. The tumor suppressor microRNA let-7 represses the HMGA2 oncogene. Genes Dev. (2007).

[132] Pierantoni, G. M, Finelli, P, Valtorta, E, Giardino, D, Rodeschini, O, Esposito, F, Losa, M, Fusco, A, & Larizza, L. High-mobility group A2 gene expression is frequently induced in non-functioning pituitary adenomas (NFPAs), even in the absence of chromosome 12 polysomy. Endocr Relat Cancer. (2005).

[133] Butz, H, Likó, I, Czirják, S, Igaz, P, Khan, M. M, Zivkovic, V, Bálint, K, Korbonits, M, Rácz, K, & Patócs, A. Down-regulation of Wee1 kinase by a specific subset of microRNA in human sporadic pituitary adenomas. J Clin Endocrinol Metab. (2010). E, 181-91.

[134] Stenvang, J, Petri, A, Lindow, M, Obad, S, & Kauppinen, S. Inhibition of microRNA function by antimiR oligonucleotides. Silence. (2012).

[135] Ebert, M. S, Neilson, J. R, & Sharp, P. A. MicroRNA sponges: competitive inhibitors of small RNAs in mammalian cells. Nat Methods. (2007).

[136] Lennox, K. A, & Behlke, M. A. Chemical modification and design of anti-miRNA oligonucleotides. Gene Ther. (2011).

[137] Esau, C. C. Inhibition of microRNA with antisense oligonucleotides. Methods. (2008).

[138] Corsten, M. F, Miranda, R, Kasmieh, R, Krichevsky, A. M, Weissleder, R, & Shah, K. MicroRNA-21 knockdown disrupts glioma growth in vivo and displays synergistic cytotoxicity with neural precursor cell delivered S-TRAIL in human gliomas. Cancer Res. (2007).

[139] Würdinger, T, Tannous, BA, Saydam, O, Skog, J, Grau, S, Soutschek, J, Weissleder, R, Breakefield, XO, Krichevsky, AM, & mi, . -296 regulates growth factor receptor overexpression in angiogenic endothelial cells. Cancer Cell. 2008,14(5):382-393.

Section 6

Pediatric Brain Tumors

Chapter 19

Carbonic Anhydrase IX in Adult and Pediatric Brain Tumors

Kristiina Nordfors, Joonas Haapasalo,
Hannu Haapasalo and Seppo Parkkila

Additional information is available at the end of the chapter

http://dx.doi.org/10.5772/52358

1. Introduction

Carbonic anhydrases (CAs) are zinc-containing metalloenzymes present in prokaryotes and eukaryotes (Sly and Hu 1995). CAs have been investigated since 1930's (Meldrum and Roughton 1933). They are important in normal human physiology, e.g., in gluconeogenesis, lipogenesis, ureagenesis, bone resorption, and formation of gastric juice and cerebrospinal fluid (Sly and Hu 1995, Pastoreková et al. 2004). There are at least 15 members in human alpha-CA family: Five active family members are cytosolic (CA I-III, VII, and XIII), four are membrane associated (CA IV, IX, XII, and XIV), two are mitochondrial (CA VA and VB), and one is a secretory form (CA VI). In addition, there are three acatalytic forms, which are called CA-related protein (CARPs). CAs can be categorized to catalytically active or inactive, intracellular or extracellular, and wide-spread or restricted to few tissues.

Their main physiological fuction is to catalyze the conversion of CO2 to bicarbonate ion and proton, as described by the following reaction:

$$CO_2 + H_2O \xleftrightarrow{CA} HCO_3^- + H^+$$

In addition to their functions in normal physiology, the roles of CAs in different diseases have been extensively investigated during the last decades. They are involved in certain neurological and hereditary disorders, oedema, and most importantly, in cancer. There are at least three tumor associated isoforms; CA II, IX and XII. Especially carbonic anhydrase IX (CA IX) has been associated to neoplastic growth and cancer. The following chapter will discuss the role of CA IX in brain tumors.

2. Carbonic anhydrase IX

Carbonic anhydrase IX was first found by Pastroreková et al. (1992) and the *CA9* gene was cloned by the Pastrorek et al. (1994). Previously, a research group from Netherlands described a monoclonal antibody, named G250, which stained cell membranes of renal cell carcinoma, but did not stain normal epithelium (Oosterwijk et al. 1986). They continued their studies to establish G250 as a tool in cancer diagnostics and treatment. Afterwards, the protein recognized by the G250 antibody was characterized to be CA IX (Grabmaier et al. 2000).

CA 9 gene was originally located to the chromosome 17q21.2 by fluorescence in situ hybridization (Opavský et al. 1996), but it was later localized to the chromosome 9p13-p12 by radiation hybrid mapping (http://www.ncbi.nlm.nih.gov/gene/768). *CA9* gene consists of eleven exons and ten introns (Opavský et al. 1996), and encodes a protein containing 466 amino acids. It has a proteoglycan (PG) domain, central catalytic (CA) domain, transmembrane anchor, and short COOH- terminal cytoplasmic tail. CA IX was initially called MN, found from human carcinoma cell line, and later associated to neoplastic growth in carcinomas of ovary, uterine cervix and endometrium (Závada et al. 1993). A detailed characterisation of human CA IX protein has has shown that the recombinant CA IX protein exhibits the highest catalytic activity ever measured for any CA isozyme (Hilvo et al. 2008).

3. Carbonic anhydrase IX in normal tissue

The expression of CA IX in normal tissues has been thoroughly investigated. In mouse tissues, the highest expression has been detected in gastric mucosa, moderate expression in colon and brain, whereas low expression has been reported in pancreas and small intestine (Hilvo et al. 2004). The similar distribution pattern has been detected in human tissues; high CA IX staining has been discovered in GI-tract, especially in the epithelia of the gallbladder and gastric mucosa (Pastorek et al. 1994, Pastoreková et al. 1997, Saarnio et al. 1998a). Furthermore, Saarnio et al. (1998b) have reported the most intensive signals of CA IX in the epitelium of the duodenum and jejunum, whereas the expression diminishes towards the large intestine. Mesothelium, epithelial cells of the esophagus, and pancreatic and biliary ducts express CA IX (Turner et al. 1997, Pastoreková et al. 1997, Kivelä et al. 2000, Ivanov et al. 2001). CA IX has been detected in the male reproductive organs, whereas the female reproductive tract express only low amounts of CA IX (Liao et al. 1994; Karhumaa et al. 2001). Generally, expression of CA IX is generally low in the human brain, although positive signal has been reported in the epithelial cells of the choroid plexus (Ivanov et al. 2001, Proescholdt et al. 2005). Similarly, lower levels of CA IX mRNA have been reported in the normal brain as compared to brain neoplasms (Said et al. 2007a).

http://dx.doi.org/10.5772/52358

4. Carbonic anhydrase IX in neoplastic tissue

The von Hippel–Lindau (*VHL*) tumor suppressor gene was the first link to the major pathway controlling CA IX expression (Wykoff et al. 2000). Importantly, CA IX turned out to be one of the enzymes regulated by the hypoxia pathway, in which hypoxia inducible factor 1 (HIF-1) plays a role as a key transcription factor, especially in hypoxic tumors. Under normoxia, the encoded VHL protein (pVHL) binds to hydroxylated hypoxia inducible factor 1 – alpha and causes degradation by the ubiquitin-mediated proteasome system, inactivating the downstream target genes. (Ivanov et al.1998). HIF-1 is stabilized under hypoxic conditions and binds to hypoxia-responsive elements in many genes, e.g VEGF, erythropoietin, and glucose transporter. This leads to the induction of erythropoiesis, angiogenesis, and glycolysis (Carmeliet et al. 1998). HIF-1 also activates *CA9* gene and CA IX expression level increases dramatically in hypoxic conditions. In line with this, high CA IX expression is often found in perinecrotic regions of tumors (Wykoff et al. 2000). The similar induction of CA IX has been proposed to take place in brain tumors. CA IX mRNA has been studied in human malignant glioma cell lines and distinct patterns of hypoxic expression of CA IX have been observed (Said et al. 2007b). The finding indicated that low oxygen concentration is probably the driving force for the increased CA IX expression due to the presence of a hypoxia responsive element (HRE) in the *CA9* promoter (Wykoff et al. 2000). The activation of hypoxia-inducible genes is illustrated in Figure 1.

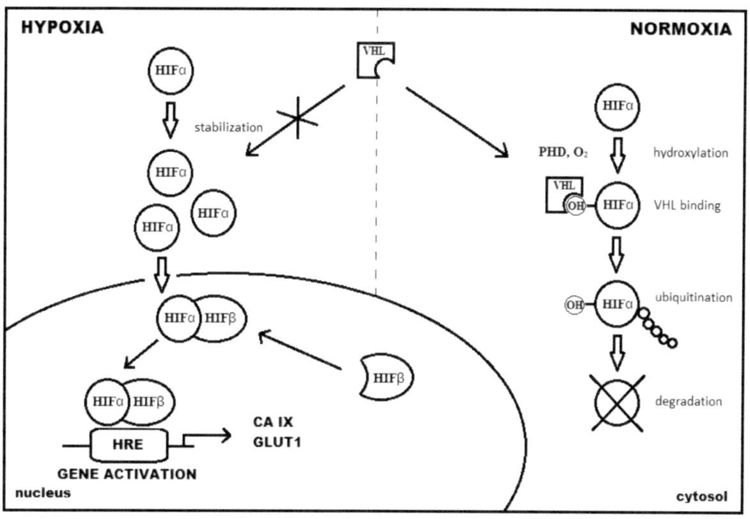

Figure 1. Activation of hypoxia-inducible genes. Under normoxia, HIFα is degraded by ubiquitin-proteasome system. Prolyl-4-hydroxylases (PHD) hydroxylate two conserved proline residues of HIF-1α, then von Hippel-Lindau protein (VHL) binds to the hydroxylated HIF-1α. Under hypoxia, PHDs are inactive in the absence of dioxygen, and HIF-1α is not recognized by VHL protein. HIF-1α accumulates and is translocated to the nucleus. HIF-1β constitutive subunit dimerizes with HIF-1α, resulting in the active transcription factor, which binds to hypoxia response element (HRE). Therefore the transcription of target genes, such as *CA9* and *GLUT1*, is induced. Adapted from Pastoreková et al. (2008) and Haapasalo (2011).

The overexpression of CAIX in majority of renal cell carcinomas (RCCs) is due to the loss of functional VHL protein, which causes the stabilization of HIF-1. (Gnarra et al. 1994, Wykoff et al. 2000). In other words, the CAs are no longer regulated by hypoxia. On the contrary, the majority of tumors do not contain VHL mutations, and in these, CA IX is usually found in focal perinecrotic areas, supporting the role of hypoxia in CA IX regulation (Wykoff et al. 2000). Furthermore, it has been suggested that HIF activates genes that change the expression profile of tumor cells suffering from hypoxia; thus, either leading to adaptation to the hypoxic stress or resulting in cell death. If this adaptation is successful, the surviving tumor cell population is associated with increasingly aggressive behaviour involving invasion and metastases, resistance to anti-cancer treatment, and finally, worse patient prognosis. (Harris 2002). This mechanism is supported by various immunohistochemical studies in which the CA IX expression is located in in the perinecrotic regions of solid tumors.

The mechanisms behind the role of CA IX in cancer have been studied widely. The hypoxia, measured by needle electrores, has been shown to correlate with CA IX expression in cervical cancer (Loncaster et al. 2001). This finding has been further clarified in genetic analysis, showing that *CA9* was the most induced gene among the 32 identified hypoxia responsive genes, which included *VEGF*, in human solid tumors (Lal et al. 2002). *In vitro*, *CA9* has been shown to be hypoxia-regulated in glioblastoma cells (Said et al. 2008).

The pivotal feature of the malignant tumor cells is their capability to maintain the normal intracellular pH, whereas the extracellular pH is significantly acidic. CA IX increases the extracellular acidification by shifting the site of CO_2 hydration from intra- to extracellular (Svastová et al. 2004). This in turn increases the capability of tumor cells to survive and invade, and the selective sulfonamide inhibitors disturb this process. Acetazolamide, a potent CA inhibitor, has been shown to suppress the invasion of renal cancer cells *in vitro* (Parkkila et al. 2000b). Interestingly, CA IX has an optimal catalytic activity for CO_2 hydration to bicarbonate and proton in acidic pH (Innocenti et al. 2009). Furthermore, when studied in cancer-derived cell lines, CA IX diminishes the intracellular pH gradient in the hypoxic core of three-dimensional tumor spheroids (Swietach et al. 2008). These findings support the theory that CA IX is an essential factor for tumor cells in adaptation to hypoxia and their survival, and is illustared in Figure 2.

Even though the expression of CA IX is mainly regulated by hypoxia, it has been shown that acidosis increases CA IX expression via a hypoxia-independent mechanism (Ihnatko et al. 2006). CA IX has been proposed to be regulated by low oxygen concentrations or constitutive, oncogene-related mechanisms (Said et al. 2007a). Furthermore, CA IX modulates E-cadherin mediated cell adhesion by decreasing the binding of this cell adhesion molecule to beta-catenin (Svastová et al. 2003). This, in turn, could possibly benefit the cancer cells by an increase in cell motility and invasion. As mentioned before, acetazolamide can suppress the invasion of renal cancer cells *in vitro* (Parkkila et al. 2000b). However, the inhibition of CA IX in RNAi-treated breast cancer cells reduced the invasion capacity only slightly (Robertson et al. 2004). There is also evidence that CA IX expression is a negative predictive factor when evaluating the treatment efficacy in oestrogen receptor-positive tumors treated with adjuvant tamoxifen after

http://dx.doi.org/10.5772/52358

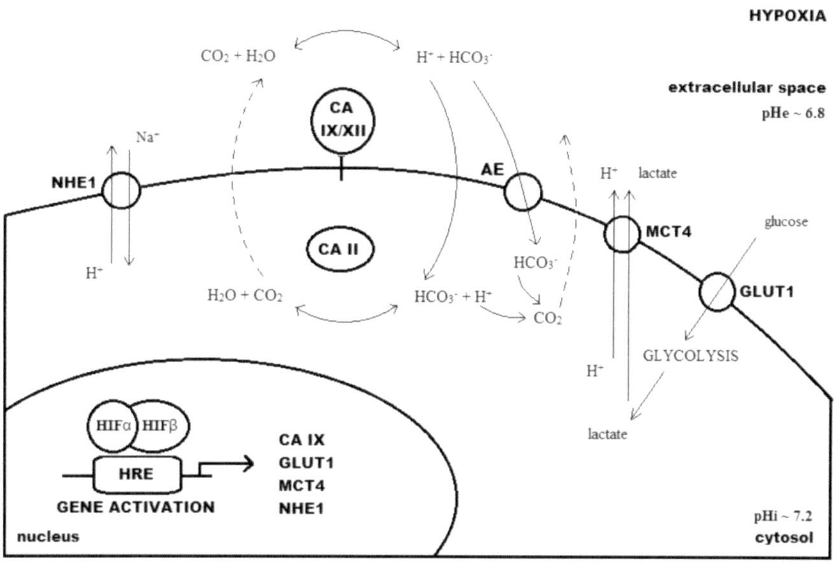

Figure 2. Example of pH regulation in a cancer cell under hypoxia. This is controlled by HIF-1 mediated gene activation. The rapid metabolic rate requires glucose which is transported to the cell by the glucose transporter (GLUT1). Glycolysis produces lactate and protons, which are transported to extracellular space by the H^+/monocarboxylate transporter 4 (MCT4). The transmebrane CA IX (and XII), and cytosolic CA II prevent intracellular acidification and maintain the physiological pH. Anion exchangers (AE) transport bicarbonate to cytosol, which then buffers the protons produced by the active metabolism. Resulting CO_2 is secreted from the cell by diffusion. The Na^+/H^+ exchanger 1 (NHE1) participates in the secretion of proton. The HIF-mediated machinery and oncogenic pathways result in secretion of protons and CO_2 to extracellular space, thus promoting the breakdown of the extracellular matrix and invasion of tumor cells. Adapted from Pastoreková et al. (2008) and Haapasalo (2011).

primary chemo-endocrine therapy (Generali et al. 2006). The role of CA IX in resistance to chemotherapy could be explained by the effects of pH on tamoxifen uptake.

Ectopic expression of CA IX is induced in various tumors. These include the malignancies of breast, cervix uteri, esophagus, kidney, and lung (Liao et al. 1994, McKiernan et al. 1997, Liao et al. 1997, Turner et al. 1997, Vermylen et al. 1999, Bartosová et al. 2002). When these tumors are considered, CA IX is absent in the corresponding normal tissue. Conversely, CA IX expression is usually absent or reduced in tumors which have originated from CA IX-positive tissues. These include carcinomas of stomach and gallbladder (Saarnio et al. 2001, Leppilampi et al. 2003). This makes the CA IX a promising molecule as a prognostic factor as well as a potential target for therapeutic methods.

In cervical cancer, the CA IX expression correlates to tumor hypoxia and poor patient prognosis, and could be used in the selection of suitable patients for hypoxia-modification therapies (Loncaster et al. 2001). In lung cancer CA IX is a marker of poor prognosis (Swinson et al. 2003, Kim et al. 2004), and it has been associated to proteins linked to angiogenesis, disruption of cell-cell adhesion and inhibition of apoptosis (Giatromanolaki et al. 2001). CA IX could also been used as a differentiation tool between preneoplastic lesions and lung cancer (Vermylen et al. 1998) and a high concentration of CA IX in plasma serves as a independent prognostic biomarker in patients with non-small cell lung cancer (Ilie et al. 2010). CA IX expression is sensitive for diagnostics of mesothelioma and metastatic clear cell renal cell carcinoma of the lung (Ramsey et al. 2012). Furthermore, CA IX expression has been associated with poor prognosis for patients with head and neck cancer (Beasley et al. 2001, Koukourakis et al. 2001), esophageal cancer (Birner et al. 2011), ovarian cancer (Hynninen et al. 2006, Choschzick et al. 2011), soft tissue sarcoma (Måseide et al. 2004), and bladder carcinoma (Hoskin et al. 2003). It has been confirmed in several studies that CA IX correlates with poor prognosis in breast cancer (Chia et al. 2001, Brennan et al. 2006, Hussain et al. 2007) and is related to overexpression of c-erbB2 (Bartosová et al. 2002).

The most widely investigated tumor type, considering CA IX, is renal cell carcinoma (RCC) in which CA IX represents a useful marker (Liao et al. 1997, McKiernan et al. 1997, Parkkila et al. 2000a). In its most common subtype, clear cell carcinoma, CA IX expression is higher than in other renal cell cancer types (Sandlund et al. 2007). In addition, patients with both conventional renal cell cancer and low CA IX expression had a less favourable prognosis. In renal cancer CA IX is a promising therapeutic target for novel oncological applications, including immunotherapy and radioisotopic methods (Pastoreková et al. 2006, Bleumer et al. 2006). CA IX and CA XII are functionally involved in tumor growth (Chiche et al. 2009). Renal cell cancer *in vivo* experiments showed that *CA9* gene silencing alone led to a 40% reduction in xenograft tumor volume, and silencing of both *CA9* and *CA12* resulted in an 85% reduction in tumor volume.

5. Carbonic anhydrases in adult brain tumors

The incidence of brain tumors is similar in different countries and rather stable over the past two decades (Pollack et al. 2011). There are about 50 new pediatric and 1000 adult brain tumors every year in Finland with five million habitants (Statistics Finland 2011). The etiology of brain tumors has been under intense investigation but no clear evidence between different environmental, nutritional or lifestyle and carcinogenesis have been found (Baldwin et al. 2004). Most common primary CNS tumors of the adult are gliomas and meningiomas. Glioblastoma is a highly malignant and unfortunately common, glial tumor and the 5-year survival of the patients is less than 10 % (Stupp et al. 2009). On the other hand, almost all (90-98%) patients with meningioma are alive after five years (Statistics Finland 2011).

The expression of carbonic anhydrases in brain tumors has been previously reported (Parkkila AK et al. 1995). The first findings assessed CA II, which was stained positively by immunohistochemistry in astrocytic tumors, oligodendrogliomas and medulloblastomas. The expression of CA IX was first reported by Ivanov et. al (2001). In this first study, they screened tumors of different genetic background as well as several malignant cell lines for the expression of CA IX. mRNA analysis revealed high-to-moderate levels of expression of *CA9* and *CA12* in glioma cell lines. Immunolocalization of CA IX was further studied in 11 gliomas; low-grade gliomas were not stained for CA IX, whereas grade III-IV gliomas were all CA IX positive. In addition, 3 oligodendrogliomas were included in the analysis and they failed to express CA IX. Furthermore, all hemangioblastomas (3 tumors), meningiomas (5 tumors), and two out of three choroid plexus tumors were positive for CA IX.

This overview of different tumors was followed by a study of Proescholdt et al. (2005) on CA IX and CA XII, which combined brain tumors of different histology and grade of malignancy. The material consisted of total of 112 tumor samples (grade I-IV astrocytomas, meningiomas, metastases, primitive neuroectodermal tumors (PNETs), and hemangioblastomas). Generally, low-grade astrocytomas did not show any positive staining for CA IX and the expression increased with increasing WHO grade. The strongest staining of all glioma samples was observed in the glioblastomas, and almost all of the samples (97%) were positive. In these, the staining was detected around necrotic areas. However, more diffuse staining pattern without any association to necrosis was detected and CA IX expression was found in almost all tumor cells, including those near blood vessels, suggesting the induction also without the hypoxia-inducible mechanism. In the meningiomas, increased CA IX staining, with diffuse and evenly distributed pattern, was found in comparison to the normal brain. The authors found the most widespread CA IX and XII staining of all tumors in hemangioblastoma samples.

As to brain tumors, the first large study to describe the expression of CA IX in human diffusely infiltrating astrocytomas was published year after (Haapasalo et al. 2006). The study material consisted of 362 diffusely infiltrating astrocytoma samples (grades II-IV), which were obtained from surgically operated patients. Cellular CA IX immunopositivity was observed in 78% of diffusely infiltrating astrocytomas and the percentages according the WHO grade were as follows; 65% of grade II astrocytomas, 73% of grade 3 astrocytomas, and 82% of grade 4 astrocytomas. The immunohistochemial results were verified by mRNA analysis. The statistical comparison of cytoplasmic CA IX intensity and tumor grade revealed significantly higher CA IX intensity in tumors of higher malignancy grade. Again, CA IX was expressed in areas close to the necrotic regions and cytoplasmic staining was seen in the neoplastic cells of the infiltrative zone. When important clinicopathologial features were assessed, CA IX showed no association with p53 expression nor did it correlate with epidermal growth factor receptor–amplification, apoptosis, or cell proliferation by Ki-67/MIB-1. There was a significant correlation between increasing CA IX intensity and increasing patient age. For the first time, CA IX positivity was associated to shortened patient survival in univariate analysis: CA IX intensity divided the tumors into four significantly differing prognostic subsets (Figure 3). The survival difference was even significant within grade II and grade IV tumors separately. Most importantly, statistical analysis of the data revealed that the patient age, tumor grade, and CA IX intensity all had independent prognostic value when evaluated by Cox multivariate analysis.

The finding that CA IX predicts poor prognosis has been confirmed by others. Korkolopoulou et al. (2007) showed that increasing CA IX immunopositivity was associated with a shortened survival in univariate analysis. Furthermore, they reported similar independent prognosticators in multivariate analysis including CA IX, tumor grade and patient age. The perinecrotic distribution of CA IX immunostaining was detected and intensity increased in parallel with the extent of necrosis and histological grade. In concordance, Sathornsumetee et al. (2008) conducted a trial, in which patients with recurrent malignant astrocytomas treated with a combination of VEGF -neutralizing antibodies were retrospectively evaluated. Survival

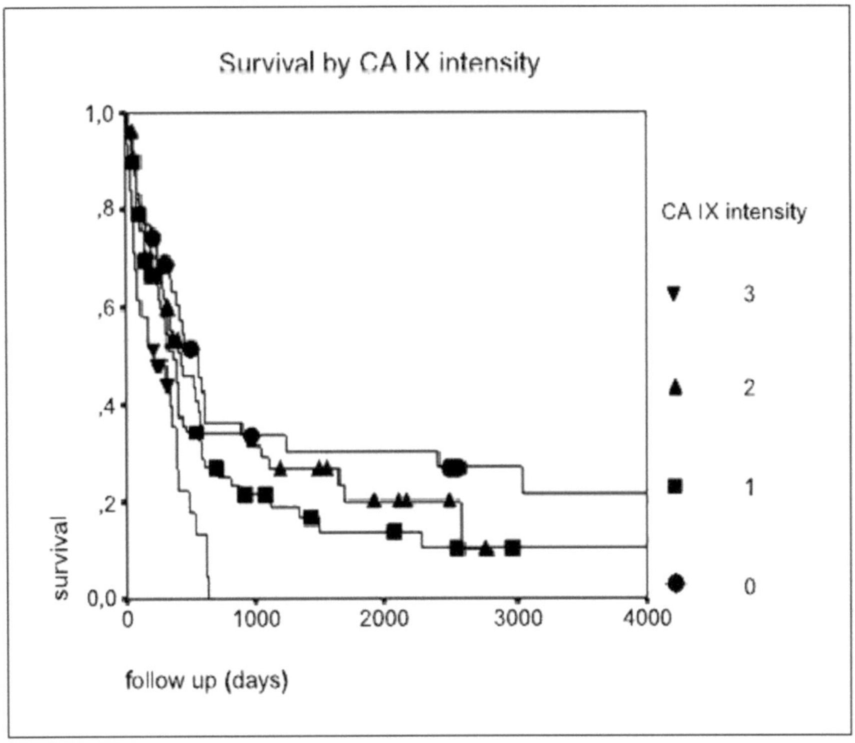

Figure 3. Prognostic significance of CA IX in diffusely infiltrating astrocytomas (grades II-IV). Kaplan-Meier curves are shown ($p = 0.0011$, log-rank test). Haapasalo J et al. (2006)

analysis revealed that high CA IX expression was associated with poor survival outcome. VEGF was associated with radiographic response but not with survival. Interestingly, they tested both CA IX and HIF simultaneously in a Cox model as separate factors, and only CA IX remained as a statistically significant factor. One opposite result has been published in glioma patient cohort (Flynn et al. 2008). In this study, no significant correlations between the CA IX expression and patient survival or tumor grade were found, although the patients with CA IX-positive tumors seemed to have a trend towards a worse prognosis. This might be due to different immunostaining method used. The most reliable method for CA IX immunostaining having no cross-reactivity with other CAs (Saarnio et al. 1998b), is based on M75 antibodies used by us and e.g. Korkolopoulou et al. (2007). Flynn et al. (2008) had also smaller number of patients. Yoo et. al (2010) assessed the issue again, and showed that CA IX expression was a predictive factor for poor survival and correlated positively with increasing WHO grade.

The expression of CA IX has been studied in other gliomas as well. Järvelä et al. (2008) showed by immunohistochemistry that 80% of studied 86 oligodendroglial tumors stained positively for CA IX. In addition, CA IX predicted poor prognosis in univariate analysis and in multivariate analysis CA IX expression, patient age and histological component (pure oligodendroglioma vs. mixed oligoastrocytoma) showed independent prognostic values. Abraham et al. (2012) have recently assessed the expression of all hypoxia related molecules HIF-1, VEGF, Glut-1, and CA IX, in oligodendrogliomas. They found that all these proteins were statistically significantly different between grade II and III oligodendrogliomas, anaplastic oligodendrogliomas having stronger expression. Ingterestingly, low CA IX expression predicted better prognosis in anaplastic oligodendrogliomas but not in grade II oligodendrogliomas, whereas the prognostic significance was not reported in the whole tumor material.

As for mostly benign tumors, Yoo et al. (2007) showed that 50% of all meningiomas contained regions of hypoxia as judged by expression of CA IX. CA IX expression was significantly associated with higher-grade histology and tended to be more common in recurrent tumors. Futhermore, Korhonen et al. (2009) reported 11.6% cytosolic CA IX expression in meningiomas. CA IX positivity was neither associated with the studied clinicopathological factors nor survival.

Recently, Jensen et al. (2012) assessed the molecular markers of hypoxia, vascularity, and proliferation in meningeomas, including CA IX. As expected, VEGF, HIF, CA IX, and Glut-1 were positively correlated. There was an association between higher-grade tumors with higher scores for CA IX, VEGF, and HIF-1alpha, but CA IX was not associated to overall survival.

CA IX is also significantly upregulated in craniopharyngiomas and is associated with increased cyst size (Proescholdt et al. 2011). The mechanisms of CA IX regulation remain unknown, since neither hypoxia nor p53 appear to play a role in these tumors. The authors state, that inhibition of CA IX may be a potential target for the adjuvant treatment in patients with cystic craniopharyngiomas.

6. CA IX in pediatric brain tumors

Pediatric cancers are still the main cause of death in children aged 1-14 years in the UK and Finland (Gatta et al. 2005, Statistics Finland 2011). After leukemia brain tumors are the second most common tumor group. Approximately 60-70% of the patients with brain tumors are alive five years from the diagnosis (Pokhrel and Hakulinen 2009). The most common pediatric brain tumors are pilocytic astrosytoma, medulloblastoma and ependymoma. Neurosurgical operation is the most important treatment modality. Inoperable or highly malignant tumors are treated also with radio- and chemotherapy. CNS is vulnerable, especially when evolving. Most of the patients do survive but the tumor and the different treatment modalities can cause side effects that reduce the quality of life. Supratentorial tumors, tumor reoperations, shunt revisions and chemotherapy increase the risk of these problems (Reimers et al. 2003, Pietilä et al. 2012). There is only a limited scope for improvement with conventional chemotherapy and thus, there is an urgent need of therapeutic agents for these patients. CA IX is one novel molecule that might serve as a prognostic/diagnostic tool, and perhaps, a target for various therapeutic methods.

Some publications have assessed the CA IX expression in pediatric brain tumors. Ivanov et al. (2001) screened a small amount of brain tumors and found the following inmmunohistochemistry results: most of the 7 central/peripheral PNETs expressed the CA IX, all of 6 studied epedymomas were posivive. Preusser et al. (2005) assessed the CA IX in intracranial ependymomas. 84 out of 100 tumors expressed CA IX, and it was associated with a bizarre angiogenesis and necrosis. However, CA IX failed to reach a prognostic significance in univariate analysis. The most common, solid, extracranial pediatric nervous tumor is neuroblastoma. Dungwa et al. (2012) found positive membranous/cytoplasmic CA IX expression in 21 (23%) of 91 neuroblastomas but was absent in ganglioneuromas. Neuroblastomas with 1p deletion and MYCN amplification had even stronger membranous expression. 18% of the neuroblastomas showed nuclear CA IX expression in 10% or more tumoral cells. Nuclear CA IX expression associated with worse overall –and event-free survival.

We have previously studied CA IX in 39 medulloblastomas and PNETs (Nordfors et al. 2010). CA IX positivity was found in 23% of tumors and the expression was linked to necrosis. CA IX expression was analysed in concordance with various clinical features and molecular markers. Proliferation (Ki-67/MIB-1), apoptosis or expression of Bcl-2, p53 or c-erbB-2 were not associated with CA IX in any of the groups except for the correlation between positive c-erbB-2 and positive CA IX expression in PNETs. CA IX was also positively associated with female gender. There was no significant difference in the expression of CA IX between primary and recurrent tumors in any of the groups. Moreover, there was no correlation between the tumor type (MBs/PNETs) and CA IX intensity. Interestingly, CA IX-positivity was a marker of worse outcome in patients with MB/PNET in univariate and multivariate analyses (Figure 4). Generally, CA IX is associated with higher grade, necrosis, and worse CA IX seems to have several inductors. CA IX is often found in perinecrotic areas. Because necrosis is an uncommon feature and is not considered to be a significant prognostic factor in MBs, the induction of CA IX in MBs/PNETs may also involve hypoxia-independent mechanisms. In addition, there is the evidence that CA IX is expressed in grade I pilocytic astrocytomas, and the immunopositivity for CA IX is associated to histopathological features of degeneration and increased proliferation (our unpublished results).

In children, possible side-effects of therapeutic interventions may be more severe and the exact biology of hypoxia and its clinical relevance in childhood tumors is still unclear. Thus, further studies will be needed before novel agents concerning hypoxia can be introduced into pediatric oncology.

7. Future aspects

The tumor tissue specific CA IX expression has led researchers to propose several novel treatment strategies. A promising treatment strategy is to use CA selective inhibitors (Pastoreková et al. 2004). Tumor cells probably use CAs as key enzymes to adapt to the hostile environment caused by metabolic stress of cancer cells, and thus, acidification facilitates the spread and invasion of cancer cells (Svastová et al. 2004). High CA IX expression might increase the capability of cells to infiltrate the neighboring tissue. The inhibition of this process would potentially disturb the invasion processes of cancer cells.

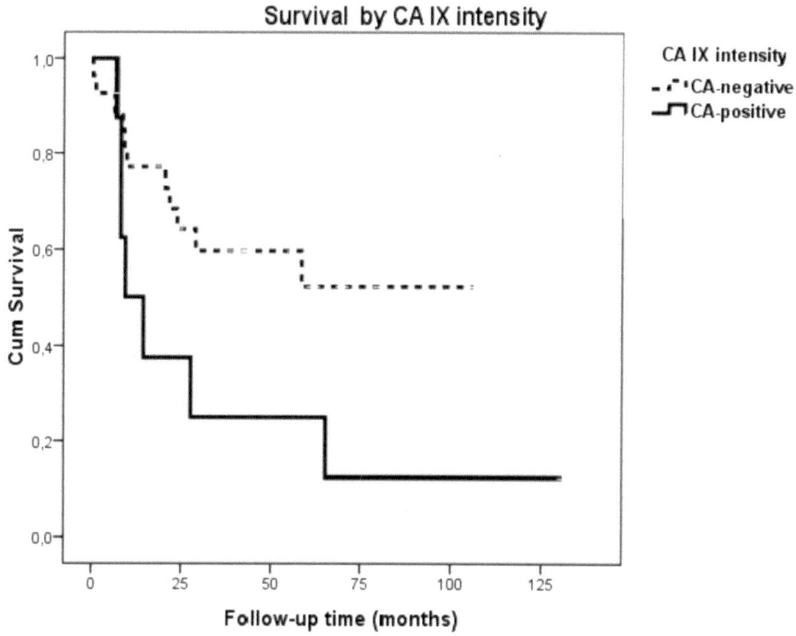

Figure 4. Prognostic significance of CA IX in medulloblastomas/PNETs. Kaplan-Meier curves are shown (P = 0.041, log-rank test). Nordfors et al. (2010)

Another possible treatment option is to use cancer-specific antibodies. The CA and proteoglycan domains give the molecule a unique extracellular structure. CA IX expression is high in renal cell carcinoma (Liao et al. 1997) and this has enabled therapeutic trials with high-dose radiolabeled CA IX antibody (cG250) and CA IX-loaded dendritic cells. Unfortunately, a significant breakthrough in clinical trials remains to be achieved and in RCC trials are still in phase II (Stillebroer et al. 2010).

CA IX could also be used as a potential target for immune therapy. Greiner et al. (2006) found a significant correlation between high mRNA levels of CA IX and a longer overall survival in acute myeloid leukemia. This might be due to the induction of a strong antileukemic immune response by CA IX. Similar findings have been found in metastatic RCC patients (Uemura et al. 2006). Vaccination with tumor-RNA pulsed dendritic cells led to increased numbers of CA IX peptide-specific cytotoxic T76 lymphocytes and IgG levels without any major adverse event. Metastasis of three patients shrank or even disappeared and the overall survival was longer for six patients. However, further studies are required to confirm these findings in larger study cohorts.

Bevacizumab, an anti-VEGF antibody, inhibits the developing vasculature of tumors, but resistance is common. Antiangiogenic therapy induces hypoxia and thus, CA IX. Curiously, McIntyre et al. (2012) knocked down CAIX expression in a colon cancer and a glioblastoma cell lines and combined the results with bevacizumab. They found that CAIX expression was associated with increased necrosis and apoptosis *in vivo* and *in vitro*. Added to this, acidity seemed to inhibit CAIX activity, and this may be the mechanism whereby excess acid self-limits the build-up of extracellular acid. It seems that inhibition of the hypoxic adaptation to antiangiogenic therapy enhances bevacizumab treatment and highlights the value of developing small molecules or antibodies which inhibit CAIX for combination therapy.

8. Conclusions

CA IX has been linked to several cancer tissues, whereas the normal tissue is mostly negative. This seems to be the case also when different brain tumors are concerned. Malignant astrocytomas and oligodendrogliomas express CA IX and it has been shown as a useful prognosticator. Being a hypoxia/necrosis marker, CA IX can be used as a diagnostic tool in the grading of astrocytomas and oligodendrogliomas. Tumor biopsies containing a small amount of tissue for diagnosis, are especially good targets. In addition, CA IX is associated to more malignant phenotype in meningiomas and some other mostly benign brain tumors.

CA IX is present in the most common malignant brain tumor of children, medulloblastoma, as well as in PNETs. Interestingly, in these tumors CA IX predicts poor prognosis and could be used as a marker when planning the cancer therapy. Added to this, CA IX has been shown to be expressed in other pediatric brain tumors, such as ependymomas and pilocytic astrocytomas, where it is linked to degenerative histopathological features.

CA IX is associated with hypoxia, necrosis, and angiogenesis – features traditionally linked to the tumorigenesis of brain tumors. Several studies show that CA IX could be used as a target molecule in adult and pediatric brain tumors. Further clinical trials for cancer treatment are needed aiming to either eradicate the tumor cell population or turn the tumor into a more chronic and stable disease.

Author details

Kristiina Nordfors[1], Joonas Haapasalo[2], Hannu Haapasalo[3] and Seppo Parkkila[4]

1 Department of Pediatrics, Tampere University Hospital, Tampere, Finland

2 Unit of Neurosurgery, Tampere University Hospital, Tampere, Finland

3 Department of Pathology, Fimlab Ltd and Tampere University Hospital, Tampere, Finland

4 Department of Anatomy, Tampere University, Fimlab Ltd and Tampere University Hospital, Tampere, Finland

References

[1] Abraham S, Hu N, Jensen R (2012); Hypoxia-inducible factor-1-regulated protein expression and oligodendroglioma patient outcome: comparison with established biomarkers and preoperative UCSF low-grade scoring system. J Neurooncol. 108:459-68.

[2] Baldwin RT, Preston-Martin S (2004); Epidemiology of brain tumors in childhood – a review. Toxicol Appl Pharmacol 199:118-31.

[3] Bartosová M, Parkkila S, Pohlodek K, Karttunen TJ, Galbavý S, Mucha V, Harris AL, Pastorek J, Pastoreková S (2002); Expression of carbonic anhydrase IX in breast is associated with malignant tissues and is related to overexpression of c-erbB2. J. Pathol. 197:314-21.

[4] Beasley NJ, Wykoff CC, Watson PH, Leek R, Turley H, Gatter K, Pastorek J, Cox GJ, Ratcliffe P, Harris AL (2001); Carbonic anhydrase IX, an endogenous hypoxia marker, expression in head and neck squamous cell carcinoma and its relationship to hypoxia, necrosis, and microvessel density. Cancer Res. 61:5262-7.

[5] Birner P, Jesch B, Friedrich J, Riegler M, Zacherl J, Hejna M, Wrba F, Schultheis A, Schoppmann SF (2011); Carbonic Anhydrase IX Overexpression is Associated with Diminished Prognosis in Esophageal Cancer and Correlates with Her-2 Expression; Ann. Surg. Oncol. 18:3330-7.

[6] Bleumer I, Oosterwijk E, Oosterwijk-Wakka JC, Völler MC, Melchior S, Warnaar SO, Mala C, Beck J, Mulders PF (2006); A clinical trial with chimeric monoclonal antibody WX-G250 and low dose interleukin-2 pulsing scheme for advanced renal cell carcinoma. J. Urol. 175:57-62.

[7] Brennan DJ, Jirstrom K, Kronblad A, Millikan RC, Landberg G, Duffy MJ, Rydén L, Gallagher WM, O'Brien SL (2006); CA IX is an independent prognostic marker in premenopausal breast cancer patients with one to three positive lymph nodes and a putative marker of radiation resistance. Clin. Cancer Res. 12:6421-31.

[8] Carmeliet P, Dor Y, Herbert JM, Fukumura D, Brusselmans K, Dewerchin M, Neeman M, Bono F, Abramovitch R, Maxwell P, Koch CJ, Ratcliffe P, Moons L, Jain RK, Collen D, Keshert E, Keshet E (1998); Role of HIF-1alpha in hypoxia-mediated apoptosis, cell proliferation and tumour angiogenesis. Nature 394:485-490.

[9] Chia SK, Wykoff CC, Watson PH, Han C, Leek RD, Pastorek J, Gatter KC, Ratcliffe P, Harris AL (2001); Prognostic significance of a novel hypoxia-regulated marker, carbonic anhydrase IX, in invasive breast carcinoma. J. Clin. Oncol. 19:3660-8.

[10] Chiche J, Ilc K, Laferrière J, Trottier E, Dayan F, Mazure NM, Brahimi-Horn MC, Pouysségur J (2009); Hypoxia-inducible carbonic anhydrase IX and XII promote tumour cell growth by counteracting acidosis through the regulation of the intracellular pH. Cancer Res. 69:358-68.

[11] Choschzick M, Oosterwijk E, Müller V, Woelber L, Simon R, Moch H, Tennstedt P (2011); Overexpression of carbonic anhydrase IX (CAIX) is an independent unfavorable prognostic marker in endometrioid ovarian cancer. Virchows Arch. 459:193-200.

[12] Dungwa JV, Hunt LP, Ramani P (2012); Carbonic anhydrase IX up-regulation is associated with adverse clinicopathologic and biologic factors in neuroblastomas. Hum Pathol. 43:1651-60.

[13] Flynn JR, Wang L, Gillespie DL, Stoddard GJ, Reid JK, Owens J, Ellsworth GB, Salzman KL, Kinney AY, Jensen RL (2008); Hypoxia-regulated protein expression, patient characteristics, and preoperative imaging as predictors of survival in adults with glioblastoma multiforme. Cancer 113:1032-42.

[14] Gatta G, Capocaccia R, Stiller C, Kaatsch P, Berrino F and Terenziani M; EUROCARE Working Group (2005); Childhood cancer survival trends in Europe: a EUROCARE Working Group study. J Clin Oncol 23:3742-3751.

[15] Generali D, Fox SB, Berruti A, Brizzi MP, Campo L, Bonardi S, Wigfield SM, Bruzzi P, Bersiga A, Allevi G, Milani M, Aguggini S, Dogliotti L, Bottini A, Harris AL (2006); Role of carbonic anhydrase IX expression in prediction of the efficacy and outcome of primary epirubicin/tamoxifen therapy for breast cancer. Endocr. Relat. Cancer 13:921-30.

[16] Giatromanolaki A, Kukourakis MI, Sivridis E, Pastorek J, Wykoff CC, Gatter KC, Harris AL (2001); Expression of hypoxia-inducible carbonic anhydrase-9 relates to angiogenic pathways and independently to poor outcome in non-small cell lung cancer. Cancer Res. 61:7992-8.

[17] Gnarra JR, Tory K, Weng Y, Schmidt L, Wei MH, Li H, Latif F, Liu S, Chen F, Duh FM, et al. (1994); Mutations of the VHL tumour suppressor gene in renal carcinoma. Nat Genet. 7:85-90.

[18] Grabmaier K, Vissers JL, De Weijert MC, Oosterwijk-Wakka JC, Van Bokhoven A, Brakenhoff RH, Noessner E, Mulders PA, Merkx G, Figdor CG, Adema GJ, Oosterwijk E (2000); Molecular cloning and immunogenicity of renal cell carcinoma-associated antigen G250. Int J Cancer. 85:865-70.

[19] Haapasalo J (2011); Carbonic Anhydrases II, IX and XII in Astrocytic Gliomas: Their relationship with clinicopathological features and proliferation. PhD thesis. Acta Universitatis Tamperensis; 1647, Tampere University Press, Tampere.

[20] Haapasalo JA, Nordfors KM, Hilvo M, Rantala IJ, Soini Y, Parkkila AK, Pastoreková S, Pastorek J, Parkkila SM, Haapasalo HK (2006); Expression of carbonic anhydrase IX in astrocytic tumours predicts poor prognosis. Clin Cancer Res. 12:473-7.

[21] Harris AL (2002); Hypoxia–a key regulatory factor in tumour growth. Nature Rev. Cancer. 2: 38–47.

[22] Hilvo M, Baranauskiene L, Salzano AM, Scaloni A, Matulis D, Innocenti A, Scozzafava A, Monti SM, Di Fiore A, De Simone G, Lindfors M, Jänis J, Valjakka J, Pastoreko-

vá S, Pastorek J, Kulomaa MS, Nordlund HR, Supuran CT, Parkkila S. (2008); Biochemical characterization of CA IX: one of the most active carbonic anhydrase isozymes. J. Biol. Chem. 283:27799-809.

[23] Hoskin PJ, Sibtain A, Daley FM and Wilson GD (2003); GLUT1 and CAIX as intrinsic markers of hypoxia in bladder cancer: relationship with vascularity and proliferation as predictors of outcome of ARCON. J Cancer 89:1290-1297.

[24] Hussain SA, Ganesan R, Reynolds G, Gross L, Stevens A, Pastorek J, Murray PG, Perunovic B, Anwar MS, Billingham L, James ND, Spooner D, Poole CJ, Rea DW, Palmer DH (2007); Hypoxia-regulated carbonic anhydrase IX expression is associated with poor survival in patients with invasive breast cancer. Br. J. Cancer 96:104-9.

[25] Hynninen P, Vaskivuo L, Saarnio J, Haapasalo H, Kivelä J, Pastoreková S, Pastorek J, Waheed A, Sly WS, Puistola U, Parkkila S (2006); Expression of transmembrane carbonic anhydrases IX and XII in ovarian tumors. Histopathology 49:594-602.

[26] Ihnatko R, Kubes M, Takacova M, Sedlakova O, Sedlak J, Pastorek J, Kopacek J, Pastoreková S (2006); Extracellular acidosis elevates carbonic anhydrase IX in human glioblastoma cells via transcriptional modulation that does not depend on hypoxia. Int. J. Oncol. 29:1025-33.

[27] Ilie M, Mazure NM, Hofman V, Ammadi RE, Ortholan C, Bonnetaud C, Havet K, Venissac N, Mograbi B, Mouroux J, Pouysségur J, Hofman P (2010); High levels of carbonic anhydrase IX in tumour tissue and plasma are biomarkers of poor prognostic in patients with non-small cell lung cancer. Br J Cancer. 102:1627-35.

[28] Innocenti A, Pastoreková S, Pastorek J, Scozzafava A, De Simone G, Supuran CT (2009); The proteoglycan region of the tumor-associated carbonic anhydrase isoform IX acts as anintrinsic buffer optimizing CO2 hydration at acidic pH values characteristic of solid tumors. Bioorg Med Chem Lett. 19:5825-8.

[29] Ivanov SV, Kuzmin I, Wei M-H, Pack S, Geil L, Johnson BE, Stanbridge EJ, Lerman MI (1998); Down-regulation of transmembrane carbonic anhydrases in renal cell carcinoma cell lines by wild-type von Hippel-Lindau transgenes. Proc Natl Acad Sci USA 95:12596-12601.

[30] Ivanov S, Liao SY, Ivanova A, Danilkovitch-Miagkova A, Tarasova N, Weirich G, Merrill MJ, Proescholdt MA, Oldfield EH, Lee J, Zavada J, Waheed A, Sly W, Lerman MI and Stanbridge EJ (2001); Expression of hypoxia-inducible cell-surface transmembrane carbonic anhydrases in human cancer. Am J Pathol 158:905-919.

[31] Jensen R, Lee J (2012); Predicting outcomes of patients with intracranial meningiomas using molecular markers of hypoxia, vascularity, and proliferation. Neurosurgery. 71:146-56.

[32] Järvelä S, Parkkila S, Bragge H, Kähkönen M, Parkkila AK, Soini Y, Pastorekova S, Pastorek J, Haapasalo H (2008); Carbonic anhydrase IX in oligodendroglial brain tumors. BMC Cancer. 4;8:1.

[33] Karhumaa P, Kaunisto K, Parkkila S, Waheed A, Pastoreková S, Pastorek J, Sly WS, Rajaniemi H (2001); Expression of the transmembrane carbonic anhydrases, CA IX and CA XII, in the human male excurrent ducts. Mol Hum Reprod. 7:611-6.

[34] Kim SJ, Rabbani ZN, Vollmer RT, Schreiber EG, Oosterwijk E, Dewhirst MW, Vujaskovic Z, Kelley MJ (2004); Carbonic anhydrase IX in early-stage non-small cell lung cancer. Clin. Cancer Res. 10:7925-33.

[35] Kivelä AJ, Parkkila S, Saarnio J, Karttunen TJ, Kivelä J, Parkkila A-K, Pastoreková S, Pastorek J, Waheed A, Sly WS, Rajaniemi H (2000); Expression of transmembrane carbonic anhydrase isoenzymes IX and XII in normal human pancreas and pancreatic tumours. Histochem. Cell Biol. 114: 197-204.

[36] Korhonen K, Parkkila AK, Hélen P, Välimäki R, Pastoreková S, Pastorek J, Parkkila S, Haapasalo H (2009); Carbonic anhydrases in meningiomas: association of endothelial carbonic anhydrase II with aggressive tumor features. J Neurosurg. 111:472-7.

[37] Korkolopoulou P, Perdiki M, Thymara I, Boviatsis E, Agrogiannis G, Kotsiakis X, Angelidakis D, Rologis D, Diamantopoulou K, Thomas-Tsagli E, Kaklamanis L, Gatter K, Patsouris E (2007); Expression of hypoxia-related tissue factors in astrocytic gliomas. A multivariate survival study with emphasis upon carbonic anhydrase IX. Hum. Pathol. 38:629-38.

[38] Koukourakis MI, Giatromanolaki A, Sivridis E, Simopoulos K, Pastorek J, Wykoff CC, Gatter KC and Harris AL (2001); Hypoxia-regulated carbonic anhydrase-9 (CA9) relates to poor vascularization and resistance of squamous cell head and neck cancer to chemoradiotherapy. Clin Cancer Res 7:3399-3403.

[39] Lal A, Peters H, St Croix B, Haroon ZA, Dewhirst MW, Strausberg RL, Kaanders JH, van der Kogel AJ, Riggins GJ (2001); Transcriptional response to hypoxia in human tumors. J Natl Cancer Inst. 93:1337-43.

[40] Liao SY, Brewer C, Závada J, Pastorek J, Pastoreková S, Manetta A, Berman ML, DiSaia PJ, Stanbridge EJ (1994); Identification of the MN antigen as a diagnostic biomarker of cervical intraepithelial squamous and glandular neoplasia and cervical carcinomas. Am. J. Pathol. 145:598-609.

[41] Liao SY, Aurelio ON, Jan K, Zavada J, Stanbridge EJ (1997); Identification of the MN/CA9 protein as a reliable diagnostic biomarker of clear cell carcinoma of the kidney. Cancer Res 57:2827-31.

[42] Loncaster JA, Harris AL, Davidson SE, Logue JP, Hunter RD, Wycoff CC, Pastorek J, Ratcliffe PJ, Stratford IJ, West CM (2001); Carbonic anhydrase (CA IX) expression, a potential new intrinsic marker of hypoxia: correlations with tumor oxygen measure-

ments and prognosis in locally advanced carcinoma of the cervix. Cancer Res. 61:6394-9.

[43] Liao SY, Brewer C, Závada J, Pastorek J, Pastoreková S, Manetta A, Berman ML, DiSaia PJ, Stanbridge EJ (1994); Identification of the MN antigen as a diagnostic biomarker of cervical intraepithelial squamous and glandular neoplasia and cervical carcinomas. Am. J. Pathol. 145:598-609.

[44] Liao SY, Aurelio ON, Jan K, Zavada J, Stanbridge EJ (1997); Identification of the MN/CA9 protein as a reliable diagnostic biomarker of clear cell carcinoma of the kidney. Cancer Res 57:2827-31.

[45] Loncaster JA, Harris AL, Davidson SE, Logue JP, Hunter RD, Wycoff CC, Pastorek J, Ratcliffe PJ, Stratford IJ, West CM (2001); Carbonic anhydrase (CA IX) expression, a potential new intrinsic marker of hypoxia: correlations with tumor oxygen measurements and prognosis in locally advanced carcinoma of the cervix. Cancer Res. 61:6394-9.

[46] McIntyre A, Patiar S, Wigfield S, Li JL, Ledaki I, Turley H, Leek R, Snell C, Gatter K, Sly WS, Vaughan-Jones RD, Swietach P, Harris AL. Carbonic Anhydrase IX Promotes Tumor Growth and Necrosis In Vivo and Inhibition Enhances Anti-VEGF Therapy (2012); Clin Cancer Res. 18:3100-11.

[47] McKiernan JM, Buttyan R, Bander NH, Stifelman MD, Katz AE, Chen MW, Olsson CA, Sawczuk IS (1997); Expression of the tumor-associated gene MN: a potential biomarker for human renal cell carcinoma. Cancer Res. 57:2362-5.

[48] Meldrum NU and Roughton FJW (1933); Carbonic anhydrase. Its preparation and properties. J Physiol (London) 80:113-142.

[49] Måseide K, Kandel RA, Bell RS, Catton CN, O'Sullivan B, Wunder JS, Pintilie M, Hedley D, Hill RP (2004); Carbonic anhydrase IX as a marker for poor prognosis in soft tissue sarcoma. Clin. Cancer Res. 10:4464-71.

[50] Nordfors K, Haapasalo J, Korja M, Niemelä A, Laine J, Parkkila AK, Pastorekova S, Pastorek J, Waheed A, Sly WS, Parkkila S, Haapasalo H (2010); The tumour-associated carbonic anhydrases CA II, CA IX and CA XII in a group of medulloblastomas and supratentorial primitive neuroectodermal tumours: an association of CA IX with poor prognosis. BMC Cancer. 18;10:148.

[51] Oosterwijk E, Ruiter DJ, Hoedemaeker PJ, Pauwels EK, Jonas U, Zwartendijk J, Warnaar SO (1986); Monoclonal antibody G 250 recognizes a determinant present in renal-cell carcinoma and absent from normal kidney. Int J Cancer 38:489-94.

[52] Opavský R, Pastoreková S, Zelník V, Gibadulinová A, Stanbridge EJ, Závada J, Kettmann R, Pastorek J (1996); Human MN/CA9 gene, a novel member of the carbonic anhydrase family: structure and exon to protein domain relationships. Genomics. 33:480-7.

[53] Parkkila AK, Herva R, Parkkila S, Rajaniemi H (1995); Immunohistochemical demonstration of human carbonic anhydrase isoenzyme II in brain tumours. Histochem J. 27:974-82.

[54] Parkkila S, Parkkila AK, Saarnio J, Kivelä J, Karttunen TJ, Kaunisto K, Waheed A, Sly WS, Türeci O, Virtanen I, Rajaniemi H (2000a); Expression of the membrane-associated carbonic anhydrase isozyme XII in the human kidney and renal tumors. J Histochem Cytochem. 48:1601-8.

[55] Parkkila S, Rajaniemi H, Parkkila AK, Kivela J, Waheed A, Pastoreková S, Pastorek J, Sly WS (2000b); Carbonic anhydrase inhibitor suppresses invasion of renal cancer cells in vitro. Proc. Natl. Acad. Sci. U S A 97:2220-4.

[56] Pastorek J, Pastoreková S, Callebaut I, Mornon JP, Zelník V, Opavsky R, Zat'ovicová M, Liao S, Portetelle D, Stanbridge EJ, Závada J, Burny A, Kettman R (1994); Cloning and characterization of MN, a human tumor-associated protein with a domain homologous to carbonic anhydrase and a putative helix- loop-helix DNA binding segment. Oncogene 9: 2877–2888.

[57] Pastoreková S, Parkkila S, Parkkila A-K, Opavský R, Zelnik V, Saarnio J, Pastorek J (1997); Carbonic anhydrase IX, MN/CA IX: Analysis of stomach complementary DNA sequence and expression in human and rat alimentary tracts. Gastroenterology 112:398-408.

[58] Pastoreková S, Parkkila S, Pastorek J, Supuran CT (2004); Carbonic anhydrases: current state of the art, therapeutic applications and future prospects. J. Enzyme Inhib. Med. Chem. 19:199-229.

[59] Pastoreková S, Parkkila S, Zavada J (2006); Tumor-associated carbonic anhydrases and their clinical significance. Adv. Clin. Chem. 42:167-216.

[60] Pastoreková S, Ratcliffe PJ, Pastorek J (2008); Molecular mechanisms of carbonic anhydrase IX-mediated pH regulation under hypoxia. BJU Int. 101:8-15.

[61] Pastoreková S, Závadová Z, Kost'ál M, Babusiková O, Závada J (1992); A novel quasi-viral agent, MaTu, is a two-component system. Virology 187:620-626.

[62] Pietilä S, Korpela R, Lenko HL, Haapasalo H, Alalantela R, Nieminen P, Koivisto AM, Mäkipernaa A (2012); Neurological outcome of childhood brain tumor survivors. J Neurooncol. 108:153-61.

[63] Pokhrel A and Hakulinen T (2009); Age-standardisation of relative survival ratios of cancer patients in a comparison between countries, genders and time periods. Eur J Cancer 45:642-647.

[64] Pollack IF, Jakacki RI (2011); Childhood brain tumors: epidemiology, current management and future directions. Nature Rev Neurol 7:495-506.

[65] Preusser M, Wolfsberger S, Haberler C, Breitschopf H, Czech T, Slavc I, Harris AL, Acker T, Budka H, Hainfellner JA. Vascularization and expression of hypoxia-related

tissue factors in intracranial ependymoma and their impact on patient survival (2005); Acta Neuropathol. 109:211-6.

[66] Proescholdt MA, Mayer C, Kubitza M, Schubert T, Liao SY, Stanbridge EJ, Ivanov S, Oldfield EH, Brawanski A, Merrill MJ (2005); Expression of hypoxia-inducible carbonic anhydrases in brain tumors. Neuro Oncol. 7:465-75.

[67] Proescholdt M, Merrill M, Stoerr EM, Lohmeier A, Dietmaier W, Brawanski A. Expression of carbonic anhydrase IX in craniopharyngiomas (2011); J Neurosurg. 115:796-801.

[68] Ramsey ML, Yuh BJ, Johnson MT, Yeldandi AV, Zynger DL. Carbonic anhydrase IX is expressed in mesothelioma and metastatic clear cell renal cell carcinoma of the lung (2012); Virchows Arch;460:89-93.

[69] Reimers TS, Ehrenfels S, Mortensen EL, Schmiegelow M, Sønderkaer S, Carstensen H, Schmiegelow K and Müller J (2003); Cognitive deficits in long-term survivors of childhood brain tumors: Identification of predictive factors. Med Pediatr Oncol 40:26-34.

[70] Robertson N, Potter C, Harris AL (2004); Role of carbonic anhydrase IX in human tumor cell growth, survival, and invasion. Cancer Res. 64:6160-5.

[71] Saarnio J, Parkkila S, Parkkila A-K, Haukipuro K, Pastoreková S, Pastorek J, Kairaluoma MI, Karttunen TJ (1998a); Immunohistochemical study of colorectal tumors for expression of a novel transmembrane carbonic anhydrase, MN/CA IX, with potential value as a marker of cell proliferation. Am. J. Pathol. 153: 279-285.

[72] Saarnio J, Parkkila S, Parkkila A-K, Waheed A, Casey MC, Zhou ZY, Pastoreková S, Pastorek J, Karttunen T, Haukipuro K, Kairaluoma MI, Sly WS (1998b); Immunohistochemistry of carbonic anhydrase isozyme IX (MN/CA IX) in human gut reveals polarized expression in the epithelial cells with the highest proliferative capacity. J. Histochem. Cytochem. 46: 497-504.

[73] Saarnio J, Parkkila S, Parkkila A-K, Pastoreková S, Haukipuro K, Pastorek J, Juvonen T, Karttunen TJ (2001); Transmembrane carbonic anhydrase, MN/CA IX, is a potential biomarker for biliary tumours. J. Hepatol. 35:643-649.

[74] Said HM, Hagemann C, Staab A, Stojic J, Kühnel S, Vince GH, Flentje M, Roosen K, Vordermark D (2007a); Expression patterns of the hypoxia-related genes osteopontin, CA9, erythropoietin, VEGF and HIF-1alpha in human glioma in vitro and in vivo. Radiother Oncol. 83:398-405.

[75] Said HM, Staab A, Hagemann C, Vince GH, Katzer A, Flentje M, Vordermark D (2007b); Distinct patterns of hypoxic expression of carbonic anhydrase IX (CA IX) in human malignant glioma cell lines. J. Neurooncol 81:27-38.

[76] Said HM, Polat B, Staab A, Hagemann C, Stein S, Flentje M, Theobald M, Katzer A, Vordermark D (2008); Rapid detection of the hypoxia-regulated CA-IX and NDRG1 gene expression in different glioblastoma cells in vitro. Oncol Rep. 20:413-9.

[77] Sandlund J, Oosterwijk E, Grankvist K, Oosterwijk-Wakka J, Ljungberg B, Rasmuson T (2007); Prognostic impact of carbonic anhydrase IX expression in human renal cell carcinoma. BJU Int. 100:556-60.

[78] Sathornsumetee S, Cao Y, Marcello JE, Herndon JE 2nd, McLendon RE, Desjardins A, Friedman HS, Dewhirst MW, Vredenburgh JJ, Rich JN (2008); Tumor angiogenic and hypoxic profiles predict radiographic response and survival in malignant astrocytoma patients treated with bevacizumab and irinotecan. J. Clin. Oncol. 26:271-8.

[79] Sly WS, Hu PY (1995); Human carbonic anhydrases and carbonic anhydrase deficiencies. Annu. Rev. Biochem. 64:375-401.

[80] Statistics Finland (2011); Statistical databases for cause of death in years 2003-2009.

[81] Stupp R, Hegi ME, Mason WP, van den Bent MJ, Taphoorn MJ, Janzer RC, Ludwin SK, Allgeier A, Fisher B, Belanger K, Hau P, Brandes AA, Gijtenbeek J, Marosi C, Vecht CJ, Mokhtari K, Wesseling P, Villa S, Eisenhauer E, Gorlia T, Weller M, Lacombe D, Cairncross JG, Mirimanoff RO; European Organisation for Research and Treatment of Cancer Brain Tumour and Radiation Oncology Groups; National Cancer Institute of Canada Clinical Trials Group (2009); Effects of radiotherapy with concomitant and adjuvant temozolomide versus radiotherapy alone on survival in glioblastoma in a randomised phase III study: 5-year analysis of the EORTC-NCIC trial. Lancet Oncol. 10:459-66.

[82] Svastová E, Zilka N, Zat'ovicová M, Gibadulinová A, Ciampor F, Pastorek J, Pastoreková S (2003); Carbonic anhydrase IX reduces E-cadherin-mediated adhesion of MDCK cells via interaction with beta-catenin. Exp. Cell. Res. 290:332-45.

[83] Swietach P, Wigfield S, Supuran CT, Harris AL, Vaughan-Jones RD (2008); Cancer-associated, hypoxia-inducible carbonic anhydrase IX facilitates CO2 diffusion. BJU Int. 101:22-4.

[84] Swinson DE, Jones JL, Richardson D, Wykoff C, Turley H, Pastorek J, Taub N, Harris AL, O'Byrne KJ (2003); Carbonic anhydrase IX expression, a novel surrogate marker of tumor hypoxia, is associated with a poor prognosis in non-small-cell lung cancer. J Clin Oncol. 21:473-82.

[85] Turner JR, Odze RD, Crum CP, Resnick MB (1997); MN antigen expression in normal, preneoplastic, and neoplastic esophagus: a clinicopathological study of a new cancer-associated biomarker. Hum. Pathol. 28: 740-744.

[86] Vermylen P, Roufosse C, Burny A, Verhest A, Bosschaerts T, Pastoreková S, Ninane V, Sculier JP (1999); Carbonic anhydrase IX antigen differentiates between preneoplastic malignant lesions in non-small lung carcinoma. Eur Respir J. 14:806-11.

[87] Wykoff CC, Beasley NJ, Watson PH, Turner KJ, Pastorek J, Sibtain A, Wilson GD, Turley H, Talks KL, Maxwell PH, Pugh CW, Ratcliffe PJ, Harris AL (2000); Hypoxia-inducible expression of tumor-associated carbonic anhydrases. Cancer Res. 60:7075-83.

[88] Yoo H, Baia GS, Smith JS, McDermott MW, Bollen AW, Vandenberg SR, Lamborn KR, Lal A.Expression of the hypoxia marker carbonic anhydrase 9 is associated with anaplastic phenotypes in meningiomas (2007); Clin Cancer Res. 13:68-75.

[89] Yoo H, Sohn S, Nam BH, Min HS, Jung E, Shin SH, Gwak HS, Lee SH (2010); The expressions of carbonic anhydrase 9 and vascular endothelial growth factor in astrocytic tumors predict a poor prognosis. Int J Mol Med. 26:3-9.

[90] Závada J, Závadová Z, Pastoreková S, Ciampor F, Pastorek J, Zelník V (1993); Expression of MaTu-MN protein in human tumor cultures and in clinical specimens. Int J Cancer. 54:268-74.

Chapter 20

New Molecular Targets and Treatments for Pediatric Brain Tumors

Claudia C. Faria, Christian A. Smith and James T. Rutka

Additional information is available at the end of the chapter

http://dx.doi.org/10.5772/53300

1. Introduction

The outstanding progress in advanced molecular technologies has provided a tremendous amount of data that has altered the way in which we classify and categorize pediatric brain tumors. From the initial identification of chromosomal aberrations by karyotyping and comparative genomic hybridization, we have rapidly moved to expression array studies and to integrative genomic approaches which allowed the stratification of several pediatric brain tumors into molecular subgroups. These data have not only increased our understanding of the molecular pathogenesis of pediatric brain tumors, but have also identified prognostic markers and opened new avenues for targeted therapies.

One of the most important discoveries in pediatric astrocytomas was the duplication and the mutation of the v-raf murine sarcoma viral oncogene homolog B1 *(BRAF)* gene, found in pilocytic astrocytomas and malignant astrocytomas, respectively. Clinical trials using BRAF signaling pathway inhibitors are currently ongoing.

Until recently, the biology of diffuse intrinsic pontine glioma (DIPG) was poorly understood. Overexpression of epidermal growth factor receptor (*EGFR*) and platelet-derived growth factor receptor alpha (*PDGFRα*) amplification have now been reported in multiple studies in DIPG and clinical trials with the respective inhibitors (nimotuzumab for *EGFR* and dasatinib for PDGFRα), alone or in combination with other drugs, are in progress.

Integrated genomics has shown that medulloblastoma, the most common malignant pediatric brain tumor, comprises four distinct molecular and clinical variants. The stratification of patients into the Wnt subgroup, the sonic hedgehog (SHH) subgroup, Group 3 and Group 4 may lead to the identification of those patients that will most likely benefit from targeted therapies, like SMO inhibitors. Moreover, this molecular classification may help identify patients predicted to have a poor prognosis, who may benefit from intensified therapies, and patients with a favorable prognosis that potentially benefit from reduced radiation and chemotherapy regimens. It is already known from four independent studies that the Wnt subgroup patients have a very good prognosis while patients in Group 3 have a high incidence of metastasis and a dismal prognosis.

The transcriptional profiling of two large independent cohorts of posterior fossa ependymomas also identified two groups with distinct molecular and clinical features. Group A ependymomas have a balanced genome, occur in younger patients and tumors are located laterally. These patients have a worse clinical outcome and higher incidence of metastasis and recurrence. In contrast, Group B ependymomas occur in the midline and have a better prognosis. Since ependymomas are usually refractory to current chemotherapeutic agents, these discoveries may shed some light into the pathways involved in tumor initiation and progression and also identify new targets for therapy.

We are now facing the next-generation (Next-Gen) sequencing era which will provide further insights into the dysregulated signaling pathways in each tumor type. The identification of driver mutations will allow a better understanding of tumorigenesis and lead to the development of more accurate preclinical models. Moreover, the profiling of transcriptomes, genetic and epigenetic events of large cohorts of tumors will eventually shed some light into the cells of origin of specific subgroups and also the important driver events for tumor initiation, maintenance and progression. On the clinical side, this knowledge will allow the stratification of patients into appropriate risk groups and the tailoring of treatments according to each tumor's genomic landscape. In this chapter we describe the latest advances in molecular genomics of the most common pediatric brain tumors as well as its prognostic significance and relevance to the clinic. We also highlight the most recent clinical trials using molecular targeted therapies and discuss further possible avenues in the treatment of pediatric brain cancer.

2. Astrocytomas

Astrocytomas are a common brain tumor in children. According to the 2007 classification of the World Health Organization (WHO) they can be classified into four grades (WHO grade I-IV), which reflect their biological and clinical behavior. Pilocytic astrocytomas (WHO grade I) represent the most frequent brain tumor in the pediatric population and have excellent survival rates over 95% [1]. On the other hand, glioblastomas (WHO grade IV) are aggressive tumors, often non-responsive to treatments and with survival rates ranging from 10% to 30% [1]. We will focus on the molecular biology of these two types of pediatric astrocytomas.

2.1. Pilocytic astrocytoma

The first-line treatment for pilocytic astrocytoma (PA) is surgical resection. Although most children with these tumors survive for a long time, some will experience tumor recurrence, especially if the tumor resection is incomplete. Recurrent and progressive tumors are treated with radiation and/or chemotherapy but, until recently, the mechanisms of recurrence and malignant transformation were poorly understood.

Early studies on chromosomal aberrations in PAs showed normal karyotypes in most cases. Trisomy of chromosomes 5 and 7 and 7q gains were some of the few cytogenetic abnormalities found [2]. Using an array-based comparative genomic hybridization (array-CGH), Pfister *et al.* studied a large series of pediatric low-grade astrocytomas and uncovered mechanisms of mitogen-activated protein kinase (MAPK) activation in these tumors. The authors identified a tandem duplication of the *BRAF* gene locus (7q34) in more than 50% of the PAs and, in a smaller percentage (~6%) of tumors, a *BRAF* activating mutation V600E (a valine to glutamate change at hotspot codon 600) [3]. Later, it was demonstrated that the constitutive activation of BRAF was due to a fusion between a novel gene *(KIAA1549)* and the *BRAF* oncogene and also that this fusion was related to a better clinical outcome in incompletely resected low-grade astrocytomas [4]. Other, less frequent, reported gene fusions in PAs include the fusion of *BRAF* with the *FAM131B* gene and the fusion between a Raf kinase family member (*RAF1*) and SLIT-ROBO Rho GTPase-activating protein 3 *(SRGAP3)* gene [5]. The combined analysis of *BRAF* and isocitrate dehydrogenase 1 (*IDH1)* was shown to be both sensitive and specific to separate PAs from diffuse astrocytomas (WHO grade II). PAs contained the *KIAA1549:BRAF* fusion in 70% of cases but no *IDH2* or *IDH2* mutations while diffuse astrocytomas exhibited 76% of cases with *IDH1* mutations but no *BRAF* fusion [6]. There is also an interesting correlation between tumor location and the type of MAPK alteration. Posterior fossa tumors usually have increased incidence of *KIAA1549:BRAF* fusion while supratentorial tumors have high frequency of $BRAF^{V600E}$ mutation. Approximately 80-90% of PA cases reported in the literature have at least one alteration in the MAPK pathway. Interestingly, all the alterations described in the MAPK pathway seem to be mutually exclusive suggesting that a single hit may be sufficient to induce transformation [5].

With the discovery of constitutive activation of MAPK pathway and BRAF alterations in most PAs, there has been an increasing interest in using these targets for novel therapeutic approaches. A number of phase I and phase II clinical trials are ongoing to test small molecule inhibitors of MAPK and related pathways (Table 1).

Drug		Clinical Trial	Reference (http://clinicaltrials.gov)
Group	**Name**		
MEK inhibitor	AZD6244	Phase I	NCT01386450, NCT01089101
RAF inhibitor (multikinase inhibitor)	Sorafenib	Phase II	NCT01338857 (suspended)
mTOR inhibitor	Everolimus	Phase II	NCT01158651, NCT00782626

Table 1. Pediatric clinical trials for pilocytic astrocytomas using targeted therapies

2.2. Glioblastoma multiforme

Glioblastoma multiforme (GBM) is the most common brain tumor in adults and is less frequent in the pediatric population. Despite improvements in neurosurgery and neuro-oncology, children diagnosed with GBM still have a dismal outcome with low survival rates even with aggressive therapeutic regimens. Although the histology of pediatric and adult GBMs appears identical, the molecular biology of these tumors is different. Therefore, the development of effective therapies for GBM in children should probably not rely on advances made in adult tumors.

Mutations in phosphatase and tensin homolog (*PTEN*) and amplifications of *EGFR* are common in adult malignant gliomas but less frequent in the pediatric setting. However, when compared to pediatric low-grade gliomas, pediatric GBMs have a significant higher expression of *EGFR*, although with no reported mutations and few deletions (~17%) in *EGFRvIII* [7]. While in adult GBMs the activation of the AKT pathway is a result of *PTEN* mutations, in pediatric tumors these are infrequent, although overexpression of AKT and its association with poor survival has been reported [8,9]. In a study with a large cohort of pediatric high-grade gliomas (HGGs) (37 GBMs out of 63 tumor samples), Bax *et al.* identified *PDGFRα* amplification and cyclin-dependent kinase inhibitor 2A/B (*CDKN2A/B)* deletion as the most frequent focal events. Interestingly, the patients with high-grade tumors and a stable genomic profile had a better survival, independent of the histological grade or type [10]. Several studies showed that *IDH1* mutations, common in adult secondary GBM (98%), are rare in pediatric GBM [7]. *TP53 (*tumor protein 53*)* mutations were reported in pediatric high-grade tumors with an increased frequency in older children (40%) when compared to those less than 3 years (12%) [11]. Overexpression of p53, but not *TP53* mutations, was also associated with a significant reduction in the 5 year progression-free survival [12]. A recent study used high resolution single nucleotide polymorphism (SNP) arrays to identify novel chromosomal alterations in pediatric GBM, including amplifications of 7q21-22 and 1q43-44 and loss of heterozygosity (LOH) in15q15.1-15q23 and 17p13-17p11.2. Genes involved in cell-cycle regulation and cell death pathways were the predominant targets of LOHs [13].

It has been shown that overexpression of O^6-methylguanine-DNA methyltransferase (MGMT) is rare in HGGs but it has also been reported that it is associated with a poor overall survival in children. The *MGMT* gene encodes a DNA-repair enzyme that can reduce the efficacy of alkylating agents. When the *MGMT* gene is silenced by promoter methylation, DNA repair in tumor tissue is compromised and patients have a better survival [7].

Finaly, a very recent study uncovered an interesting interplay between genetic and epigenetic events in pediatric GBM. The authors performed whole-exome sequencing in 48 pediatric GBMs and identified 44% of tumors harbouring somatic mutations in genes involved in the chromatin remodeling pathway, including the histone H3 gene (*H3F3A*), the α-thalassaemia/mental retardation syndrome X-linked *(ATRX*) gene and the death-domain associated protein (*DAXX*) gene [14]. Interestingly, the *H3F3A* mutations were found to be specific of GBMs and more prevalent in the pediatric population. Moreover, 54% of all cases and 86% of patients with *H3F3A* and/or *ATRX* mutations, also showed *TP53* somatic mutations [14].

The novel targeted therapies that are currently under clinical investigation for high-grade gliomas, including GBM, are reviewed in reference [15].

3. Diffuse intrinsic pontine glioma

Despite decades of clinical research, the prognosis of diffuse intrinsic pontine glioma (DIPG) remains dismal with more than 90% of affected children dying within two years of diagnosis [16]. The only known effective treatment is radiation therapy although in most patients it has a transient effect. Different combinations of chemotherapy, radiation and radiosensitizers were attempted but failed to improve long-term survival [17]. The indication for biopsy in DIPG has been reserved for atypical tumors (prominent enhancement in magnetic ressonance imaging (MRI), low T2/FLAIR signal and/or high signal on diffuse imaging). However, the recognition that it is crucial to understand the biology of DIPG in order to design more rational drug treatments, led to a plea for routine biopsies in these patients. Some groups are already performing regular image-guided stereotactic biopsies in patients with DIPGs [18,19] and, furthermore, biopsies have been included in a clinical trial to decide which patients with DIPG would benefit from targeted therapy with erlotinib, an *EGFR* inhibitor [20]. Autopsies became another important source of DIPG tissue collection. Recent studies showed that up to 50% of parents agree with the autopsy and, if done within a short period of time after death, it is possible to obtain good quality DNA and RNA and even culture primary DIPG cell lines [21-23].

The paradigm shift to obtain tissue from patients with DIPG not only increased our knowledge in the molecular biology of the disease but also raised important clinical considerations. Paugh *et al.* described differences at the copy number and expression level in both adult and pediatric HGGs, including DIPGs. They showed that gain of chromosome 1q and *PDGFRα* amplification were frequent in children while chromosome 7 gain, 10q loss and *EGFR* amplification were characteristic of adult HGGs [24]. The identification of these two distinct biological entities has important clinical implications since pediatric clinical trials over the past decades have been designed with drugs known to have some activity in adult HGGs. It is now clear that DIPG has to be considered and treated as a separate disease. The same group compared the copy number alterations (CNAs) in DIPGs and nonbrainstem pediatric glioblastomas concluding that they are also genomically distinct. They identified receptor tyrosine kinase and retinoblastoma protein (*RB*) amplifications in 47% and 30% of DIPG cases, respectively, and found high frequency of focal amplifications of *PDGFRα, MET* and insuline-like growth factor receptor 1 *(IGF1R)* [25]. Furthermore, Zarghooni *et al.*, using SNP arrays, showed that DIPGs have distinct CNAs from pediatric supratentorial high-grade astrocytomas, with gains in *PDGFRα* and poly (ADP-ribose) polymerase-1 *(PARP-1)* amongst the most frequent [26]. Another group showed other differences between these tumors including frequent losses of 17p and 14q in DIPGs [27]. A very recent study used DNA from tumor tissue obtained at diagnosis by steriotactic biopsies and identified oncogenic mutations in *TP53* (40%), *PI3KCA* (15%) and *ATM/MPL* (5%). In fact, *PI3KCA* represents the first mutated oncogene described in DIPG [28].

Another level of gene expression regulation in DIPG occurs through epigenetic mechanisms, including histone modifications. Very recent sudies used whole-genome sequencing in large cohorts of DIPGs to identify somatic mutations in the *H3F3A* gene. Khuong-Quang *et al.* reported mutations in H3.3 that resulted in the substitution of lysine by methionine at amino acid 27 (K27M-H3.3) in 71% of cases and the presence of these mutations were associated with a worse survival independent of patient age and histological grade [29]. Furthermore, gains or amplifications in *PDGFRα* and *MYC/PVT1* were exclusively seen in K27M-H3.3 mutants. The authors also described *TP53* mutations in 77% and *ATRX* mutations in 9% of DIPGs [29]. Interestingly, both the mutated and wild-type H3.3 subgroups showed high frequency of *TP53* mutation. In another study, Wu *et al.* identified mutations in *H3F3A* (encodes histone H3.3) and *HIST1H3B* (encodes histone H3.1) in 78% of DIPGs and 22% of nonbrainstem pediatric glioblastomas [30]. The different H3 mutations were mutually exclusive and seemed to be a feature of pediatric HGGs.

The discoveries from the molecular biology of DIPGs identified several drugable targets allowing the development of molecular target-based trials that are summarized in Table 2. Some of these trials have shown a subset of patients with survival longer than expected and, therefore, several other trials are ongoing, some of them including combined therapies [17,31].

Finally, DIPG treatment involves another challenge which is drug distribution. Probably due to an intact blood-brain barrier, penetration of drugs in the pons seems to be poor, a fact demonstrated by the lack of gadolinium enhancement in the MRI in most DIPGs. Therefore, it is crucial to improve drug delivery either by disrupting the blood-brain barrier (e.g. focused ultrasound or drugs that increase permeability such as manitol), by local delivery (tumor injection or convection enhanced delivery) or even nanoparticles [17]. These techniques may promote high drug concentrations in the pons, including agents that normally don't cross the blood-brain barrier.

Drug	Clinical Trial	1 year Overall Survival (OS)	Reference
Imatinib	Phase I	45.5%	2007 [32]
Tipifarnib	Phase I	36.4%	2008 [33]
Gefitinib	Phase I	48%	2010 [34]
Vandetanib	Phase I	37%	2010 [35]
Erlotinib	Phase I	50%	2011 [20]
Gefitinib	Phase II	56%	2011 [36]
Nimotuzumab	Phase II	Median OS 9.6 months	2011 [37]

Table 2. Clinical trials for diffuse intrinsic pontine glioma (DIPG) using targeted therapies

4. Medulloblastoma

Medulloblastoma, the commonest malignant brain tumor in the pediatric population, is no longer considered a single disease. Recent efforts of multiple independent groups have reached to a consensus that medulloblastoma comprises four distinct molecular variants named WNT, SHH, Group 3 and Group 4 [38]. The subgroups have different demographics, genetic profiles and prognosis [39]. This may explain why patients with the same histological disease have different clinical outcomes and a variable response to current treatments including surgery, whole-brain radiation and intensive chemotherapy. Figure 1 summarizes the main features of the four medulloblastoma subgroups.

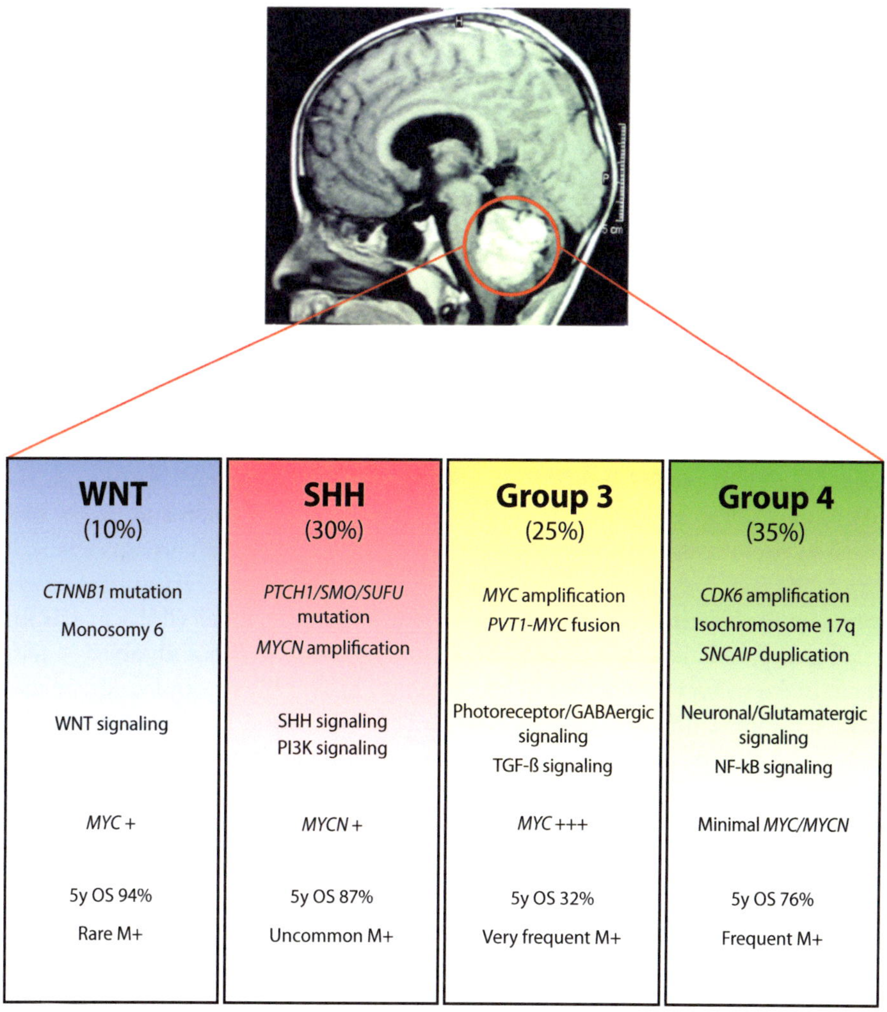

Figure 1. Features of the four medulloblastoma subgroups, including molecular genetics and clinical outcome

4.1. WNT medulloblastomas

WNT medulloblastomas are frequent in older children and teenagers and are rarely seen in infants. Patients within this subgroup have usually an excellent outcome with survival rates over 90%. However, Remke *et al.* showed that this is only true for pediatric cases as adult WNT patients exhibit survival rates of approximately 80% [40]. Histologically, WNT tumors are almost always of the classic variant and they rarely disseminate.

This subgroup is enriched in genes of the WNT pathway. Although few gains and losses were reported in the WNT genome, mutations in *CTNNB1* are frequent and usually occur with deletion of one copy of chromosome 6 (monosomy 6). Patients with *CTNNB1* mutation have accumulation of β-catenin in the nucleus and better survival rates. Positive nuclear immunostaining for β-catenin is now currently accepted as a marker of WNT medulloblastomas [41,42], although DKK1 and DKK2 were also proposed as markers for this subgroup [42,43]. The overall good outcome of WNT tumors suggests that this subgroup may be a good candidate for de-escalation therapy in future clinical trials.

4.2. SHH medulloblastomas

SHH medulloblastomas are frequently found in infants and adults (approximately 60% of cases in each age group) but are rare in childhood. In the SHH subgroup, prognostic factors such as M-stage and desmoplasia are age-dependent. Metastasis at presentation represents a negative prognostic factor only in adults while desmoplasia is associated with worse outcome only in pediatric cases [44]. From a histological point of view this subgroup is unique since it includes tumors of the four main variants (classic, nodular desmoplastic, large-cell anaplastic and medulloblastoma with extensive nodularity).

SHH medulloblastomas are characterized by aberrant expression of SHH pathway genes including *SMO, PTCH1, SUFU* and *GLI2*. Amplifications of *MYCN* and *YAP1* are also seen in this subgroup. Additionally, deletion of chromosome 9q is a common and highly restricted event in SHH tumors, most likely secondary to *PTCH1* mutation on chromosome 9q22 [45]. Of notice is the fact that the transcriptomes of pediatric and adult SHH tumors have different expression profiles with increased levels of genes related to extracellular matrix function in the first group and elevated levels of *HOX* family genes and genes involved in tissue development in the second group [44,46]. In an attempt to simplify the molecular subgrouping of medulloblastomas, different laboratories used formalin-fixed paraffin-embedded tissues (FFPE) to test a variety of markers for SHH medulloblastomas including SFRP1, GLI1 and GAB1 [42,43,47].

The clinical and molecular distinction of infant and adult SHH medulloblastomas suggests a disparate underlying biology and raises the question of possible different responses to current targeted therapies.

4.3. Group 3 medulloblastomas

Group 3 medulloblastomas are restricted to pediatric patients. Indeed, two recent studies concluded that Group 3 tumors are extremely rare in adults [40,48]. Another feature of this subgroup is its aggressive behavior with high incidence of metastasis, frequent large-cell anaplastic histology and an invariable dismal prognosis (approximately 20 to 30% overall survival). It has been shown that Group 3 medulloblastomas consist of two distinct subtypes one of which harbors frequent amplifications of the *MYC* gene and has the worse outcome [49]. Although Group 3 and 4 have some common genetic features, including gain of chromosome 7, losses of chromosomes 5q and 10q and gain of chromosome 1q are more frequent in Group 3 tumors. NPR3 and KCNA1 were proposed as biomarkers for Group 3 and Group 4, respectively [42].

Until recently, there were no known targetable pathways in Group 3 medulloblastomas and the suggested intensification of treatment for these patients would necessarily result in increased toxicity and morbidity (see below).

4.4. Group 4 medulloblastomas

Group 4 tumors represent simultaneously the most common and the less well-understood subgroup of medulloblastomas. They are found across all age groups and have an intermediate prognosis although the adult patients show a reduced survival when compared to their pediatric counterparts. Group 4 medulloblastomas are usually of the classic variant and they rarely present with metastasis. The most frequent genetic aberration in Group 4 tumors, present in up to 80% of cases, is isochromosome 17q (i17q) although *MYCN* amplifications were also reported. The expression of follistatin-related protein 5 (*FSTL5)* was identified as a marker of high-risk Group 4 patients [50].

4.5. From genomic revolution to clinical trials in medulloblastoma

Despite important advances in medulloblastoma treatment, approximately 40% of children will have recurrence and 30% will die from the disease. Moreover, the survivors are often left with significant disabilities due to cytotoxic side effects of chemotherapy and radiation to the developing central nervous system (CNS). Identifying the genetic events that drive medulloblastoma is, therefore, critical to develop more effective and less toxic therapies.

Except for SHH inhibitors that have shown some promise in SHH patients [51], there were no other targetable genes or pathways for WNT, Group 3 and Group 4 medulloblastomas. However, very recently published studies from four independent groups dissected the genomic landscape of medulloblastoma using large cohorts of patients and the latest high-throughput technology.

Using SNP arrays in a large cohort of over 1,000 medulloblastoma samples, Northcott *et al.* reported that somatic CNAs are a common event in medulloblastoma and are subgroup-specific [52]. In Group 3 tumors the authors identified recurrent *PVT1* gene fusions with *MYC* and *NDRG1* through chromothripsis, a process of erroneous DNA repair after chromosome shattering. This process of catastrophic DNA rearrangement has been previously shown in SHH medulloblastomas with *TP53* mutations [53]. The most frequent somatic CNA was a duplication of *SNCAIP*, a gene on chromosome 5q23.2 involved in Parkinson's disease. Interestingly, *SNCAIP* duplication is restricted to Group 4α, a subtype of Group 4 with a relatively balanced genome when compared to Group 4β [52]. The authors also reported novel targetable pathways that could be the basis for future clinical trials, including PI3K pathway in SHH, TGF-β pathway in Group 3 and NF-κB pathway in Group 4 [52].

Another interesting observation, consistent with the first published study using genome sequencing in medulloblastoma [54], is the low number of somatic mutations found in these tumors when compared to adult solid tumors and the increased mutation frequency with age [52,55-57]. Jones *et al.* also identified tetraploidy as an early event in Group 3 and Group 4 medulloblastomas, concomitant with *TP53* mutations in some tumors [55].

The genome sequencing of independent cohorts of medulloblastoma samples and matched blood, identified previously known mutated genes (*CTNNB1, PTCH1, MLL2, SMARCA4, TP53*) but also allowed the discovery of new recurrent somatic mutations (*DDX3X, CTDNEP1, KDM6A, TBR1, GPS2, BCOR, LDB1, EZH2, CHD7, ZMYM3*), often subgroup-specific [52,55-57]. Notably, these studies identified genes involved in histone modification and chromatin remodeling complexes across all subgroups, which may explain the complexity and heterogeneity seen in medulloblastoma.

The ongoing genomic revolution in medulloblastoma is moving the next generation of clinical trials towards targeted treatments according to the molecular subgroup. SHH inhibitors, including GDC-0449 and NVP-LDE225, already proved its efficacy in tumor growth reduction but the reported acquired resistance suggests that a combination of targeted therapies may be a key approach to improve response [58]. Phase II clinical trials using GDC-0449 are now recruiting pediatric and adult patients with recurrent or refractory medulloblastoma and phase I trials with NVP-LDE225 are recruiting patients with advanced solid tumors including medulloblastoma. Under debate is the de-escalation of therapy in WNT patients and the intensification of treatment and/or targeted therapy for Group 3 patients [59,60]. Finaly, the discovery of a significant number of chromatin modifier genes across medulloblastoma subgroups suggests that histone deacetylase inhibitors may constitute a good therapeutic option in the future.

5. Ependymoma

Ependymoma, the third most common brain tumor in childhood, is still incurable in up to 45% of patients [61]. The gold standard of treatment is maximal safe surgical resection followed by radiation since chemotherapy is usually ineffective. Ependymomas can arise in different regions of the CNS including the cerebral hemispheres, the posterior fossa and the spinal cord. This diversity is extended to its demographic, genetic, clinical and prognostic characteristics. Both children and adults can be affected although posterior fossa tumors are more common in children and supratentorial and spinal tumors occur more frequently in adults. The clinical behavior of ependymoma is variable with some patients experiencing a fatal clinical course while others have a long recurrence-free survival. The lack of novel targeted treatments for ependymoma can be explained by the paucity of cell lines and animal models of the disease.

The genetic heterogeneity of ependymoma has been highlighted by different studies with some cohorts of tumors showing frequent chromosomal alterations and others displaying a balanced genome. Korshunov *et al.* identified gain of chromosome 1q, *CDKN2A* homozygous deletion and age at diagnosis as independent factors of worse prognosis in ependymoma [62]. Johnson *et al.* described subgroups of ependymoma clustered by their CNAs, messenger RNA (mRNA) and microRNA (miRNA) profiles and, interestingly, tumors were segregated by their CNS location [63]. Furthermore, the authors were able to generate a mouse model of supratentorial ependymoma presenting strong evidence that the radial glial cells are likely the cells of origin of this tumor [63]. More recently, Witt *et al.* transcriptionaly profiled two large independent cohorts of posterior fossa tumors identifying two distinct subgroups, Group A and Group B ependymomas [64]. Group A tumors comprise only posterior fossa ependymomas while Group B tumors include posterior fossa tumors that clustered with spinal ependymomas. Patients with Group A ependymomas are younger (median age 2.5 years), with the majority of tumors located laterally and with a balanced genome. These patients have higher incidence of recurrence and metastasis and a worse prognosis (5 year overall survival of 69%). Patients with Group B ependymomas are older (median age 20 years), with tumors in the midline (95%) and a high degree of genomic instability (Figure 2). Although several cytogenetic abnormalities were found in this group, including loss of chromosomes 1, 2, 3, 6, 8, 10, 14q, 17q, 22q, and gain of chromosomes 4, 5q, 7, 9, 11, 12, 15q, 18, 20, and 21q, patients have a good prognosis (5 year overall survival of 95%). The genes that characterize Group B ependymomas are involved in microtubule assembly and oxidative metabolism while Group A tumors include several pathways associated with cancer. The authors identified *LAMA2* and *NELL2* as markers of Group A and Group B ependymomas, respectively [64]. Using unsupervised cluster analysis of gene expression signatures, others also described two groups of infratentorial ependymomas (Group 1 and Group 2) that overlap with Group A and Group B of Witt *et al.*, respectively [65]. The distinct genetic profiles of posterior fossa ependymomas suggest that novel targeted therapies against subgroup-specific pathways maybe the key strategy to improve survival, particularly in Group A patients.

The interesting observation that up to 50% of pediatric ependymomas have a balanced genome [62] raises the possibility that epigenetic mechanisms may play a role in ependymoma pathogenesis. Most studies have focused on promoter hypermethylation of candidate genes known to be tumor suppressor genes in ependymoma or frequently methylated in other cancers. *HIC-1* and *RASSF1A* promoter hypermethylation were described in 83% and 86% of ependymomas, respectively. They are known to be tumor suppressor genes, silenced by hypermethylation in many human cancers [66]. Promoter hypermethylation of other genes, including *CDKN2A* (21%), *CDKN2B* (32%), *p14ARF* (21%), and *MGMT* (27%) were also reported in studies with large cohorts of tumor samples [66]. More recently, Rogers *et al.* used an array-based analysis to determine the methylation profile of 98 ependymomas [67]. The authors found that supratentorial and spinal ependymomas have a hypermethylated phenotype and that the genes identified are involved in cell growth and apoptosis. The increase in promoter methylation of CpG islands across a large number of genes has been described in other cancers as CpG island methylator phenotype (CIMP). Although it has been correlated to a worse outcome in other cancers, the authors could not find an association between methylation and prognosis in ependymomas [67].

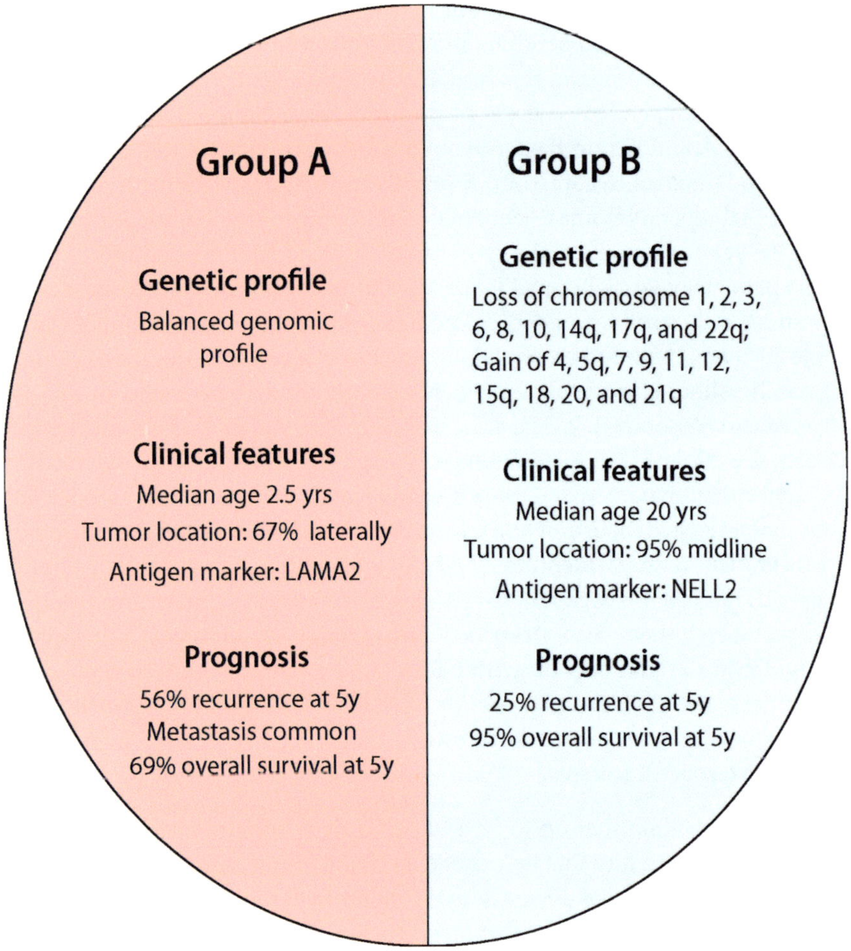

Figure 2. Features of the posterior fossa ependymoma subgroups, including genetic profile, clinical features and prognosis.

Another less frequent epigenetic event in cancer genomes is hypomethylation. This loss of DNA methylation occurs mainly in repetitive elements (Alu repeats). In a recent study, Xie *et al.* used a genome-wide approach to study the methylation profiles of Alu repeat sequences in pediatric intracranial ependymomas [68]. Notably, they identified a global loss of methylation in the regions flanking, rather than within, Alu sequences, and this was corre-

http://dx.doi.org/10.5772/53300

lated with a more agressive tumor phenotype. The biological significance of this finding is yet to be unraveled.

The increased knowledge of the genetic and epigenetic events that drive ependymoma may lead to more effective targeted therapies aimed to repair molecular functions and dysregulated pathways. However, there are currently no clinical trials evaluating specific molecular therapies in ependymoma. Despite the recent achievements in ependymoma research, greater progress is needed to decifer the molecular and biological mechanisms of this disease and, ultimately, to improve patient's clinical outcome.

6. Conclusion

Major steps have been made to a better understanding of the molecular genetics underlying the most common pediatric brain tumors. An important advance was to recognize that adult and pediatric brain tumors are distinct and, therefore, need different therapeutic approaches. This knowledge opened new avenues for targeted therapies and clinical trials based on tumor-specific molecular subgrouping are currently ongoing. When compared to standard chemotherapy and radiation, the use of biological agents has several advantages. They can target cancer cells and spare normal cells in the developing CNS of children and also be used to delay radiotherapy, which is responsible for long-term side effects of treatment. Many of the newer agents are small molecules, with low molecular weight, which facilitates blood-brain barrier penetration. However, despite the enthusiasm with the phase I and phase II clinical trials using biological agents as monotherapy, mainly for progressive and recurrent brain tumors, efficacy has not yet been proven. In the future, combination therapies will likely be needed to target multiple pathways involved in tumorigenesis and to overcome the cytostatic effect of several biological agents. As the amount of data generated by high-throughput studies increases the drugable targets for each pediatric brain tumor, the number of clinical trials will continue to expand aiming a better control of the disease with less morbidity and extended survival.

Acknowledgments

Claudia Faria was supported by a fellowship from The Hospital for Sick Children Research Training Centre and the Garron Family Cancer Centre. She is a PhD candidate from The Programme for Advanced Medical Education, supported by Fundação Gulbenkian, Fundação Champalimaud, Ministério da Saúde e Fundação para a Ciência e Tecnologia, Portugal. This work was also supported by grants from the Canadian Cancer Society Research Institute (grant no. 019073), the Wiley fund, the Laurie Berman Fund for Brain Tumour Research, Pediatric Brain Tumour Foundation of the United States, and B.r.a.i.n.child.

Author details

Claudia C. Faria[1], Christian A. Smith[2] and James T. Rutka[1]

1 Division of Neurosurgery and Labatt Brain Tumour Research Centre, The Hospital for Sick Children, University of Toronto, Canada

2 Labatt Brain Tumour Research Centre, The Hospital for Sick Children, University of Toronto, Canada

References

[1] Ohgaki H, Kleihues P. Population-based studies on incidence, survival rates, and genetic alterations in astrocytic and oligodendroglial gliomas. J Neuropathol Exp Neurol. 2005 Jun;64(6):479-89.

[2] Dubuc AM, Northcott PA, Mack S, Witt H, Pfister S, Taylor MD. The genetics of pediatric brain tumors. Curr Neurol Neurosci Rep. 2010 May;10(3):215-23.

[3] Pfister S, Janzarik WG, Remke M, Ernst A, Werft W, Becker N, et al. BRAF gene duplication constitutes a mechanism of MAPK pathway activation in low-grade astrocytomas. J Clin Invest. 2008 May;118(5):1739-49.

[4] Hawkins C, Walker E, Mohamed N, Zhang C, Jacob K, Shirinian M, et al. BRAF-KIAA1549 fusion predicts better clinical outcome in pediatric low-grade astrocytoma. Clin Cancer Res. 2011 Jul 15;17(14):4790-8.

[5] Jones DT, Gronych J, Lichter P, Witt O, Pfister SM. MAPK pathway activation in pilocytic astrocytoma. Cell Mol Life Sci. 2012 Jun;69(11):1799-811.

[6] Korshunov A, Meyer J, Capper D, Christians A, Remke M, Witt H, et al. Combined molecular analysis of BRAF and IDH1 distinguishes pilocytic astrocytoma from diffuse astrocytoma. Acta Neuropathol. 2009 Sep;118(3):401-5.

[7] MacDonald TJ, Aguilera D, Kramm CM. Treatment of high-grade glioma in children and adolescents. Neuro Oncol. 2011 Oct;13(10):1049-58.

[8] Faury D, Nantel A, Dunn SE, Guiot MC, Haque T, Hauser P, et al. Molecular profiling identifies prognostic subgroups of pediatric glioblastoma and shows increased YB-1 expression in tumors. J Clin Oncol. 2007 Apr 1;25(10):1196-208.

[9] Pollack IF, Hamilton RL, Burger PC, Brat DJ, Rosenblum MK, Murdoch GH, et al. Akt activation is a common event in pediatric malignant gliomas and a potential adverse prognostic marker: a report from the Children's Oncology Group. J Neurooncol. 2010 Sep;99(2):155-63.

[10] Bax DA, Mackay A, Little SE, Carvalho D, Viana-Pereira M, Tamber N, et al. A distinct spectrum of copy number aberrations in pediatric high-grade gliomas. Clin Cancer Res. 2010 Jul 1;16(13):3368-77.

[11] Pollack IF, Finkelstein SD, Burnham J, Holmes EJ, Hamilton RL, Yates AJ, et al. Age and TP53 mutation frequency in childhood malignant gliomas: results in a multi-institutional cohort. Cancer Res. 2001 Oct 15;61(20):7404-7.

[12] Pollack IF, Finkelstein SD, Woods J, Burnham J, Holmes EJ, Hamilton RL, et al. Expression of p53 and prognosis in children with malignant gliomas. N Engl J Med. 2002 Feb 7;346(6):420-7.

[13] Qu HQ, Jacob K, Fatet S, Ge B, Barnett D, Delattre O, et al. Genome-wide profiling using single-nucleotide polymorphism arrays identifies novel chromosomal imbalances in pediatric glioblastomas. Neuro Oncol. 2010 Feb;12(2):153-63.

[14] Schwartzentruber J, Korshunov A, Liu XY, Jones DT, Pfaff E, Jacob K, et al. Driver mutations in histone H3.3 and chromatin remodelling genes in paediatric glioblastoma. Nature. 2012 Feb 9;482(7384):226-31.

[15] Nageswara Rao AA, Scafidi J, Wells EM, Packer RJ. Biologically targeted therapeutics in pediatric brain tumors. Pediatr Neurol. 2012 Apr;46(4):203-11.

[16] Hargrave D, Bartels U, Bouffet E. Diffuse brainstem glioma in children: critical review of clinical trials. Lancet Oncol. 2006 Mar;7(3):241-8.

[17] Jansen MH, van Vuurden DG, Vandertop WP, Kaspers GJ. Diffuse intrinsic pontine gliomas: a systematic update on clinical trials and biology. Cancer Treat Rev. 2012 Feb;38(1):27-35.

[18] Roujeau T, Machado G, Garnett MR, Miquel C, Puget S, Geoerger B, et al. Stereotactic biopsy of diffuse pontine lesions in children. J Neurosurg. 2007 Jul;107(1 Suppl):1-4.

[19] Pirotte BJ, Lubansu A, Massager N, Wikler D, Goldman S, Levivier M. Results of positron emission tomography guidance and reassessment of the utility of and indications for stereotactic biopsy in children with infiltrative brainstem tumors. J Neurosurg. 2007 Nov;107(5 Suppl):392-9.

[20] Geoerger B, Hargrave D, Thomas F, Ndiaye A, Frappaz D, Andreiuolo F, et al. Innovative Therapies for Children with Cancer pediatric phase I study of erlotinib in brainstem glioma and relapsing/refractory brain tumors. Neuro Oncol. 2011 Jan;13(1):109-18.

[21] Angelini P, Hawkins C, Laperriere N, Bouffet E, Bartels U. Post mortem examinations in diffuse intrinsic pontine glioma: challenges and chances. J Neurooncol. 2011 Jan;101(1):75-81.

[22] Broniscer A, Baker JN, Baker SJ, Chi SN, Geyer JR, Morris EB, et al. Prospective collection of tissue samples at autopsy in children with diffuse intrinsic pontine glioma. Cancer. 2010 Oct 1;116(19):4632-7.

[23] Caretti V, Jansen MH, van Vuurden DG, Lagerweij T, Bugiani M, Horsman I, et al. Implementation of a Multi-Institutional Diffuse Intrinsic Pontine Glioma Autopsy Protocol and Characterization of a Primary Cell Culture. Neuropathol Appl Neurobiol. 2012 Jul 27.

[24] Paugh BS, Qu C, Jones C, Liu Z, Adamowicz-Brice M, Zhang J, et al. Integrated molecular genetic profiling of pediatric high-grade gliomas reveals key differences with the adult disease. J Clin Oncol. 2010 Jun 20;28(18):3061-8.

[25] Paugh BS, Broniscer A, Qu C, Miller CP, Zhang J, Tatevossian RG, et al. Genome-wide analyses identify recurrent amplifications of receptor tyrosine kinases and cell-cycle regulatory genes in diffuse intrinsic pontine glioma. J Clin Oncol. 2011 Oct 20;29(30):3999-4006.

[26] Zarghooni M, Bartels U, Lee E, Buczkowicz P, Morrison A, Huang A, et al. Whole-genome profiling of pediatric diffuse intrinsic pontine gliomas highlights platelet-derived growth factor receptor alpha and poly (ADP-ribose) polymerase as potential therapeutic targets. J Clin Oncol. 2010 Mar 10;28(8):1337-44.

[27] Barrow J, Adamowicz-Brice M, Cartmill M, MacArthur D, Lowe J, Robson K, et al. Homozygous loss of ADAM3A revealed by genome-wide analysis of pediatric high-grade glioma and diffuse intrinsic pontine gliomas. Neuro Oncol. 2011 Feb;13(2):212-22.

[28] Grill J, Puget S, Andreiuolo F, Philippe C, MacConaill L, Kieran MW. Critical oncogenic mutations in newly diagnosed pediatric diffuse intrinsic pontine glioma. Pediatr Blood Cancer. 2012 Apr;58(4):489-91.

[29] Khuong-Quang DA, Buczkowicz P, Rakopoulos P, Liu XY, Fontebasso AM, Bouffet E, et al. K27M mutation in histone H3.3 defines clinically and biologically distinct subgroups of pediatric diffuse intrinsic pontine gliomas. Acta Neuropathol. 2012 Sep;124(3):439-47.

[30] Wu G, Broniscer A, McEachron TA, Lu C, Paugh BS, Becksfort J, et al. Somatic histone H3 alterations in pediatric diffuse intrinsic pontine gliomas and non-brainstem glioblastomas. Nat Genet. 2012 Mar;44(3):251-3.

[31] Bartels U, Hawkins C, Vezina G, Kun L, Souweidane M, Bouffet E. Proceedings of the diffuse intrinsic pontine glioma (DIPG) Toronto Think Tank: advancing basic and translational research and cooperation in DIPG. J Neurooncol. 2011 Oct;105(1):119-25.

[32] Pollack IF, Jakacki RI, Blaney SM, Hancock ML, Kieran MW, Phillips P, et al. Phase I trial of imatinib in children with newly diagnosed brainstem and recurrent malignant gliomas: a Pediatric Brain Tumor Consortium report. Neuro Oncol. 2007 Apr;9(2):145-60.

[33] Haas-Kogan DA, Banerjee A, Kocak M, Prados MD, Geyer JR, Fouladi M, et al. Phase I trial of tipifarnib in children with newly diagnosed intrinsic diffuse brainstem glioma. Neuro Oncol. 2008 Jun;10(3):341-7.

[34] Geyer JR, Stewart CF, Kocak M, Broniscer A, Phillips P, Douglas JG, et al. A phase I and biology study of gefitinib and radiation in children with newly diagnosed brain stem gliomas or supratentorial malignant gliomas. Eur J Cancer. 2010 Dec;46(18): 3287-93.

[35] Broniscer A, Baker JN, Tagen M, Onar-Thomas A, Gilbertson RJ, Davidoff AM, et al. Phase I study of vandetanib during and after radiotherapy in children with diffuse intrinsic pontine glioma. J Clin Oncol. 2010 Nov 1;28(31):4762-8.

[36] Pollack IF, Stewart CF, Kocak M, Poussaint TY, Broniscer A, Banerjee A, et al. A phase II study of gefitinib and irradiation in children with newly diagnosed brain-stem gliomas: a report from the Pediatric Brain Tumor Consortium. Neuro Oncol. 2011 Mar;13(3):290-7.

[37] Massimino M, Bode U, Biassoni V, Fleischhack G. Nimotuzumab for pediatric diffuse intrinsic pontine gliomas. Expert Opin Biol Ther. 2011 Feb;11(2):247-56.

[38] Taylor MD, Northcott PA, Korshunov A, Remke M, Cho YJ, Clifford SC, et al. Molecular subgroups of medulloblastoma: the current consensus. Acta Neuropathol. 2012 Apr;123(4):465-72.

[39] Northcott PA, Korshunov A, Pfister SM, Taylor MD. The clinical implications of medulloblastoma subgroups. Nat Rev Neurol. 2012 Jun;8(6):340-51.

[40] Remke M, Hielscher T, Northcott PA, Witt H, Ryzhova M, Wittmann A, et al. Adult medulloblastoma comprises three major molecular variants. J Clin Oncol. 2011 Jul 1;29(19):2717-23.

[41] Fattet S, Haberler C, Legoix P, Varlet P, Lellouch-Tubiana A, Lair S, et al. Beta-catenin status in paediatric medulloblastomas: correlation of immunohistochemical expression with mutational status, genetic profiles, and clinical characteristics. J Pathol. 2009 May;218(1):86-94.

[42] Northcott PA, Korshunov A, Witt H, Hielscher T, Eberhart CG, Mack S, et al. Medulloblastoma comprises four distinct molecular variants. J Clin Oncol. 2011 Apr 10;29(11):1408-14.

[43] Thompson MC, Fuller C, Hogg TL, Dalton J, Finkelstein D, Lau CC, et al. Genomics identifies medulloblastoma subgroups that are enriched for specific genetic alterations. J Clin Oncol. 2006 Apr 20;24(12):1924-31.

[44] Northcott PA, Hielscher T, Dubuc A, Mack S, Shih D, Remke M, et al. Pediatric and adult sonic hedgehog medulloblastomas are clinically and molecularly distinct. Acta Neuropathol. 2011 Aug;122(2):231-40.

[45] Northcott PA, Dubuc AM, Pfister S, Taylor MD. Molecular subgroups of medulloblastoma. Expert Rev Neurother. 2012 Jul;12(7):871-84.

[46] Al-Halabi H, Nantel A, Klekner A, Guiot MC, Albrecht S, Hauser P, et al. Preponderance of sonic hedgehog pathway activation characterizes adult medulloblastoma. Acta Neuropathol. 2011 Feb;121(2):229-39.

[47] Ellison DW, Dalton J, Kocak M, Nicholson SL, Fraga C, Neale G, et al. Medulloblastoma: clinicopathological correlates of SHH, WNT, and non-SHH/WNT molecular subgroups. Acta Neuropathol. 2011 Mar;121(3):381-96.

[48] Kool M, Korshunov A, Remke M, Jones DT, Schlanstein M, Northcott PA, et al. Molecular subgroups of medulloblastoma: an international meta-analysis of transcriptome, genetic aberrations, and clinical data of WNT, SHH, Group 3, and Group 4 medulloblastomas. Acta Neuropathol. 2012 Apr;123(4):473-84.

[49] Cho YJ, Tsherniak A, Tamayo P, Santagata S, Ligon A, Greulich H, et al. Integrative genomic analysis of medulloblastoma identifies a molecular subgroup that drives poor clinical outcome. J Clin Oncol. 2011 Apr 10;29(11):1424-30.

[50] Remke M, Hielscher T, Korshunov A, Northcott PA, Bender S, Kool M, et al. FSTL5 is a marker of poor prognosis in non-WNT/non-SHH medulloblastoma. J Clin Oncol. 2011 Oct 10;29(29):3852-61.

[51] Rudin CM, Hann CL, Laterra J, Yauch RL, Callahan CA, Fu L, et al. Treatment of medulloblastoma with hedgehog pathway inhibitor GDC-0449. N Engl J Med. 2009 Sep 17;361(12):1173-8.

[52] Northcott PA, Shih DJ, Peacock J, Garzia L, Morrissy AS, Zichner T, et al. Subgroup-specific structural variation across 1,000 medulloblastoma genomes. Nature. 2012 Aug 2;488(7409):49-56.

[53] Rausch T, Jones DT, Zapatka M, Stutz AM, Zichner T, Weischenfeldt J, et al. Genome sequencing of pediatric medulloblastoma links catastrophic DNA rearrangements with TP53 mutations. Cell. 2012 Jan 20;148(1-2):59-71.

[54] Parsons DW, Li M, Zhang X, Jones S, Leary RJ, Lin JC, et al. The genetic landscape of the childhood cancer medulloblastoma. Science. 2011 Jan 28;331(6016):435-9.

[55] Jones DT, Jager N, Kool M, Zichner T, Hutter B, Sultan M, et al. Dissecting the genomic complexity underlying medulloblastoma. Nature. 2012 Aug 2;488(7409):100-5.

[56] Pugh TJ, Weeraratne SD, Archer TC, Pomeranz Krummel DA, Auclair D, Bochicchio J, et al. Medulloblastoma exome sequencing uncovers subtype-specific somatic mutations. Nature. 2012 Aug 2;488(7409):106-10.

[57] Robinson G, Parker M, Kranenburg TA, Lu C, Chen X, Ding L, et al. Novel mutations target distinct subgroups of medulloblastoma. Nature. 2012 Aug 2;488(7409):43-8.

[58] Metcalfe C, de Sauvage FJ. Hedgehog fights back: mechanisms of acquired resistance against Smoothened antagonists. Cancer Res. 2011 Aug 1;71(15):5057-61.

[59] Ramaswamy V, Northcott PA, Taylor MD. FISH and chips: the recipe for improved prognostication and outcomes for children with medulloblastoma. Cancer Genet. 2011 Nov;204(11):577-88.

[60] Leary SE, Olson JM. The molecular classification of medulloblastoma: driving the next generation clinical trials. Curr Opin Pediatr. 2012 Feb;24(1):33-9.

[61] Merchant TE, Li C, Xiong X, Kun LE, Boop FA, Sanford RA. Conformal radiotherapy after surgery for paediatric ependymoma: a prospective study. Lancet Oncol. 2009 Mar;10(3):258-66.

[62] Korshunov A, Witt H, Hielscher T, Benner A, Remke M, Ryzhova M, et al. Molecular staging of intracranial ependymoma in children and adults. J Clin Oncol. 2010 Jul 1;28(19):3182-90.

[63] Johnson RA, Wright KD, Poppleton H, Mohankumar KM, Finkelstein D, Pounds SB, et al. Cross-species genomics matches driver mutations and cell compartments to model ependymoma. Nature. 2010 Jul 29;466(7306):632-6.

[64] Witt H, Mack SC, Ryzhova M, Bender S, Sill M, Isserlin R, et al. Delineation of two clinically and molecularly distinct subgroups of posterior fossa ependymoma. Cancer Cell. 2011 Aug 16;20(2):143-57.

[65] Wani K, Armstrong TS, Vera-Bolanos E, Raghunathan A, Ellison D, Gilbertson R, et al. A prognostic gene expression signature in infratentorial ependymoma. Acta Neuropathol. 2012 May;123(5):727-38.

[66] Dubuc AM, Mack S, Unterberger A, Northcott PA, Taylor MD. The epigenetics of brain tumors. Methods Mol Biol. 2012;863:139-53.

[67] Rogers HA, Kilday JP, Mayne C, Ward J, Adamowicz-Brice M, Schwalbe EC, et al. Supratentorial and spinal pediatric ependymomas display a hypermethylated phenotype which includes the loss of tumor suppressor genes involved in the control of cell growth and death. Acta Neuropathol. 2012 May;123(5):711-25.

[68] Xie H, Wang M, Bonaldo Mde F, Rajaram V, Stellpflug W, Smith C, et al. Epigenomic analysis of Alu repeats in human ependymomas. Proc Natl Acad Sci U S A. 2010 Apr 13;107(15):6952-7.

Section 7

Radioresistance of Brain Tumors

Chapter 21

In silico Analysis of Transcription Factors Associated to Differentially Expressed Genes in Irradiated Glioblastoma Cell Lines

P. R. D. V. Godoy, S. S. Mello, F. S. Donaires,
E. A. Donadi, G. A. S. Passos and
E. T. Sakamoto-Hojo

Additional information is available at the end of the chapter

http://dx.doi.org/10.5772/53299

1. Introduction

Glioblastoma multiforme (GBM) is one of the most frequent tumors in the central nervous system and the most malignant tumor among gliomas. In the past two decades, cytogenetic and molecular genetic studies have identified a number of recurrent chromosomal abnormalities and genetic alterations in malignant gliomas, particularly in GBM [1]. It was already described that GBM harbors combinations of the following genetic alterations: loss of heterozygozity of 10q, *EGFR* amplification, *TP53* mutations, p16^{INK4a} deletion and PTEN mutations [2]. New integrative genomics studies provided a comprehensive view of the complicated genomic landscape of GBM, revealing a set of core signaling pathways commonly activated in GBM involving TP53, RB, and RTK (receptor tyrosine kinase) pathways [3, 4]. The majority of GBM tumors present genetic alterations in all three pathways, which helps to stimulate cell proliferation and enhance cell survival while allowing tumor cells to escaping from cell-cycle checkpoints, senescence, and apoptosis. This approach also identified previously unknown genetic alterations in *IDH1/2, NF1, ERBB2*, and *NFKBIA* genes [1].

The current GBM treatment involves aggressive management including surgery, adjuvant temozolomide-based chemotherapy, and radiotherapy [5], but GBM patients still present a dismal prognosis, and the median survival is 14.6 months from diagnosis [6]. Although radiotherapy has been found to significantly prolong survival rates for GBM patients, radioresistance is a typical characteristic of this tumor [7].

Current genome-wide studies and the molecular characterization of GBM have allowed the identification of potential new targets, development of novel therapeutic small molecules and monoclonal antibodies and initiation of clinical trials with these targets [6, 8-10]. However, there is a wide molecular diversity and heterogeneity associated with the aberrantly GBM signaling pathways, culminating in the relative lack of success of these new approaches [10]. Recently, an alternative strategy involves the selective targeting of GBM stem cells, which are resistant to chemo- and radiotherapy. But still, almost all small-molecule inhibitors designed to target these cells failed to demonstrate the effectiveness of this strategy, compared with the conventional therapy [11].

Considering that most of the treatment protocols are still ineffective, novel approaches are needed towards killing of GBM cells. Transcription machinery, as well as its regulatory elements is also a feasible new target for the application of molecular therapies. Transcription of DNA is dependent on the spatially and temporally coordinated interaction between transcriptional machinery involving RNA polymerase II, transcription factors (TFs)) and transcriptional regulatory components (promoter elements, enhancers, silencers and locus control regions) [12, 13]. The low level of transcription, directed by the general transcription factors associated to RNA polymerase core enzyme, is known as basal transcription [14]. However, there is a rapidly expanding number of 'context-dependent' transcription factors that bind DNA and these TFs are capable of positively or negatively regulating the transcription process depending on the context of their binding sites, the complement of protein interactions and other environmental influences [15].

Postgenomic analyses of major transcription factor families, in both malignant and nonmalignant cell types, have opened new discussions about TF function. The mechanisms by which TFs act in cancer cell systems appear to exhibit a restricted repertoire of skills and plasticity displayed by normal cell systems [16]. The evolution of a restricted malignant transcriptome can be seen clearly in the nuclear receptor superfamily, but is also apparent in the MYC and AP-1 networks [17]. Oncogenic transcriptional rigidity reflects the simultaneous deregulation of target loci such that proliferative and survival signals are enhanced and antimitotic inputs are either limited or lost. Co-repressor proteins significantly contribute with the disruption of these processes [16]. Therefore, understanding mechanisms involved in gene regulation and transcriptional network may lead to a better knowledge about the crucial functions of TFs, providing information to explore possibilities of their application as molecular targets in cancer therapy [18].

A valuable tool to study the transcription machinery is the DNA microarray technology [19], which measures the transcript expression of thousands of genes to identify changes in expression profiles at different biological conditions [20-24], thus allowing to compare different cell types under diverse treatment conditions. The influence of *TP53* status on transcriptional profiles was previously described in tumor cell lines [25, 26]. Expression signatures of irradiated GBM cells were already performed for cell lines that are proficient and deficient for *TP53* [27, 28].

Recently, information on the regulation of gene expression can also be used within the context of functional enrichment tests, and different databases containing TFs binding sites and other regulatory motifs are available, allowing to scan promoter regions of genes to detect the presence of target motifs [29]. This information allow to determining whether a set of pre-selected genes is under control of TFs. FatiGO + [30] is a web-based tool capable of associating TFs that are common to a gene set used as parameters. This TF prediction method was already applied to a GBM dataset obtained from public repositories of microarray experiments, and the up-regulation of two predicted TFs, E2F1 and E2F4, was validated for several GBM cell lines [31], demonstrating the suitability of this method.

In the current study, we aimed to identify TFs that could be predicted from significant differentially expressed genes (previously obtained in microarray experiments in irradiated GBM cells) using an *in silico* analysis.

We found few predicted TFs that were common between GBM cell lines, while several exclusive TFs were found for each cell line, indicating that the transcriptional response to ionizing radiation is very particular to each cell line examined in our microarray study, a fact that can be due to the genetic heterogeneity inherent to GBM cells. In spite of this, there was a convergence of biological functions among cell lines; the most relevant processes were related to apoptosis, cell proliferation, cell cycle, DNA repair, oxidative stress, among others. Furthermore, the present results also showed several TFs that were already reported as associated to cancer and stress responses.

2. Materials and methods

2.1. Briefly characterization of the experiment that provided the statistically modulated genes used for TF prediction

2.1.1. Cell culture and irradiation

Human GBM T98G and U87MG cell lines were supplied by the American Type Culture Collection (ATCC) (Rockville, Maryland, USA) and gently donated by Dr. Mari C. Sogayar (Universidade de São Paulo, Brazil). U343MG-a (U343), a cell line established from a primary malignant astrocytoma in an adult [32], was kindly donated by Dr. James T. Rutka (The Arthur and Sonia Labatt Brain Tumour Research Center, Canada); U251MG cell lines was also purchased from the ATCC (Rockville, MD, USA) and gently donated by Dr. Guido Lenz (Universidade Federal do Rio Grande do Sul, Brazil) [33]. All cell lines grown in the presence of DMEM + HAM F10 medium (Sigma-Aldrich, St. Louis, USA) plus 10% fetal calf serum (Cultilab, Campinas, Brazil), and kept at 37°C and 5% CO2, until they reach semi-confluency. Cells were sub-cultured and $1 x 10^6$ cells were seeded in 25 cm^2 flasks, being incubated at 37°C for 48 h, and irradiated with 8 Gy of gamma-rays (^{60}Co source, dose rate of 2.0 Gy / min., Unit Gammatron S-80, Siemens, 1.25 MeV, HC-FMRP/USP).

2.1.2. cDNA microarrays method and analysis

Two experiments with irradiated and sham-irradiated GBM cells were carried out using a glass slide microarrays containing ~4300 clones of cDNA probe (in replicates) from the human IMAGE Consortium cDNA library [34]; kindly provided by Dr. Catherine Nguyen (INSERM-CNRS, Marseille, France)], and prepared according to the protocol described by Hegde et al [35]. Microarrays were spotted onto glass slides (Corning, Lowell, MA, USA) by using a Generation III Array Spotter (Amersham Molecular Dynamics, Sunnyvale, USA) according to the manufacturer's instructions.

Total RNA extraction was performed for all cell lines, 30 min. and 6 h after irradiation, using the Trizol reagent (Invitrogen, Carlsbad, USA) according to manufacturer's instructions. Each cDNA sample was spotted twice in the slide (duplicate spots). The cDNA complex probes were prepared using the CyScribe Post Labeling Kit (Amersham Biosciences, Buckinghamshire, UK) as previously described [23]. Hybridizations were carried out using an automatic system (Automatic Slide Processor, Amersham Biosciences, UK) and signals were immediately captured after the final wash procedure, using a Generation III laser scanner (Amersham Biosciences, UK). This array platform was already used in several studies [22-26, 36].

2.1.3. Data acquisition and gene expression analysis

The provided microarray data was filtered and normalized [25, 36]. Following the normalization procedure, microarray data was exported to tab-delimited tables in MEV format and analyzed in MEV (v. 3.1) software [37].

The gene set submitted to SAM (Significance Analysis of Microarray [20]) were previously obtained by a t-test (α=5%) comparing irradiated (8 Gy) *versus* unirradiated (controls) T98G, U251MG, U343MG-a and U87MG cell lines, separately, considering two time points (30 min. and 6 h). The overall results are displayed in Table 1. The complete gene lists are available at http//www.rge.fmrp.usp.br/passos/genesgbm01/

Condition	**Number of genes**		**Fold Change variation**
	up-regulated	**down-regulated**	
U343MG-a (30 min.)	7	116	+1.53 to -2.42
U343MG-a (6 h)	3	11	+1.83 to -1.39
U87MG (30 min.)	56	73	+1.88 to - 2.95
U87MG (6 h)	86	54	+1.68 to -1.95
T98G (30 min)	32	0	+2.26 to +1.13
T98G (6 h)	16	7	+2.70 to -1.63
U251MG (30 min.)	12	69	+1.85 to -1.40
U251MG (6 h)	17	20	+2.28 to -2.18

Table 1. Overall quantitative results on significant differentially expressed genes obtained by the DNA microarray method, and analysis performed by SAM – Significance Analysis of Microarray (FDR < 5 %), for the comparison irradiated *versus* un-irradiated cells.RNA samples from U87, U343, T98 and U251 cells were collected at 30 min. and 6 h following irradiation with 8 Gy of gamma-rays. Fold-change (+) or (-) means up- and down-regulation in transcript expression, respectively.

The list of significantly modulated genes was obtained for a FDR < 5%. U343 cells showed 123 and 14 significantly differentially expressed genes at 30 min and 6 h after irradiation, respectively, whereas U87 showed 129 genes at 30 min and 140 genes at 6 h; T98G cell line displayed 32 and 23 significantly up-regulated genes at 30 min. and 6 h, respectively, whereas U251 showed 81 genes at 30 min. and 37 genes at 6 h (Table 2).

2.2. Transcriptional factor analysis

The analysis of TFs related to the significant differentially expressed genes (SAM) was performed by applying the FatiGO + [30]. This program uses the TRANSFAC [38], and CisRed [39] transcription factors database, including their respective binding sites and regulated genes.

FatiGO + analyzes if the pre –selected set of genes (provided after SAM analysis), are under control of the same TF, and search for significant enrichments to each TF that is associated to the gene list compared to the complete reference list, containing ~4300 clones that were spotted onto the microarray slide [29].

The p-values obtained in the analysis of regulatory elements have been established by the program using the Fisher's exact test for multiple comparisons (unadjusted p-value). The Enrichment Index (EI) calculated for each TF corresponds to the increment obtained regarding the number of genes (%) statistically modulated (SAM) that are associated to a specific TF (List #1) divided by the total number of genes (%) in the array set that were predicted as targets for the same TF (List #2):

EI = % gene List #1/ % gene list #2

The TFs were selected according to unadjusted p-values < 0.05. The genes were submitted to FatiGO + v3.2, using the Gene symbol identifier and the selected gene distance of 10 kb. After selecting the TFs associated to modulated genes (SAM), a search was conducted in PubMed (http://www.ncbi.nlm. Nih.gov / sites / entrez /) looking for biological functions of those TFs.

2.3. Quantitative real-time PCR (qPCR)

We analyzed the transcript expression of HEB, a predict TF that was found associated to 57.7% of up-regulated genes in U87 cells, 30 min. after IR. The reverse transcription step was carried out in the remaining RNA samples from microarray experiments, with the Superscript III Reverse Transcriptase kit (Invitrogen, USA), according to manufacturer's instructions. The integrity of cDNA samples was validated by the amplification of the endogenous B2M gene and visualization in agarose gel electrophoresis. qPCR was carried out using SYBR green master mix (Applied Biosystems, Foster City, USA) and the expression levels were estimated by the Relative Expression Software Tool (REST) [49], using 10000 interactions as setup parameter. All primers (Integrated DNA Technologies, Coralville, USA) were designed in Primer3 software [50] and are displayed on Table 2. The reactions were carried out in the Applied Biosystems 7500 Real-Time PCR System (Applied

Biosystems, USA) equipment, using primer sets with an annealing temperature near 60°C and an amplicon of 100–120 bp. The PCR cycle was the following: pre-heating at 50°C for 2 min., 10 min. at 95°C (denaturation step), followed by 40 cycles at 95°C for 15 sec., and at 60°C for 60 sec. The dissociation curves were set up as following: 95°C for 15 sec., 60°C for 20 sec. and 95°C for 15 sec.

Primer	Sequence	PCR product size (pb)
B2M – forward	5'- AGGCTATCCAGCGTACTCCA - 3'	112
B2M – reverse	5' - TCAATGTCGGATGGATGAAA - 3'	
HEB – forward	5' - CCGCTTGAGTTATCCTCCAC - 3'	116
HEB – reverse	5' - GTGAGGCAGCAACGTAAGGT - 3'	

Table 2. Primer sequences used in Real Time qPCR; the housekeeping B2M gene was used as internal control.

2.4. Western Blot (WB)

Protein extraction was performed with the Trizol reagent (Invitrogen, Carlsbad-USA) according to the manufacturer's instructions, using the same samples for RNA extraction. These samples were obtained from U87 cells collected at 30 min. post-irradiation. The expression of HEB was analyzed by Western blot, using ACTB as internal control. Samples were prepared with 30 µg of total protein. After electrophoresis, proteins were transferred from the gel to the membrane Invitrolon PVDF using the XCell IITM Blot Module system (Invitrogen, Carlsbad - USA). The immunodetection and protein visualization were conducted with the WesternBreeze Chromogenic kit (Invitrogen, Carlsbad - USA). The antibodies used in this study were anti-HEB (Santa Cruz, Santa Cruz, USA), and anti-ACTB (Cell Signaling, Danvers, USA), dilution of 1:1000.

We performed densitometric analysis of WB bands using the GelPro Analyzer (MediaCybernetics, Rockville, USA) 4.0, and the relative expression of HEB was calculated relatively to ACTB.

3. Results

In the FatiGO + analysis, the lists of statistically modulated genes (SAM) were up-loaded in order to find TFs that were significantly associated with up-regulated and down-regulated genes for non-adjusted p-values < 0.05 (Table 3).

A Venn diagram was constructed based on the numbers of predicted TFs from data set previously obtained for each cell line (microarray experiments) (Fig. 1). TFs predicted for 30 min and 6 h were pooled together. Each cell line showed a number of exclusive TFs, but we also observed common TFs between cell lines. Out of 18 exclusive TFs found for U87MG cell line, PEBP (p = 0.008), Bach2 (p = 0.007), Freac-4 (p = 0.003), HLV (p = 0.006), Evi-1 (p = 0.009) displayed the lowest p-values, while PPARG and SEF-1 displayed the highest EI (31.3). U343 presented 9 exclusive TFs; High values of EI were found for MAF (33.1), E2F:DP-1 (22.0), PR (45.5) and STAT3 (38.5), and ARP-1 was the TF presenting the lowest p-value (0.009). T98G cells displayed only 6 exclusive TFs: EBF, Pax, Pbx1b, C/EBP, Poly A downstream element and Pax-9; two of them, EBF and PolyA showed low p-values, 0.005 and 0.007, respectively. Regarding U251MG cells, 13 TFs were predicted, and only APOLYA presented a high EI (27.8) (Table 3).

Interestingly, STAT3 was the common TF found for TP53 wild-type cells; however, this TF was associated with up-regulated genes in U87, and with down-regulated genes in U343. Only one TF (VBP) was common among three cell lines (U87, U343 and U251), being associated with down-regulated genes. Among the *TP53* mutant cell lines, ATF4 was common between T98 and U251, associated with up-regulated genes (30 min. and 6 h). Two TFs were found common between U343 and U251, TEF (associated to down-regulated genes, 30 min.) and MAF (associated to up-regulated, 6 h). Finally, C/BPGamma was commonly predicted for up-regulated genes in U87 (30 min.) and U251 (6 h) cell lines (Fig. 1).

Therefore, our results showed that most of the predicted TFs were exclusive to each cell line and few TFs were common among the GBM cell lines; these results indicate that the transcriptional response to ionizing radiation is very particular to each cell line, and most probably this can be due to the genetic heterogeneity of GBM cells.

By using the real time qPCR method, we confirmed the expression of HEB to validate the *in silico* prediction for this TF. By using the REST 2009 software, we found that HEB was statistically up-regulated (+2.6) when comparing irradiated and sham-irradiated U87 cell lines (30 min.) (Fig. 2A). Primer efficiency was also determined for B2M (0.9615) and HEB (0.9652).

We also look for HEB protein expression by Western Blot; both ACTB and HEB antibodies were used for irradiated and sham-irrradiated U87, 30 min after irradiation (Fig.2B). The relative expression values calculated by densitometric analysis showed that HEB expression was 1.7 higher in irradiated (8 Gy) cells, relatively to the control value (Fig. 2C).

U343MG-a					
Collection time	**Transcription factor**	**% of genes (List 1)**	**% of genes (List 2)**	**EI**	**p-value**
30 min. (↓)	ARP-1	14.8	6.7	2.2	0.009
	TEF	37.5	25.3	1.5	0.013
	VBP	19.3	10.4	1.9	0.013
	Imperfect Hogness/Goldberg BOX	2.3	0.2	14.2	0.016
	Muscle initiator sequence-20	20.5	12.2	1.7	0.031

U343MG-a					
Collection time	**Transcription factor**	**% of genes (List 1)**	**% of genes (List 2)**	**EI**	**p-value**
	Elk-1	44.3	33.1	1.3	0.038
	Sox-5	4.6	1.5	3.1	0.048
	ACAAT	12.5	6.7	1.9	0.049
6 h (↑)	MAF	50.0	1.5	33.1	0.031
	E2F-4:DP-1	50.0	2.3	22.0	0.046
6 h (↓)	ICSBP	40.0	3.7	10.9	0.013
	PR	20.0	0.4	45.5	0.024
	STAT3	20.0	0.5	38.5	0.028
	ARP-1	40.0	6.7	6.0	0.040

U87 MG					
Collection time	**Transcription factor**	**% of genes (List 1)**	**% of genes (List 2)**	**EI**	**p-value**
30 min. (↑)	C/EBPgamma	85.0	64.4	1.3	0.007
	AP-1	80.0	61.1	1.3	0.014
	HEB	57.5	38.5	1.5	0.021
	SREBP-1	97.5	84.5	1.2	0.024
	FOXP3	87.5	72.0	1.2	0.032
	PPARG	2.5	0.1	31.3	0.046
	SEF-1	2.5	0.1	31.3	0.046
30 min. (↓)	Bach2	63.5	43.9	1.4	0.007
	PEBP	28.9	14.4	2.0	0.008
	COUP-TF:HNF-4	11.5	3.7	3.1	0.014
	MEF-3	5.8	1.2	5.0	0.026
	FOX	78.9	64.8	1.2	0.039
6 h (↑)	DEC	45.6	31.9	1.4	0.032
	STAT3	3.5	0.5	6.8	0.042
6 h (↓)	Freac-4	10.5	1.6	6.8	0.003
	HLF	50.0	28.2	1.8	0.006
	Evi-1	97.4	81.6	1.2	0.009
	VBP	23.7	10.4	2.3	0.015
	TCF-4	55.3	37.2	1.5	0.028

U343MG-a					
Collection time	**Transcription factor**	**% of genes (List 1)**	**% of genes (List 2)**	**EI**	**p-value**
	AP-1	79.0	61.1	1.3	0.028
	Gfi-1	10.5	3.1	3.4	0.031
	CRE-BP1	15.8	6.6	2.4	0.039
	HNF-4alpha	29.0	16.4	1.8	0.047

T98G					
Collection time	**Transcription factor**	**% of genes (List 1)**	**% of genes (List 2)**	**EI**	**p-value**
30 min. (↑)	EBF	29.6	10.5	2.8	0.005
	ATF4	22.2	8.4	2.6	0.023
	Pax	92.6	75.3	1.2	0.041
6 h (↑)	Pbx1b	14.3	1.8	8.2	0.026
6 h (↓)	C/EBP	100.0	20.0	5.0	0.002
	Poly A downstream element	75.0	12.6	6.0	0.007
	Pax-9	75.0	23.8	3.2	0.045

U251MG					
Collection time	**Transcription factor**	**% of genes (List 1)**	**% of genes (List 2)**	**EI**	**p-value**
30 min. (↑)	SMAD-4	40.0	10.4	3.9	0.015
	PTF1-beta	20.0	2.7	7.4	0.030
	APOLYA	10.0	0.4	27.8	0.039
30 min. (↓)	VBP	21.7	10.4	2.1	0.025
	HNF-6	6.5	1.4	4.7	0.030
	E2F	52.2	36.0	1.4	0.030
	TEF	39.1	25.3	1.5	0.040
	TTF1	23.9	13.3	1.8	0.047
	CDP CR1	54.4	39.7	1.4	0.049
	POU1F1	54.4	39.7	1.4	0.049
6 h (↑)	MAF	15.4	1.5	10.2	0.017
	CREB	46.2	17.8	2.6	0.018
	ATF4	30.8	8.4	3.7	0.020
	MEIS1B:HOXA9	15.4	1.9	8.2	0.025

U343MG-a					
Collection time	**Transcription factor**	**% of genes (List 1)**	**% of genes (List 2)**	**EI**	**p-value**
	C/EBPgamma	92.3	64.4	1.4	0.041
6 h (↓)	HES1	45.5	15.6	2.9	0.019
	Lmo2 complex	27.3	6.0	4.5	0.026
	ATATA	18.2	2.9	6.2	0.041

Table 3. Transcription factors associated with statistically modulated genes (SAM, FDR ≤ 5 %), as predicted by the FATIGO + v3.2., analysis performed for U343MG-a, U87MG, T98G and U251MG cell lines (30 min. and 6 h post-irradiation). We used gene lists that showed patterns of repression (↓) and induction (↑) in irradiated cells compared with mock-irradiated. The Enrichment Index (EI) calculated for each TF corresponds to the increment regarding the number of genes (%) statistically modulated (SAM) that are associated to a specific TF (List #1) divided by the total number of genes (%) in the array set that were predicted as targets for the same TF (List #2). The gene distance for the analysis of the TFs was 10 kb.

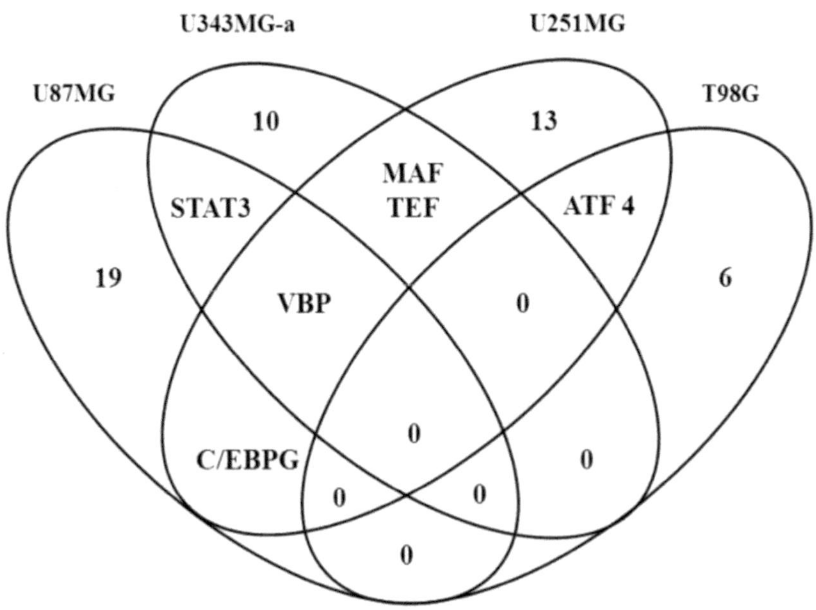

Figure 1. Venn diagram showing predicted TFs associated with significant differentially expressed genes (from micro-array experiments) selected for four GBM cell lines, comparing irradiated *versus* sham-irradiated cells, collected at 30 min. and 6 h following irradiation. TF prediction was carried out using FatiGO + v3.2.

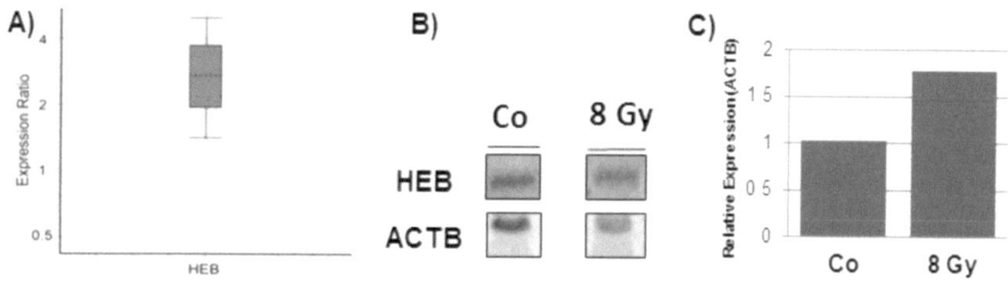

Figure 2. HEB expression. A) HEB expression levels obtained by the qPCR method. This TF was found associated with up-regulated genes in U87 cells, 30 min. after irradiation. Boxes represent the interquartile range; the dotted line represents the median value; whiskers represent the minimum and maximum observations. B) Protein expression analyzed by Western Blot using antibodies for HEB (Santa Cruz) and ACTB (Cell Signalling) as endogenous control. C) Densitometric analysis of Western Blot bands using the Gel Pro Analyzer 4.0 software displayed for HEB expression relatively to ACTB.

4. Discussion

Recently, genome wide technologies, such as DNA microarrays, provide a huge amount of information about gene expression, but require additional bioinformatics analyses for data interpretation. In order to reduce complex signatures to a small number of activated transcriptional elements, new bioinformatics tools have been developed. To date, genome-wide TF-binding regions and sites were identified using a variety of indirect methods and data sets, revealing abundant binding sites for different TFs in mammalian cells [40-43]. Using lists of differentially expressed genes that were generated by microarray experiments, it is possible to predict TFs that can target common binding sites to a gene set. In the current study, we performed an *in silico* analysis (FatiGO + v3.2.) to identify TFs from a list of significant differentially expressed genes selected for irradiated GBM cell lines in microarray experiments. Only few predicted TFs were common to GBM cell lines, while several TFs were exclusive to each cell line, indicating that the transcriptional response to ionizing radiation is very peculiar to each cell line examined in our microarray study. The most relevant predicted TFs are discussed below. While few predicted TFs were shared between different cell lines, several TFs were found exclusive to each cell line, except U251.

4.1. Commonly predicted TFs for two or three GBM cell lines

We found few TFs that were predicted for more than one cell line: MAF, TEF, ATF4, STAT3, VBP and C/EBPGamma. Most of these TFs (STAT3, TEF and VBP) are related to apoptosis, while other biological classes were also found, such as oxidative stress (ATF4), differentiation (MAF) and nucleotide excision repair (C/EBPGamma).

STAT3, *signal transducer and activator of transcription 3* (acute-phase response factor), is part of the STAT family of cytoplasmic latent transcription factors, and was predicted for the TP53 wild type cells, U87 (up-regulated genes, 6 h) and U343 (down-regulated genes, 6 h).

Phosphorylated STAT3 leads to transcriptional activation of downstream genes involved in processes such as cell proliferation, suppression of apoptosis, and angiogenesis [44, 45]. It was demonstrated that STAT3 is constitutively activated and overexpressed in human gliomas; STAT3 activation correlates with malignancy [46, 47], while STAT3 inhibition reduces the lethality of GBM tumors *in vivo* [48], and its inhibition have been tested in phase 0 trial in head and neck cancers [49].

Thyrotroph embryonic factor (TEF) and human hepatic leukemia factor (HLF) are members of the PAR (*proline and acidic amino acid-rich*) subfamily of basic region/leucine zipper (bZIP) transcription factors. The chicken vitellogenin gene-binding protein (VBP) is also a bZIP TF member and is considered as the chicken homologue of TEF. TEF was predicted from down-regulated genes in U343 and U251 (30 min.), and its homolog, VBP, from down-regulated genes in U87 (6 h), U343 (30 min.) and U251 (30 min.). PAR bZIP proteins have recently been shown to be involved in amino acid and neurotransmitter metabolism in both liver and brain [50]. PAR bZIP proteins are also able to transactivate the promoter of bcl-gS which is directly involved in apoptosis induction. Consistently, transfection of TEF induces the expression of endogenous bcl-gS in cancer cells, independently on TP53 [51].

Activating transcription factor 4 (*tax-responsive enhancer element B67*); activating transcription factor 4C (ATF4) belongs to the large ATF/CREB family of transcription factors [52] and was predicted from up-regulated genes in T98 (30 min) and U251 (6 h). Up-regulation of ATF4 is directly involved in the endoplasmic reticulum (ER) stress through induction of CHOP in GBM treated with Nelfinavir (protease inhibitor class of drugs) [53] or in concert with PERK, GADD34 and EIF2alpha in Hela cells submitted to hypoxia [54]. Therefore, activation of ATF4 was already reported in GBM treated cells.

MAF, the v-maf musculoaponeurotic fibrosarcoma oncogene homolog (avian) is a unique subclass of bZIP proteins and was predicted from up-regulated genes in U343 and U251 at 6 h. Depending on the binding site and binding partner, the encoded protein can be a transcriptional activator or repressor. Members of the MAF family appear to play important roles in the regulation of differentiation [55]. MAF was found up-regulated in various cancers, such as colon cancer (but only in tumors that presented high levels of COX-2 expression) [56], a small subset of myelomas, hairy cell leukemia, T- and NK-cell neoplasms and small cell lymphomas [57].

C/EBPGamma, a member of the CCAAT/enhancer-binding protein (C/EBP) family of transcription factors was predicted from up-regulated genes in U87 (30 min.) and U251 (6 h). This TF regulates the expression of ERCC5 [58], and is a participant of DNA repair [59], particularly in the nucleotide excision repair [60].

The predicted TFs represent the overall GBM response to irradiation, since they were selected for more than one cell line, and as mentioned above, their functions are directly associated with stress responses involving apoptosis, DNA repair and ER stress. Moreover, as an example of STAT3, which is in clinical trial [49], predicted TFs may constitute potential targets to be investigated and validated in cancer treatment.

http://dx.doi.org/10.5772/53299

4.2. Exclusively predicted TFs for irradiated U343 cell line

Few predicted TFs (PR, E2F4:DP-1, and ARP-1) associated with statistically significant modulated genes in irradiated U343 cells were found exclusive to this cell line. The functions of these TFs are mainly associated with cell cycle/ tumor growth, being involved in various types of cancer. The overexpression of E2F4 and its binding partner DP-1 revealed a dual function of E2F4, which acts as an activator as well as a repressor, being implicated in positive regulation of the cell cycle [61]. In a previous work, the up-regulation of E2F4 was confirmed for several GBM cell lines [31], demonstrating the potential of this TF as molecular target in cancer therapy.

Progesterone receptor (PR), a nuclear receptor transcription factor was associated with down-regulated genes in U343 cells (6 h). Steroid hormones participate in several physiological and pathological processes in the brain, including the regulation of tumor cell growth [62-64]. Progesterone exerts many of its effects by the interaction with specific intracellular receptors [62, 65].

ARP-1, also known as orphan nuclear receptor chicken ovalbumin upstream promoter transcription factor II (COUP-TFII) is a member of the steroid/thyroid nuclear hormone receptor superfamily [66] and can act as transcriptional repressor or activator. ARP-1 plays critical roles in organogenesis [67-70], and is a major angiogenesis regulator within the tumor microenvironment during pancreatic tumor progression and metastasis [71]. Besides, ARP-1 was associated with therapy response in oligodendroglial tumors with 1p/19q loss [72]. In the present study, this TF was predicted from down-regulated genes (30 min. and 6 h), indicating its possible involvement in radiation responses restricted to U343 cell line.

4.3. Exclusively predicted TFs for irradiated U87 cell line

A high number of TFs with low p-value (Bach2, PEBP, Freac-4, HLF and Evi-1) and high EI (PPARG and SEF-1) was associated with significant expressed genes in U87 cell line.

PPARG is a member of the peroxisome proliferator activated receptor (PPAR) family, a subfamily of the nuclear receptor superfamily [73]. The protein level of this receptor has been recently identified as a significant prognostic marker [74]. Interestingly, recent studies have shown that PPARG is expressed in normal and malignant human brain, and the treatment with PPARG agonists induces growth arrest and apoptosis in brain tumor cells *in vitro* and in animal models *in vivo* [75-77]. Recent findings show that PPARG agonists regulate growth and expansion of brain tumor stem cells [78] and also altered the expression of stemness genes [79]. Unfortunately, clinical trials also failed to demonstrate the effectiveness of such agonists as a monotherapy for cancer treatment, a fact which stimulates the search for combination treatments to enhance their effects [80].

Basic leucine zipper transcription factor 2 (Bach2) is an evolutionarily related member of the BTB-basic region leucine zipper transcription factor family. Bach2 can function as transcriptional activator and repressor [81]. This TF down-regulates cell proliferation of the neuroblastoma cell line N1E-115 and negatively affects their potential to differentiate, being considered as gatekeeper of the differentiated status [82]. Bach2 presents high frequency of loss of heterozygosity of the Bach2 gene in human B cell lymphomas [83]. Consistent with its putative role as a tumor suppressor, Bach2 enhances apoptosis in response to oxidative stress [84, 85].

The transcription Factor PEBP, also called Raf kinase inhibitor protein (RKIP) is a member of the phosphatidylethanolamine-binding protein (PEBP) family. RKIP plays a pivotal modulatory role in several protein kinase signaling cascades. RKIP regulates the activity of the Raf/MEK/ERK, which is responsible for proliferation and differentiation of diverse cell types [86]. It has been reported that RKIP was poorly expressed in primary tumors, being absent in various metastatic cancers; its induction sensitize resistant tumor cells to apoptosis by various chemo- and immunotherapeutic drugs, as well as inhibitors of metastasis [87].The absence of RKIP is also associated with highly malignant behavior and poor survival of patients [88].

The forkhead domain is a monomeric DNA binding motif that defines a rapidly growing family of eukaryotic transcriptional regulators. We found Freac-4, also known as Forkhead Box D1 (FOXD1) associated with down-regulated genes in U87 cells (6 h). This gene was found repressed in chemoresistant tumors, as analyzed by microarrays [89]. However, FOXD1 and FOXD2 were highly expressed in prostate cancer and lymph node metastases, among various cancer types [90]. In another study, using kidney-derived cell lines, it was suggested that FOXD1 may be regulated by TP53, WTAR (a mutated form of WT1) and WT1 [91].

As already mentioned, HLF is a member of PAR bZIP transcription factors, and was associated with down-regulated genes, 6 h after irradiation in U87. PAR bZIP proteins are also involved in apoptosis induction [51].The fused gene *E2A-HLF* was responsible for the development of lymphoid malignancies in 60 % of the transgenic mice [92].

Activator protein one (AP1) transcription factors are a family of jun and fos proteins, whose subunits present diverse pro/anti-cancer effects, like inhibition or increase in proliferation, inhibition of apoptosis and angiogenesis [93, 94]. AP-1 is one of the genes early activated after radiation in primary human B cells [95]. The inhibition of AP-1 blocks the proliferation of breast tumor cells by suppressing the growth factor signaling [96]. The modulation of AP-1 activity may be a new attempt to reduce the malignant transformation. However, only the function involved with malignancy should be targeted [97], since AP-1 presents oncogenic and anti-oncogenic properties. This TF was associated to U87 cells (up-regulated genes, 30 min.) and (down-regulated genes, 6 h).

The EVI1 gene encodes a zinc finger transcription factor with important roles in normal development and leukemogenesis. Reports in animal model and findings in *in vitro* studies. showed that EVI1 affected cellular proliferation, differentiation, and apoptosis [98]. EVI-1 was also found overexpressed in infratentorial ependymomas, it can promote proliferation of ependymal tumor cells, and its expression indicates an unfavorable prognosis [99].

U87 cell line presented several predicted TFs with significant p values and higher enrichment index than other cell lines. Most of the predicted TFs are related to apoptosis (PPARG, Batch2, PEBP, HLF, AP1 and EVI1), but they were associated with up- or down-regulated genes. Overall, the biological functions of these TFs are related to cell proliferation, differentiation and tumor growth, indicating the relevance of their deregulation in cancer development and malignancy, and possibly, in tumor responses to anti-cancer therapies.

4.4. Exclusively predicted TFs for irradiated T98G cell line

Only two TFs were predicted for T98G cells: EBF and C/EBP. The early B-cell factors (EBF) are a family of four highly conserved DNA-binding transcription factors with an atypical zinc-finger and helix-loop-helix motif. Zardo and colleagues found that the EBF3 locus on the human chromosome 10q is deleted or methylated in brain tumors [100]. Functional studies revealed that EBF3 activates genes involved in cell cycle arrest and apoptosis, while in opposite, it represses genes involved in cell survival and proliferation [101]. Therefore, EBFs represent a novel tumor suppressor whose inactivation blocks normal development and contributes to tumorigenesis of diverse types of human cancer [102].

CEBP is also known as basic leucine zipper transcription factor, CCAAT/enhancer binding protein alpha (CEBPA), which directly interacts with CDK2 and CDK4 and arrests cell proliferation by inhibition of these kinases [103]. CEBPA is crucial for normal granulopoiesis, and dominant-negative mutations of CEBPA gene were found in patients with myeloblastic subtypes (M1 and M2) of acute myeloid leukemia [104]. CEBPA also plays a role in DNA damage response dependent on TP53, as observed in keratinocytes [105]. C/EBPA was found silenced in human squamous cell carcinoma (SCC), and loss of C/EBPA confers susceptibility to UVB-induced skin SCCs involving defective cell cycle arrest in response to UVB [106]. Interestingly, these findings indicate the role of CEBP in DNA damage responses, and possibly, the potential of this TF to be explored as therapeutic molecular target.

4.5. Validation of TF prediction

As a predicted TF associated with up-regulated genes, HEB (p-value = 0.021 and EI = 1.5) was chosen to be studied in terms of expression levels, aiming to validate the *in silico* analysis, although for a single TF. Interestingly, we showed that HEB transcript expression was up-regulated (+2.6) in irradiated U87 cell line, 30 min. after irradiation, while HEB protein expression analyzed by Western blot was 1.7 higher in irradiated (8 Gy) cells, relatively to un-exposed controls.

HEB is a member of the class A basic helix-loop-helix (bHLH) family that participates in the nervous system development [107, 108]. According to O'Neil et al. [109], the repression of E47/HEB has been associated with the induction of leukemia in mice. In another study, it was demonstrated the induction of HEB in gliomas compared with non-neoplastic brain tissue [110]. Moreover, HEB seems to be involved in cell proliferation control of neural stem cells and also progenitor cells, being important to sustain their undifferentiated state during embryonic and adult neurogenesis [108]. Although HEB expression has not yet been correlated with radiation responses in GBM cells, in the present study, we found its association with significant differentially expressed genes at 30 min. following irradiation in U87 cell line; interestingly, we also showed that HEB transcript and protein expression was induced in irradiated U87 cell line, 30 min. after irradiation. This finding, although restrict to one TF, indicates the validity of the TF prediction by *in silico* analysis.

5. Conclusions: Lessons from TF prediction in irradiated GBM cells

The present findings about prediction of TFs associated to differentially expressed genes in GBM cell lines showed that few TFs were shared among different GBM cell lines, while several TFs were found exclusive to each cell line, indicating that the transcriptional response to ionizing radiation is very particular to each cell line, probably due to the genetic heterogeneity, which is characteristic of GBM cell lines. In spite of this observation, several biological functions were similar among cell lines, such as apoptosis, cell proliferation, cell cycle control, DNA repair, ER stress, and differentiation. Furthermore, most of the predicted TFs were already reported as differentially expressed, deleted or mutated in cancer, including GBM. However, apart the similarity of biological functions, different pathways seems to be associated to the predicted TFs. Interestingly, we could not find TP53 as a TF associated to the data set (List #1) analyzed in the present study, even for the GBM cells that were wild-type for *TP53* gene, and even considering the presence of *TP53* cDNA clone in the microarray slide. It is possible that the TP53 protein could not be activated in GBM cells, impairing its action as transcription factor, as previously suggested by other authors [111].

The most intriguing finding refers to apoptotic related TFs. Probably, predicted TFs related to apoptosis control, and found associated with expressed genes at early time (30 minutes) following irradiation, are related to survival in GBM cells; this is supported by reports showing that in general, these cells are very resistant to undergo apoptosis, even under conditions of drug treatment or radiation exposure [112-114]. In fact, GBM cells seem to be capable of activating several pathways to escaping from cell killing by anticancer therapies.

Even considering the relevance of our findings, some methodological limitations should be mentioned regarding *in silico* prediction of TFs. Despite the great advancement in terms of DNA binding sites detection, it is hard to determine which sites are functional regulatory elements that influence transcription. It is possible that a considerable fraction of these binding sites are nonfunctional and may constitute biological noise [115]. Other choices, such as ChIP experiments, may overcome this concern by detecting indirect TF-DNA interactions through protein/protein interaction [116].

In spite of the limitation mentioned above, in a previous study, we validated the expression of E2F [31] and the HEB expression was confirmed in the present study, both of them in GBM cell lines. In addition, we selected predicted TFs that were associated with stress response genes, and importantly, the TFs were reported as deregulated or mutated in different cancer types, thus indicating the relevance of further studies to better exploring the role of TFs in the context of therapeutic strategies based on molecular targets.

Author details

P. R. D. V. Godoy[1], S. S. Mello[1], F. S. Donaires[1], E. A. Donadi[2], G. A. S. Passos[3] and E. T. Sakamoto-Hojo[1,4]

1 Department of Genetics, Faculty of Medicine, University of São Paulo, Ribeirão Preto, SP, Brazil

2 Department of Medic Clinic, Faculty of Medicine, University of São Paulo, Ribeirão Preto, SP, Brazil

3 Department of Genetics, Faculty of Medicine and Faculty of Dentistry, University of São Paulo, Ribeirão Preto, SP, Brazil

4 Department of Biology, Faculty of Philosophy, Sciences and Letters-USP, University of São Paulo, Ribeirão Preto, SP, Brazil

References

[1] Chen, J, RM McKay, and LF Parada, Malignant glioma: lessons from genomics, mouse models, and stem cells. Cell, 2012. 149(1): p. 36-47.

[2] Ohgaki, H, Genetic pathways to glioblastomas. Neuropathology, 2005. 25(1): p. 1-7.

[3] McLendon, R et al., Comprehensive genomic characterization defines human glioblastoma genes and core pathways. Nature, 2008. 455(7216): p. 1061-8.

[4] Parsons, DW, et al., An integrated genomic analysis of human glioblastoma multiforme. Science, 2008. 321(5897): p. 1807-12.

[5] Stupp, R, et al., Radiotherapy plus concomitant and adjuvant temozolomide for glioblastoma. N Engl J Med, 2005. 352(10): p. 987-96.

[6] Ohka, F, A Natsume, and T Wakabayashi, Current trends in targeted therapies for glioblastoma multiforme. Neurol Res Int, 2012. 2012: p. 878425.

[7] Stupp, R, et al., Chemoradiotherapy in malignant glioma: standard of care and future directions. J Clin Oncol, 2007. 25(26): p. 4127-36.

[8] Sathornsumetee, S, et al., Molecularly targeted therapy for malignant glioma. Cancer, 2007. 110(1): p. 13-24.

[9] Perry, J, et al., Novel therapies in glioblastoma. Neurol Res Int, 2012. 2012: p. 428565.

[10] Polivka, J, Jr., et al., New molecularly targeted therapies for glioblastoma multiforme. Anticancer Res, 2012. 32(7): p. 2935-46.

[11] Natsume, A, et al., Glioma-initiating cells and molecular pathology: implications for therapy. Brain Tumor Pathol, 2011. 28(1): p. 1-12.

[12] Thomas, MC and CM Chiang, The general transcription machinery and general co-factors. Crit Rev Biochem Mol Biol, 2006. 41(3): p. 105-78.

[13] Maston, GA, SK Evans, and MR Green, Transcriptional regulatory elements in the human genome. Annu Rev Genomics Hum Genet, 2006. 7: p. 29-59.

[14] Hampsey, M, Molecular genetics of the RNA polymerase II general transcriptional machinery. Microbiol Mol Biol Rev, 1998. 62(2): p. 465-503.

[15] Gaston, K and PS Jayaraman, Transcriptional repression in eukaryotes: repressors and repression mechanisms. Cell Mol Life Sci, 2003. 60(4): p. 721-41.

[16] Battaglia, S, O Maguire, and MJ Campbell, Transcription factor co-repressors in cancer biology: roles and targeting. Int J Cancer, 2010. 126(11): p. 2511-9.

[17] Thorne, JL, MJ Campbell, and BM Turner, Transcription factors, chromatin and cancer. Int J Biochem Cell Biol, 2009. 41(1): p. 164-75.

[18] Mees, C, J Nemunaitis, and N Senzer, Transcription factors: their potential as targets for an individualized therapeutic approach to cancer. Cancer Gene Ther, 2009. 16(2): p. 103-12.

[19] Kel, A, et al., Beyond microarrays: find key transcription factors controlling signal transduction pathways. BMC Bioinformatics, 2006. 7 Suppl 2: p. S13.

[20] Tusher, VG, R Tibshirani, and G Chu, Significance analysis of microarrays applied to the ionizing radiation response. Proc Natl Acad Sci U S A, 2001. 98(9): p. 5116-21.

[21] Sakamoto-Hojo, ET, et al., Gene expression profiles in human cells submitted to genotoxic stress. Mutat Res, 2003. 544(2-3): p. 403-13.

[22] Fachin, AL, et al., Gene expression profiles in human lymphocytes irradiated in vitro with low doses of gamma rays. Radiat Res, 2007. 168(6): p. 650-65.

[23] Fachin, AL, et al., Gene expression profiles in radiation workers occupationally exposed to ionizing radiation. J Radiat Res (Tokyo), 2009. 50(1): p. 61-71.

[24] Carminati, PO, et al., Alterations in gene expression profiles correlated with cisplatin cytotoxicity in the glioma U343 cell line. Genet Mol Biol, 2010. 33(1): p. 159-68.

[25] Godoy, PRDV, et al. Portrait of transcriptional expression profiles displayed by different glioblastoma cell lines. in: M Garami. (ed.) Molecular Targets of CNS Tumors. Rijeka: InTech; 2011. p. 277-300.

[26] da Silva, GN, et al., Expression of genes related to apoptosis, cell cycle and signaling pathways are independent of TP53 status in urinary bladder cancer cells. Mol Biol Rep, 2011. 38(6): p. 4159-70.

[27] Otomo, T, et al., Microarray analysis of temporal gene responses to ionizing radiation in two glioblastoma cell lines: up-regulation of DNA repair genes. J Radiat Res (Tokyo), 2004. 45(1): p. 53-60.

[28] Godoy, PRDV, et al., Glioblastoma cell lines differing in TP53 status (mutant or wild-type) display different molecular signaling responses to gamma-irradiation Submitted, 2013.

[29] Al-Shahrour, F, et al., FatiGO +: a functional profiling tool for genomic data. Integration of functional annotation, regulatory motifs and interaction data with microarray experiments. Nucleic Acids Res, 2007. 35(Web Server issue): p. W91-6.

[30] Al-Shahrour, F, et al., BABELOMICS: a suite of web tools for functional annotation and analysis of groups of genes in high-throughput experiments. Nucleic Acids Res, 2005. 33(Web Server issue): p. W460-4.

[31] Donaires, FS, et al., Transcriptional factors associated to over-expressed genes in glioblastoma multiforme, as predicted by in silico analysis on publicly microarray data-set Submitted, 2013.

[32] Dirks, PB, et al., Retinoic acid and the cyclin dependent kinase inhibitors synergistically alter proliferation and morphology of U343 astrocytoma cells. Oncogene, 1997. 15(17): p. 2037-48.

[33] Filippi-Chiela, EC, et al., Autophagy interplay with apoptosis and cell cycle regulation in the growth inhibiting effect of resveratrol in glioma cells. PLoS ONE, 2011. 6(6): p. e20849.

[34] Lennon, G, et al., The I.M.A.G.E. Consortium: An Integrated Molecular Analysis of Genomes and Their Expression. Genomics, 1996. 33(1): p. 151-152.

[35] Hegde, P, et al., A concise guide to cDNA microarray analysis. Biotechniques, 2000. 29(3): p. 548-50, 552-4, 556 passim.

[36] Mello, SS, et al., Delayed effects of exposure to a moderate radiation dose on transcription profiles in human primary fibroblasts. Environ Mol Mutagen, 2011. 52(2): p. 117-29.

[37] Saeed, AI, et al., TM4: a free, open-source system for microarray data management and analysis. Biotechniques, 2003. 34(2): p. 374-8.

[38] Wingender, E, et al., TRANSFAC: an integrated system for gene expression regulation. Nucleic Acids Res, 2000. 28(1): p. 316-9.

[39] Robertson, G, et al., cisRED: a database system for genome-scale computational discovery of regulatory elements. Nucleic Acids Res, 2006. 34(Database issue): p. D68-73.

[40] Ferretti, V, et al., PReMod: a database of genome-wide mammalian cis-regulatory module predictions. Nucleic Acids Res, 2007. 35(Database issue): p. D122-6.

[41] Bieda, M, et al., Unbiased location analysis of E2F1-binding sites suggests a widespread role for E2F1 in the human genome. Genome Res, 2006. 16(5): p. 595-605.

[42] Birney, E, et al., Identification and analysis of functional elements in 1% of the human genome by the ENCODE pilot project. Nature, 2007. 447(7146): p. 799-816.

[43] Cawley, S, et al., Unbiased mapping of transcription factor binding sites along human chromosomes 21 and 22 points to widespread regulation of noncoding RNAs. Cell, 2004. 116(4): p. 499-509.

[44] Bowman, T, et al., Stat3-mediated Myc expression is required for Src transformation and PDGF-induced mitogenesis. Proc Natl Acad Sci U S A, 2001. 98(13): p. 7319-24.

[45] Brennan, C, et al., Glioblastoma subclasses can be defined by activity among signal transduction pathways and associated genomic alterations. PLoS ONE, 2009. 4(11): p. e7752.

[46] Lo, HW, et al., Constitutively activated STAT3 frequently coexpresses with epidermal growth factor receptor in high-grade gliomas and targeting STAT3 sensitizes them to Iressa and alkylators. Clin Cancer Res, 2008. 14(19): p. 6042-54.

[47] Weissenberger, J, et al., IL-6 is required for glioma development in a mouse model. Oncogene, 2004. 23(19): p. 3308-16.

[48] Doucette, TA, et al., Signal transducer and activator of transcription 3 promotes angiogenesis and drives malignant progression in glioma. Neuro Oncol, 2012.

[49] Sen, M, et al., First-in-Human Trial of a STAT3 Decoy Oligonucleotide in Head and Neck Tumors: Implications for Cancer Therapy. Cancer Discov, 2012. 2(8): p. 694-705.

[50] Gachon, F, et al., The loss of circadian PAR bZip transcription factors results in epilepsy. Genes Dev, 2004. 18(12): p. 1397-412.

[51] Benito, A, et al., A novel role for proline- and acid-rich basic region leucine zipper (PAR bZIP) proteins in the transcriptional regulation of a BH3-only proapoptotic gene. J Biol Chem, 2006. 281(50): p. 38351-7.

[52] De Angelis, R, et al., Functional interaction of the subunit 3 of RNA polymerase II (RPB3) with transcription factor-4 (ATF4). FEBS Lett, 2003. 547(1-3): p. 15-9.

[53] Tian, X, et al., Modulation of CCAAT/enhancer binding protein homologous protein (CHOP)-dependent DR5 expression by nelfinavir sensitizes glioblastoma multiforme cells to tumor necrosis factor-related apoptosis-inducing ligand (TRAIL). J Biol Chem, 2011. 286(33): p. 29408-16.

[54] Blais, JD, et al., Activating transcription factor 4 is translationally regulated by hypoxic stress. Mol Cell Biol, 2004. 24(17): p. 7469-82.

[55] Blank, V and NC Andrews, The Maf transcription factors: regulators of differentiation. Trends Biochem Sci, 1997. 22(11): p. 437-41.

[56] Asting, AG, et al., COX-2 gene expression in colon cancer tissue related to regulating factors and promoter methylation status. BMC Cancer, 2011. 11: p. 238.

[57] Natkunam, Y, et al., Characterization of c-Maf transcription factor in normal and neoplastic hematolymphoid tissue and its relevance in plasma cell neoplasia. Am J Clin Pathol, 2009. 132(3): p. 361-71.

[58] Crawford, EL, et al., CEBPG regulates ERCC5/XPG expression in human bronchial epithelial cells and this regulation is modified by E2F1/YY1 interactions. Carcinogenesis, 2007. 28(12): p. 2552-9.

[59] Mullins, DN, et al., CEBPG transcription factor correlates with antioxidant and DNA repair genes in normal bronchial epithelial cells but not in individuals with bronchogenic carcinoma. BMC Cancer, 2005. 5: p. 141.

[60] O'Donovan, A, et al., Isolation of active recombinant XPG protein, a human DNA repair endonuclease. J Biol Chem, 1994. 269(23): p. 15965-8.

[61] Lee, BK, AA Bhinge, and VR Iyer, Wide-ranging functions of E2F4 in transcriptional activation and repression revealed by genome-wide analysis. Nucleic Acids Res, 2011. 39(9): p. 3558-73.

[62] Graham, JD and CL Clarke, Physiological action of progesterone in target tissues. Endocr Rev, 1997. 18(4): p. 502-19.

[63] Grunberg, SM, et al., Treatment of unresectable meningiomas with the antiprogesterone agent mifepristone. J Neurosurg, 1991. 74(6): p. 861-6.

[64] Schrell, UM, et al., Hormonal dependency of cerebral meningiomas. Part 1: Female sex steroid receptors and their significance as specific markers for adjuvant medical therapy. J Neurosurg, 1990. 73(5): p. 743-9.

[65] Mahesh, VB, DW Brann, and LB Hendry, Diverse modes of action of progesterone and its metabolites. J Steroid Biochem Mol Biol, 1996. 56(1-6 Spec No): p. 209-19.

[66] Tsai, SY and MJ Tsai, Chick ovalbumin upstream promoter-transcription factors (COUP-TFs): coming of age. Endocr Rev, 1997. 18(2): p. 229-40.

[67] Lee, CT, et al., The nuclear orphan receptor COUP-TFII is required for limb and skeletal muscle development. Mol Cell Biol, 2004. 24(24): p. 10835-43.

[68] Takamoto, N, et al., COUP-TFII is essential for radial and anteroposterior patterning of the stomach. Development, 2005. 132(9): p. 2179-89.

[69] You, LR, et al., Suppression of Notch signalling by the COUP-TFII transcription factor regulates vein identity. Nature, 2005. 435(7038): p. 98-104.

[70] You, LR, et al., Mouse lacking COUP-TFII as an animal model of Bochdalek-type congenital diaphragmatic hernia. Proc Natl Acad Sci U S A, 2005. 102(45): p. 16351-6.

[71] Qin, J, et al., COUP-TFII regulates tumor growth and metastasis by modulating tumor angiogenesis. Proc Natl Acad Sci U S A, 2010. 107(8): p. 3687-92.

[72] Shaw, EJ, et al., Gene expression in oligodendroglial tumors. Cell Oncol (Dordr), 2011. 34(4): p. 355-67.

[73] Issemann, I and S Green, Activation of a member of the steroid hormone receptor superfamily by peroxisome proliferators. Nature, 1990. 347(6294): p. 645-50.

[74] Robbins, GT and D Nie, PPAR gamma, bioactive lipids, and cancer progression. Front Biosci, 2012. 17: p. 1816-34.

[75] Cellai, I, et al., Antineoplastic effects of rosiglitazone and PPARgamma transactivation in neuroblastoma cells. Br J Cancer, 2006. 95(7): p. 879-88.

[76] Grommes, C, et al., Inhibition of in vivo glioma growth and invasion by peroxisome proliferator-activated receptor gamma agonist treatment. Mol Pharmacol, 2006. 70(5): p. 1524-33.

[77] Strakova, N, et al., Peroxisome proliferator-activated receptors (PPAR) agonists affect cell viability, apoptosis and expression of cell cycle related proteins in cell lines of glial brain tumors. Neoplasma, 2005. 52(2): p. 126-36.

[78] Chearwae, W and JJ Bright, PPARgamma agonists inhibit growth and expansion of CD133+ brain tumour stem cells. Br J Cancer, 2008. 99(12): p. 2044-53.

[79] Pestereva, E, S Kanakasabai, and JJ Bright, PPARgamma agonists regulate the expression of stemness and differentiation genes in brain tumour stem cells. Br J Cancer, 2012. 106(10): p. 1702-12.

[80] Veliceasa, D, FT Schulze-Hoepfner, and OV Volpert, PPARgamma and Agonists against Cancer: Rational Design of Complementation Treatments. PPAR Res, 2008. 2008: p. 945275.

[81] Oyake, T, et al., Bach proteins belong to a novel family of BTB-basic leucine zipper transcription factors that interact with MafK and regulate transcription through the NF-E2 site. Mol Cell Biol, 1996. 16(11): p. 6083-95.

[82] Shim, KS, et al., Bach2 is involved in neuronal differentiation of N1E-115 neuroblastoma cells. Exp Cell Res, 2006. 312(12): p. 2264-78.

[83] Sasaki, S, et al., Cloning and expression of human B cell-specific transcription factor BACH2 mapped to chromosome 6q15. Oncogene, 2000. 19(33): p. 3739-49.

[84] Hoshino, H, et al., Oxidative stress abolishes leptomycin B-sensitive nuclear export of transcription repressor Bach2 that counteracts activation of Maf recognition element. J Biol Chem, 2000. 275(20): p. 15370-6.

[85] Muto, A, et al., Identification of Bach2 as a B-cell-specific partner for small maf proteins that negatively regulate the immunoglobulin heavy chain gene 3' enhancer. Embo J, 1998. 17(19): p. 5734-43.

[86] Yeung, K, et al., Suppression of Raf-1 kinase activity and MAP kinase signalling by RKIP. Nature, 1999. 401(6749): p. 173-7.

[87] Wu, K and B Bonavida, The activated NF-kappaB-Snail-RKIP circuitry in cancer regulates both the metastatic cascade and resistance to apoptosis by cytotoxic drugs. Crit Rev Immunol, 2009. 29(3): p. 241-54.

[88] Martinho, O, et al., Downregulation of RKIP is associated with poor outcome and malignant progression in gliomas. PLoS ONE, 2012. 7(1): p. e30769.

[89] Ju, W, et al., Identification of genes with differential expression in chemoresistant epithelial ovarian cancer using high-density oligonucleotide microarrays. Oncol Res, 2009. 18(2-3): p. 47-56.

[90] van der Heul-Nieuwenhuijsen, L, NF Dits, and G Jenster, Gene expression of forkhead transcription factors in the normal and diseased human prostate. BJU Int, 2009. 103(11): p. 1574-80.

[91] Pierrou, S, et al., Cloning and characterization of seven human forkhead proteins: binding site specificity and DNA bending. Embo J, 1994. 13(20): p. 5002-12.

[92] Smith, KS, et al., Disrupted differentiation and oncogenic transformation of lymphoid progenitors in E2A-HLF transgenic mice. Mol Cell Biol, 1999. 19(6): p. 4443-51.

[93] Shaulian, E and M Karin, AP 1 in cell proliferation and survival. Oncogene, 2001. 20(19): p. 2390-400.

[94] Schreiber, M, et al., Control of cell cycle progression by c-Jun is p53 dependent. Genes Dev, 1999. 13(5): p. 607-19.

[95] Wilson, RE, et al., Early response gene signalling cascades activated by ionising radiation in primary human B cells. Oncogene, 1993. 8(12): p. 3229-37.

[96] Liu, Y, et al., Inhibition of AP-1 transcription factor causes blockade of multiple signal transduction pathways and inhibits breast cancer growth. Oncogene, 2002. 21(50): p. 7680-9.

[97] Libermann, TA and LF Zerbini, Targeting transcription factors for cancer gene therapy. Curr Gene Ther, 2006. 6(1): p. 17-33.

[98] Wieser, R, The oncogene and developmental regulator EVI1: expression, biochemical properties, and biological functions. Gene, 2007. 396(2): p. 346-57.

[99] Koos, B, et al., The transcription factor evi-1 is overexpressed, promotes proliferation, and is prognostically unfavorable in infratentorial ependymomas. Clin Cancer Res, 2011. 17(11): p. 3631-7.

[100] Zardo, G, et al., Integrated genomic and epigenomic analyses pinpoint biallelic gene inactivation in tumors. Nat Genet, 2002. 32(3): p. 453-8.

[101] Zhao, LY, et al., An EBF3-mediated transcriptional program that induces cell cycle arrest and apoptosis. Cancer Res, 2006. 66(19): p. 9445-52.

[102] Liao, D, Emerging roles of the EBF family of transcription factors in tumor suppression. Mol Cancer Res, 2009. 7(12): p. 1893-901.

[103] Wang, H, et al., C/EBPalpha arrests cell proliferation through direct inhibition of Cdk2 and Cdk4. Mol Cell, 2001. 8(4): p. 817-28.

[104] Pabst, T, et al., Dominant-negative mutations of CEBPA, encoding CCAAT/enhancer binding protein-alpha (C/EBPalpha), in acute myeloid leukemia. Nat Genet, 2001. 27(3): p. 263-70.

[105] Yoon, K and RC Smart, C/EBPalpha is a DNA damage-inducible p53-regulated mediator of the G1 checkpoint in keratinocytes. Mol Cell Biol, 2004. 24(24): p. 10650-60.

[106] Thompson, EA, et al., C/EBPalpha expression is downregulated in human nonmelanoma skin cancers and inactivation of C/EBPalpha confers susceptibility to UVB-induced skin squamous cell carcinomas. J Invest Dermatol, 2011. 131(6): p. 1339-46.

[107] Ravanpay, AC and JM Olson, E protein dosage influences brain development more than family member identity. J Neurosci Res, 2008. 86(7): p. 1472-81.

[108] Uittenbogaard, M and A Chiaramello, Expression of the bHLH transcription factor Tcf12 (ME1) gene is linked to the expansion of precursor cell populations during neurogenesis. Brain Res Gene Expr Patterns, 2002. 1(2): p. 115-21.

[109] O'Neil, J, et al., TAL1/SCL induces leukemia by inhibiting the transcriptional activity of E47/HEB. Cancer Cell, 2004. 5(6): p. 587-96.

[110] Riemenschneider, MJ, TH Koy, and G Reifenberger, Expression of oligodendrocyte lineage genes in oligodendroglial and astrocytic gliomas. Acta Neuropathol, 2004. 107(3): p. 277-82.

[111] Shu, HK, et al., The intrinsic radioresistance of glioblastoma-derived cell lines is associated with a failure of p53 to induce p21(BAX) expression. Proc Natl Acad Sci U S A, 1998. 95(24): p. 14453-8.

[112] Rubel, A, et al., The membrane targeted apoptosis modulators erucylphosphocholine and erucylphosphohomocholine increase the radiation response of human glioblastoma cell lines in vitro. Radiat Oncol, 2006. 1: p. 6.

[113] Honda, N, et al., Radiosensitization by overexpression of the nonphosphorylation form of IkappaB-alpha in human glioma cells. J Radiat Res, 2002. 43(3): p. 283-92.

[114] Yamagishi, N, J Miyakoshi, and H Takebe, Enhanced radiosensitivity by inhibition of nuclear factor kappa B activation in human malignant glioma cells. Int J Radiat Biol, 1997. 72(2): p. 157-62.

[115] Struhl, K, Gene regulation. A paradigm for precision. Science, 2001. 293(5532): p. 1054-5.

[116] Chen, X, et al., Integration of external signaling pathways with the core transcriptional network in embryonic stem cells

Section 8

Stem Cells

Chapter 22

Brain Tumor Stemness

Andrés Felipe Cardona and León Darío Ortíz

Additional information is available at the end of the chapter

http://dx.doi.org/10.5772/52633

1. Introduction

The incidence of primary tumors of the central nervous system (CNS) has been estimated in 15.8/100,000 and 17.2/100,000 individuals for men and women, respectively [1,2], which globally represents approximately 190,000 new cases per year. They represent the 3rd most common cause of death from cancer in middle-aged men, and the 4th most common in women between 15 and 34 years of age [3,4]. The most frequent tumors called gliomas exhibit glial characteristics on pathologic examination [1,3]. Despite advances in the knowledge of the molecular biology of gliomas, effective therapeutic strategies remain elusive. After multimodality treatment with surgery, radiation and chemotherapy, the overall survival (OS) of patients with Glioblastoma (GB), the most frequent glioma, is around 14.6 months and the survival at 2 years is 26% [5, 6, 7, 8]. Although it is recognized that there are progenitor cells that can differentiate into neuronal and glial cells, the concept of a brain tumor stem cells is more controversial. In 2002, Altman and colleagues proposed the theory of post-natal neurogenesis that, associated with the finding of progenitor cells in glial tumors, suggested that these cells could be targeted for more effective therapies[9]. One of the difficulties is that there are no specific phenotypic markers for these cancer stem cells, and, therefore, their identification is limited to a functional characterization.

Nonetheless, pluripotent cells obtained from human brain tumors that express the CD133 surface marker (or Prominin 1; PROM1 is the founding member of pentaspantransmembrane glycoproteins) have the ability for sustained self-renewal, proliferation and tumor initiation/propagation. Furthermore, this functionally defined glioma stem cells form a niche around the blood vessels, being highly pro- angiogenic; those are regulated by hypoxia and are resistant to conventional oncologic treatment like radiotherapy and/or chemotherapy [10, 11]. In addition, they have important migration and invasion capabilities while actively interacting with the immune system. Therefore, therapeutic opportunities include targeting of stem cell specific pathways, induction of differentiation of stem cells, blocking microenvironment signals (including angiogenesis factors), and harnessing the immune system to recognize and attack stem cells. Significant challenges continues since the presence of cancer stem cells within the tumor is highly heterogenous, they can remain quiescent for years, and they may share biological features with normal stem cells [12, 13].

We present here a detailed review of the published literature on cancer stem cells of gliomas and meduloblastomas, and their possible relationships with the response to chemo-radiotherapy and to future therapeutic interventions. Similarly, we discuss their role in the progression of the disease, and we provide an analysis of the functional properties of neuronal progenitor cells and of their tumor homologues that lose their regulatory capacity during the process of neurogenesis.

2. Identification of progenitor cells in the brain and the relationship with glial tumors

Cancer only develops after mutations occurs in a few cells. These abnormal cells lose the capacity for self -regulation and have the potential for uncontrolled proliferation [12]. Two hypothetical models have been invoked to explain this phenomenon. The first is the "stochastic" which predicts that all cells have a homogeneous capacity to initiate a neoplasm with areas in which the elements are activated in a synchronic and constitutive manner [12]. The second model is the "hierarchic" which assumes that only a sub-group of cells in the tumor has the potential to proliferate and to generate new neoplasic focus; the other cells act as support or representate well-differentiated or terminal tumor cells. This model explains the findings of the pluripotent progenitor cells in acute myeloid leukemia, in cerebral tumors, and in cancer of the breast, prostate and colon [13, 14]. Nevertheless, those two models are not exclusive and it is likely that there is a combination of both scenarios in most types of cancer. Fig. (1) Summarizes the principal molecular alterations of cerebral tumors of glial origin.

Early studies by Nottebohm et al. reported the discovery of neural embryonic tissue in the cerebral parenchyma of birds [15],followed by reports of similar findings in rodents, primates and humans [16]. As a consequence, it is generally accepted that neurogenesis persists during adulthood, particularly at the level of the dentate gyrus of the hippocampus (in the hilus and in several planes of the granular laminae) and in the upper region of the deep lateral ventricles, neighboring the striated body, as shown in Fig. (2).These cells constitute about 0.2% of the elements forming the encephalon, primitively associated with the telencephalon and generally expressing the glial fibrillary acidic protein (GFAP) [16, 17]. They have a putative role in, and are capable of regenerating the neurogenetic structure in vivo and in vitro; generally enjoying a state of relative quiescence with a cell cycle of about 28 days (type B cells or pluripotent astrocytes) [18].

Usually, the pluripotent progenitor cells have a capacity of generating other second-order progenitor elements that divide every 12 hours (rapid proliferation phase). These cells, termed type C (immature precursors), maintain multipotent capacity and generate other neuronal precursors with greater maturity, termed type A cells (migrant neuroblasts). This type A cells are capable of migrating in groups across the rostral portion of the lateral ventricle up to the olfactory bulb where they are integrated as new interneurons in different layers of the cortex (Fig. 2) [19].The subventricular stem cells are conserved in eutherian mammals, but only in man is the cellular displacement not grouped, but rather individual; and follow a destiny that, as-yet, has not been clarified [20]. Analogously to the subventricular zone, the hippocampus granular region amplifies some lesser-known precursor cells termed type D, which have limited migratory capacity (short distances) [20].

From the neurochemical perspective, the type B cells express intermediate filaments such as vimentin and nestin, and are characteristically negative for the neuronal markers PSA-NCAM (Poly-Sialated Neural Cell Adhesion Molecule) and TuJ1 (class III beta-tubulin) [21]. They frequently express PDGFR-α (platelet-derived growth factor receptor) which appears to act as a regulator of balance for the differentiation between the oligodendrocytes and neurons during the phase of asymmetric neurogenesis. The type B cells, while being highly sensitive to stimulation by epidermal growth factor (EGF) and FGF2 (fibroblast growth factor type 2) [20], show constitutive positivity for CD133.

The expression of CD133 marker has been observed in normal progenitor cells, glial tumors and central nervous system neoplasms ("neurosphere" model) [22, 23]. CD133 is a 130 KDa surface glycoprotein with 5 transmembrane domains [24]. There are several isoforms of CD133 regulated by methylation, but their specific regulatory roles in transcription are still unknown [24]. Some reports suggest that their position in the membrane has some relationship with the dynamic organization of cell structure and, as such, determines cell polarity, migration and interaction with other neighboring cells, especially with those belonging to the tumor endothelium [21, 25]. The CD133 positive (CD133+) cells have a series of mechanisms that contribute to preferential activation of regulatory points of the cell cycle, increasing its resistance to standard chemotherapy and radiation therapy. [26]. This finding and other routes of abnormal activation such as Wnt/β-catenin (Wnt was coined as a combination of Wg and Int and can be pronounced as 'wint'), Notch (The notch signaling pathway is a highly conserved cell signaling system present in most multicellular organism), SHh (sonic-hedgehog), PTEN (phosphatase and tensin homolog) and Bmi-1 (polycomb ring finger oncogene) explain, at least in part, why progenitor cells of glial tumors are resistant to radiotherapy [26, 27]. In addition, these cells exhibit primary resistance to chemotherapy agents like carboplatin, paclitaxel and etoposide [28, 29].

GB are remarkably heterogeneous tumors, both phenotypically and genetically, and it is very unlikely that a single antigen will selectively identify a single population of uniquely tumorigenic cells that is common to all GBs. It is important to note that CD133-negative brain tumor cells can also generate tumors in murine cancer models, and those new cells can express CD133 in celular membrane [30]. In human tissue, another investigation have shown that A2B5, a glial progenitor marker, is expressed in human gliomas, up to 61.7% of tumoral cells, viewed on flow cytometry [31]. It would be considered that the role of CD133+ cells, versus the rest of the cell population, in brain tumor initiation and progression is still uncertain, but most of studies and models agree with the importance of CD133+ cells in tumorgenesis on the brain [16-29].

A study that evaluated the genetic expression of the BCRP1/ABCG2 (also known as Abcg2 murine/ABCG2 human) and MGMT (O-6-methylguanine-DNA methyltransferase) in glial progenitors found a significant increase in their activity, similar to various apoptosis suppressors such as Bcl-2 (B-cell lymphoma 2, apoptosis checkpoint), FLIP (inhibitory protein), BCL-XL ("B-cell lymphoma-extra large", involved in the signal transduction pathway of the FAS-L.) and of some inhibitors of pro-apoptosis proteins such as XIAP (Co-chaperone of The hsp90, immunophilin homolog XAP2), cIAP1 (cellular inhibitor of apoptosis 1), cIAP2 (cellular inhibitor of apoptosis 2), NAIP (neuronal apoptosis inhibitory protein) and survivin (baculoviral inhibitor of apoptosis repeat-containing 5 or BIRC5) [23]. Furthermore, the inhibition of the caspases 3, 7 and 9 is significantly higher in recurrent GB rich in CD133+ cells than in its counterpart in which lower counts are observed [32].

Nestin, an intermediate class IV filament that is produced in considerable quantities in normal and tumor progenitor cells during brain development and in glial neoplasms [33, 34], is a constituent part of the cytoskeleton, has the responsibility for the maintenance of the cell morphology and facilitates adhesion, proliferation and migration. In adults, nestin is expressed in the subventricular progenitor cells, in some remnants near the choroid plexus and in the prosencephalon [35]. As in high grade gliomas, nestin is re-expressed in multiple cell lines of the brain during other circumstances such as acute ischemia, trauma and meningo-encephalitis [36]. In neoplasms, the co-expression of nestin and vimentin is related to substantial increase in invasive capacity (associated with multifocality), the facility to repair external attack (nuclear nestin regulates chromatin), and motility. This combination of markers could be useful in assessing the prognosis, especially since its presence is associated to a more aggressive tumor phenotype, rich in progenitor cells [37].

The normal and tumor precursor cells share the expression of multiple markers, the capacity of unlimited regeneration, exponential proliferation and open differentiation. Additionally, they have similar telomerase activity and resistance to apoptosis, as well as a higher capacity to transport substances to membrane level [38]. The latter characteristic facilitates the exocyte of anti-neoplastic molecules via proteins of the ABC family, such as MDR-1 (Gene that encodes P-glycoprotein; ABCB1, ATP-binding cassette, sub-family B member 1), MRP-1 (human multidrug resistance protein or ABCC1), ABCA2, ABCA3 and ABCG2 (Genes that encodes the ATP-binding cassette sub-family A member 2 protein, sub-family A member 3 protein and sub-family G member 2 protein; respectively) [21, 38, 39].

3. Molecular changes that favor tumor progenitor cells

The progenitor cells of brain tumors have certain characteristics that differentiate them from their normal counterparts. By definition, the cancer stem cells need to have the capacity to develop tumors following orthotopic implantation (if the tumor is an identical phenotypic copy of the original tumor). They exhibit a sustained capacity for self-renewal and are capable of showing polyclonality [33]. Reilly et al. established a murine model that combined mutations in the p53 gene and in the gene specific for neurofibromatosis (Nf1, neurofibromin 11), capable of activating the Ras (a protein superfamily of small GTPases) pathway to favor the formation of astrocytomas. They found that the deletion of any tumor suppressor gene and/or the activation of oncogenes such as Ras and Akt (serine/threonine protein kinase) in the undifferentiated cells that express CD133 or nestin, resulted in the formation of glial tumors [40].

Another important alteration is view on PDGF. The effect of PDGF on the nestin-positive progenitor cells is equivalent to that which occurs when the loss of CDKN2A (cyclin-dependent kinase inhibitor 2A), which codes for the INK4a (tumour suppressor protein) and ARF (ADP-ribosylation factor 11) is combined with the increase in the expression of EGFR in the immature and in the mature cells [36,41]. Further, during embryogenesis neural progenitors have been shown to express the A isoform of the PDGFR, while its mature homologue (glia and neurons) is expressed on the PDGF surface. PDGFR-B is found in small quantities in pluriultipotent cells, but only increases as the cells differentiate and mature, especially into oligodendrocytes, and in the presence of phosphorylated PDGFR-A [42]. Infusion of PDGF-A in the subventricular region of certain rodents suppresses the production of neuroblasts and generates a hyperplasia of type B cells which frequently results in the development of astrocytomas and oligodendrogliomas. Additionally, activation, via the PDGF signaling, in the regions of the brain rich in precursor cells contributes to tumorigenesis, which seems to be favored by autocrine and paracrine stimulation of PDGF-A, PDGF-B and the OLIG2 (oligodendrocyte lineage transcription factor 2) transcription factors [42, 43].

Some of the signaling pathways included in the evolution of progenitor cells and in their differentiation are altered in the gliomas. The Notch pathway is essential for the maintenance of tumor cell architecture. It is expressed from embryogenesis and interacts, normally or abnormally, with multiple ligands such as DLL-1, 3 and 4 (delta-like 1, 3 and 4 respectively), together with the Jag-1 and Jag-2 proteins (jagged 1 and 2 respectively). The Notch signaling pathway controls neural differentiation and is known to maintain CNS character and to inhibit neurogenesis. The Notch–Hes (Hairy and enhancer of split) pathway is necessary for self-renewing cell division and, thus, maintenance of the neural precursor population [44-47]. Another recent studies have shown that Fbw7 acts as a molecular switch that antagonizes Notch activity and JNK/c-Jun signaling to enable neural stem cell differentiation and progenitor survival [48]. In tumor progenitors, the Notch receptors has been shown acting as a trigger for stimulation of differentiation [49] and, in preclinical studies, it has been shown experimental therapeutic implications [50]. Differentiation is mediated by tumor necrosis factor- α (TNF-α) activator enzyme and by the C-secretase, which is responsible for the signal transcription to the nucleus for unlinking responses via transcription factor CBF1/Su(H)/LAG1 (CSL) (homologous Drosophila gene Suppressor of Hairless /Longevity assurance gene 1 or cardiolipinsynthetase) [49]. This interaction results in the activation of target genes responsible for preempting differentiation and apoptosis [49] and gives the opportunity for developing therapeutic options [49, 50]. The Notch signaling pathway prevents the degradation and ubiquitous distribution of nestin in the progenitor cells, and cooperates with K-Ras (v-Ki-ras2; Kirsten rat sarcoma viral oncogene homolog) in promoting colony formation [49-51].

A study demonstrated that the inhibition of the Notch-1 receptor induces apoptosis and inhibits the proliferation of glial cell tumors that express CD133 [52]. This provides an opportunity to modulate the pathways responsible of treatment resistance, since there are compounds available that act as decoys, as inhibitors of ϒ-secretase, as intracellular bait directed against MAML-1 (mastermind-like 1), or simply as inhibitors of the Ras pathway [53, 54].

Epithelial Growth Factor is another important issue in the molecular changes on progenitor cells. Using the model of the neurosphere [22], Singh et al. inoculated cells isolated from high grade glioma into the cranium of immuno-suppressed rodents and observed that the minimum number of cells required to produce a neoplasm was 1x105. However, when the experiment was repeated using CD133+ cells stimulated by EGF, the number required was reduced to 100-fold [25, 55]. It is important to note that CD133 expression occurs not only in the neural and neoplastic progenitor cells but also in endothelial stem cells that participate in blood vessel formation necessary for the development of normal brain and for tumorigenesis [55, 56]. In preclinical models, activated EGFR signaling induce behaviors characteristic of GB on stem cells, including enhanced proliferation, survival and migration, even in the absence of EGF ligand. wtEGFR block neuronal differentiation and is associated with a dramatic increase in chemotaxis in the presence of EGF. EGFRvIII expression lead to an increase in neural stem cells proliferation and survival, while it simultaneously blocked neuronal differentiation and promoted glial fate. It gives an opportunity for terapeutic development on this EGF field [57].

4. The micro-environment of progenitor cells and glial tumors

The presence of progenitor cells in Acute Myeloid Leukemia highlights the importance of the micro-environment in maintaining its function, and the quiescent state [9, 12, 14]. The perivascular niche of the glial tumor progenitor cells is highly specialized and depends, in great part, on the capillaries that are similar to those in the periventricular region of the human brain. At the proximity to the endothelial cells, enables inter-cellular communication that causes enrichment with brain derived neurotrophic factor (BDNF), vascular endothelial growth factor C (VEGF-C) and pigment factor derived from the endothelium (PEDF) [9]; molecules that facilitate, principally, migration and neoplasic proliferation. Even more, there is consistent evidence that the extra-cellular matrix is responsible for key points in the regulation of tumor precursors via the tenascin-C gene. Expression of this gene by the cells of the neural crest translates into anti-adhesive properties that block the interaction of fibronectin with the syndecans [58]. Further, chondroitin sulfate continues stimulating the progenitor cell to maintain its primitive state, and impedes evolution of its progeny.

Although the niche affects the biology of the progenitor cells in the tumor, the communication is not unidirectional. Several studies have demonstrated that the precursors are able to promote the replication of endothelial cells, including the necessary stimulus for the forma-

http://dx.doi.org/10.5772/52633

tion of complex neovascular structures [59, 60] by increasing the concentrations of VEGF and BDNF [9, 60, 61]. Complementing these data, Calabrese et al. found, using multi-photon laser scanning microscopy, that the CD133+/nestin+ cells were always found in the intimal layer proximal to the vascular endothelium of GB, medulloblastomas, ependymomas and oligodendrogliomas [61].

Classically, pathology of high-grade gliomas describes a disorganized and aberrant vascular growth randomly generated to supply the voracity of the tumor. However, several recently published reviews explain that this architecture is available in the altered form to serve as lodging for the tumor precursors and their vascular analogues [9, 14].

Glial progenitor cells and their descendants are capable of interfering with the blood vessels of the brain, using the effect known as "perivascular satellitosis". Nevertheless, it is infrequent to find extra-axial lesions. Clinically, the microvascular density of GB correlates with prognosis [62]; a factor that contributes to the response observed in anti-angiogenesis, possibly dependent on VEGF generated in elevated quantities by the CD133+ cells [63, 64]. Further, the observation that CD133+ GB cells lose their ability to recruit endothelial cells and form blood vessels after being exposed to low concentrations of bevacizumab suggests that this effect is controlled, at least in part, by the decrease in the expression of VEGF, VEGFR2 and angiopoietin-2 (Ang-2) [9].

Data from pre-clinical studies and clinical trials indicate that three drugs that block angiogenesis may be promising therapy for high-grade gliomas, due to their inhibitory potential on the niche of tumor progenitors. An estudy demonstrated that endothelial cells increase brain tumor stem cell survival and targeting the tumor vasculature with bevacizumab reduces the number of cancer stem cells in treated tumors [65]. Bevacizumab (humanized monoclonal antibody against VEGF receptors 1 and 2) and cediranib (AZD2171, potent inhibitor of VEGF receptor tyrosine kinases type 1, 2 and 3) are being evaluated currently in clinical trials. [65, 66, 67]Those are agents that act on the VEGF 1, 2 and 3 receptors, suggesting an improvement in progression- free survival (PFS) and OS in patients with recurrent high grade gliomas. Cilengitide blocks the $\alpha v\beta 6$, $\alpha v\beta 5$ y $\alpha v\beta 3$ integrins [68] and has been evaluated in clinical trials [69, 70]. As previously mentioned, the effect of these molecules is the normalization of the tumor vessels, or the depletion of the blood flow, that interferes with the maintenance and survival of the precursor and terminal cells of the tumor, thus, anti-angiogenic therapy may function as a therapy against Glioma Stem Cells. A further nuance has come from early studies that suggest that glioblastoma cells can form parts of the tumor vasculature [71]. It is likely that anti-angiogenic drugs might not only inhibit tumor vascularization to suppress GB growth, but also directly disrupt the niches for the maintenance of GSCs, therefore weakening the "tumor roots".

5. Role of progenitor cells in meduloblastomas

The two germinal epithelia of the cerebellum are found in the deep ventricular zone of the velum of the posterior medulla and in the outermost layer of the metencephalon [72]. The matrix of the first of these regions gives rise to several neuronal and glial cell lines, and the second, only produces granular cells which are the most numerous elements in all of the prosencephalon [73]. In humans, peak growth of the cerebellum occurs later in comparison with the remainder of the CNS, and its principal stage of development is in the third trimester of gestation. In other more rudimentary mammalians this event occurs during the two weeks following birth [74]. Nevertheless, evolution of this neural structure is observed in children up to the end of the first year of life, and appears to be dependent on the presence of the CD133+ cells, which are concentrated principally in the white matter and in the rhombic lips [75].

The evidence that connects the pluripotent neural cells with the tumor elements of the meduloblastoma is merely correlative and is supported by the expression of the calbindin-D (calcium binding protein D) among the precursors of normal cerebellum and, as well as being found in 50% of the meduloblastomas, especially in those of the classical type. In contrast, nodular lesions or desmoplasias express the marker p75, which suggests a dual tumor origin. This hypothesis is supported by the behavior of the meduloblastomas induced in murine models that frequently express CD133+ but which have a specific dissimilar evolution such as, among other aspects, the aberrant activation of the Hedgehog (Hh) gene [76].

The Hh pathway regulates the development of the cerebellum in many species, but has cardinal importance among humans, where it promotes migration of precursors of granular cells, and their proliferation incited by the production of the Hh ligand in Purkinje cells. The mutation in the PTCH (patched homolog 1) receptor which results in constitutive activation of the Hh pathway is found in a great number of patients with sporadic meduloblastoma, as well as in those with Gorlin syndrome, an autosomal dominant entity characterized by coexistence of basal cell carcinomas and primitive neuroectodermal tumors [73, 75]. Approximately 14% of the mice heterozygous for the PTCH mutation develop medulobastomas, in which primary alterations of the precursors of the granular cells are frequently found, as well as changes in the SMO (smoothened) and SUFU (suppressor of fused homolog) genes, which are generators of this type of neoplasia in vivo [77]. Other animal models have demonstrated that meduloblastomas initiated by genetic changes in the different pathways of Hh also result in the activation of this signaling pathway; in particular, the inactivation of the CXCR6 (chemokine receptor CXCR6) that results in the expression of Gli1, Gli2 (GLI family zinc finger 1 and 2), Ptc2 (Hh receptor Patched type 2) and Sfrp1(secreted frizzled-related protein 1) proteins evident in the meduloblastomas, and which are susceptible to inhibition of Hh with molecules such as cyclopamine, or with specific inhibitors such as Hh-antagonist [78].

Another signaling pathway altered in sporadic and inherited meduloblastomas is the Wingless/Wnt (wingless-type MMTV integration site family member) that regulates the proliferation of progenitor cells in the deep ventricular region and in the hippocampus [9]. The loss of Wnt1, a key effector of β-catenin, causes several abnormalities in the midbrain and in the cerebellum, and is found over-expressed in classical meduloblastomas [79, 80]. Although its role in the regulation of the pluripotent progenitors of the cerebellum is not clear, it appears to depend on similar mutations to those identified in the patients with Turcot syndrome; an autosomal recessive condition caused by the loss of function of the adenomatous polyposis gene, and which is present in 5% of meduloblastomas [80]. The mutations have also been observed in a small subgroup of patients with primitive neuroectoderm tumors and results in the decrease in expression of Axin-2 (plays an important role in the regulation of the stability of beta-catenin in the Wnt signaling pathway); the gene that acts as negative regulator of Wnt and which has been detected in a small group of patients with meduloblastoma [81].

The nuclear translocation of the β-catenin resulting in the activation of the Wnt pathway is observed in 25% of the patients with meduloblastoma and, usually, corresponds to an elevated presence of the CD133 cells. Paradoxically, and in contrary to what occurs in high-grade gliomas, their presence is associated with a favorable clinical evolution, related to the absence of alterations in Hh and aberrations in chromosome 17 [82].

The Notch signaling pathway is observed to be active in the progenitor cells of the deep ventricular region and in the rhombic region. It promotes proliferation and survival and inhibits cellular differentiation. The four isoforms of the receptor do not result in the same changes in the cerebellum. For example, Notch-2 stimulates the proliferation of progenitors of the granular neuromas, while Notch-1 is associated with their differentiation; a consistent finding in the classical forms of meduloblastomas [82]. Some primitive neuroectoderm tumors show increase in the Notch-2 loci and in co-expression of the Hes1 pathway, that correlate clinically with adverse prognosis; while other studies have provided evidence for alternative and abnormal regulation Notch Hh pathway [72]. Finally, hypoxia and the protein products that this activity generates, promote the proliferation of progenitor cells of the cerebellum stimulated by the Notch pathway; a finding that has been confirmed in meduloblastomas [83]. Fig. (3) summarizes the principal signaling pathways of the neural precursors of the cerebellum and of meduloblastomas.

Several subordinate pathways can promote the generation of meduloblastomas from neural progenitor cells. The REN (renin) gene located on chromosome 17 promotes the differentiation of granular precursors, suppressing the Hh signals, an alteration that frequently results in meduloblastoma [73]. The N-myc oncogene (v-mycmyelocytomatosis viral related oncogene, neuroblastoma derived), which plays an essential role in cerebellum growth, is a primary constituent of white matter of the Hh pathway in meduloblastoma and is observed to be amplified in large cell variants, which favor a negative clinical outcome. Other transcription factors associated with the more primitive processes of progenitor cells of the cerebellum and tumor development are RE-1 (RE1-Silencing Transcription factor), OTX2 (orthodenticle homolog 2) and BMI1 (BMI1 polycomb ring finger oncogene) [72, 73]. A recent report described the substantial role of molecular alterations of CD15+/CD133– in the induction of primitive neuroectoderm brain tumors [84].

6. Therapeutic implications of tumor progenitors

The prognostic implications of the presence of stem cells in gliomas has been examined in a few clinical trials. A study that included 44 patients with GB treated surgically followed by radiotherapy and temozolamide (TMZ), evaluated the prognostic value of CD133 expression and of the capacity of the tumor to generate CD133+ cells in culture. The CD133 status, as determined by immunohistochemistry, had no prognostic value, but the in vitro capacity to generate precursors was associated to a significant reduction in OS (HR: 2.50; 95%CI: 1.04-6.06; P = 0.004) of 8 (95%CI: 4.0-11.5) and 15 months (95%CI: 11.0-19.0) for tumors with higher and lower quantity of CD133+ cells, respectively (P = 0.0002). Similarly, the PFS was also associated to the ability to generate precursors from the tumor (3.5 months for high versus 9.0 months for low grade; P = 0.0001). The CD133+ count was also associated with a higher mortality risk (HR: 1.65; 95%CI: 1.05-2.60; P = 0.0285) [85]. A similar study examining high grade oligodendrogliomas found that tumors without CD133+ cells had an improved prognosis, and this marker predicted clinical outcome better than histological assessment [86]. Another immunohistochemical analysis for nestin and CD133 of both, low grade and high grade gliomas, revealed that their expression correlates with survival, with tumors that co-express nestin+/CD133+ carrying a shorter survival [87]. These findings have stimulated the active search for new therapeutic strategies directed against the precursors of cerebral tumors, and their microenvironment.

Therapeutic interventions directed against cerebral tumor progenitor cells can be divided into three groups: firstly, directed towards provoking differentiation of the precursors; secondly, designed to eliminate the progenitor cells inhibiting their multi-potentiality and quiescence; thirdly, directed towards attacking the tumor microenvironment [88, 89].

The therapies that provoke differentiation of the progenitors focus on the capacity to reverse the malignant state and, essentially, to recover the auto-regenerative property [90]. To-date, two groups of medications affect differentiation: derivatives of retinoic acid and compounds directed against epigenetic changes (histone deacetylators).

Among the compounds directed towards eliminating progenitor cells, the therapies of note are those that are directed against tumor markers of progenitor cells expressed in cellular membrane (antibodies against CD133+) [9], the inhibitors of the Hh pathway (cyclopamine, NBT-272) [91], PPAR-γ agonists [92], TMZ [93], inhibitors of mTOR (sirolimus, everolimus, temsirolimus, deforolimus) [94], derivatives of bone morphogenetic protein (BMP) [95], target molecules directed against check-points that avoid damage induced by radiotherapy in the progenitors (Chk1 and Chk2, checkpoint homolog type 1 and 2) [15], imatinib [96, 97] and inhibitors of the ABCB super-family [98]. Similarly, it is important to mention the drugs that modify the micro-environment, among which are the angiogenesis blocking drugs such as bevacizumab [65], cediranib [67] and cilengitide [68, 69] and, equally, the inhibitors of PI3K (phosphoinositide-3-kinase) that could act turning the medulloblastoma progenitors closest to the vascular niche more sensitive to irradiation, as in vitro studies show for human endothelial cells precursors [99]. Fig. (4) highlights some strategies directed against the cell precursors of brain tumors.

The effect of retinoic acid on the CD133+ cells appears to be related to the repression of the Wnt/β-catenin pathway that slows the proliferation accompanying over-expression of Axin [100]. The same strategy is used in a preclinical model to test the effectiveness of combining 13-cis-retenoic acid with vorinostat (SAHA) in medulloblastoma cells in culture. Retinoic acid acts on the transcriptional activation of BMP-2 (Bone morphogenetic protein 2), and SAHA facilitates the apopotosis controlling chromatin; effects that lead to an increase in the sensitivity to cisplatin and etoposide [101]. Heat shock protein 90 (HSP90) operates as a supplier of β-catenin during its conformational maturation phase. The inhibitor 17-allylamino-17-demethoxygeldanamycin (17-AAG) modifies the HSP90 phenotype and affects the aberrant expression of the β-catenin. This enables the inhibition (in vivo and in vitro) of the growth of several cell lines of glioma and their progenitors CD133+, and translates into an increase in the effect of radiation on the GB; a finding that is more evident during exposure to TMZ [102].

With respect to the preponderant role of Hh in the development of normal and tumor progenitor cells, Bar et al explored the effectiveness of cyclopamine in a subpopulation of primordial GB cells [103]. In the study, 26% of the samples showed Gli (transcription factors mediating the Hh pathway isolated from Glioblastoma) over-expression, a target function of this pathway that was inhibited satisfactorily in 60% of the cases. The outcome was a significant decrease in the CD133+ progenitor growth. In parallel, the administration of cyclopamine on neurospheres inhibited the generation of new colonies, suggesting a regression of the clonogenic capacity of the glioma progenitors.

Beier et al. demonstrated that TMZ is incapable of inducing death of the CD133+ cells. Proliferation was effectively inhibited by reducing its metabolism in vitro by 72% following 7 days of incubation [93]. Depending on the subtype of cells, TMZ induces arrest in the G2-M transition or delay in the cell cycle at G2. However, in all the cultures, the cells at sub-G0 peak of apoptosis, was <8%. Genetical analysis shows that the pattern of presentation of the promoter of the MGMT gene was greater among the negative cells, which does not explain the susceptibility of the progenitors to the alkylating agent [93].

Glial progenitors and their progeny conserve a mechanism of homogeneous differentiation promoted by BMP (bone morphogenetic protein) and its ligands, reducing slightly the quantity of CD133+ cells and favoring the increase in the astroglia and of the cellular elements, similar to neurons. An study observed in some in vivo models that the therapeutic stimulus of the different isoforms of BMP delays tumor growth and the potential for vascular invasion of the GB [104].

Cancer stem cells from GB specimens seems to be immune suppressive as they inhibit mitogen T cell proliferation from normal donors [105].Therefore targeting specifically cancer stem cells may revert the immune suppressive microenvironment induced by these cells, allowing a synergistic effect when combined with immune therapy. On the other hand GB derived stem cells may be a source of unique antigens that can be used for dendritic cell vaccination, as has been demonstrated in the animal model [106].

As previously mentioned, the use of bevacizumab attenuates the capacity of the tumor progenitors to promote angiogenesis, and it will be seen not only following the regulation of acidosis and hypoxia but also by the activation of oncogenes such as PTEN and EGFR [64, 107]. Cediranib, a pan-inhibitor of VEGF receptor, normalizes the blood vessels of the tumor in patients with recurrent GB; the perilesional edema is alleviated and the capacity for pre-production of the CD133+ progenitors and the endothelium precursor cells is reduced [66]. Cilengitide reduces the expression of αvβ3 integrin in the tumor micro-environment. The migratory and proliferative capacity of the precursors is reduced by up to 60%; an effect that appears to be dependent on the dose and on the co-expression of other surface antigens of the endothelial cells (CD144 and von Willebrand factor) [68-70].

Aldehyde dehydrogenase function is used by cancer stem cells to repopulate a tumor mass after chemotherapy cytoreduction. As in hematopoyetic stem cells, it would be spected that inhibition of Aldehyde dehydrogenase helps differentiate cells. With the inhibition of aldehyde dehydrogenase, stem cell division to non-stem daughter cells tends to become blocked. Exist potent aldehyde dehydrogenase inhibitors on the market: chloral hydrate, chloramphenicol, and disulfiram, that could be useful [108].

7. Conclusion

Our understanding about cancer and the relationship with the theory of stem cells is growing up as the tumoral incidence around the world does.

Advances in molecular cell biology will give to the oncology physicians and scientist the tools for understanding the processes underlying tumorgenesis and intracelullar processes for viability, serving as possible targets in oncotherapy, diagnosis and prognosis.

Molecular characteristics that give susceptibility for brain tumors to some therapies encourage the clinicians to become experts for giving the best therapeutic choices according to molecular guidance for radio/chemotherapy or other alternatives, like biological therapy, immunotherapy and experimental treatment options.

Future about stem cells as a chapter of brain tumors is on the road for establish individualized treatment profiles, depending on clinical, pathological and molecular characteristics of patients and tumors, a traslational analysis from the molecules to the patients.

Author details

Andrés Felipe Cardona[1,2*] and León Darío Ortíz[2,3]

*Address all correspondence to: a_cardonaz@yahoo.com andres.cardona@fsfb.org.co

1 Clinical and Translational Oncology Group, Institute of Oncology, Fundación Santa Fe de Bogotá, Bogotá D.C., Colombia

2 Red LANO/ONCOL Group, Colombia

3 Neuro-Oncology Group, Institute of Oncology, Clínicalas Américas, Medellín, Colombia

http://dx.doi.org/10.5772/52633

References

[1] CBTRUS 2000-2004 data. United States population estimates by 5-year age group were obtained from United States census; estimates available at www.census.gov.

[2] Ries LAG, Melbert D, Krapcho M, et al (eds). SEER Cancer Statistics Review, 1975–2004, National Cancer Institute. Bethesda, MD, http://seer.cancer.gov/csr/1975_2004/, based on November 2006 SEER data submission, posted to the SEER web site, 2008

[3] Ferlay J, Bray F, PisaniP,et al. GLOBOCAN 2002: Cancer Incidence, Mortality and PrevalenceWorldwide, Version 2.0. IARC CancerBase No. 5. Lyon, IARCPress, 2004. Limited version available from: URL: http://www_depdb.iarc.fr/globocan2002.htm

[4] Stupp R, Roila F; ESMO Guidelines Working Group. Malignant glioma: ESMO clinical recommendations for diagnosis, treatment and follow-up. Ann Oncol. 2008; 19 (Suppl 2): 83-5.

[5] Gilbert MR. Designing clinical trials for brain tumors: the next generation. CurrOncol Rep 2007; 9: 49-54.

[6] Buckner JC. Factors influencing survival in high grade gliomas. SeminOncol 2003; 30: 10-4.

[7] Stupp R, MasonWP, van den Bent MJ, et al. Radiotherapy plus concomitant and adjuvant temozolomide for glioblastoma. N Engl J Med 2005; 352: 987-96.

[8] Wong ET, Hess KR, Gleason MJ, et al. Outcomes and prognostic factors in recurrent glioma patients enrolled onto phase II clinical trials. J ClinOncol 1999; 17: 2572-8.

[9] Gilbertson RJ, Rich JN. Making a tumour's bed: glioblastoma stem cells and the vascular niche. Nat Rev Cancer 2007; 7: 733-6.

[10] Nam DH, Park K, Suh YL, et al. Expression of VEGF and brain specific angiogenesis inhibitor-1 in glioblastoma: prognostic significance. Oncol Rep 2004; 11: 863-9.

[11] Knizetova P, Darling JL, Bartek J. Vascular endothelial growth factor in astroglioma stem cell biology and response to therapy. J Cell Mol Med 2008; 12: 111-25.

[12] Reya T, Morrison SJ, Clarke MF, et al. Stem cells, cancer, and cancer stem cells. Nature 2001; 414: 105-11.

[13] Sell S. Stem cell origin of cancer and differentiation therapy. Crit Rev OncolHematol 2004; 51: 1-28.

[14] Bonnet D, Dick JE. Human acute myeloid leukemia is organized as a hierarchy that originates from a primitive hematopoietic cell. Nature Med 1997; 3: 730-7.

[15] Nottebohm F. Neuronal replacement in adulthood. Ann NY AcadSci 1985; 457:143-161.

[16] Lie DC, Song H, Colamarino SA, et al. Neurogenesis in the adult brain: new strategies for central nervous system diseases. Annu Rev PharmacolToxicol 2004; 44: 399-421.

[17] Ming GL, Song H. Adult neurogenesis in the mammalian central nervous system. Annu Rev Neurosci 2005; 28: 223-50.

[18] Doetsch F, Caille I, Lim DA, et al. Subventricular zone astrocytes are neural stem cells in the adult mammalian brain. Cell 1999; 97: 703-16.

[19] Morshead CM. Neural stem cells in the adult mammalian forebrain: a relatively quiescent subpopulation of subependymal cells. Neuron 1994; 13: 1071-82.

[20] Sanai N, Tramontin AD, Quiñones-Hinojosa A, et al. Unique astrocyte ribbon in adult human brain contains neural stem cells but lacks chain migration. Nature 2004; 427: 740-4.

[21] Doetsch F, Garcia-Verdugo JM, Alvarez-Buylla A. Cellular composition and three-dimensional organization of the subventricular germinal zone in the adult mammalian brain. J Neurosci 2007; 17: 5046-61.

[22] Guerrero H, Chaichana K, Quiñones A et al. Neurosphere Culture and Human Organotypic Model to Evaluate Brain Tumor Stem Cells. Can St Cell; 2009;568(6):73-83.

[23] Galli R, Binda E, Orfanelli U, et al. Isolation and characterization of tumorigenic, stem-like neural precursors from human glioblastoma. Cancer Res 2004; 64: 7011-21.

[24] Kania G, Corbeil D, Fuchs J. Somatic stem cell marker prominin-1/CD133 is expressed in embryonic stem cell derived progenitors. Stem Cells 2001; 23: 791-804.

[25] Singh SK, Hawkins C, Clarke ID. Identification of human brain tumour initiating cells. Nature 2004; 432: 396-401.

[26] Bao S, Wu Q, McLendon RE. Glioma stem cells promote radioresistance by preferential activation of the DNA damage response. Nature 2006; 444: 756-60.

[27] Rich JN. Cancer stem cells in radiation resistance. Cancer Res 2007; 67:8980-4.

[28] Liu G, Yuan X, Zeng Z. Analysis of gene expression and chemoresistance of CD133+ cancer stem cells in glioblastoma. Mol Cancer 2006; 5: 67-78.

[29] Jin F, Zhao L, Guo YJ et al. Influence of Etoposide on anti-apoptotic and multidrug resistance-associated protein genes in CD133 positive U251 glioblastoma stem-like cells. Brain Res. 2010;8(1336):103-11.

[30] Wang J, Sakariassen P, Tsinkalovsky O et al. CD133 negative glioma cells form tumors in nude rats and give rise to CD133 positive cells. Int J Can. 2008;122:761–8.

[31] Ogden A, Waziri A, Lochhead R. Identification of A2B5+CD133- tumor-initiating cells in adult human gliomas. Neurosurgery. 2008;62:505–15.

[32] Schimmer AD. Inhibitor of apoptosis proteins: translating basic knowledge into clinical practice. Cancer Res 2004; 64: 7183-90.

[33] Vescovi AL, Galli R, Reynolds BA. Brain tumour stem cells. Nat Rev Cancer 2006; 426: 425-36.

[34] Dell'Albani P. Stem cell markers in gliomas. Neurochem Res 2008; 33: 2407-15.

[35] Gu H, Wang S, Messam CA, et al. Distribution of nestinimmunoreactivity in the normal adult human forebrain. Brain Res 2002; 943: 174-80.

[36] Holmin S, Almquist P, Lendahl U. Adult nestin expressing subependymal cells differentiate to astrocytes in response to brain injury. Eur J NeuroSci 1997; 9: 65-75.

[37] Dahlstrand J, Collins VP, Lendahl U. Expression of the class VI intermediate filament nestin in human central nervous system tumors. Cancer Res 1992; 52: 5334-41.

[38] Zhenju J, Lenhard R. Telomeres and telomerase in cancer stem cell. Eur J Cancer 2006; 42: 1197-203.

[39] Bi C, Fang J, Chen F et al. Chemoresistance of CD133(+) tumor stem cells from human brain glioma. Zhong Nan Da. 2007;32(4):568-73.

[40] Reilly K, Loisel D, Bronson R et al. Nf1; Trp53 mutant mice develop glioblastoma with evidence of strain-specific effects. Nat Genet. 2000;26:109–13.

[41] Bachoo RM, Maher EA, Ligon KL, et al. Epidermal growth factor receptor and Ink4a/Arf: convergent mechanisms governing terminal differentiation and transformation along the neural stem cell to astrocyte axis. Cancer Cell 2002; 1:269-77.

[42] Erlandsson A, Enarsson M, Forsberg-Nilsson K. Immature neurons from CNS stem cells proliferate in response to platelet-derived growth factor. J Neurosci 2001; 21: 3483-91.

[43] Ligon KL, Huillard E, Mehta S, et al. Olig2-regulated lineage-restricted pathway controls replication competence in neural stem cells and malignant glioma. Neuron 2007; 53: 503-17.

[44] Yoon K. Mind bomb 1-expressing intermediate progenitors generate notch signaling to maintain radial glial cells. Neuron. 2008;58:519–31.

[45] Mizutani K, Yoon K, Dang L et al. Differential Notch signalling distinguishes neural stem cells from intermediate progenitors. Nature. 2007;449:351–5.

[46] Corbin J. Regulation of neural progenitor cell development in the nervous system. J Neurochem. 2008;106:2272–87.

[47] Yoon K, Gaiano N. Notch signaling in the mammalian central nervous system: insights from mouse mutants. Nat Neurosci. 2005;8:709–15.

[48] Hoeck J, Jandke A, Blake S et al. Fbw7 controls neural stem cell differentiation and progenitor apoptosis via Notch and c-Jun. Nat Neurosc. 2010;13:1365–72.

[49] Hitoshi S, Seaberg RM, Koscik C, et al. Primitive neural stem cells from the mammalian epiblastdifferentiate to definitive neural stem cells under the control of Notch signalling. Genes Dev 2004; 18: 1806-11.

[50] Ferrari G, Bonini S, Uberti D et al. Targeting Notch pathway induces growth inhibition and differentiation of neuroblastoma cells. NeuroOncol. 2010;12(12):1231-43.

[51] Tanigaki K, Nogaki F, Takahashi J. Notch1 and Notch3 instructively restrict bFGF-responsive multipotent neural progenitor cells to an astroglial fate. Neuron 2001; 29: 45-55.

[52] Zhang XP, Zheng G, Zou L. Notch activation promotes cell proliferation and the formation of neural stem-like colonies in human glioma cells. Mol Cell Bioch 2008; 307:101-8.

[53] Purow BW, Haque RM, Noel MW, et al. Expression of Notch-1 and its ligands, Delta-like-1 and Jagged-1, is critical for glioma cell survival and proliferation. Cancer Res 2005; 65: 2353-63.

[54] Miele L. Notch Signaling. Clin Can Res 2006; 12: 1074-79.

[55] Singh SK, Clarke ID, Terasaki M, et al. Identification of a cancer stem cell in human brain tumors. Cancer Res 2003; 63: 5821-8.

[56] Assanah M. Lochhead R, Ogden A, et al. Glial progenitors in adult white matter are driven to form malignant gliomas by platelet-derived growth factor-expressing retroviruses. J Neurosci 2006; 26: 6781-90.

[57] Ayuso A, Moliterno JA, Kratovac S et al. Activated EGFR signaling increases proliferation, survival, and migration and blocks neuronal differentiation in post-natal neural stem cells. J Neurooncol. 2010;97(3):323-37.

[58] Garcion E, Halilagic A, Faissner A, et al. Generation of an environmental niche for neural stem cell development by the extracellular matrix molecule tenascin C. Development 2004; 131: 3423-32.

[59] Scadden DT. The stem-cell niche as an entity of action. Nature 2006; 441: 1075-79.

[60] Visvader JE, Lindeman GJ. Cancer stem cells in solid tumours: accumulating evidence and unresolved questions. Nat Rev Can 2008; 8: 755-68.

[61] Calabrese C, Poppleton H, Kocak M, et al. A perivascular niche for brain tumor stem cells. Cancer Cell 2007; 11: 69-82.

[62] Leon SP, Folkerth RD, Black PM. Microvessel density is a prognostic indicator for patients with astroglial brain tumors. Cancer 1996; 77: 362-72.

[63] Wang R, Chadalavada K, Wilshire J et al. Glioblastoma stem-like cells give rise to tumour endothelium. Nature. 2010;468:829–33.

[64] Bao S, Wu Q, Sathornsumetee S, et al. Stem cell-like glioma cells promote tumor angiogenesis through vascular endothelial growth factor. Cancer Res 2006; 66: 7843-48.

[65] Vredenburgh J, Desjardins A, Herndon JE 2nd et al. Bevacizumab plus irinotecan in recurrent glioblastomamultiforme. J ClinOncol. 2007;25(30):4722-9.

[66] Batchelor TT, Sorensen AG, di Tomaso E, et al. AZD2171, a pan-VEGF receptor tyrosine kinase inhibitor, normalizes tumor vasculature and alleviates edema in glioblastoma patients. Cancer Cell 2007; 11: 83-95.

[67] Batchelor T, Duda D, di Tomaso E et al. Phase II Study of Cediranib, an Oral Pan–Vascular Endothelial Growth Factor Receptor Tyrosine Kinase Inhibitor, in Patients With Recurrent Glioblastoma. J ClinOncol. 2007;25(30):4722-9.

[68] Loges S, Butzal M, Otten J, et al. Cilengitide inhibits proliferation and differentiation of human endothelial progenitor cells in vitro. BiochemBiophys Res Commun 2007; 357: 1016-20.

[69] Stupp R, Hegi ME, Neyns B et al. Phase I/IIa study of cilengitide and temozolomide with concomitant radiotherapy followed by cilengitide and temozolomide maintenance therapy in patients with newly diagnosed glioblastoma. J ClinOncol. 2010;28:2712-8.

[70] Tabatabai G, Weller M, Nabors B et al. Targeting integrins in malignant glioma. Target Oncol. 2010;5(3):175-81.

[71] Shaifer CA, Huang J, Lin PC. Glioblastoma cells incorporate into tumor vasculature and contribute to vascular radioresistance. Int J Cancer. 2010;127(9):2063-75.

[72] Sotelo C. Cellular and genetic regulation of the development of the cerebellar system. ProgNeurobiol 2004; 72: 295-339.

[73] Fan X, Eberhart CG. Medulloblastoma Stem Cells. J ClinOncol 2008; 26:2821-7.

[74] Wang VY, Rose MF, Zoghbi HY. Math1 expression redefines the rhombic lip derivatives and reveals novel lineages within the brainstem and cerebellum. Neuron 2005; 48: 31-43.

[75] Lee Y, Miller HL, Jensen P. A molecular fingerprint for medulloblastoma. Cancer Res 2003; 63: 5428-37.

[76] Dahmane N, Sanchez P, Gitton Y. The Sonic Hedgehog-Gli pathway regulates dorsal brain growth and tumorigenesis. Development 2001; 128: 5201-12.

[77] Yang Z, Ellis T, Markant S et al. Medulloblastoma Can Be Initiated by Deletion of Patched in Lineage-Restricted Progenitors or Stem Cells. Can Cell. 2008;14(2):135-45.

[78] Sasai K, Romer JT, Kimura H. Medulloblastomas derived from CXCR6 mutant mice respond to treatment with a smoothened inhibitor. Cancer Res 2007; 67: 3871-7.

[79] Schuller U, Rowitch DH. Beta-catenin function is required for cerebellar morphogenesis. Brain Res 2007; 1140: 161-9.

[80] Koch A, Hrychyk A, Hartmann W. Mutations of the Wnt antagonist AXIN2 (conductin) result in TCF-dependent transcription in medulloblastomas. Int J Cancer 2007; 121: 284-91.

[81] Clifford SC, Lusher ME, Lindsey JC. Wnt/Wingless pathway activation and chromosome 6 loss characterize a distinct molecular sub-group of medulloblastomas associated with a favorable prognosis. Cell Cycle 2006; 5: 2666-70.

[82] Dakubo GD, Mazerolle CJ, Wallace VA. Expression of Notch and Wnt pathway components and activation of Notch signaling in meduloblastomas from heterozygous patched mice. J Neurooncol 2006; 79: 221-7.

[83] Keith B, Simon MC. Hypoxia-inducible factors, stem cells, and cancer. Cell 2007; 129: 465-72.

[84] Read T, Fogarty M, Markant S et al. Identification of CD15 as a Marker for Tumor-Propagating Cells in a Mouse Model of Medulloblastoma. Can Cell. 2009:15:135–47.

[85] Beier D, Wischhusen J, Dietmaier W, et al. CD133 expression and cancer stem cells predict prognosis in high-grade oligodendroglial tumors. Brain Pathol 2008;18: 370-7.

[86] Zhang M, Song T, Yang L, et al. Nestin and CD133: valuable stem cell-specific markers for determining clinical outcome of glioma patients. J ExpClin Cancer Res 2008; 27: 85.

[87] Pallini R, Ricci L, Banna G et al.Cancer Stem Cell Analysis and Clinical Outcome in Patients with GlioblastomaMultiforme. ClinCancer Res 2008;14:8205-12.

[88] Spira AI, Carducci MA. Differentiation therapy. CurrOpinPharmacol 2003; 3: 338-43.

[89] Massard C, Deutsch E, Soria JC. Tumour stem cell-targeted treatment: elimination or differentiation. Ann Oncol 2006; 17: 1620-4.

[90] Nicolis SK. Cancer stem cells and "stemness" genes in neuro-oncology. Neurobiol Dis 2007; 25: 217-29.

[91] Clement V, Sanchez P, de Tribolet N, et al. HEDGEHOG–GLI1 signaling regulates human glioma growth, cancer stem cell self-renewal, and tumorigenicity. CurrBiol 2007; 17: 165-72.

[92] Chearwae W, Bright JJ. PPARgamma agonists inhibit growth and expansion of CD133+ brain tumour stem cells. Br J Cancer 2008; 99:2044-53.

[93] Beier D, Röhrl S, Pillai DR, et al. Temozolomide preferentially depletes cancer stem cells in glioblastoma. Cancer Res 2008; 68: 5706-15.

[94] Guzman ML. The sesquiterpene lactone parthenolide induces apoptosis of human acute myelogenous leukemia stem and progenitor cells. Blood 2005; 105: 4163-9.

[95] Piccirillo SG, Reynolds BA, Zanetti N, et al. Bone morphogenetic proteins inhibit the tumorigenic potential of human brain tumour-initiating cells. Nature 2006; 444: 761-5.

[96] Dresemann G, Hosius C, Lilienthal J, et al. Treatment failure due to intracerebral stem cell-like behavior of glioblastoma (GB) cells: A reason for targeted maintenance therapy with imatinib (I) and hydroxyurea (H)? An analysis of study DE21 and DE40 (Ambrosia). J ClinOncol 2008; 26: 2048[Abstr].

[97] Abouantoun TJ, Macdonald TJ. Imatinib blocks migration and invasion of medulloblastoma cells by concurrently inhibiting activation of platelet-derived growth factor receptor and transactivation of epidermal growth factor receptor. Mol Cancer Ther. 2009;5:1-19.

[98] Schatton T, Murphy GF, Frank NY, et al. Identification of cells initiating human melanomas. Nature 2008; 451: 345-9.

[99] Hambardzumyan D, Becher OJ, Rosenblum MK, et al. PI3K pathway regulates survival of cancer stem cells residing in the perivascular niche following radiation in medulloblastoma in vivo. Genes Dev 2008; 22: 436-48.

[100] Lu J, Zhang F, Zhao D, et al. ATRA-inhibited proliferation in glioma cells is associated with subcellular redistribution of beta-catenin via up-regulation of Axin. J Neurooncol 2008; 87: 271-7.

[101] Spiller SE, Ditzler SH, Pullar BJ, et al. Response of preclinical medulloblastoma models to combination therapy with 13-cis retinoic acid and suberoylanilidehydroxamic acid (SAHA). J Neurooncol 2008; 87: 133-41.

[102] Elisabeth CM, Leigh J, Kesari S, et al. Efficacy of the HSP90 inhibitor 17-AAG in human glioma cell lines and tumorigenic glioma stem cells. NeuroOncol 2009; 11: 109-21.

[103] Bar EE, Chaudhry A, Lin A, et al. Cyclopamine-mediated hedgehog pathway inhibition depletes stem-like cancer cells in glioblastoma. Stem Cells 2007; 25: 2524-33.

[104] Lee J, Son MJ, Woolard K, et al. Epigenetic-mediated dysfunction of the bone morphogenetic protein pathway inhibits differentiation of glioblastoma-initiating cells. Cancer Cell 2008; 13: 69-80.

[105] Di Tomaso T, Mazzoleni S, Wang E, et al. Immunobiological characterization of cancer stem cells isolated from glioblastoma patients. Clin Cancer Res 2010; 16: 800-13.

[106] Xu Q, Liu G, Yuan X, et al. Antigen-specific T-cell response from dendritic cell vaccination using cancer stem-like cell-associated antigens. Stem Cells 2009; 27: 1734-40.

[107] Castellino R, Muh C, Durden D. PI-3 Kinase-PTEN Signaling Node: An Intercept Point for the Control of Angiogenesis. Curr Pharm Des. 2009;15(4):380-8.

[108] Kast R, Belda C. Suppressing Glioblastoma Stem Cell Function by Aldehyde Dehydrogenase Inhibition with Chloramphenicol or Disulfiram as a New Treatment Adjunct. Curr St Cell Res Ther. 2009;4:314-7.

Chapter 23

Nestin: Neural Stem/Progenitor Cell Marker in Brain Tumors

Yoko Matsuda, Hisashi Yoshimura,
Taeko Suzuki and Toshiyuki Ishiwata

Additional information is available at the end of the chapter

http://dx.doi.org/10.5772/52634

1. Introduction

Glioblastomas are the most common primary malignant neoplasms in the adult brain, and have the characteristics of glial cells [1]. The WHO histopathological classification guidelines categorize gliomas according to their histopathological grades; low-grade gliomas are not anaplastic and are associated with a favorable patient prognosis, while high-grade gliomas exhibit increased cellularity, nuclear atypia, mitotic activity, microvascular proliferation, and necrosis. Glioblastomas are the highest grade of the gliomas. Surgical treatment is the main therapy used for glioblastomas, with radiotherapy and chemotherapy performed as adjuvant care. Despite intensive research and recent advances in treatment, the prognosis for patients with glioblastoma remains poor, with a five-year survival rate of approximately 3% [2, 3]. In addition to having rapid growth rates, glioblastomas aggressively invade the adjacent normal brain tissues, they are often surgically unresectable, and recurrent glioblastomas are resistant to conventional radiotherapy and chemotherapy.

Nestin is a class VI intermediate filament protein that was first described as a neural stem/progenitor cell marker [4, 5]. Neuroepithelial stem cells can differentiate into neurons, oligodendrocytes, and astrocytes, and nestin has been shown to be down-regulated or to completely disappear during such differentiation. Nestin-positive neuroepithelial stem cells are detected in the subventricular zone of the human adult brain and they remain mitotically active throughout adulthood [6]. Unlike other intermediate filament proteins, nestin plays important roles in cellular processes, including stemness, migration, and cell cycle regulation.

Nestin expression has been reported in various types of tumor cells originating from the central nervous system, including glioblastomas. Several reports have indicated a close relationship between neuroepithelial stem cells and glioblastoma cells at their origin because both cell types express the same stem cell markers, such as CD133 and nestin. High-grade gliomas express higher nestin levels compared to low-grade gliomas [7, 8]. We have reported that knockdown of nestin using short hairpin RNA (shRNA) suppressed cell growth, migration, and invasion [9]; therefore, nestin may serve as a novel candidate for molecular targeted therapy for glioblastomas. In the present chapter, we summarize the available data regarding the expression and roles of nestin in normal brain tissues and brain tumor tissues, and discuss the possibility of using nestin as a novel therapeutic target in brain tumors, mainly for glioblastomas.

2. Structure and characterization of nestin

Nestin is a large protein (>1600 amino acids) that contains a short N-terminal and an unusually long C-terminal. It interacts with other intermediate filament proteins, including vimentin, desmin, and internexin, to form heterodimers and mixed polymers; however, in contrast to other intermediate filament proteins, nestin cannot form homopolymers [10]. The nestin gene has four exons and three introns; in humans, neural cell-specific expression is reportedly regulated by the second intron, whereas nestin expression in tumor endothelium is enhanced by the first intron [11]. Nestin is known to be phosphorylated on Thr316 by cdc2 kinase [12] and/or cyclin-dependent kinase 5 [13], and to modulate mitosis-associated cytoplasmic reorganization during mitosis. However, the roles of glycosylation of nestin have not been closely examined [14].

During early stages of development, nestin is expressed in dividing cells in the central nervous system (CNS), peripheral nervous system, and in myogenic and other tissues. During differentiation in normal brain tissue, nestin expression is downregulated and replaced by expression of tissue-specific intermediate filament proteins; therefore, nesting is widely used as a neuronal stem cell marker. Nestin is also expressed in immature non-neuronal cells and progenitor cells in normal tissues [15-17]. High levels of nestin expression have been detected in oligodendroglial lineage cells, ependymocytes, Sertoli cells, enteroglia, hair follicle cells, podocytes of renal glomeruli, pancreatic stellate cells, pericytes, islets, optic nerve, and odontoblasts [18-23].

In pathological conditions, nestin is re-expressed during repair processes, as well as in various neoplasms and proliferating endothelial cells. Nestin expression has been observed in repair processes in the CNS, muscle, liver, and infarcted myocardium [24-26]. Furthermore, increased nestin expression has been reported in various tumor cells, including CNS tumors, pancreatic cancer, gastrointestinal stromal tumors (GISTs), prostate cancers, breast cancers, malignant melanomas, dermatofibrosarcoma protuberances, and thyroid tumors [27-31]. In several tumors, expression of nestin has been reported to be closely correlated with poor prognosis. Nestin is specifically expressed in proliferating small-sized vascular endothelial cells in glioblastomas and in colorectal, prostate, and pancreatic cancers [7, 32-34].

http://dx.doi.org/10.5772/52634

3. Nestin in normal fetal and adult brain tissues

Many lines of evidence have shown nestin-positive brain cells to be neural stem/progenitor cells; therefore, a great deal of research has involved the use of nestin to detect neural stem cells [35-37]. Children, but not adult humans, exhibit nestin-positive cells in the subventricular zone of the third ventricle [6], and the human embryonic midbrain stem cell line NGC-407 showed degradation of nestin after induction of differentiation [38]. However, in adult mice, nestin-positive cells were detected in CA2 lesions of the hippocampus after transient ischemia [39]. Another study reported that nestin-positive neuroepithelial stem cells are detected in the subventricular zone of the human adult brain and remain mitotically active throughout adulthood [40]. Nestin has been used for research in the field of neural progenitor cells; for example, neural progenitor cell-specific gene transfection was successfully performed using a nestin-driven gene transfection system [41-46]. A recent study has shown that nestin is also a stem/progenitor cell marker in the pituitary gland [47].

4. Nestin in various types of brain tumors

Nestin expression in brain tumor cells has been reported in schwannomas [48], ependymomas [49, 50], neurocytomas [51], adamantinomatous craniopharyngiomas [52], pituitary adenomas [53], medulloblastomas [54-59], oligodendrogliomas [60], and glioblastomas [7, 8, 48, 61] (Table 1). Tissue microarrays of 257 brain tumors have revealed frequent nestin expression in gliomas and schwannomas [48]. Another analysis included 379 tumors, and the results further revealed that nestin immunoreactivity is associated with poor outcome in intracranial ependymomas, and that nestin is an independent marker for poor progression-free survival and overall survival [49].

Expression of nestin has also been reported in tanycytic ependymoma, a rare variant of ependymoma [50], and central neurocytoma cases express nestin, as determined by PCR [51]. Co-expression of nestin, microtubule-associated protein 2 (MAP2), and GFAP has been reported in adamantinomatous craniopharyngiomas [52]. In pituitary adenomas, CD133-positive cells ubiquitously co-express CD34, nestin, and VEGFR2, and may play a role in the neovascularization of tumors [53]. Human medulloblastoma cell lines [54] and medulloblastoma stem cells [55-58] express nestin, and secreted protein acidic and rich in cysteine (SPARC) has been shown to induce neuronal differentiation in medulloblastoma cells with elevations of nestin, NeuN, and neurofilament [59]. One study found that oligodendrogliomas express no or weak nestin, but high Olig2 and alpha-internexin [60]. Oligoastrocytomas moderately express nestin, while astrocytoma and glioblastoma strongly express nestin. Nestin is an intermediate filament protein and is localized in the cytoplasm in most brain tumors; however, in human neuroblastoma and medulloblastoma cell lines, nestin has been observed in nuclei [62], suggesting that nestin may directly bind to DNA or intranucleic proteins. Altogether, these findings demonstrate that nestin is expressed in a wide variety of brain tumors and that this expression correlates with their functions or cell behaviors.

Brain tumors	Expression pattern and roles
Schwannomas	Frequent nestin expression [48]
Ependymomas	Poor progression-free survival and overall survival [49]
Neurocytomas [51]	N/D
Adamantinomatous craniopharyngiomas	Expressed in the invasion niche [52]
Pituitary adenomas	Coexpressed with CD133 [53]
Medulloblastomas	Expressed in tumor stem cells [55-58]
Oligodendrogliomas [60]	N/D
Gliomas	High grade [7,8]
	Worse overall survival [48,61]
Glioblastomas	Infiltration into surrounding tissue [8]
	Tumor stem cells [72-77]
N/D: Not determined.	

Table 1. Expression and roles of nestin in brain tumors

5. Nestin in glioblastoma

5.1. Nestin in low-grade gliomas and glioblastomas

Immunohistochemical analysis has demonstrated nestin expression in the cytoplasm of glioblastoma cells (Figure 1). Large-scale and multicenter studies have shown high immunoreactivity of nestin in glioma cases to be correlated with high grade [7, 8] and worse overall survival [48, 61] (Table 1). Furthermore, expression of nestin and MIB-1 labeling indices in immunohistochemical analyses may correlate with aggressiveness of pilocytic astrocytoma and pilomyxoid astrocytoma [63]. An analysis of several stem cell markers—including CD133, nestin, B lymphoma Mo-MLV insertion region 1 homolog (BMI-1), Maternal embryonic leucine zipper kinase (MELK), and Notch 1-4—was performed using quantitative RT-PCR in 42 glioblastoma samples; MELK was most upregulated, followed by nestin [64]. In contrast, others have reported that nestin immunoreactivity is mostly due to an acute glial reaction and is not specific to the neoplasm [65], and that nestin expression in gliomas does not correlate with prognosis [66].

http://dx.doi.org/10.5772/52634

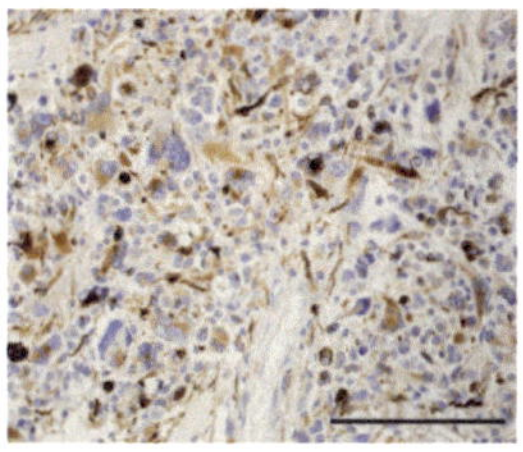

Figure 1. Expression of nestin in glioblastomas. Bar, 100 μm

Immunostaining of nestin in glioblastoma cells has been demonstrated to delineate between invading tumor and the adjacent gray and white matter; therefore, nestin is considered to be a useful marker for examining the infiltration of glioblastomas into surrounding tissues [8]. Furthermore, knockdown of nestin in human glioblastoma cells has been shown to suppress cell migration and invasion, and to increase F-actin expression and cell adhesion to extracellular matrices [9].

Nestin-positive non-tumorous brain cells migrate into the glioblastoma cells and delay astrocytic or elongated bipolar morphology and glomerulus-like microvasculature [67]; therefore, nestin-positive cells have been considered an important component of the tumor microenvironment. CD133-positive and nestin-positive niches are perivascularly localized in all glioma tissues, and the presence of these niches increases significantly with increasing tumor grade [68]. Mice were engineered to co-express platelet-derived growth factor B receptor and Bcl-2 under the control of the glioneuronal-specific nestin promoter, and this resulted in the development of low- and high-grade gliomas [69]. Another study found that human glioblastoma subclones characterized by high nestin levels formed tumors in vivo at a significantly faster rate than subclones with low nestin expression, suggesting that induction of nestin plays an important role in glioblastoma carcinogenesis [70]. However, the opposite result has also been reported [71].

5.2. Nestin in glioma stem cells

Cancer stem cells appear to be responsible for tumor metastasis, resistance to radiotherapy and chemotherapy, and disease relapse; thus, their analysis and therapeutic targeting are believed to be crucial. Many studies have shown that there is a small population of cancer stem cells in glioblastomas, and that nestin is one of the stem/progenitor cell markers of glioblastomas [72-77]. CD133, Oct4, Sox2, and Nanog have also been considered to be stem cell markers in glioblastomas [78, 79]. However, CD133-negative and nestin-negative glioblastoma cells show tumorigenic potential in vivo [71]; thus, there remains some controversy over which specific markers should be used to detect glioblastoma stem cells. An in vitro study has shown that neurospheres of glioblastoma cells exhibit high expressions of nestin, CD133, and Oct4 compared to the expressions in monolayer cells [80]. One study reported that radiation induces increased expressions of stem cell markers, including nestin, CD133, and Musashi [81]; in contrast, another study has shown that radiation induced accumulation of CD133-positive glioblastoma cells, but not nestin [82]. Glioblastoma stem cells are maintained in vivo in a niche characterized by hypoxia, and hypoxia reportedly increases the expressions of nestin, CD133, podoplanin, and Bmi-1 [83]. Together, these available data suggest that there is close relationship between nestin and stemness in glioblastoma.

Expression of nestin in cancer stem cells of glioblastoma may indicate the origin and function of these cells. Potential cancer stem cell origins include migration of neural stem cells toward the tumor, migration of mesenchymal stem cells from bone marrow, or dedifferentiation of tumor cells [84]; each of these hypotheses have been proven experimentally. In brain tumors, long-term cultured human neural stem cells undergo spontaneous transformation to tumor-initiating cells [37]. In contrast, Nanog promotes dedifferentiation of p53-deficient mouse astrocytes into glioblastoma stem cells [85]. These results indicate that glioblastoma stem cells may arise from both the transformation of nestin-positive neural stem cells and differentiated astrocytes. Retinoic acid treatment for glioblastoma stem cells was demonstrated to reduce the expression of neural stem cell markers, such as nestin, CD133, Msi-1, and Sox-2 [86].

Xenografts developed from human anaplastic astrocytoma and glioblastoma tumor-derived spheres in the brain of a nude mouse revealed co-expression of PCNA, VCAM-1, caspase-3, and nestin [87]. Cells positive for both caspase-3 and nestin were located adjacent to or around the blood vessels. Glioblastoma stem cells expressed nestin/CD31 or CD133/CD31, and these cells were capable of differentiating into endothelial cells [88]. Dong et al. have shown that human glioma stem/progenitor cells transdifferentiate into vascular endothelial cells in vitro and in vivo [89]. Glioblastoma stem cells have close relationships with the angiogenic switch, intratumor hypoxia, and the neoplastic microvascular network. These findings provide new insights for targeted therapy against glioblastomas.

5.3. Regulation of nestin in glioblastoma cells

Glioblastomas usually show hyperactivation of the PI3K-Akt pathway. Exogeneous expression of the Akt-binding domain of Girdin inhibits its Akt-mediated phosphorylation, and reportedly diminishes migration and the expression of the stem cell markers nestin and SOX2 [90]. Nestin expression in glioblastomas is correlated with proangiogenic chemokines (CXCL12 and its receptor CXCR4) and growth factors (VEGF and PDGF-B and its receptor PDGFRbeta) [91]. Hypoxia and radiation are both inducers of stem cells, and were associated with increased expression of nestin [81, 83]. In glioblastoma cases, a 9-gene profile that included podoplanin and insulin-like growth factor binding protein 2 was found to predict the prognosis, and was also positively associated with expressions of nestin and CD133 [92]. Additionally, the enhancer lesion of nestin is known to be located in the second intron in neural cells, and this lesion is highly conserved in mouse, rat, and human [93].

5.4. Nestin in interstitial tissues and angiogenesis of glioblastoma

Glioblastoma-conditioned medium has been shown to induce human mesenchymal stem cells (hMSCs) to increase expressions of nestin, CD151, VE-cadherin, desmin, α-smooth muscle actin, and nerval/glial antigen 2—indicating pericyte-like differentiation, rather than differentiation to endothelial cells or smooth muscle cells [94]. hMSCs migrate towards glioblastoma and are incorporated into tumor microvessels.

Much evidence has shown that expression of nestin in vascular endothelial cells is associated with proliferation and angiogenesis [32, 95-98]. In glioblastomas, expression of nestin in both tumor cells and endothelial cells was increased according to increasing tumor grade [7]. A recent study has indicated that the capillaries in gliomas may come from the differentiation of glioblastoma stem cells, and that the glioblastoma stem cells are accumulated around the capillaries [99]. In contrast, CD105 has been proposed to be a more useful marker of tumor angiogenesis in glioblastomas than nestin [100]. The morphology of nestin-positive cells in brain tumors is reportedly more typical of neural stem cells, and less than 0.1% of these cells co-express the endothelial marker CD34 [101].

5.5. Nestin as a therapeutic target for glioblastoma

We have reported that knockdown of nestin using shRNA suppresses cell migration and invasion [9]. Lu et al. demonstrated that blocking the expression of nestin in glioblastomas via intratumor injection of shRNA significantly slowed tumor growth and volume [70]; therefore, nestin may serve as a novel candidate for molecular targeted therapy for glioblastomas [9]. The phytoalexin resveratrol suppresses cell growth, migration, invasion, and expression of nestin in glioblastoma cells [102]. It has been shown that peptides can bind to a nestin isotype that is specifically expressed in glioma stem cells, which enables them to target nestin-positive cells in human glioma tissue [103]. Future studies should focus on developing delivery systems to target these anti-nestin reagents to brain tumors, and on the estimation of the side-effects for normal brain stem cells that express nestin.

6. Conclusion

The neuronal stem cell marker nestin regulates cell growth, migration, invasion, and stemness, and has been found to be expressed in a wide variety of brain tumors. Nestin may be a candidate for the development of promising therapeutic and diagnostic modalities for glioblastoma.

Acknowledgements

The authors thank Dr. Zenya Naito, Mr. Yuji Yanagisawa, Ms. Yoko Kawamoto, Ms. Kiyoko Kawahara, and Ms. Megumi Murase (Departments of Pathology and Integrative Oncological Pathology) for helpful discussions, and Ms. Yuko Ono (Departments of Pathology and Integrative Oncological Pathology) for preparing the manuscript.

Author details

Yoko Matsuda, Hisashi Yoshimura, Taeko Suzuki and Toshiyuki Ishiwata*

*Address all correspondence to: ishiwata@nms.ac.jp

Departments of Pathology and Integrative Oncological Pathology, Nippon Medical School, Bunkyo-ku, Toky, Japan

References

[1] Louis DN, Ohgaki H, Wiestler OD, Cavenee WK, Burger PC, Jouvet A, Scheithauer BW, Kleihues P. The 2007 WHO classification of tumours of the central nervous system. Acta Neuropathol 2007;114(2):97-109.

[2] Bondy ML, Scheurer ME, Malmer B, Barnholtz-Sloan JS, Davis FG, Il'yasova D, Kruchko C, McCarthy BJ, Rajaraman P, Schwartzbaum JA, Sadetzki S, Schlehofer B, Tihan T, Wiemels JL, Wrensch M, Buffler PA. Brain tumor epidemiology: consensus from the Brain Tumor Epidemiology Consortium. Cancer 2008;113(7 Suppl):1953-68.

[3] Brem SS, Bierman PJ, Black P, Blumenthal DT, Brem H, Chamberlain MC, Chiocca EA, DeAngelis LM, Fenstermaker RA, Fine HA, Friedman A, Glass J, Grossman SA, Heimberger AB, Junck L, Levin V, Loeffler JJ, Maor MH, Narayana A, Newton HB, Olivi A, Portnow J, Prados M, Raizer JJ, Rosenfeld SS, Shrieve DC, Sills AK, Jr., Spence AM, Vrionis FD. Central nervous system cancers: Clinical Practice Guidelines in Oncology. J Natl Compr Canc Netw 2005;3(5):644-90.

[4] Lendahl U, Zimmerman LB, McKay RD. CNS stem cells express a new class of intermediate filament protein. Cell 1990;60(4):585-95.

[5] Ishiwata T, Matsuda Y, Naito Z. Nestin in gastrointestinal and other cancers: effects on cells and tumor angiogenesis. World J Gastroenterol 2011;17(4):409-18.

[6] Dahiya S, Lee da Y, Gutmann DH. Comparative characterization of the human and mouse third ventricle germinal zones. J Neuropathol Exp Neurol 2011;70(7):622-33.

[7] Hlobilkova A, Ehrmann J, Knizetova P, Krejci V, Kalita O, Kolar Z. Analysis of VEGF, Flt-1, Flk-1, nestin and MMP-9 in relation to astrocytoma pathogenesis and progression. Neoplasma 2009;56(4):284-90.

[8] Kitai R, Horita R, Sato K, Yoshida K, Arishima H, Higashino Y, Hashimoto N, Takeuchi H, Kubota T, Kikuta K. Nestin expression in astrocytic tumors delineates tumor infiltration. Brain Tumor Pathol 2010;27(1):17-21.

[9] Ishiwata T, Teduka K, Yamamoto T, Kawahara K, Matsuda Y, Naito Z. Neuroepithelial stem cell marker nestin regulates the migration, invasion and growth of human gliomas. Oncol Rep 2011;26(1):91-9.

[10] Steinert PM, Chou YH, Prahlad V, Parry DA, Marekov LN, Wu KC, Jang SI, Goldman RD. A high molecular weight intermediate filament-associated protein in BHK-21 cells is nestin, a type VI intermediate filament protein. Limited co-assembly in vitro to form heteropolymers with type III vimentin and type IV alpha-internexin. J Biol Chem 1999;274(14):9881-90.

[11] Aihara M, Sugawara K, Torii S, Hosaka M, Kurihara H, Saito N, Takeuchi T. Angiogenic endothelium-specific nestin expression is enhanced by the first intron of the nestin gene. Lab Invest 2004;84(12):1581-92.

[12] Sahlgren CM, Mikhailov A, Hellman J, Chou YH, Lendahl U, Goldman RD, Eriksson JE. Mitotic reorganization of the intermediate filament protein nestin involves phosphorylation by cdc2 kinase. J Biol Chem 2001;276(19):16456-63.

[13] Sahlgren CM, Mikhailov A, Vaittinen S, Pallari HM, Kalimo H, Pant HC, Eriksson JE. Cdk5 regulates the organization of Nestin and its association with p35. Mol Cell Biol 2003;23(14):5090-106.

[14] Grigelioniene G, Blennow M, Torok C, Fried G, Dahlin I, Lendahl U, Lagercrantz H. Cerebrospinal fluid of newborn infants contains a deglycosylated form of the intermediate filament nestin. Pediatr Res 1996;40(6):809-14.

[15] Sejersen T, Lendahl U. Transient expression of the intermediate filament nestin during skeletal muscle development. J Cell Sci 1993;106 (Pt 4):1291-300.

[16] Frojdman K, Pelliniemi LJ, Lendahl U, Virtanen I, Eriksson JE. The intermediate filament protein nestin occurs transiently in differentiating testis of rat and mouse. Differentiation 1997;61(4):243-9.

[17] Terling C, Rass A, Mitsiadis TA, Fried K, Lendahl U, Wroblewski J. Expression of the intermediate filament nestin during rodent tooth development. Int J Dev Biol 1995;39(6):947-56.

[18] Yang J, Bian W, Gao X, Chen L, Jing N. Nestin expression during mouse eye and lens development. Mech Dev 2000;94(1-2):287-91.

[19] Almazan G, Vela JM, Molina-Holgado E, Guaza C. Re-evaluation of nestin as a marker of oligodendrocyte lineage cells. Microsc Res Tech 2001;52(6):753-65.

[20] Amoh Y, Li L, Yang M, Moossa AR, Katsuoka K, Penman S, Hoffman RM. Nascent blood vessels in the skin arise from nestin-expressing hair-follicle cells. Proc Natl Acad Sci U S A 2004;101(36):13291-5.

[21] Lardon J, Rooman I, Bouwens L. Nestin expression in pancreatic stellate cells and angiogenic endothelial cells. Histochem Cell Biol 2002;117(6):535-40.

[22] Takano T, Rutka JT, Becker LE. Overexpression of nestin and vimentin in ependymal cells in hydrocephalus. Acta Neuropathol 1996;92(1):90-7.

[23] Ishizaki M, Ishiwata T, Adachi A, Tamura N, Ghazizadeh M, Kitamura H, Sugisaki Y, Yamanaka N, Naito Z, Fukuda Y. Expression of nestin in rat and human glomerular podocytes. J Submicrosc Cytol Pathol 2006;38(2-3):193-200.

[24] Niki T, Pekny M, Hellemans K, Bleser PD, Berg KV, Vaeyens F, Quartier E, Schuit F, Geerts A. Class VI intermediate filament protein nestin is induced during activation of rat hepatic stellate cells. Hepatology 1999;29(2):520-7.

[25] Lin RC, Matesic DF, Marvin M, McKay RD, Brustle O. Re-expression of the intermediate filament nestin in reactive astrocytes. Neurobiol Dis 1995;2(2):79-85.

[26] El-Helou V, Dupuis J, Proulx C, Drapeau J, Clement R, Gosselin H, Villeneuve L, Manganas L, Calderone A. Resident nestin+ neural-like cells and fibers are detected in normal and damaged rat myocardium. Hypertension 2005;46(5):1219-25.

[27] Yamada H, Takano T, Ito Y, Matsuzuka F, Miya A, Kobayashi K, Yoshida H, Watanabe M, Iwatani Y, Miyauchi A. Expression of nestin mRNA is a differentiation marker in thyroid tumors. Cancer Lett 2009;280(1):61-4.

[28] Strojnik T, Rosland GV, Sakariassen PO, Kavalar R, Lah T. Neural stem cell markers, nestin and musashi proteins, in the progression of human glioma: correlation of nestin with prognosis of patient survival. Surg Neurol 2007;68(2):133-43; discussion 43-4.

[29] Brychtova S, Fiuraskova M, Hlobilkova A, Brychta T, Hirnak J. Nestin expression in cutaneous melanomas and melanocytic nevi. J Cutan Pathol 2007;34(5):370-5.

[30] Tsujimura T, Makiishi-Shimobayashi C, Lundkvist J, Lendahl U, Nakasho K, Sugihara A, Iwasaki T, Mano M, Yamada N, Yamashita K, Toyosaka A, Terada N. Expression of the intermediate filament nestin in gastrointestinal stromal tumors and interstitial cells of Cajal. Am J Pathol 2001;158(3):817-23.

[31] Li H, Cherukuri P, Li N, Cowling V, Spinella M, Cole M, Godwin AK, Wells W, DiRenzo J. Nestin is expressed in the basal/myoepithelial layer of the mammary gland and is a selective marker of basal epithelial breast tumors. Cancer Res 2007;67(2): 501-10.

[32] Gravdal K, Halvorsen OJ, Haukaas SA, Akslen LA. Proliferation of immature tumor vessels is a novel marker of clinical progression in prostate cancer. Cancer Res 2009;69(11):4708-15.

[33] Teranishi N, Naito Z, Ishiwata T, Tanaka N, Furukawa K, Seya T, Shinji S, Tajiri T. Identification of neovasculature using nestin in colorectal cancer. Int J Oncol 2007;30(3):593-603.

[34] Yamahatsu K, Matsuda Y, Ishiwata T, Uchida E, Naito Z. Nestin as a novel therapeutic target for pancreatic cancer via tumor angiogenesis. Int J Oncol 2012;40(5):1345-57.

[35] Liu L, Shi M, Wang L, Hou S, Wu Z, Zhao G, Deng Y. Ndrg2 expression in neurogenic germinal zones of embryonic and postnatal mouse brain. J Mol Histol 2012; 43 (1): 27-35.

[36] Romero-Grimaldi C, Murillo-Carretero M, Lopez-Toledano MA, Carrasco M, Castro C, Estrada C. ADAM-17/tumor necrosis factor-alpha-converting enzyme inhibits neurogenesis and promotes gliogenesis from neural stem cells. Stem Cells 2011;29(10):1628-39.

[37] Wu W, He Q, Li X, Zhang X, Lu A, Ge R, Zhen H, Chang AE, Li Q, Shen L. Long-term cultured human neural stem cells undergo spontaneous transformation to tumor-initiating cells. Int J Biol Sci 2011;7(6):892-901.

[38] Khan Z, Akhtar M, Ekstrom TJ. HDAC inhibitor 4-phenylbutyrate preserves immature phenotype of human embryonic midbrain stem cells: implications for the involvement of DNA methyltransferase. Int J Mol Med 2011;28(6):977-83.

[39] Wang H, Imamura Y, Ishibashi R, Chandana EP, Yamamoto M, Noda M. The Reck tumor suppressor protein alleviates tissue damage and promotes functional recovery after transient cerebral ischemia in mice. J Neurochem 2010;115(2):385-98.

[40] Kaneko Y, Sakakibara S, Imai T, Suzuki A, Nakamura Y, Sawamoto K, Ogawa Y, Toyama Y, Miyata T, Okano H. Musashi1: an evolutionally conserved marker for CNS progenitor cells including neural stem cells. Dev Neurosci 2000;22(1-2):139-53.

[41] Seok SH, Na YR, Han JH, Kim TH, Jung H, Lee BH, Emelyanov A, Parinov S, Park JH. Cre/loxP-regulated transgenic zebrafish model for neural progenitor-specific oncogenic Kras expression. Cancer Sci 2010;101(1):149-54.

[42] Goto J, Talos DM, Klein P, Qin W, Chekaluk YI, Anderl S, Malinowska IA, Di Nardo A, Bronson RT, Chan JA, Vinters HV, Kernie SG, Jensen FE, Sahin M, Kwiatkowski DJ. Regulable neural progenitor-specific Tsc1 loss yields giant cells with organellar dysfunction in a model of tuberous sclerosis complex. Proc Natl Acad Sci U S A 2011;108(45):E1070-9.

[43] Nagy JI, Lynn BD, Tress O, Willecke K, Rash JE. Connexin26 expression in brain parenchymal cells demonstrated by targeted connexin ablation in transgenic mice. Eur J Neurosci 2011;34(2):263-71.

[44] Wey A, Knoepfler PS. c-myc and N-myc promote active stem cell metabolism and cycling as architects of the developing brain. Oncotarget 2010;1(2):120-30.

[45] Tanori M, Santone M, Mancuso M, Pasquali E, Leonardi S, Di Majo V, Rebessi S, Saran A, Pazzaglia S. Developmental and oncogenic effects of insulin-like growth factor-I in Ptc1+/- mouse cerebellum. Mol Cancer 2010;9:53.

[46] See WL, Miller JP, Squatrito M, Holland E, Resh MD, Koff A. Defective DNA double-strand break repair underlies enhanced tumorigenesis and chromosomal instability in p27-deficient mice with growth factor-induced oligodendrogliomas. Oncogene 2010;29(12):1720-31.

[47] Florio T. Adult pituitary stem cells: from pituitary plasticity to adenoma development. Neuroendocrinology 2011;94(4):265-77.

[48] Arai H, Ikota H, Sugawara KI, Nobusawa S, Hirato J, Nakazato Y. Nestin expression in brain tumors: its utility for pathological diagnosis and correlation with the prognosis of high-grade gliomas. Brain Tumor Pathol 2012; 29 (3): 160-7.

[49] Milde T, Hielscher T, Witt H, Kool M, Mack SC, Deubzer HE, Oehme I, Lodrini M, Benner A, Taylor MD, von Deimling A, Kulozik AE, Pfister SM, Witt O, Korshunov A. Nestin Expression Identifies Ependymoma Patients with Poor Outcome. Brain Pathol 2012.

[50] Zhang S, Wang X, Zhang Z, Chen Y. Tanycytic ependymoma arising from the right lateral ventricle: a case report and review of the literature. Neuropathology 2008;28(4):427-32.

[51] Paek SH, Shin HY, Kim JW, Park SH, Son JH, Kim DG. Primary culture of central neurocytoma: a case report. J Korean Med Sci 2010;25(5):798-803.

[52] Burghaus S, Holsken A, Buchfelder M, Fahlbusch R, Riederer BM, Hans V, Blumcke I, Buslei R. A tumor-specific cellular environment at the brain invasion border of adamantinomatous craniopharyngiomas. Virchows Arch 2010;456(3):287-300.

[53] Yunoue S, Arita K, Kawano H, Uchida H, Tokimura H, Hirano H. Identification of CD133+ cells in pituitary adenomas. Neuroendocrinology 2011;94(4):302-12.

[54] Kim YH, Cho SH, Lee SJ, Choi SA, Phi JH, Kim SK, Wang KC, Cho BK, Kim CY. Growth-inhibitory effect of neurotrophin-3-secreting adipose tissue-derived mesenchymal stem cells on the D283-MED human medulloblastoma cell line. J Neurooncol 2012;106(1):89-98.

[55] Huang X, Ketova T, Litingtung Y, Chiang C. Isolation, enrichment, and maintenance of medulloblastoma stem cells. J Vis Exp 2010(43).

[56] Pistollato F, Rampazzo E, Persano L, Abbadi S, Frasson C, Denaro L, D'Avella D, Panchision DM, Della Puppa A, Scienza R, Basso G. Interaction of hypoxia-inducible factor-1alpha and Notch signaling regulates medulloblastoma precursor proliferation and fate. Stem Cells 2010;28(11):1918-29.

[57] Yu CC, Chiou GY, Lee YY, Chang YL, Huang PI, Cheng YW, Tai LK, Ku HH, Chiou SH, Wong TT. Medulloblastoma-derived tumor stem-like cells acquired resistance to TRAIL-induced apoptosis and radiosensitivity. Childs Nerv Syst 2010;26(7):897-904.

[58] Sutter R, Shakhova O, Bhagat H, Behesti H, Sutter C, Penkar S, Santuccione A, Bernays R, Heppner FL, Schuller U, Grotzer M, Moch H, Schraml P, Marino S. Cerebellar stem cells act as medulloblastoma-initiating cells in a mouse model and a neural stem cell signature characterizes a subset of human medulloblastomas. Oncogene 2010;29(12):1845-56.

[59] Bhoopathi P, Chetty C, Dontula R, Gujrati M, Dinh DH, Rao JS, Lakka SS. SPARC stimulates neuronal differentiation of medulloblastoma cells via the Notch1/STAT3 pathway. Cancer Res 2011;71(14):4908-19.

[60] Durand K, Guillaudeau A, Pommepuy I, Mesturoux L, Chaunavel A, Gadeaud E, Porcheron M, Moreau JJ, Labrousse F. Alpha-internexin expression in gliomas: relationship with histological type and 1p, 19q, 10p and 10q status. J Clin Pathol 2011;64(9):793-801.

[61] Wan F, Herold-Mende C, Campos B, Centner FS, Dictus C, Becker N, Devens F, Mogler C, Felsberg J, Grabe N, Reifenberger G, Lichter P, Unterberg A, Bermejo JL, Ahmadi R. Association of stem cell-related markers and survival in astrocytic gliomas. Biomarkers 2011;16(2):136-43.

[62] Krupkova O, Jr., Loja T, Redova M, Neradil J, Zitterbart K, Sterba J, Veselska R. Analysis of nuclear nestin localization in cell lines derived from neurogenic tumors. Tumour Biol 2011;32(4):631-9.

[63] Nagaishi M, Yokoo H, Hirato J, Yoshimoto Y, Nakazato Y. Clinico-pathological feature of pilomyxoid astrocytomas: three case reports. Neuropathology 2011;31(2): 152-7.

[64] Yoshimoto K, Ma X, Guan Y, Mizoguchi M, Nakamizo A, Amano T, Hata N, Kuga D, Sasaki T. Expression of stem cell marker and receptor kinase genes in glioblastoma tissue quantified by real-time RT-PCR. Brain Tumor Pathol 2011;28(4):291-6.

[65] Idoate MA, Diez Valle R, Echeveste J, Tejada S. Pathological characterization of the glioblastoma border as shown during surgery using 5-aminolevulinic acid-induced fluorescence. Neuropathology 2011;31(6):575-82.

[66] Kim KJ, Lee KH, Kim HS, Moon KS, Jung TY, Jung S, Lee MC. The presence of stem cell marker-expressing cells is not prognostically significant in glioblastomas. Neuropathology 2011;31(5):494-502.

[67] Najbauer J, Huszthy PC, Barish ME, Garcia E, Metz MZ, Myers SM, Gutova M, Frank RT, Miletic H, Kendall SE, Glackin CA, Bjerkvig R, Aboody KS. Cellular host responses to gliomas. PLoS One 2012;7(4):e35150.

[68] He H, Li MW, Niu CS. The pathological characteristics of glioma stem cell niches. J Clin Neurosci 2012;19(1):121-7.

[69] Kong LY, Wu AS, Doucette T, Wei J, Priebe W, Fuller GN, Qiao W, Sawaya R, Rao G, Heimberger AB. Intratumoral mediated immunosuppression is prognostic in genetically engineered murine models of glioma and correlates to immunotherapeutic responses. Clin Cancer Res 2010;16(23):5722-33.

[70] Lu WJ, Lan F, He Q, Lee A, Tang CZ, Dong L, Lan B, Ma X, Wu JC, Shen L. Inducible expression of stem cell associated intermediate filament nestin reveals an important role in glioblastoma carcinogenesis. Int J Cancer 2011;128(2):343-51.

[71] Prestegarden L, Svendsen A, Wang J, Sleire L, Skaftnesmo KO, Bjerkvig R, Yan T, Askland L, Persson A, Sakariassen PO, Enger PO. Glioma cell populations grouped by different cell type markers drive brain tumor growth. Cancer Res 2010;70(11): 4274-9.

[72] Zhu G, Su W, Jin G, Xu F, Hao S, Guan F, Jia W, Liu F. Glioma stem cells targeted by oncolytic virus carrying endostatin-angiostatin fusion gene and the expression of its exogenous gene in vitro. Brain Res 2011;1390:59-69.

[73] Bulnes S, Garcia-Blanco A, Bengoetxea H, Ortuzar N, Argandona EG, Lafuente JV. Glial stem cells and their relationship with tumour angiogenesis process. Rev Neurol 2011;52(12):743-50.

[74] Xiao ZY, Tang H, Xu ZM, Yan ZJ, Li P, Cai YQ, Jiang XD, Xu RX. An experimental study of dendritic cells transfected with cancer stem-like cells RNA against 9L brain tumors. Cancer Biol Ther 2011;11(11):974-80.

[75] Tomuleasa C, Soritau O, Rus-Ciuca D, Ioani H, Susman S, Petrescu M, Timis T, Cernea D, Kacso G, Irimie A, Florian IS. Functional and molecular characterization of glioblastoma multiforme-derived cancer stem cells. J BUON 2010;15(3):583-91.

[76] Qin K, Jiang X, Zou Y, Wang J, Qin L, Zeng Y. Study on the proliferation and drug-resistance of human brain tumor stem-like cells. Cell Mol Neurobiol 2010;30(6): 955-60.

[77] Michelakis ED, Sutendra G, Dromparis P, Webster L, Haromy A, Niven E, Maguire C, Gammer TL, Mackey JR, Fulton D, Abdulkarim B, McMurtry MS, Petruk KC. Metabolic modulation of glioblastoma with dichloroacetate. Sci Transl Med 2010;2(31): 31ra4.

[78] Guo Y, Liu S, Wang P, Zhao S, Wang F, Bing L, Zhang Y, Ling EA, Gao J, Hao A. Expression profile of embryonic stem cell-associated genes Oct4, Sox2 and Nanog in human gliomas. Histopathology 2011;59(4):763-75.

[79] Wookey PJ, McLean CA, Hwang P, Furness SG, Nguyen S, Kourakis A, Hare DL, Rosenfeld JV. The expression of calcitonin receptor detected in malignant cells of the brain tumour glioblastoma multiforme and functional properties in the cell line A172. Histopathology 2012;60(6):895-910.

[80] Binello E, Qadeer ZA, Kothari HP, Emdad L, Germano IM. Stemness of the CT-2A Immunocompetent Mouse Brain Tumor Model: Characterization In Vitro. J Cancer 2012;3:166-74.

[81] Kim RK, Yoon CH, Hyun KH, Lee H, An S, Park MJ, Kim MJ, Lee SJ. Role of lymphocyte-specific protein tyrosine kinase (LCK) in the expansion of glioma-initiating cells by fractionated radiation. Biochem Biophys Res Commun 2010;402(4):631-6.

[82] Tamura K, Aoyagi M, Wakimoto H, Ando N, Nariai T, Yamamoto M, Ohno K. Accumulation of CD133-positive glioma cells after high-dose irradiation by Gamma Knife surgery plus external beam radiation. J Neurosurg 2010;113(2):310-8.

[83] Kolenda J, Jensen SS, Aaberg-Jessen C, Christensen K, Andersen C, Brunner N, Kristensen BW. Effects of hypoxia on expression of a panel of stem cell and chemoresistance markers in glioblastoma-derived spheroids. J Neurooncol 2011;103(1):43-58.

[84] Schiffer D, Annovazzi L, Caldera V, Mellai M. On the origin and growth of gliomas. Anticancer Res 2010;30(6):1977-98.

[85] Moon JH, Kwon S, Jun EK, Kim A, Whang KY, Kim H, Oh S, Yoon BS, You S. Nanog-induced dedifferentiation of p53-deficient mouse astrocytes into brain cancer stem-like cells. Biochem Biophys Res Commun 2011;412(1):175-81.

[86] Ying M, Wang S, Sang Y, Sun P, Lal B, Goodwin CR, Guerrero-Cazares H, Quinones-Hinojosa A, Laterra J, Xia S. Regulation of glioblastoma stem cells by retinoic acid: role for Notch pathway inhibition. Oncogene 2011;30(31):3454-67.

[87] Zarnescu O, Brehar FM, Bleotu C, Gorgan RM. Co-localization of PCNA, VCAM-1 and caspase-3 with nestin in xenografts derived from human anaplastic astrocytoma and glioblastoma multiforme tumor spheres. Micron 2011;42(8):793-800.

[88] He H, Niu CS, Li MW. Correlation between glioblastoma stem-like cells and tumor vascularization. Oncol Rep 2012;27(1):45-50.

[89] Dong J, Zhao Y, Huang Q, Fei X, Diao Y, Shen Y, Xiao H, Zhang T, Lan Q, Gu X. Glioma stem/progenitor cells contribute to neovascularization via transdifferentiation. Stem Cell Rev 2010;7(1):141-52.

[90] Natsume A, Kato T, Kinjo S, Enomoto A, Toda H, Shimato S, Ohka F, Motomura K, Kondo Y, Miyata T, Takahashi M, Wakabayashi T. Girdin maintains the stemness of glioblastoma stem cells. Oncogene 2012;31(22):2715-24.

[91] Maderna E, Salmaggi A, Calatozzolo C, Limido L, Pollo B. Nestin, PDGFRbeta, CXCL12 and VEGF in glioma patients: different profiles of (pro-angiogenic) molecule expression are related with tumor grade and may provide prognostic information. Cancer Biol Ther 2007;6(7):1018-24.

[92] Colman H, Zhang L, Sulman EP, McDonald JM, Shooshtari NL, Rivera A, Popoff S, Nutt CL, Louis DN, Cairncross JG, Gilbert MR, Phillips HS, Mehta MP, Chakravarti A, Pelloski CE, Bhat K, Feuerstein BG, Jenkins RB, Aldape K. A multigene predictor of outcome in glioblastoma. Neuro Oncol 2010;12(1):49-57.

[93] Lothian C, Lendahl U. An evolutionarily conserved region in the second intron of the human nestin gene directs gene expression to CNS progenitor cells and to early neural crest cells. Eur J Neurosci 1997;9(3):452-62.

[94] Birnbaum T, Hildebrandt J, Nuebling G, Sostak P, Straube A. Glioblastoma-dependent differentiation and angiogenic potential of human mesenchymal stem cells in vitro. J Neurooncol 2011;105(1):57-65.

[95] Matsuda Y, Fujii T, Suzuki T, Yamahatsu K, Kawahara K, Teduka K, Kawamoto Y, Yamamoto T, Ishiwata T, Naito Z. Comparison of Fixation Methods for Preservation of Morphology, RNAs, and Proteins From Paraffin-embedded Human Cancer Cell-implanted Mouse Models. J Histochem Cytochem 2010; 59 (1): 68-75.

[96] Yamahatsu K, Matsuda Y, Ishiwata T, Uchida E, Naito Z. Nestin as a novel therapeutic target for pancreatic cancer via tumor angiogenesis. Int J Oncol 2012; 40 (5): 1345-57.

[97] Mokry J, Nemecek S. Angiogenesis of extra- and intraembryonic blood vessels is associated with expression of nestin in endothelial cells. Folia Biol (Praha) 1998;44(5): 155-61.

[98] Mokry J, Nemecek S. Cerebral angiogenesis shows nestin expression in endothelial cells. Gen Physiol Biophys 1999;18 Suppl 1:25-9.

[99] Li MW, Niu CS. [Correlative study of distribution of brain tumor stem cell with micro-vascular system]. Zhonghua Yi Xue Za Zhi 2010;90(5):305-9.

[100] Sica G, Lama G, Anile C, Geloso MC, La Torre G, De Bonis P, Maira G, Lauriola L, Jhanwar-Uniyal M, Mangiola A. Assessment of angiogenesis by CD105 and nestin expression in peritumor tissue of glioblastoma. Int J Oncol 2011;38(1):41-9.

[101] Calabrese C, Poppleton H, Kocak M, Hogg TL, Fuller C, Hamner B, Oh EY, Gaber MW, Finklestein D, Allen M, Frank A, Bayazitov IT, Zakharenko SS, Gajjar A, Davidoff A, Gilbertson RJ. A perivascular niche for brain tumor stem cells. Cancer Cell 2007;11(1):69-82.

[102] Castino R, Pucer A, Veneroni R, Morani F, Peracchio C, Lah TT, Isidoro C. Resveratrol reduces the invasive growth and promotes the acquisition of a long-lasting differentiated phenotype in human glioblastoma cells. J Agric Food Chem 2011;59(8): 4264-72.

[103] Beck S, Jin X, Yin J, Kim SH, Lee NK, Oh SY, Kim MK, Kim EB, Son JS, Kim SC, Nam DH, Kang SK, Kim H, Choi YJ. Identification of a peptide that interacts with Nestin protein expressed in brain cancer stem cells. Biomaterials 2011;32(33):8518-28.